VENTRICULAR TACHYCARDIAS

DEVELOPMENTS IN CARDIOVASCULAR MEDICINE

Recent volumes

Hanrath P, Bleifeld W, Souquet, J. eds: Cardiovascular diagnosis by ultrasound. Transesophageal, computerized, contrast, Doppler echocardiography. 1982. ISBN 90-247-2692-1.
Roelandt J, ed: The practice of M-mode and two-dimensional echocardiography. 1983. ISBN 90-247-2745-6.
Meyer J, Schweizer P, Erbel R, eds: Advances in noninvasive cardiology. 1983. ISBN 0-89838-576-8.
Morganroth J, Moore EN, eds: Sudden cardiac death and congestive heart failure: Diagnosis and treatment. 1983. ISBN 0-89838-580-6.
Perry HM, ed: Lifelong management of hypertension. 1983. ISBN 0-89838-582-2.
Jaffe EA, ed: Biology of endothelial cells. 1984. ISBN 0-89838-587-3.
Surawicz B, Reddy CP, Prystowsky EN, eds: Tachycardias. 1984. ISBN 0-89838-588-1.
Spencer MP, ed: Cardiac Doppler diagnosis. 1983. ISBN 0-89838-591-1.
Villarreal H, Sambhi MP, eds: Topics in pathophysiology of hypertension. 1984. ISBN 0-89838-595-4.
Messerli FH, ed: Cardiovascular disease in the elderly. 1984. ISBN 0-89838-596-2.
Simoons ML, Reiber JHC, eds: Nuclear imaging in clinical cardiology. 1984. ISBN 0-89838-599-7.
Ter Keurs HEDJ, Schipperheyn JJ, eds: Cardiac left ventricular hypertrophy. 1983. ISBN 0-89838-612-8.
Sperelakis N, ed: Physiology and pathophysiology of the heart. 1984. ISBN 0-89838-615-2.
Messerli FH, ed: Kidney in essential hypertension. 1984. ISBN 0-89838-616-0.
Sambhi MP, ed: Fundamental fault in hypertension. 1984. ISBN 0-89838-638-1.
Marchesi C, ed: Ambulatory monitoring: Cardiovascular system and allied applications. 1984. ISBN 0-89838-642-X.
Kupper W, MacAlpin RN, Bleifeld W, eds: Coronary tone in ischemic heart disease. 1984. ISBN 0-89838-646-2.
Sperelakis N, Caulfield JB, eds: Calcium antagonists: Mechanisms of action on cardiac muscle and vascular smooth muscle. 1984. ISBN 0-89838-655-1.
Godfraind T, Herman AS, Wellens D, eds: Calcium entry blockers in cardiovascular and cerebral dysfunctions. 1984. ISBN 0-89838-658-6.
Morganroth J, Moore EN, eds: Interventions in the acute phase of myocardial infarction. 1984. ISBN 0-89838-659-4.
Abel FL, Newman WH, eds: Functional aspects of the normal, hypertrophied, and failing heart. 1984. ISBN 0-89838-665-9.
Sideman S, Beyar R, eds: Simulation and imaging of the cardiac system. 1985. ISBN 0-89838-687-X.
Van der Wall E, Lie KI, eds: Recent views on hypertrophic cardiomyopathy. 1985. ISBN 0-89838-694-2.
Beamish RE, Singal PK, Dhalla NS, eds: Stress and heart disease. 1985. ISBN 0-89838-709-4.
Beamish RE, Panagio V, Dhalla NS, eds: Pathogenesis of stress-induced heart disease. 1985. ISBN 0-89838-710-8.
Morganroth J, Moore EN, eds: Cardiac arrhythmias. 1985. ISBN 0-89838-716-7.
Mathes E, ed: Secondary prevention in coronary artery disease and myocardial infarction. 1985. ISBN 0-89838-736-1.
Lowell Stone H, Weglicki WB, eds: Pathology of cardiovascular injury. 1985. ISBN 0-89838-743-4.
Meyer J, Erbel R, Rupprecht HJ, eds: Improvement of myocardial perfusion. 1985. ISBN 0-89838-748-5.
Reiber JHC, Serruys PW, Slager CJ: Quantitative coronary and left ventricular cineangiography. 1986. ISBN 0-89838-760-4.
Fagard RH, Bekaert IE, eds: Sports cardiology. 1986. ISBN 0-89838-782-5.
Reiber JHC, Serruys PW, eds: State of the art in quantitative coronary arteriography. 1986. ISBN 0-89838-804-X.
Roelandt J, ed: Color Doppler Flow Imaging. 1986. ISBN 0-89838-806-6.
Van der Wall EE, ed: Noninvasive imaging of cardiac metabolism. 1986. ISBN 0-89838-812-0.
Liebman J, Plonsey R, Rudy Y, eds: Pediatric and fundamental electrocardiography. 1986. ISBN 0-89838-815-5.
Hilger HH, Hombach V, Rashkind WJ, eds: Invasive cardiovascular therapy. 1987. ISBN 0-89838-818-X
Serruys PW, Meester GT, eds: Coronary angioplasty: a controlled model for ischemia. 1986. ISBN 0-89838-819-8.
Tooke JE, Smaje LH: Clinical investigation of the microcirculation. 1986. ISBN 0-89838-819-8.
Van Dam RTh, Van Oosterom A, eds: Electrocardiographic body surface mapping. 1986. ISBN 0-89838-834-1.
Spencer MP, ed: Ultrasonic diagnosis of cerebrovascular disease. 1987. ISBN 0-89838-836-8.
Legato MJ, ed: The stressed heart. 1987. ISBN 0-89838-849-X.
Roelandt J, ed: Digital techniques in echocardiography. 1987. ISBN 0-89838-861-9.
Sideman S, Beyar R, eds: Activation, metabolism and perfusion of the heart. 1987. ISBN 0-89838-871-6.
Safar ME et al., eds: Arterial and venous systems in essential hypertension. 1987. ISBN 0-89838-857-0.
Ter Keurs HEDJ, Tyberg JV, eds: Mechanics of the circulation. 1987. ISBN 0-89838-870-8
Aliot E, Lazzara R, eds: Ventricular tachycardias. 1987. ISBN 0-89838-881-3.

VENTRICULAR TACHYCARDIAS
from Mechanism to Therapy

edited by

ETIENNE ALIOT MD, F.A.C.C.
Professor of cardiology
Department of Cardiology, Hôpital Central, Nancy, France

RALPH LAZZARA MD, F.A.C.C.
Professor of cardiology
Department of Cardiology, Veterans Administration Medical Center
and University of Oklahoma Health Center, Oklahoma City, Oklahoma, U.S.A.

1987 **MARTINUS NIJHOFF PUBLISHERS**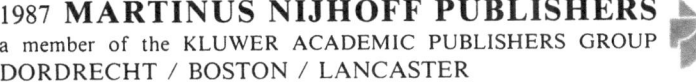
a member of the KLUWER ACADEMIC PUBLISHERS GROUP
DORDRECHT / BOSTON / LANCASTER

Distributors

for the United States and Canada: Kluwer Academic Publishers, P.O. Box 358, Accord Station, Hingham, MA 02018-0358, USA
for the UK and Ireland: Kluwer Academic Publishers, MTP Press Limited, Falcon House, Queen Square, Lancaster LA1 1RN, UK
for all other countries: Kluwer Academic Publishers Group, Distribution Center, P.O. Box 322, 3300 AH Dordrecht, The Netherlands

Library of Congress Cataloging in Publication Data

Library of Congress Cataloging-in-Publication Data

Ventricular tachycardias.

    (Developments in cardiovascular medicine ; 71)
    Based on a meeting held in Vittel, France in May
1986.
    Includes index.
    1. Ventricular tachycardia--Congresses. I. Aliot,
Etienne. II. Lazzara, Ralph. III. Series: Developments
in cardiovascular medicine ; v. 71. [DNLM: 1. Heart
Ventricle--congresses. 2. Tachycardia--physiotherapy--
congresses. 3. Tachycardia--therapy--congresses.
W1 DE997VME v. 71 / WG 330 V4668 1986]
RC685.T33V47 1987   616.1'2   87-7657

ISBN-13: 978-94-010-7992-1   e-ISBN-132: 978-94-009-3323-1
DOI: 10.1007/978-94-009-3323-1

Copyright

To our wives, Chris and Barbara,

and our children,
Delphine, Sophie, Romain, Melissa, Rosalie and Ralph Jr
for their support and understanding.

Preface

The rhythm of the heart, its normal functioning and pathologic disturbances, has been a favored subject of investigation by clinical and basic scientists in recent decades. This heightened interest and attention was stimulated by the somber and surprising revelations from epidemiologists and pathologists of the enormity of the number of sudden arrhythmic deaths in the Western world, and the concurrent advancement of technology for recording and control of electrical activity of the heart. Technological advancements have included the recording of intracellular potentials from cardiac cells, the recording of intracardiac extracellular potentials generated by specific cardiac structures, simultaneous recordings from numerous sites with computer processing for spatial mapping of activation or potential variations with time, high gain, high resolution recordings with signal averaging for detecting potentials of low amplitudes, complex stimulation protocols, various high energy stimulation modes, intracellular voltage control of multicellular preparations and single cardiac cells, and the isolation of single cardiac cells for electrophysiological study. The interest and technology have produced an increasing bounty of information and understanding, acceptable solutions to some clinical problems, and definite progress toward solutions to other problems.

Progress in research in electrophysiology and arrhythmias has been reviewed and highlighted in various meetings and books in recent years. Because the body of information has become so large, general overviews of the field have necessarily been superficial in certain aspects or have contained gaps. To have a treatment that approaches comprehensiveness and completeness, some focusing is necessary. Since ventricular arrhythmias constitute the most important problem with respect to human health, it seemed appropriate and timely to focus on this topic, and to endeavor to deal with it in a comprehensive manner from the clinical and mechanistic standpoints. Accordingly, a meeting was organized in Vittel, France, in May of 1986 where noted clinical and basic scientists from around the world, with interests and accomplishments bearing on the subject of ventricular tachyarrhythmias, were gathered to review and critique published data, summarize progress, and present new data and ideas.

Our perception of the meeting was that it was eminently successful in reviewing and critiqueing the field and it was charged with the excitement of new ideas. The participants, speakers and audience, were gratified and stimulated, experiencing that combination of enlightenment and excitement that ensues good scientific discussion. The overwhelming favorable response to the meeting prompted us to prepare a book publication with this meeting as the basis. We hope the contents of the monograph will be as valuable and stimulating to the readers as the meeting was to the participants.

Etienne ALIOT
Nancy, France
Ralph LAZZARA
Oklahoma City, OK, U.S.A.

Contents

Acknowledgements

We would like to thank all authors for their important contribution to the realization of this book.

We also want to especially thank Professor Jean-Marie GILGENKRANTZ for his continuing help and support, as well as Danielle DAVID and Claude MET-TAVANT for their efficient technical assistance.

Finally, we are grateful to the publishers for their patience.

List of contributors

ABBOTT Joseph A.
Department of Cardiology, University of California at San Francisco, 2130 Fulton Street,
San Francisco, CA 94117, USA

ALABI P.B.
Academic Department of Cardiology, Freeman Hospital, Newcastle upon Tyne, United Kingdom

ALIOT Etienne M.
Département de Cardiologie, CHRU de Nancy, Hôpital Central, 54037 Nancy Cedex, France

ALMENDRAL Jesus M.
Servicio de Cardiologia, Hospital Provincial de Madrid, Spain

ANTON P.M.
Department of Cardiology, Academic Hospital of Maastricht, University of Limburg, Maastricht,
The Netherlands

ATALLAH G.
Hôpital Cardiovasculaire et Pneumologique Louis Pradel, BP Lyon Montchat, 69394 Lyon
Cedex 03, France

BAILEY J.C.
Krannert Institute of Cardiology, 1001 W. 10th Street, Indianapolis, IN 46202, USA

BARAKA M.
Service de Rythmologie et de Stimulation Cardiaque, Hôpital Jean Rostand, 39, rue Le Galleu,
94200 Ivry, France

BERBARI Edward J.
Veterans Administration Medical Center, Cardiology Research Service (151-F), 921 Northeast 13th
Street, Oklahoma City, OK 73104, USA

BIANCHI Marina
Département de Cardiologie, CHRU de Nancy, Hôpital Central, 54037 Nancy Cedex, France

BORGGREFE M.
Hospital of the University of Düsseldorf, Department of Cardiology, Pneumology and Angiology,
Düsseldorf, West Germany

BOTVINICK Elias H.
University of California at San Francisco, 3rd and Parnassus Avenues, San Francisco, CA 94143, USA

BOURGUIGNON M.
Service Frédéric Joliot, Département de Biologie du C.E.A., 91400 Orsay, France

BREITHARDT Gunter
Hospital of the University of Düsseldorf, Department of Cardiology, Pneumology and Angiology, Düsseldorf, West Germany

BREMBILLA-PERROT Béatrice
Service de Cardiologie, CHRU de Nancy-Brabois, 54500 Vandoeuvre-les Nancy, France

BROUSTET J.P.
Department of Exercise Testing, Hôpital Cardiologique de Haut Lévêque, 33604 Pessac, France

BRUGADA Pedro
Department of Cardiology, Academic Hospital of Maastricht, University of Limburg, Maastricht, The Netherlands

BUXTON Alfred E.
Cardiovascular Section, Room 658 Ravdin Building, Hospital of the University of Pennsylvania, 3400 Spruce Street, Philadelphia, PA 19104, USA

CABROL C.
Service de Chirurgie Cardiovasculaire, CHU Pitié-Salpêtrière, 93, boulevard de l'Hôpital, 75013 Paris, France

CAMPBELL R.W.F.
Academic Department of Cardiology, Freeman Hospital, Newcastle Upon Tyne, United Kingdom

CAUCHEMEZ B.
Département de Cardiologie, Hôpital Lariboisière, 2, rue Ambroise Paré, 75010 Paris, France

CHOMETTE G.
Service d'Anatomo-Pathologie, CHU Pitié-Salpêtrière, 47, boulevard de l'Hôpital, 75013 Paris, France

CORABOEUF E.
Laboratoire de Physiologie Comparée et Laboratoire de Biomembranes et des Ensembles Neuronaux associé au Centre National de la Recherche Scientifique, Université Paris XI, 91405 Orsay, France

COUMEL P.
Département de Cardiologie, Hôpital Lariboisière, 2, rue Ambroise Paré, 75010 Paris, France

DAE Michael W.
Department of Cardiology, University of California at San Francisco, 2130 Fulton Street, San Francisco, CA 94117, USA

DAVIS J.C.
Department of Cardiology, University of California at San Francisco, 2130 Fulton Street, San Francisco, CA 94117, USA

DAVY J.M.
Service de Cardiologie, Hôpital Antoine Béclère, 157, rue de la Porte de Trivaux, 92140 Clamart, France

DeCARLO Leonard
Veterans Administration Medical Center, Cardiology Research Service (151-F), 921 Northeast 13th
Street, Oklahoma City, OK 73104, USA

DONETTI Joël
Service de Cardiologie, CHRU de Nancy-Brabois, 54500 Vandoeuvre-les-Nancy, France

DOUARD H.
Department of Exercise Testing, Hôpital Cardiologique du Haut Lévêque, 33604 Pessac, France

DUBOIS Ch.
Service de Cardiologie, CHU de Liège, Hôpital de Bavière, 66 bvd de la Constitution,
4020, Liège, Belgium

ESCANDE D.
Laboratoire de Physiologie Comparée et Laboratoire de Biomembranes et des Ensembles
Neuronaux associé au Centre National de la Recherche Scientifique, Université Paris XI,
91405 Orsay, France

FARENQ G.
Service de Rythmologie et de Stimulation Cardiaque, Hôpital Jean Rostand, 39, rue Le Galleu,
94200 Ivry, France

FONTAINE Guy
Service de Rythmologie et de Stimulation Cardiaque, Hôpital Jean Rostand, 39, rue Jean Le
Galleu, 94200 Ivry, France

FONTALIRAN F.
Service d'Anatomo-Pathologie, CHU Pitié Salpêtrière, 47, boulevard de l'Hôpital, 75013 Paris,
France

FRANK R.
Service de Rythmologie et de Stimulation Cardiaque, Hôpital Jean Rostand, 39, rue Le Galleu,
94200 Ivry, France

FRIDAY Karen J.
Cardiology, Room 3E-204, University of Oklahoma Health Sciences Center, PO Box 26901,
Oklahoma City, OK 73190, USA

GARSON Arthur, Jr
Section of Cardiology, Department of Pediatrics, Texas Children's Hospital, 6621 Fannin,
Houston, TX 77030, USA

GILGENKRANTZ Jean-Marie
Département de Cardiologie, CHRU de Nancy, Hôpital Central, 54037 Nancy Cedex, France

GORGELS A.P.M.
Department of Cardiology, Academic Hospital of Maastricht, University of Limburg, Maastricht,
The Netherlands

GROSGOGEAT Yves
Service de Rythmologie et de Stimulation Cardiaque, Hôpital Jean Rostand, 39, rue Jean Le
Galleu, 94200 Ivry, France

GUIRAUDON Gérard M.
University Hospital, University of Western Ontario, London, PO Box 5339, Ontario N6A 5A5,
Canada

HAERTEN K.
Hospital of the University of Düsseldorf, Department of Cardiology, Pneumology and Angiology, Düsseldorf, West Germany

HARGROVE W. Clark
Cardiovascular Section, Room 658 Ravdin Building, Hospital of the University of Pennsylvania, 3400 Spruce Street, Philadelphia, PA 19104, USA

HERMIDA 'Jean-Sylvain
Département de Cardiologie, Hôpital Lariboisière, 2, rue Ambroise Paré, 75010 Paris, France

JACKMAN Warren J.
Cardiology, Room 3E-204, University of Oklahoma Health Sciences Center, PO Box 26901, Oklahoma City, OK 73190, USA

JAILLON Patrice
Unité de Pharmacologie Clinique, Hôpital Saint-Antoine, 75012 Paris, France

JOSEPHSON Mark E.
Cardiovascular Section, Room 658 Ravdin Building, Hospital of the University of Pennsylvania, 3400 Spruce Street, Philadelphia, PA 19104, USA

JUANTEGUY Juan M.
Sinai Hospital of Baltimore, Department of Medicine, Baltimore, Maryland, 21215, USA

KARBENN U.
Hospital of the University of Düsseldorf, Department of Cardiology, Pneumology and Angiology, Düsseldorf, West Germany

KHALIFE Khalifé
Département de Cardiologie, CHRU de Nancy, Hôpital Central, 54037 Nancy Cedex, France

KIENY Jean-René
Hôpital Cardiovasculaire et Pneumologique Louis Pradel, BP Lyon Montchat, 69394 Lyon Cedex 03, France

KIRKORIAN Gilbert
Hôpital Cardiovasculaire et Pneumologique Louis Pradel, BP Lyon Montchat, 69394 Lyon Cedex 03, France

KLEIN George J.
University Hospital, University of Western Ontario, London, PO Box 5339, Ontario N6A 5A5, Canada

KLESZCZ A.
Service Frédéric Joliot, Département de Biologie du C.E.A., 91400 Orsay, France

KULBERTUS H.E.
Service de Cardiologie, CHU de Liège, Hôpital de Barière, 66 bvd de la Constitution, 4020. Liège, Belgium

KULBERTUS H.E.
Service de Cardiologie, CHU de Liège, Hôpital de Bavière, 66 bvd de la Constitution, 4020, Liège, Belgium

LACOMBE Pierre
Centre Cardiovasculaire J. Cantini, 8 bis avenue Védrines, 13009 Marseille, France

d

LAVAUD P.
Hôpital Cardiovasculaire et Pneumologique Louis Pradel, BP Lyon Montchat, 69394 Lyon Cedex 03, France

LAZZARA Ralph
Department of Cardiology, Veterans Administration Medical Center and University of Oklahoma Health Sciences Center, Oklahoma City, OK 73104, USA

LECLERCQ Jean-François
Département de Cardiologie, Hôpital Lariboisière, 2, rue Ambroise Paré, 75010 Paris, France

LE GULUDEC Dominique
Service de Cardiologie, Hôpital Antoine Béclère, 157, rue de la Porte de Trivaux, 92140 Clamart, France

LEVY Samuel
Centre Cardiovasculaire J. Cantini, 8 bis avenue Védrines, 13009 Marseille, France

MAISONBLANCHE P.
Département de Cardiologie, Hôpital Lariboisière, 2, rue Ambroise Paré, 75010 Paris, France

MARCHLINSKI Francis E.
Cardiovascular Section, Room 658 Ravdin Building, Hospital of the University of Pennsylvania, 3400 Spruce Street, Philadelphia, PA 19104, USA

MARCON François
Service de Cardiologie Infantile, CHRU de Nancy, Hôpital d'Enfants, 54511 Vandoeuvre-les-Nancy, France

MARTIN DE LA SALLE E.
Service d'Anatomo-Pathologie, CHU Pitié-Salpêtrière, 47, boulevard de l'Hôpital, 75013 Paris, France

MASON Jay W.
Cardiology Division, University of Utah, School of Medicine, Salt Lake City, UT 84112, USA

MESNILDREY P.
Service de Chirurgie Cardiovasculaire, Hôpital Lariboisière, 2, rue Ambroise Paré, 75475 Paris Cedex 10, France

MILLER John M.
Cardiovascular Section, Room 658 Ravdin Building, Hospital of the University of Pennsylvania, 3400 Spruce Street, Philadelphia, PA 19104, USA

MIROWSKI M.
Sinai Hospital of Baltimore, Department of Medicine, Baltimore, Maryland 21215, USA

MORA B.
Department of Exercise Testing, Hôpital Cardiologique du Haut Lévêque, 33604 Pessac, France

MOTTE Gilbert
Service de Cardiologie, Hôpital Antoine Béclère, 157, rue de la Porte de Trivaux, 92140 Clamart, France

MOWER Morton M.
Sinai Hospital of Baltimore, Department of Medicine, Baltimore, Maryland 21215, USA

ORISHIMO T. Franz
Cardiovascular Section, Room 658 Ravdin Building, Hospital of the University of Pennsylvania, 3400 Spruce Street, Philadelphia, PA 19104, USA

PATTERSON Eugene
Veterans Administration Medical Center, Cardiology Research Service (151-F), 921 Northeast 13th Street, Oklahoma City, OK 73104, USA

PAVIE A.
Service de Chirurgie Cardiovasculaire, CHU Pitié-Salpêtrière, 93, boulevard de l'Hôpital, 75013 Paris, France

PERNOT Claude
Service de Cardiologie Infantile, CHRU de Nancy, Hôpital d'Enfants, 54511 Vandoeuvre-les-Nancy, France

PIERARD L.
Service de Cardiologie, CHU de Liège, Hôpital de Bavière, 66 bvd de la Constitution, 4020, Liège, Belgium

PODCZECK A.
Hospital of the University of Düsseldorf, Department of Cardiology, Pneumology and Angiology, Düsseldorf, West Germany

PRYSTOWSKI Eric M.
Clinical Electrophysiology Laboratory, Duke University Medical Center, Durham, NC, USA

SCHEINMANN Melvin M.
Department of Cardiology, University of California at San Francisco, 2130 Fulton Street, San Francisco, CA 94117, USA

SCHERLAG Benjamin J.
Research Service (151-F), Veterans Medical Center, 921 Northeast 13th Street, Oklahoma City, OK 73104, USA

SCHWARZMAIER J.
Hospital of the University of Düsseldorf, Department of Cardiology, Pneumology and Angiology, Düsseldorf, West Germany

SEBAG Claude
Service de Cardiologie, Hôpital Antoine Béclère, 157, rue de la Porte de Trivaux, 92140 Clamart, France

SHARMA Arjun D.
University Hospital, University of Western Ontario, London, PO Box 5339, Ontario N6A 5A5, Canada

SIRINELLI A.
Service de Cardiologie, Hôpital Antoine Béclère, 157 rue de la Porte de Trivaux, 92140 Clamart, France

SMEETS J.P.
Service de Cardiologie, CHU de Liège, Hôpital de Bavière, 66 bvd de la Constitution, 4020, Liège, Belgium

SYROTA A.
Service Frédéric Joliot, Département de Biologie du CEA, 91400 Orsay, France

SZABO Bela
Veterans Administration Medical Center, Cardiology Research Service (151-F), 921 Northeast 13th Street, Oklahoma City, OK 73104, USA

TERRIER DE LA CHAISE Arnaud
Service de Cardiologie, CHRU de Nancy-Brabois, 54500 Vandoeuvre-les-Nancy, France

TOUBOUL Paul
Hôpital Cardiovasculaire et Pneumologique Louis Pradel, BP Lyon Montchat, 69394 Lyon Cedex 03, France

VALETTE H.
Service Frédéric Joliot, Département de Biologie du CEA, 91400 Orsay, France

VASSALLO Joseph A.
Cardiovascular Section, Room 658 Ravdin Building, Hospital of the University of Pennsylvania, 3400 Spruce Street, Philadelphia, PA 19104, USA

VELTRI Enrico P.
Sinai Hospital of Baltimore, Department of Medicine, Baltimore, Maryland 21215, USA

WELLENS Hein J.J.
Department of Cardiology, Academic Hospital of Maastricht, University of Limburg, Maastricht, The Netherlands

ZANNAD Faiez
Département de Cardiologie, CHRU de Nancy, Hôpital Central, 54037 Nancy Cedex, France

ZIMMERMANN Marc
Département de Cardiologie, Hôpital Lariboisière, 2, rue Ambroise Paré, 75010 Paris, France

1. Cellular mechanisms of ventricular arrhythmias in ischemia

RALPH LAZZARA

The elucidation of the cellular mechanisms of ventricular arrhythmias in ischemia and infarction has been impeded by the inability to monitor readily intracellular potentials in ischemically-injured myocardium in situ. Various approaches to the problem, including recording of intracellular potentials from subepicardial cells in the beating heart with floating micro-electrodes, study of excised ischemically-injured myocardium, and study of excised normal tissues exposed to simulated ischemic conditions, all have limitations and the liability of generation of misleading data and wrong conclusions. Nevertheless, intriguing and perhaps relevant and significant observations have been made of the electrophysiological properties of cells altered by ischemia. Reviews in recent years have surveyed the burgeoning literature dealing with the cellular electrophysiological alteration due to ischemia [1, 2]. In this brief review, certain findings that appear at this time to be important in generation of arrhythmias will be highlighted.

The cellular elements of reentry

The prevalent informed opinion is that reentry is the dominant mechanism for ischemic ventricular tachycardia. The requisites for reentrant excitation were expounded just after the beginning of this century [3–6] 1) directionally selective propagation involving a barrier for encirclement and unidirectional propagation around the barrier; 2) conduction time in the circuit longer than the refractory period of all the components of the circuit including the site of access. Early models (exemplified by the familiar ring model of figure 1A) included a fixed barrier to propagation, i.e. an inexcitable interior; a site of unidirectional block along the circuit; and slow conduction. Recently models more relevant to the cardiac syncytium have been constructed. In the planar models of figures 1B and 1C a linear barrier is formed by a line of refractoriness and conduction proceeds around the barrier in one or two directions, depending on the spatial distribution of the refractory periods on the surface in relation to the conduction time. In the

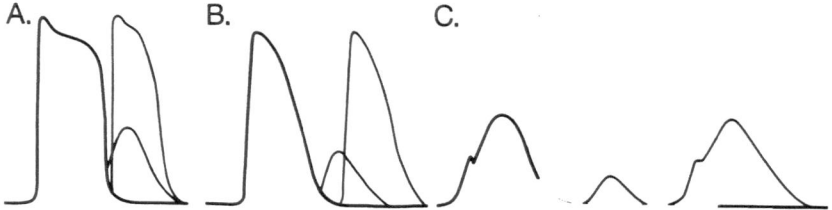

Figure 1. Models of reentry. A. The familiar ring model containing an inpenetrable inner circle as a barrier and a segment (shaded) of slow conduction and unidirectional block. In this and the other models, the dense line represents the line of block and the clear segment of the line represents the site of unidirectional block. The thinner lines represent the path of the impulse with the arrow heads denoting the direction. In the other models the thinner lines represent the wavefront of propagation. In the ring, the refractory period (RP) of the access site is 200 ms and the total conduction time around the ring is 210 ms. The times of arrival of the impulse at the various sites along the ring are represented by the numbers adjacent to the sites. B. The 'figure of eight' model contains an arc of conduction block within an abnormal region (shaded circle) where conduction is slowed and refractory properties are abnormal. The wavefront proceeds around both ends of the arc and reverses direction to cross the arc of block near the center when the refractory period of that segment recedes. C. The 'leading circle' model contains a line of block in a region of relatively prolonged refractoriness in comparison to the site of initiation of the impulse (+). The wavefront proceeds around only one end of the arc of block because the other end abuts on the boundary of the tissue (left) or because the spatial distribution of refractory periods are so asymmetical that the propagation in one direction along the line of block is much shorter to the end than the propagation in the other direction (right). Consequently, the wavefront circling in the shorter direction arrives at a site of breakthrough before the impulse circling the other end. With this gross asymmetry of refractory properties, the likelihood is that the wavefront would circle around a single line of block rather than circling around two lines of block and coalescing in a common path in the center as in the figure of eight model.

'leading circle' model of Alessie, [7] the spatial boundaries of the surface impels the impulse in one direction around the barrier (fig. 1C). A single line of block could also form if grossly asymmetric spatial distribution of refractory periods and/or conduction velocities leads at the initiation to grossly unequal lines of block and one line becomes dominant (Figure 1C, right). In the 'figure of eight' model of Wit [8] and El Sherif [9] more symmetrical spatial distribution of refractory periods and conduction velocities and lack of boundary limitations results in claw-like envelopment around both ends of the barrier and break-through near the center where refractoriness would be expected to recede earliest (fig. 1B).

The modern versions of the model incorporate the same fundamental elements of the older model: slow conduction, unidirectional block, and a barrier. The motivation for postulating slow conduction always has been the idea that the normal speed of propagation in relation to the normal refractory periods of ventricular myocardium would necessitate unrealistically long reentrant paths. In fact, the normal speed of propagation in ordinary ventricular myocardium (0.2–0.4 M/sec) would allow reentrant circuits with lengths on the order of 100 mm. In view of the size of scars of myocardial infarction in man, a circuit of this

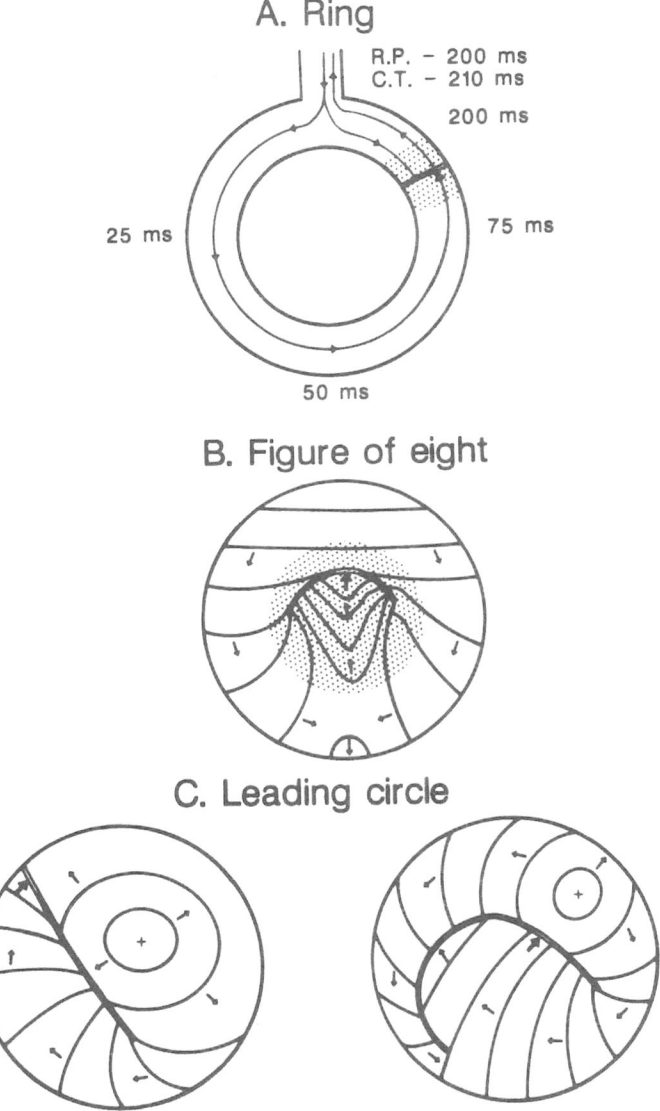

A. Ring

R.P. – 200 ms
C.T. – 210 ms

200 ms

25 ms

75 ms

50 ms

B. Figure of eight

C. Leading circle

Figure 2. Effects of ischemia on action potentials and refractoriness of ordinary ventricular myocardial cells. Drawings of typical action potentials at normal heart rates (dense traces) and with premature excitation (light traces) at the end of the absolute refractory period and the relative refractory period for normal cells (A) and for cells mildly (B) and severely (C) injured by ischemia. In the ischemically injured cells the refractory periods outlast the action potentials, especially in the more severely affected cells. In the severely affected cells the upstroke of the action potentials are frequently irregular.

magnitude around the perimeter of a scar is plausible. Nevertheless, information gained from animal models [8, 9] and humans [10] indicates that circuits often are smaller and include segments with abnormally slow conduction.

The predominant evidence up to now links slow conduction in ischemically injured myocardium to reduced fast sodium current and slowed upstrokes of action potentials, shown in figure 2. Earlier conjecture [11–13] that ischemically-injured cardiac cells might generate excitatory current solely via slow channels, so-called slow responses, has not been strongly supported, though isolated observations have been made of ischemically injured cells with slow upstrokes sensitive to slow channel blockers [14]. Indeed, studies of action potentials with severely depressed upstrokes indicate that they are unable to respond and to propagate at very high rates [1, 14]. It seems more likely that slow conduction in successful reiterative reentrant circuits is mediated by moderately depressed action potentials as in figure 2B, rather than severely depressed as in figure 3C. Sodium current is diminished because resting potential is reduced (more positive than normal) leading to inactivation of the fast channels, and because of other factors directly depressing the channel evidenced by shifts in the membrane responsiveness curves [1, 15] as shown in figure 3. The loss of resting potential of cardiac cells with acute ischemia is attributed mainly to elevation of extracellular potassium leaked from cells [16, 17]; also to activation of nonspecific cation channels by elevated cytosolic calcium [18]. The nonspecific channels would transmit depolarizing inward current. In subacute and chronic ischemic injury, the factors leading to partial depolarization are undoubtedly different and not yet fully clarified. Intracellular ionic alterations such as decrease in intracellular potassium may be important in the depolarization of later stages.

There is increasing evidence that alterations in cell-to-cell coupling in the form of reduced number of intercellular connections [19, 20] and higher resistance in ischemically injured myocardium of those connections [21] impede propagation and exaggerate the normal anisotrophy of propagation [22, 23]. The latter result might contribute to the formation of barriers and directionally selective propagation.

The property of refractoriness is affected by ischemia. The time course of repolarization is invariably changed, though the type of change varies depending on cell type, stage of ischemic injury, and other factors. In acute ischemia there is consistent abbreviation of repolarization in both myocardial cells and Purkinje fibers [24–28]. The repolarization of Purkinje fibers in the infarct zone is generally prolonged 1–4 days after coronary occlusion [29, 30], while surviving myocardial cells usually have abbreviated repolarization or little change in duration [1, 31]. These changes necessarily affect refractoriness since the gating of fast and slow channels are voltage-dependent. In addition there is a poorly understood time dependent refractoriness that outlasts repolarization. This phenomenon is variable among cells, and tends to be more prominent among more depolarized cells with more depressed action potentials (figure 2). This time dependent

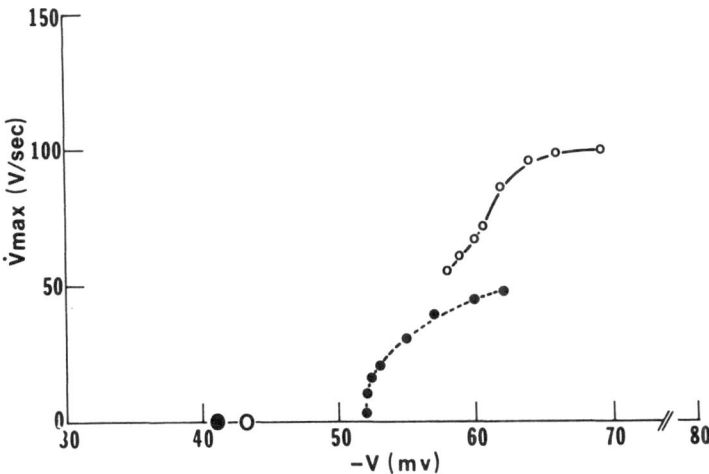

Figure 3. Depression of responsiveness by ischemia. Maximal upstroke velocity (V̇ max) plotted against membrane potentials as cells are excited during successive stages of depolarization by increasing extracellular potassium. The curve for the ischemically injured cell (solid circle) is displaced downward and to the left with respect to the curve for the cell and the normal zone (empty circles). The large circles on the abscissa represent resting membrane potentials at extracellular potassium of 24 mM.

refractoriness has been called post-repolarization refractoriness [32]. The recovery from inactivation of altered fast channels may be delayed by unidentified factors. Since refractoriness may be shortened in proportion to abbreviation of repolarization, or lengthened by prolongation of repolarization and the superimposition of post-repolarization refractoriness, the effect is to augment 'dispersion', i.e. heterogeneity, and increase the susceptibility to reentrant arrhythmias.

The formation of the reentrant circuits mapped in figures 1B and 1C is critically dependent on the spatial distribution of refractory properties. It is felt that the barrier around which the circuit forms is a line of functional block along a segment of tissue where the duration of refractoriness is longest and the spatial gradient of duration is greatest. Also the 'unidirectional block' necessary to complete the circuit derives from the recession of refractoriness, allowing the wavefront of excitation to traverse later a segment that had earlier been a site of block. Finally, slow conduction in a portion of the circuit is mainly the result of excitation of tissue during the relative refractory period, since velocity of conduction in the same regions is normal or only slightly abnormal at long cycle lengths. In the model in figure 1C, derived essentially from normal tissue, the barrier forms only if the normal dispersion and spatial heterogeneity of refractory periods is engaged by a premature impulse initiated early in a site of brief refractoriness in relation to surrounding sites. Thus it appears that abnormal properties of refractoriness can provide critical elements of circuits. However there is still the possibility that in human disease certain reentrant circuits might not have such critical dependence on the refractory properties of the tissues. For example, inexcitable regions such as scars could serve as barriers, and slow conduction could exist in abnormal regions even at long cycle lengths. On the other hand, clinical observations of the importance of short cycle lengths in the induction of ventricular arrhythmias [33] underscores the importance of refractoriness as a critical determinant of reentry in clinical ischemic heart disease.

Recently, studies of anisotropic conduction by Spach and coworkers [22, 23] have inspired the hypothesis that sparsity and increased resistance of intercellular connections in ischemic and infarcted tissues cause an enhancement of normal anisotropy and more severe slowing of conduction, expecially in directions perpendicular to the long axes of the fiber bundles. Since the safety factor is least with conduction *parallel* to the long axes of the fiber bundles, block is more likely in the longitudinal direction, and the line (or plane) of block would be transversely oriented (perpendicular to the long axes). The foundation for slow conduction, unidirectional block and barriers could lie in the basic anisotropy of conduction exaggerated and distorted by irregular loss and increased resistance of intercellular junctions. It has been suggested [19, 20] that the fractionated electrograms that are common in diseased myocardium where reentry is generated, reflect asynchronous upstrokes and irregular propagation due to the abnormalities of intercellular communications, rather than irregular upstrokes observed in severely depressed cells [1].

This hypothesis focuses on abnormalities of intercellular communication, but it is not independent of refractory properties. Increased intercellular resistance entails a reduction of transmitted excitatory current, therefore a weakened stimulus for excitation, which would interact with the refractory properties so that irregular propagation and the tendency to form unidirection block and barriers would be exaggerated at shorter cycle lengths. Thus abnormalities of intercellular communication would have the effect of further prolonging the refractory periods for the *propagated* impulse, especially for the wavefront propagating in a direction parallel to the axes of the fiber bundles. According to this hypothesis the direction of conduction of the wavefront in relation to the orientation of fiber bundles would be a major determinant of the formation of the reentrant circuits. The line of block should be generally perpendicular to the long axes of the bundles, and slow conduction also should be in the direction perpendicular to the long axes. If the spatial gradient of intrinsic refractory periods determined by direct stimulation rather than failure of conduction is the major determinant of the formation of the line of block, then the line of block should be aligned along the contours of the refractory isochromes, more or less independently of the direction of the initial wavefront and the orientation of the fiber bundles. These possibilities are illustrated in figure 4.

A process like reflection [34] has been postulated by Janse and co-workers [35, 36] to occur in very early ischemia. Electronic current flow across an 'inexcitable

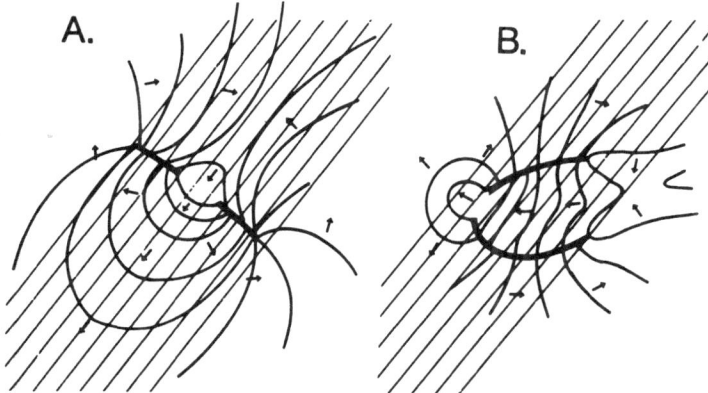

Figure 4. Postulated reentrant circuits when anisotropic conduction is the major determinant of formation of the circuit (A) and when the spatial distribution of refractoriness is the major determinant. If anisotropic conduction is the major determinant the line of block (dense line) should be perpendicular to the long axis of the fibers and the isochrones of the wavefronts of activation would tend to assume an eccentric configuration favoring an alignment along the long axes of the fibers where conduction is more rapid. If the spatial distribution of refractoriness is the major determinant (C) the line of block would tend to assume the shape of the arc of a circle which would be the general shape of the isochrones of refractoriness in a region where refractoriness is steeply approaching a maximum. The relationship of the arc of block to the long axes of the fiber bundle would not be predictable since in this model the intrinsic refractory properties determined by direct stimulation have been postulated to be the major determinant. In both schema the figure of eight model has been chosen but a leading circle model with a single line or arc of block could also be applied.

gap', excites fibers just distal to the gap with significant delay. The delayed action potential returns electrotonic current to reexcite the repolarized fibers proximal to the gap. Purkinje fibers are thought to be involved in this process. So far evidence for this mechanism is indirect.

Abnormal automaticity and triggered firing

Early studies of Purkinje fibers in infarcted regions indicated that there were enhanced diastolic depolarization and reduced diastolic potentials during the period 1–4 days after coronary occlusion [29, 30]. It has been postulated that this abnormality might be the basis for 'accelerated ventricular rhythms' or 'idio-ventricular tachycardias' that occur commonly in the early days of myocardial infarction [37], since these clinical arrhythmias are initiated by relatively late coupled complexes, are not very rapid, and rarely lead to ventricular fibrillation. This abnormal automaticity is relatively insensitive to lidocaine [38] or beta blockade [30, 39]. It appears to recede with time as the surviving Purkinje fibers are restored toward normal electrophysiological properties in general [26, 40].

Abnormal Automaticity

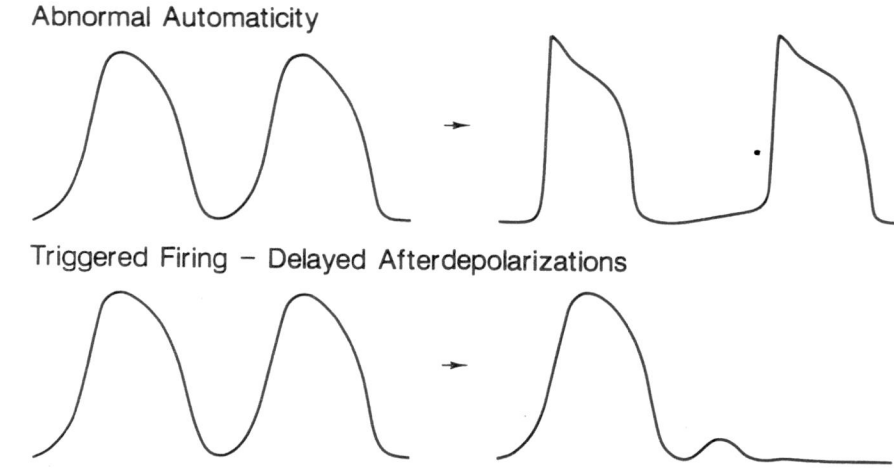

Triggered Firing – Delayed Afterdepolarizations

Figure 5. Mechanisms of abnormal impulse generation in ischemically injured Purkinje fibers. At the top (A) are shown drawings of transmembrane potentials with reduced resting potential, accelerated diastolic depolarization and pacemaker action potentials generated by an ischemically injured Purkinje fiber 24 hours after myocardial infarction. Over time (right) with superfusion the resting potentials increase toward normal and the rate of diastolic depolarization slows. At the bottom (B) transmembrane potentials indistinguishable from automatic firing, are generated by an ischemically injured Purkinje fiber. With time, the apparently automatic firing abruptly terminates disclosing delayed afterdepolarizations. Thus, the mode of termination can distinguish true automatic firing from triggered firing.

Recently El-Sherif and coworkers challenged the interpretation of abnormal automaticity, contending that all or most of the apparent automatic firing is triggered firing based on delayed afterdepolarizations [41, 42]. Delayed after-depolarizations were evident on cessation of firing in their preparations of infarcted endocardium. Their preparations differed from earlier studies in that they were much smaller. Also their superfusate contained relatively high concentrations of calcium (2.7 mM). It is possible that the trauma of dissection and the higher calcium concentration were factors promoting the generation of delayed afterdepolarizations. In vivo, neither beta blockers nor calcium entry blockers alone were notably affective in suppressing the ventricular ectopic activity. The combination of beta blockade and slow channel blockade was effective in the studies of El-Sherif and coworkers but significant hypotension resulted and this altered hemodynamic state may have played a role in the suppression of the arrhythmias. Rosen and coworkers [43], using an array of pharmacological probes in vivo, concluded that most of the ectopic activity 24 hours after coronary occlusion is due to abnormal automaticity rather than delayed afterdepolarizations.

The study of the mechanisms for generation of ventricular arrhythmias in chronic animal models is in a primitive stage, because realistic chronic models that show serious spontaneous ventricular arrhythmias have not been developed. The cellular abnormalities of a chronic cat model have been described by Myerburg and coworkers [44]. They include partial depolarization, mildly depressed upstrokes, and heterogeneity in the time course of repolarization. Since there is fibrous tissue interspersed among the myocardial cells, it is reasonable to presume that intercellular communications are reduced. However, there is very little data on the cellular factors that are important to the formation of reentry pathways and little information with respect to abnormalities of impulse generation, whether abnormal automaticity or afterdepolarizations.

There is very little basic understanding of the alterations of the sarcolemmal ionic channels in ischemia and of the intracellular ion blank distributions and movements. Most of the information so far has been derived from observation of transmembrane potentials of multicellular preparations. More fundamental understanding must await the application of newer techniques to the problem such as isolation of ischemic myocytes, membrane voltage control, and recording of individual channel currents.

References

1. Lazzara R, Scherlag BJ. 1984. Cellular electrophysiology and ischemia. In: Sperelakis, N. ed. Physiology and pathophysiology of the heart. Boston: Martinus Nijhoff 443–458.
2. Singer DH, Baumgarten CM, Ten Eick RE. 1981. Cellular electrophysiology of ventricular and other dysrhythmias: Studies on diseased and ischemic heart. Prog Cardiovasc Dis 24: 97–156.
3. Mayer AG. 1908. Rhythmical pulsation in scyphomedusae: II. Carnegie Institute. Papers. Washington Tortugas Lab 1:113–131, Carnegie Institute Publication No. 102, part VII.
4. Mines GR. 1913. On dynamic equilibrium in the heart. J Physiol 46: 350–383.
5. Mines GR. 1914. On circulating excitations in heart muscles and their possible relation to tachycarida and fibrillation. Trans R Soc Can (ser 3, sect IV) 8: 43–52.
6. Garrey WE. 1914. The nature of fibrillary contraction of the heart. Its relation to tissue mass and form. Am J Physiol 33: 397–408.
7. Allessie MA, Bonke FIM, Schopman FJG. 1977. Circus movement in rabbit atrial muscle as a mechanism of tachycardia. III. The 'leading circle' concept: A new model of circus movement in cardiac tissue without the involvement of an anatomical obstacle. Cir Res 41: 9–18.
8. Wit Al, Allessie MA, Bonke FIM, et al. 1982. Electrophysiologic mapping to determine the mechanism of experimental ventricular tachycardia initiated by premature impulses: Experimental approach and initial results demonstrating reentrant excitation. Am J Cardiol 49: 166–185.
9. El-Sherif N, Mehra R, Gough WB, et al. 1982. Ventricular activation pattern of spontaneous and induced ventricular rhythms in canine one-day-old myocardial infarction. Evidence for focal and reentrant mechanisms. Circ Res 51: 152–166.
10. Josephson M, Buxton A, Marchlinski F, et al. 1985. Sustained ventricular tachycardia in coronary artery disease – Evidence for reetrant mechanism. In: Zipes DP, Jalife J, eds. Cardiac Electrophysiology and Arrhythmias. New York: Grune and Stratton, Inc. pp 409–418.
11. Wit AL, Bigger JT. 1975. Possible electrophysiological mechanisms for lethal arrhythmias accompanying myocardial ischemia and infarction. Circulation 51 (suppl 3): 96–115.
12. Cranefield PF. 1975. The conduction of the cardiac impulse, Mount Kisco, New York, Futura.
13. Zipes DP, Besch HR, Watanabe AM. 1975. Role of the slow current in cardiac electrophysiology. Circulation 51: 761.

14. Spear JF, Horowitz LN, Hodess AB, et al. 1979. Cellular electrophysiology of human myocardial infarction 1. Abnormalities of cellular activation. Circulation 59: 247.

15. Lazzara R, Scherlag BJ. 1980. The role of the slow current in the generation of arrhythmias in ischemic myocardum. In: Zipes DP, Bailey JC, Elharrar V (eds) The slow inward current and cardiac arrhythmias. The Hague: Martinus Nijhoff, pp 399–416.

16. Moore DJ. 1938. Potassium changes in the functioning heart under conditions of ischemia and congestion. Am J Physiol 123: 443–447.

17. Hill JL, Gettes LS. 1980. Effect of acute coronary artery occlusion on local myocardial extracellular K+ activity in swine. Circulation 61: 768–778.

18. Clusin WT, Buchbinder M, Ellis AK, et al. 1984. Reduction of ischemic depolarization by the calcium channel blocker diltiazem: Correlation with improvement of ventricular conduction and early arrhythmias in the dog. Circ Res 54: 10–20.

19. Spear JF, Michelson EL, Moore EN. 1983. Reduced space constant in slowly conducting regions of chronically infarcted canine myocardium. Circ Res 53: 176.

20. Gardner PI, Ursell PC, Fenoglio JJ Jr., Wit AL. 1985. Electrophysiologic and anatomic basis for fractionated electrograms recorded from healed myocardial infarcts. Circulation 72: 596–611.

21. De Mello WC. 1982. Cell-to-cell communication in heart and other tissues. Prog Biophys Mol Biol 39: 147–182.

22. Spach MS, Miller WT III, Geselowitz DB, et al. 1981. The discontinuous nature of propagation in normal canine cardiac muscle. Circ Res 48: 39.

23. Spach MS, Kootsey JM. 1983. The nature of electrical propagation in cardiac muscle. Am J Physiol 244: H3.

24. Kardesch M, Hogancamp CE, Bing RJ. 1958. Effect of complete ischemia on the intracellular electrical activity of the whole mammaliam heart. Circ Res 6: 714–725.

25. Samson WE, Scher AM. 1960. Mechanism of S–T segment alteration during acute mycardial injury. Circ Res 3: 780–787.

26. Lazzara R, El-Sherif N, Scherlag BJ. 1973. Early and late effects of coronary artery occlusion on canine Purkinje fibers. Circ Res 33: 597–611.

27. Downar E, Janse MJ, Durrer D. 1977. The effect of acute coronary artery occlusion on subendocardial transmembrane potentials in the intact porcine heart. Circulation 56: 217–224.

28. Kleber AG, Janse MJ, Van Capelle JJL, Durrer D. 1978. Mechanism and time course of S–T and T–Q segment changes during acute regional myocardial ischemia in the pig heart determined by extracellular recordings. Circ Res 42: 603–613.

29. Friedman PL, Stewart JR, Fenoglio JJ Jr, Wit AL. 1973. Survival of subendocardial Purkinje fibers after extensive myocardial infarction in dogs: in vitro and in vivo correlation. Circ Res 33: 597–611.

30. Lazzara R, El-Sherif N, Scherlag BJ. 1973. Electrophysiological properties of Purkinje cells in one-day-old myocardial infarction. Circ Res 33: 722–734.

31. Spear JF, Michelson EL, Moore EN. 1983. Cellular electrophysiologic characteristics of chronically infarcted myocardium in dogs susceptible to sustained ventricular tachyarrhythmias. J Am Coll Cardiol 4: 1099.

32. Lazzara R, El-Sherif, Scherlag BJ. 1975. Disorders of cellular electrophysiology produced by ischemia of the canine His Bundle. Circ Res 36:444–453.

34. Antzelevitch C, Jalife J, Moe GK. 1980. Characteristics of reflection as a mechanism of reentrant arrhythmias and its relationship to parasystole. Circulation 61: 182.

35. Janse MJ, Van Capelle FJL, Morsink H, et al. 1980. Flow of 'injury' current and pattern of excitation during early ventricular arrhythmias in acute regional myocardial ischemia in isolated porcine and canine hearts: evidence for two different arrhythmogenic mechanisms. Circ Res 47: 151–165.

36. Janse MJ, Kleber AG. 1981. Electrophysiological changes and ventricular arrhythmias in the early phase of regional myocardial ischemia. Circ Res 49: 1069–1081.

37. Rothfeld EL, Zucker IR, Parsonnet V and Alinsonorin CA. 1968. Idioventricular rhythm in acute myocardial infarction. Circulation 37: 203.
38. Allen JD, Brennan JF, Wit AL. 1978. Actions of lidocaine on transmembrane potentials of subendocardial Purkinje fibers surviving in infarcted canine hearts. Circ Res 43:470.
39. Hope RR, Scherlag BJ, El-Sherif N, Lazzara R. 1976. Heirarchy of ventricular pacemakers. Circ Res 39: 883–888.
40. Friedman PL, Fenoglio JJ, Wit AL. 1975. Time course for reversal of electrophysiological and ultrastructural abnormalities in subendocardial Purkinje fibers surviving extensive myocardial infarction. Circ Res 36: 127–144.
41. El-Sherif N, Gough WB, Zeiler RH, Mehra R. 1983. Triggered ventricular rhythms in 1-day-old myocardial infarction in the dog. Circ Res 52: 566–579.
42. El-Sherif N, Mehra R, Gough WB, Zeiler RH. 1983. Reentrant vertricular arrhythmias in the late myocardial infarction period. Circulation 68: 644–656.
43. Le Marec H, Dangman KH, Danilo P Jr., et al. 1985. An evaluation of automaticity and triggered activity in the canine heart one to four days after myocardial infarction. Circulation 71: 1224–1236.
44. Myerburg RJ, Gelband H, Nilsson K, et al. 1977. Long-term electrophysiological abnormalities resulting from experimental myocardial infarction in cats. Circ Res 41: 73–84.

2. Cellular mechanisms for ectopy in non-ischemic ventricle

DENIS ESCANDE and EDOUARD CORABOEUF
Laboratoire de Physiologie Comparée et Laboratoire de Biomembranes et des Ensembles Neuronaux associé au Centre National de la Recherche Scientifique, Université Paris XI, 91405 Orsay, France

Introduction

Ventricular tachycardias may arise either (i) from the existence of an available circuit of *reentry;* (ii) from the firing of an *abnormal focus of automaticity* which may be due to *triggered activity* or may result from the development of *non-triggered spontaneously occurring abnormal automaticity* in diseased myocardium; (iii) from the existence of *dispersion of refractoriness* and resulting focal reexcitation. These mechanisms may coexist since a single properly timed ectopic premature impulse may initiate the circus movement.

The present chapter will be restricted to a consideration of the more recent advances in the understanding of the cellular and subcellular mechanisms underlying ectopy in non-ischemic ventricule. In particular, the role of intracellular Ca storage structures in the generation of oscillatory activities will be discussed. These structures, whose function is thought to be greatly modified during myocardial hypertrophy or dilatation, may also be involved in the generation of spontaneously occurring abnormal automaticity.

Triggered activity

As illustrated in Figure 1, two types of triggered activities have been described in vitro. One type is related to the appearance after the end of an action potential of a *delayed* afterdepolarization. The other type is due to an *early* afterdepolarization appearing at the stage of the final repolarization. Both types of afterdepolarizations may reach the threshold of a depolarizing current (the fast Na current or the slow inward current depending at which level of membrane potential the afterdepolarization occurs) and may thereby initiate an automatic response. The automatic response is triggered in the sense that it is evoked by an afterdepolarization that follows and is caused by the preceding action potential. Without the preceding action potential there would be no automatic response. The phe-

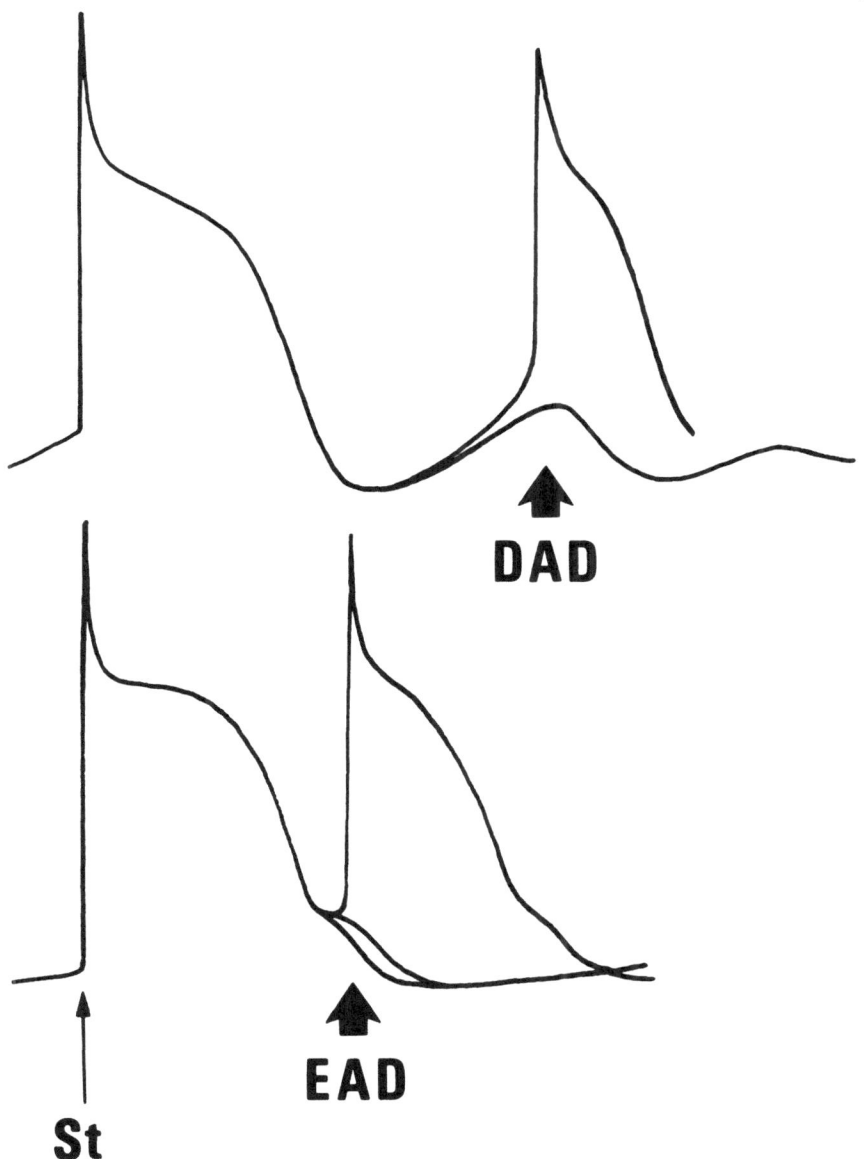

Figure 1. Schematic drawing of delayed (DAD) and early (EAD) afterdepolarizations following a stimulated (St) action potential.

nomenon may continue from one action potential to the following one and may therefore create a *sustained rhythmic activity*.

These concepts are not very new since the first description, using intracellular microelectrodes, of delayed afterdepolarizations was reported by Ferrier et al. in 1973 [1] and since early afterdepolarizations were first recognized by Coraboeuf and Boistel in 1953 [2]. During the last decade, the research engaged in different laboratories has however considerably increased our knowledge of the cellular events responsible for afterpolarizations.

Delayed afterdepolarizations (DADs)

DADs were first reported in ventricular cells poisoned with toxic concentrations of acetylstrophantidin [1]. Since this first description, many other experimental circumstances propitious for the development of DADs have been recognized: catecholamines; high rates of stimulation; increased extracellular Ca or decreased extracellular K; ventricular hypertrophy or dilatation; toxic concentrations of amrinone, milrinone, fenoximone or piroximone; caffeine at low concentrations; metabolic inhibitors ... In fact, it seems that any circumstances during which an abnormal Ca-overload of the cells exists, may lead to DADs. The intracellular Ca concentration is about 10 000 fold less than the extracellular concentration. This Ca concentration gradient is maintained by the cell membrane, which has a low permeability to charged molecules and ions and also by effective pump systems that require energy in order to maintain the cytosolic Ca concentration at these low intracellular levels. As a result of impaired energy production, injured cardiac myocytes may accumulate Ca. Decreased extracellular K and digitalis poisoning induce intracellular Ca-overload because both inhibit the Na-K pump. This inhibition induces an increase in the intracellular Na concentration which, in turn, reduces or even reverses the Na-Ca exchange. A reduction in the Na-Ca exchange may lead to an accumulation of Ca in the cells.

Under any of the above mentioned experimental circumstances, a single premature depolarization occurring at critical cycle length can induce triggered activity and terminate it [3], a property long thought to be unique to reentry.

How can an overload of the cells with Ca produce DADs? In the normal state, the following events occur for each cycle (Figure 2). At the beginning of the action potential, the activation of the Ca channels causes an amount of Ca to flow into the cell (Figure 2A). This Ca influx induces an increase in the intracellular Ca concentration that, in turn, triggers a release of Ca from sarcoplasmic reticulum (SR) stores (Figure 2B). This is the Ca-induced Ca-release as described by Fabiato in various mammals and in particular in human myocardium [4]. The Ca-release from the SR increases the intracellular Ca concentration from 10^{-7} M to about 10^{-5} M. This initiates the contraction. The invasion of the cell plasma with Ca is then rapidly corrected by a rapid reuptake of Ca by the SR (Figure 2C) and by the Na-Ca exchanger which, in the absence of any variation in the intracellular Ca stores contents, extrudes the same amount of Ca as entered via the Ca channels. Therefore, at each systole, there is a 100-fold transient increase of the intracellular Ca concentration. The use of calcium indicators and particularly of the chemilumenescent protein, *aequorin,* allows the on-line monitoring of this Ca transient [5, 6]. Aequorin is a photoprotein, extracted from the common

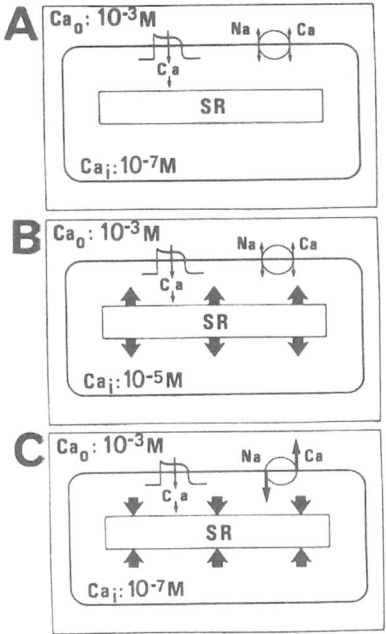
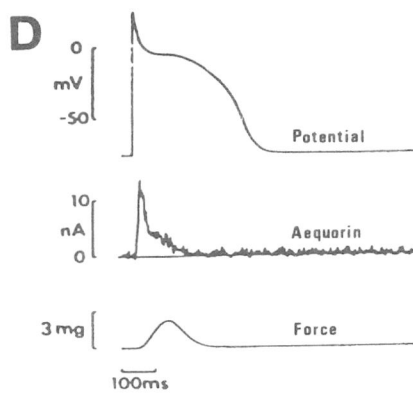

Figure 2. In A, B, and C, the different steps responsible for the Ca transient are shown. SR: sarcoplasmic reticulum. CA_o and Ca_i: extracellular and intracellular Ca concentrations respectively. See text for more details. In A and B the double arrows showing ionic movements through the Na-Ca exchanger indicate that this system can, in principle, reverse when the membrane is fully depolarized during the action potential plateau. In C (and in C, D and E of figure 3), the single arrow associated with the Na-Ca exchanger refer only to diastolic Ca movements. The size of the arrows is not related to flux intensity. D shows: (i) an action potential from a canine Purkinje strand; (ii) the aequorin signal showing the Ca transient; (iii) the contraction. Note that the Ca transient is very steep with regards to the duration of the action potential. The aequorin technique has also been applied to isolated human myocardium [5] and demonstrates similar features. D reprinted from Wier et al., J Gen Physiol 83: 395–415, 1984, by permission of Rockefeller University Press.

jellyfish, which has the feature of emitting blue light in the presence of Ca. This protein can be microinjected, by means of glass microelectrodes, into several cardiac cells. The light emitted by the injected aequorin can be recorded with a photomultiplier tube which converts the light into an electric signal: *The aequorin signal* (Figure 2D). When intracellular Ca-overloading occurs (Figure 3), the Ca reuptake by the SR may be followed by a new release (Figure 3D) since the Ca concentration remains higher than the threshold level required for triggering the release. Several spontaneous cycles release-reuptake of decreasing intensity, may follow one another. Oscillations in the intracellular Ca concentration can therefore be recorded on the aequorin signal (afterglimmers) (Figure 4).

DADs are due to an inward depolarizing current which is thought to passively follow changes in the intracellular Ca. The exact nature of this current is not

16

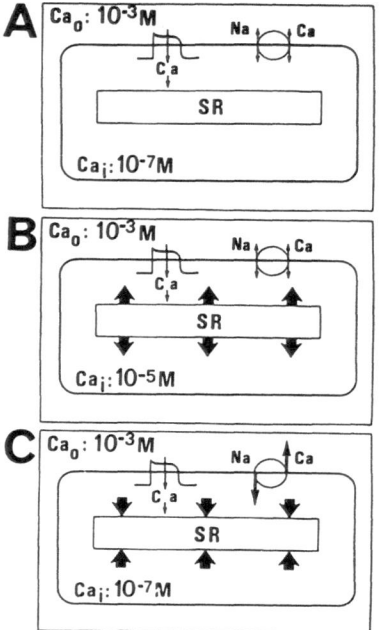

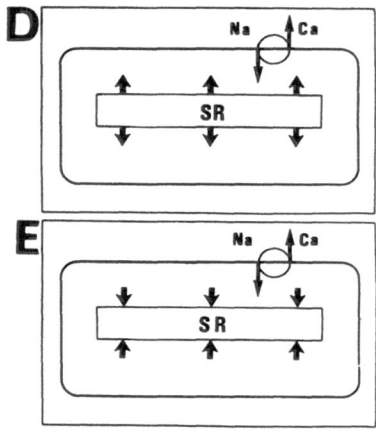

Figure 3. A, B, and C are similar as in Figure 2. When an overloading of the cells with Ca exists, the 'normal' Ca cycle (A, B, C) may be followed by a spontaneous sequence: release (D) and reuptake (E).

definitely established although it is clear that the charge carrier is mainly Na ions [7]. It may be a poorly selective channel which was discovered by Colqhoun et al. or more likely the Na-Ca exchanger itself [8] which seems to be electrogenic, exchanging at least 3 ingoing Na for 1 outgoing Ca. *In summary, DADs appear when an excess of Ca within the cell causes the oscillatory release of Ca from intracellular stores and induces a conductance change for Na in the surface membrane.*

It is well known that overdriving facilitates or inhibits DADs and resultant triggered activity [3]. Concerning *over-drive facilitation,* it is clear that high rates of stimulation result in an additional overloading of the cells with Ca, i.e. an augmentation of the causal anomaly. This additional source of Ca overload may be sufficient for DADs to reach threshold and to induce sustained rhythmic activity. It can be noted that, as the pacing cycle length is decreased between certain limits, the coupling interval of the DAD shortens. Therefore, the firing rate of the first post-drive triggered beats may depend, in some degree, on the stimulation frequency. Concerning *over-drive inhibition,* high rates of stimulation also result in an increase in the intracellular Na which stimulates the Na-K pump. Since this pump usually moves more Na outward than K inward, it generates a net outward hyperpolarizing current across the cell membrane. This hyperpolarizing

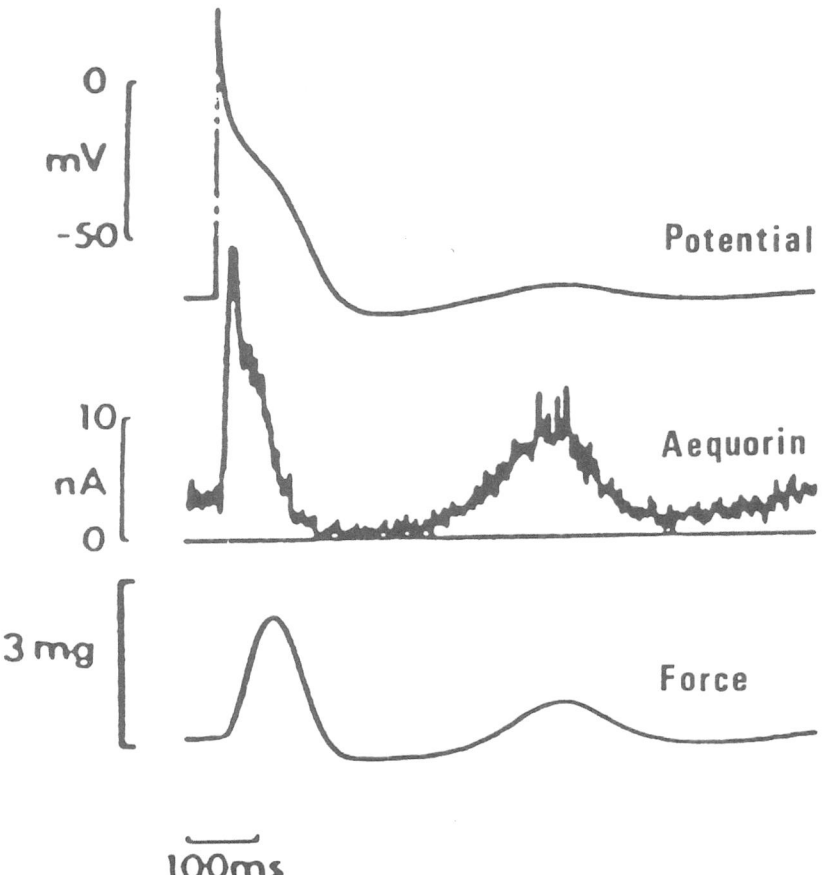

Figure 4. Ouabain-induced delayed afterdepolarizations occurred simultaneously with afterglimmers on the aequorin signal and aftercontractions on the force recordings, same preparation as illustated in Figure 2. Reprinted from Wier et al., J Gen Physiol 83: 395–415, 1984, by permission of Rockefeller University Press.

current partially counterbalances the depolarizing effects of the transient inward current, and thereby may reduce DADs amplitude. This latter mechanism may partly explain why triggered activity often ceases spontaneously. During digitalis poisoning, it is clear that spontaneous arrest of triggered activity is all the less probable as the inhibition of the Na-K pump is complete, i.e.; as the poisoning of the cells is severe.

Many inhibitors of DADs have been recognized. Increased extracellular Mg stimulates the Na-K pump and thus may reduce intracellular Na contents. The inhibition of DADs by Ca channel blockers is presumably due not to direct interference with the abnormal transient inward current but to prevention or reversal of intracellular Ca overload as a result of reduced Ca influx via the slow channel. DADs are also inhibited by quinidine, procaine amide, lidocaine,

18

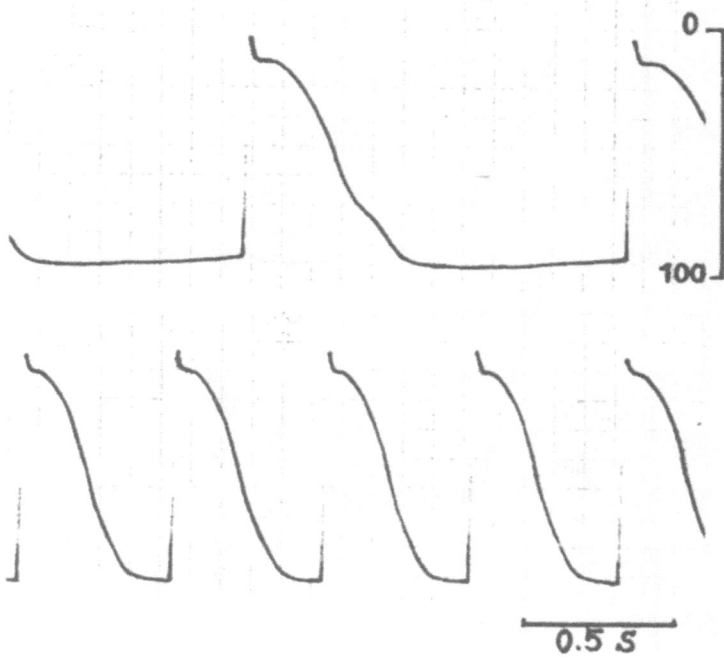

Figure 5. Inhibition of early afterdepolarizations by increasing the rate of stimulation in a canine Purkinje fiber. Reprinted from Coraboeuf et al., J Physiol, Paris, 79: 97–106, 1980, by permission of Masson.

propafenone or ethmozin. Local anesthetics inhibit DADs probably because they reduce the Na loading of the cells through a blockade of the fast inward Na current.

Early afterdepolarizations (EADs)

The mechanisms underlying EADs are not yet entirely understood. In contrast to DADs, EADs are increasingly likely to occur at slow rates of stimulation and can be suppressed by pacing (Figure 5). Experimental circumstances for EADs are acidosis, decreased extracellular K, decreased extracellular Ca, decreased extracellular Mg. EADs can be induced by sotalol, N-acetyl procainamide or cesium chloride. These experimental circumstances under which repolarization is prolonged can be compared with the etiological circumstances of the acquired long QT syndrome. The occurrence of EADs during phase 3 may worsen the prolongation of the repolarization on the surface electrogram and may explain the bizarre T or TU waves seen in patients with the long QT syndrome. Cesium chloride has been shown when injected in vivo to anesthetized dogs to prolong the

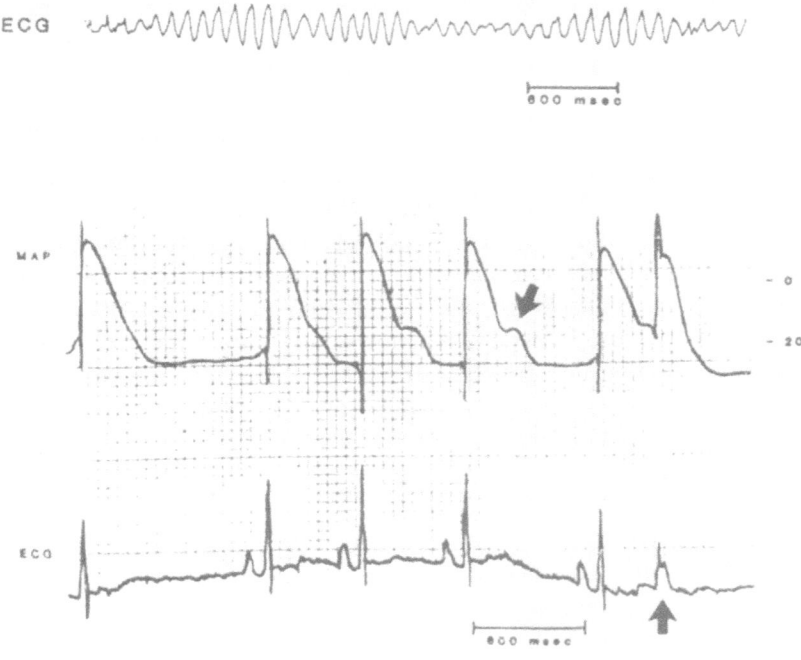

Figure 6. The upper panel shows an example of cesium chloride-induced torsades de pointes. The lower panel shows synchronous recordings of monophasic action potentials and surface ECG. Note that the coupling interval of the premature impulse approximated that of the early afterdepolarization in the previous beat. Reproduced from Levine et al. [10], by permission of the American Heart Association.

QT interval and to induce ventricular ectopy and multiform ventricular tachycardia ressembling torsades de pointes recorded in patients (Figure 6) [9, 10].

At the present time, two different hypothesis have been raised to explain EADs. One suggests that EADs might be related to the electrotonic influence of neighbouring fibers. This explanation seems unsatisfying since EADs have been recorded in isolated cells as well [11]. The other hypothesis suggests that EADs are due to an inward depolarizing current which competes with the background K current to depolarize the membrane. Any inhibition of the background K current such as induced by cesium chloride or decreased extracellular K may reveal the depolarizing effects of the inward current and may allow EADs to develop. The exact nature of the inward current is not definitely established although the fact that the current is inhibited by TTX (a specific fast Na channel inhibitor) or by low Na media suggests that it is mainly carried by Na ions. Brachmann and coworkers have reported that TTX also prevents the occurrence of cesium chloride-induced arrhythmias in the intact dog [9]. Using computer simulation of acidosis-induced

EADs, Coulombe and coworkers [12] have proposed that the inward current responsible for EADs may flow through the fast Na channel within a potential range (the Na-window) for which activation and inactivation gates are both partially open.

It has been emphasized, on the basis of *in vitro* experiments, that because low frequencies are required for EADs to reach their full development, triggered activity related to EADs should mainly occur, *in vivo,* in parasystolic foci protected from the sinus influx by an entry block [13]. *In vivo* experiments performed on dogs treated with cesium chloride indeed confirmed that in steady-state conditions, EADs were strongly attenuated when the cycle length was shortened [10]. However they also showed that in non steady-state conditions, EADs could increase in amplitude and trigger ectopic beats even at relatively short cycle lengths. This shows the complexity of EAD formation in *in vivo* conditions. EADs have been also observed in patients [14] by means of monophasic action potential recordings.

Non-triggered spontaneous activity

Oscillatory fluctuations of membrane potential

In mammalian myocardium, spontaneous oscillatory fluctuations of membrane potential have also been found in *unstimulated preparations* [15]. These spontaneous fluctuations of membrane potential are accompanied by: (i) fluctuations in force; (ii) fluctuations in the current under voltage-clamp experimental conditions; and by (iii) fluctuations in the intracellular Ca concentration as monitored with the aequorin signal [16]. Spontaneous oscillations, which frequency spectrum is similar to that of DADs, are increased in amplitude and frequency by increased extracellular Ca or by digitalis. They have also been attributed to spontaneous movements of Ca between the sarcoplasmic reticulum stores and the cytoplasm and are very likely to be due to the same current as the one generating triggered DADs. The amplitude of these spontaneous oscillations is usually too small to initiate an action potential. The relation between spontaneous oscillations of the membrane potential and ventricular fibrillation, during which regular action potentials are replaced by chaotic low amplitude electrical activity has been questioned [17]. Random summation of subcellular events could, in principle, produce the macroscopic fibrillation observed in vivo.

Abnormal automaticity

Abnormal automaticity may occur spontaneously (i.e., in the absence of any initiating beat) in partially-depolarized regular myocardium. In experiments

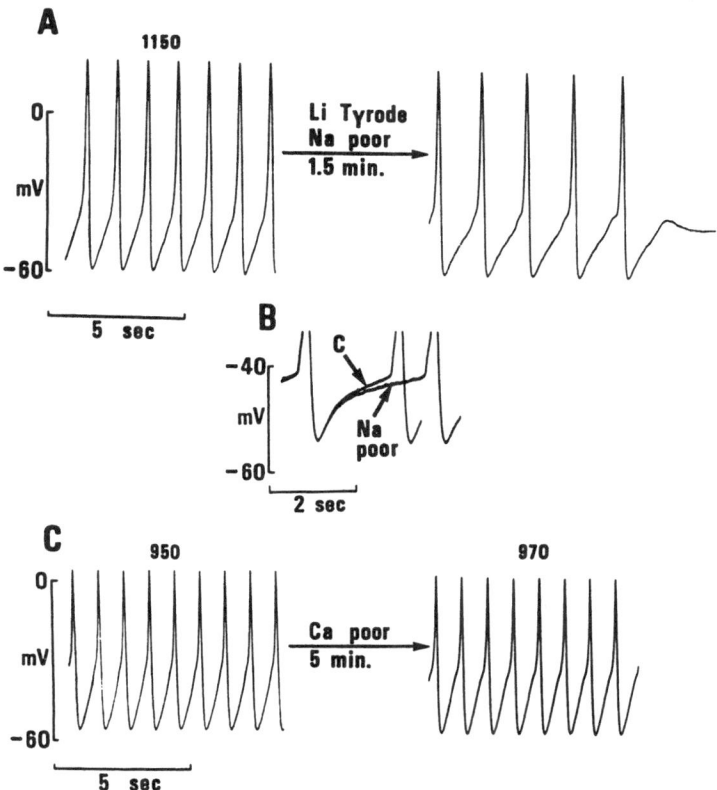

Figure 7. A: in diseased human myocardium, abnormal automaticity was rapidly suppressed by a reduction in the extracellular Na. B: expanded traces of diastolic depolarization from a different fiber in control (C) and in reduced extracellular Na are superimposed. C: a reduction in the extracellular Ca concentration failed to suppress abnormal automaticity within a short period of time. In A and C, numbers above traces indicate spontaneous basic cycle length in ms. Reproduced from Escande et al. [18] by permission of the Academic Press.

performed on human atrial myocardial strips [18], we have observed that abnormal automaticity that develops at low level of membrane potential occurs much more frequently in specimens dissected out from dilated atria than in fibers from normal atria. We have also observed that, in the human myocardium, spontaneously occurring abnormal automaticity was much more sensitive to changes in the extracellular Na than in the extracellular Ca (Figure 7). The use of SR inhibitors such as ryanodine provided us with indirect evidence that sarcoplasmic reticulum-dependent membrane currents similar to those generating DADs may also be involved in the genesis of abnormal diastolic depolarization in partially depolarized human myocardium. Figure 8A shows an irreversible slowing down of the abnormal rhythm under the influence of ryanodine. Figure 8B shows that the very slow spontaneous rhythm remaining after exposure of the fibers to ryanodine was insensitive to epinephrine although epinephrine markedly in-

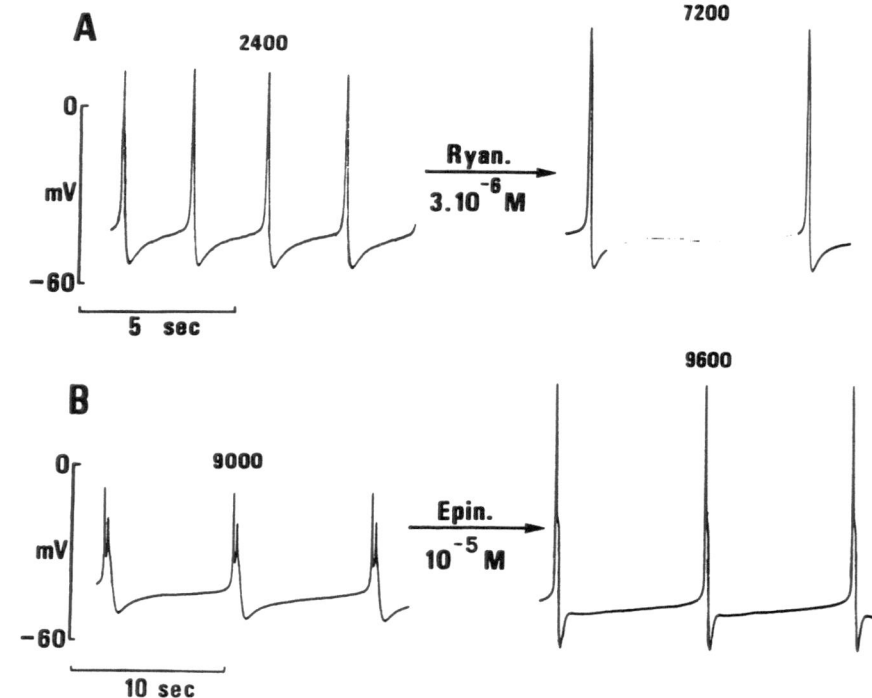

Figure 8. Human myocardium studied in vitro: A shows the irreversible effects of ryanodine on abnormal automaticity. B shows that epinephrine was ineffective to accelerate the spontaneous rhythm that remained after pretreatement of the fibers with ryanodine (different preparation from that in A). Numbers above traces indicate spontaneous basic cycle length in ms. Reproduced from Escande et al. [18] by permission of the Academic Press.

creased the amplitude and the Vmax of the slow reponses elicited at this low level of membrane potential. By contrast, adrenaline accelerates the ryanodine insensitive phase of diastolic depolarisation. Because Ca movements at the sarcoplasmic reticulum level are known to be cAMP-dependent, this and other experiments [18] suggest that sarcoplasmic reticulum- controlled currents may also participate in abnormal automaticity in the myocardium from dilated atria. The fact that the ryanodine sensitive phase of diastolic depolarization is very slow implies that the sarcoplasmic reticulum-dependent currents and therefore the intracellular Ca-transients be also very slow. In normal human myocardium this is clearly not the case [6]. However, it has been shown that the intracellular Ca transient undergoes a marked prolongation and flattening under conditions that dilate and hypertrophy the myocardium such as experimental banding of the main pulmonary artery in animals [19]. Such flattening has also been observed in the hypertrophied human myocardium [6]. These observations demonstrate that under certain pathological circumstances, intracellular Ca transient may be prolonged enough for sarcoplasmic reticulum-dependent currents to contribute towards abnormal diastolic depolarization.

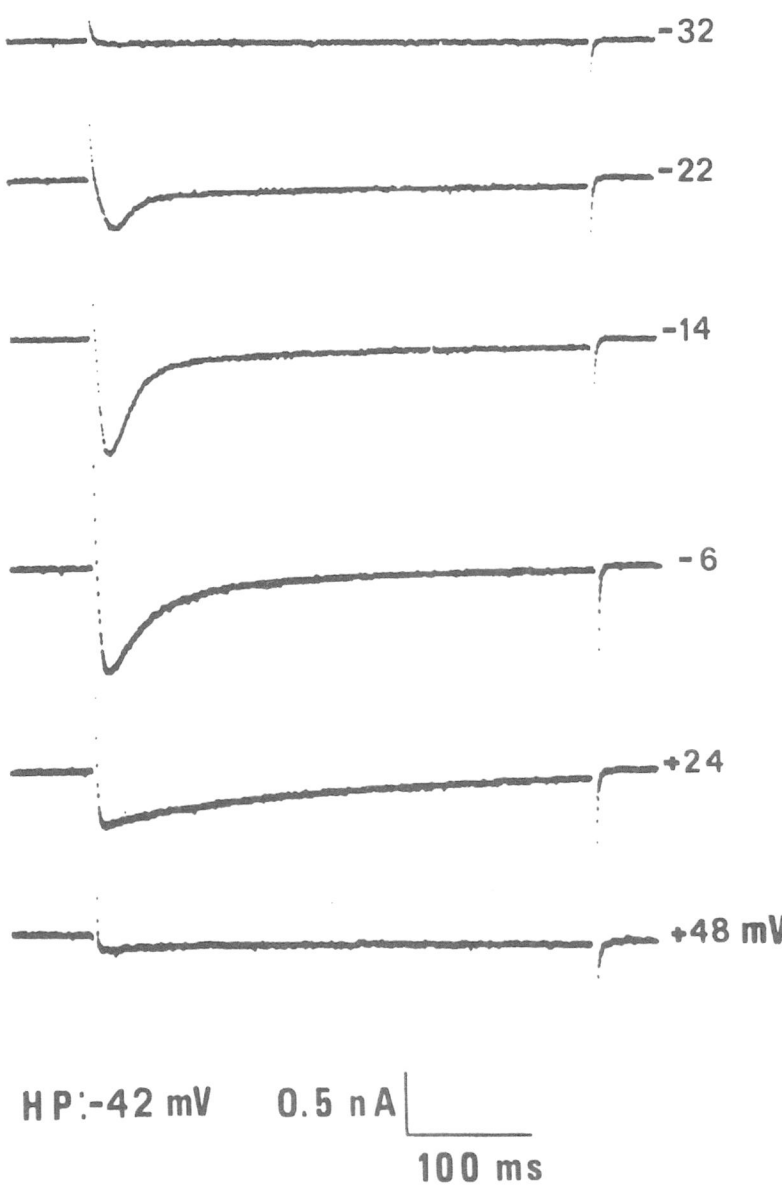

-32

-22

-14

- 6

+24

+48 mV

HP:-42 mV   0.5 nA

100 ms

Figure 9. Whole cell patch clamp recordings of the slow inward current in enzymatically-dispersed human myocytes. Currents were illicited by depolarizing steps from a holding potential of −42 mV to the indicated potential.

Conclusion

It might be stressed that most of the in vitro experimental studies performed in order to investigate the mechanisms responsible for ectopy have been realized in animal models. However, cellular mechanisms in human heart may not be readily extrapolated from findings in animals. This extrapolation may be particularly open to criticism if pathological alterations have modified to some unknown extent the physiological properties of the human cell membranes. Until recently, recordings of currents under voltage clamp in the human myocardium were quasi impossible because of the inadequate geometry of the samples obtained. The recent development of enzymatic techniques allowing the isolation of Ca-tolerant myocytes has provided a solution to this problem. By means of the patch-clamp techniques, whole cell recordings of ionic currents are now available in human heart [20, 21]. Figure 9 shows, as an example, typical recordings of the slow inward current in human cells. Although the Ca current of the human heart is the target of numerous Ca blockers drugs daily administered to thousands of patients, it has not been until now the subject of thorough studies. Clearly, the patch clamp technique will be of great interest in analyzing the normal electrophysiological properties of human myocytes as well as their physiopathological alterations. The patch clamp technique represents an interesting and promising model for evaluation of pharmacological drugs.

Acknowledgements

The authors wish to thank Edith Deroubaix for continual assistance. They also thank Paulette Richer for her help with the manuscript. This work was supported in part by a special grant A.I.85.2 from the University of Paris XI (France).

References

1. Ferrier G, Saunders J, Mendez C. 1973. A cellular mechanism for the generation of ventricular arrhythmias by acetylstrophantidin. Circ Res 32: 600–609.
2. Coraboeuf E, Boistel J. 1953. L'action des taux élevés de gaz carbonique sur le tissu cardiaque étudiée à l'aide de microélectrodes intracellulaires. C R Soc Biol (Paris) 147: 654–658.
3. Moak J, Rosen MR. 1984. Induction and termination of triggered activity by pacing in isolated canine Purkinje fibers. Circulation 69: 149–162.
4. Fabiato A, Fabiato F. 1978. Calcium-induced release of calcium from the sarcoplasmic reticulum of skinned cells from adult human, dog, cat, rabbit, rat and frog hearts and from fetal and newborn rat ventricles. Ann N Y Acad Sci 307: 491–522.
5. Morgan JP, Chesebro JH, Pluth JR, Puga FJ, Schaff HV. 1984. Intracellular calcium transients in human working myocardium as detected with aequorin. J Am Coll Cardiol 3: 410–418.
6. Morgan JP, Morgan KG. 1984. Calcium and cardiovascular function. Am J Med 77(5A): 33–46.
7. Noble D. 1984. The surprising heart: a review of recent progress in cardiac electrophysiology. J Physiol (Lond) 353: 1–49.

8. Mechmann S, Pott L. 1986. Identification of Na-Ca exchange current in single cardiac myocytes. Nature 319: 597–599.

9. Brachmann J, Scherlag BJ, Rosentshtraukh LV, Lazzara R. 1983. Bradycardia-dependent triggered activity: relevance to drug-induced multiform ventricular tachycardia. Circulation 68: 846–856.

10. Levine JH, Spear JF, Guarnieri T, Weisfeldt ML, De Langen CDJ, Becker LC, Moore EN. 1985. Cesium chloride-induced long QT syndrome: demonstration of afterdepolarizations and triggered activity in vivo. Circulation 72: 1092–1103.

11. Damiano BP, Rosen MR. 1984. Effects of pacing on triggered activity induced by early afterdepolarizations. Circulation 69: 1013–1025.

12. Coulombe A, Coraboeuf E, Malecot C, Deroubaix E. 1985. Role of the 'Na window' current and other ionic currents in triggering early after-depolarizations and resulting re-excitations in Purkinje fibers. In: Cardiac Electrophysiology and Arrhythmias. Zipes DP, Jalife J (eds), New-York, London, Toronto, Grune and Stratton, p 43–49.

13. Mendez C, Delmar M. 1985. Triggered activity: its possible role in cardiac arrhythmias. In: Cardiac Electrophysiology and Arrhythmias. Zipes DP, Jalife J (eds), New-York, London, Toronto, Grune and Stratton, p 311–313.

14. Bonatti V, Rolli A, Botti G. 1983. Recordings of monophasic action potentials of the right ventricule in the long QT syndrome complicated by severe ventricular arrhythmias. Eur Heart J 4: 168.

15. Matsuda H, Noma A, Kurachi Y, Irisawa H. 1982. Transient depolarization and spontaneous voltage fluctuations in isolated single cells from guinea-pig ventricules. Circ Res 51: 142–151.

16. Orchard CH, Eisner DA, Allen DG. 1983. Oscillations of intracellular Ca^{2+} in mammalian cardiac muscle. Nature 304: 735–738.

17. Clusin WT, Bristow MR, Karagueuzian HS, Katzung BG, Schroeder JS. 1982. Do calcium-dependent ionic currents mediate ischemic ventricular fibrilation? Am J Cardiol 49: 606–612.

18. Escande D, Coraboeuf E, Planchè C. 1987. Abnormal pacemaking is modulated by sarcoplasmic reticulum in partially-depolarized myocardium from dilated right atria in humans. J Mol Cell Cardiol 19: 231–241.

19. Gwathmey JK, DeFeo TT, Morgan JP. 1984. Hypertrophy-induced prolongation of intracellular Ca^{++} transients in mammalian working myocardium as detected with aequorin. Circulation 70 (supp II): 73.

20. Escande D, Coulombe A, Faivre JF, Coraboeuf E. 1986. Characteristics of the time-dependent slow inward current in adult human atrial single myocytes. J Mol Cell Cardiol 18: 547–551.

21. Escande D, Coulombe A, Faivre JF, Coraboeuf E. 1987. Two types of transient outward currents in adult human atrial cells. Am J Physiol 252: 142–148.

3. Mechanisms of ventricular tachycardias in experimental animal models of ischemic heart disease

BENJAMIN J. SCHERLAG, EUGENE PATTERSON, and RALPH LAZZARA
Veterans Administration Medical Center and University of Oklahoma Health Sciences Center, Oklahoma City, Oklahoma

Introduction

Since 1970 there has been a progressive accumulation of evidence in experimental animal models [1–7] and in man [8–11] of the important role of the mechanism of reentry in the initiation and maintenance of malignant ventricular tachycardias. In particular, there has been much interest in the electrophysiological properties of the substrate for sustained ventricular tachycardia occurring in the context of myocardial ischemia and infarction.

The focus of this chapter will be on the apparently contradictory character of sustained ventricular tachycardia that can be provoked by ventricular paced beats in the 4-day infarcted heart. Specifically, we addressed the question of the stability of these arrhythmias in regard to regularity and timing on the one hand and their ability to abruptly destabilize and degenerate into polymorphous forms or ventricular fibrillation.

A key feature of this presentation is the recording of continuous electrical activity and its association with sustained ventricular tachycardia under stable circumstances and in a number of cases of drug or ischemia induced transformation to an unstable and eventual malignant state.

Sustained ventricular tachycardia in the non-ischemic. Non-infarcted heart.

In our various electrophysiological studies we have utilized provocative ventricular pacing for inducing ventricular arrhythmias in the dog heart. This procedure consists of the delivery of 2–4 ventricular pacing stimuli (sometimes referred to as burst pacing) to the right ventricular outflow tract in the dog under Na-pentobarbital anesthesia. The experiments were carried out in the open-chest preparation. As a means of exacerbating any possible conduction defect that could, in conjunction with burst pacing, induce ventricular tachyarrhythmias lidocaine was injected in bolus doses of 2–6 mg/kg [12–14]. Although lidocaine is well known as a

standard anti-arrhythmic agent clinically, only recently have we begun to understand its basic electrophysiologic properties which provide explanations of its proarrhythmic actions as well [15, 16].

In 30 anesthetized mongrel dogs showing no ECG signs of myocardial ischemia
or infarction we initiated provocative ventricular pacing at rates between 240–
390/min before and after lidocaine administration. Table I describes the various
types and percent of responses. Note that in the non-ischemic, non-infarcted
heart there was a high percentage (70%) of no responses to burst pacing even at
rates as high as 390/min. Also note that there were two instances of induced
ventricular fibrillation prior to lidocaine administration. However after lidocaine
injection, Up to 6 mg/kg, there was a 73% incidence of induced tachyarrhythmias
which included multiple ventricular responses, non-sustained ventricular tachycardia, sustained ventricular tachycardia and ventricular fibrillation. Thus
even in the relatively normal heart, lidocaine, in therapeutic doses, can be used in
conjunction with provocative ventricular pacing to increase the incidence of
induced tachyarrhythmias. These mostly took benign forms such as multiple
ventricular responses and non-sustained ventricular tachycardia (60%) whereas
only 10% of the induced arrhythmias were of the malignant variety equally
divided between sustained ventricular tachycardia (3.3%) and ventricular
fibrillation (10.0%).

Ventricular tachycardia in the infarcted dog heart

Eleven dogs anesthetized with Na-pentobarbital, were studied 4 days after left
anterior descending coronary artery occlusion. Prior to permanent coronary

Tabel I. The effect of three ventricular paced beats and lidocaine on induction of sustained ventricular tachycardia in 30 normal dogs.

Ventricular paced beats (rate: 300–390/min)	% response	Ventricular pacing and lidocaine 2–6 mg/kg	% response
21 NR	70.0	7 NR	23.3
5 SVR	16.6	1 SVR	3.3
2 RVR	6.7	13 RVR	43.3
2 VF	6.7	5 NSVT	16.7
		3 VT/VF	10.0
		1 Sus VT	3.3

NR	=	no response
SVR	=	single ventricular response
RVR	=	repetitive ventricular response
NSVT	=	non-sustained ventricular tachycardia
Sus VT	=	sustained ventricular tachycardia
VT/VF	=	ventricular tachycardia/ventricular fibrillation

artery ligation each dog was pretreated with methyprednisolone, 30 mg/kg. In previous reports we have found that such pretreatment leads to a high yield of sustained ventricular tachycardia in response to provocative ventricular pacing. Table II shows a comparison of the number of inducible, sustained ventricular tachycardias in the dogs pretreated with methylprednisolone and an untreated group. Note that 9 of 11 (81%) showed sustained ventricular tachycardia in response to provocative ventricular pacing in the treated group while only 2 of 10 (20%) had a similar response in the untreated group, $p = 0.007$, Fisher's test; $p = 0.016$, corrected chi-square.

An example of an induced, sustained ventricular tachycardia is shown in figure 1. These recordings were made in a dog with a 4 day old transmural myocardial infarction. In panel A during normal sinus rhythm (NSR) a lead II (L-2) electrocardiogram, His bundle electrogram (Hbeg), electrode catheter recordings from the left ventricular endocardium near the infarct zone (IZendo), composite electrode recording overlying the infarcted epicardium (IZepi) and composite recordings from the normal epicardial zone (NZepi) are shown. Sustained ventricular tachycardia was induced by three ventricular paced beats at a rate of 240/ min delivered to the right ventricular outflow tract.

The induced tachycardia is characterized by organized, i.e. reproducible from one interectopic period to another, continuous electrical activity recorded only in the epicardium overlying the infarct zone whereas the other electrograms showed distinct isoelectric intervals in the interectopic periods. In nine dogs the rate of these monomorphic ventricular tachycardias averaged 230 beats/min. We have classified this response as a simple, single circuit reentrant ventricular tachycardia (see Discussion below). The action of lidocaine on these single circuit reentrant tachycardias was to slow the tachycardia; the degree of slowing being related to dose. In the majority of dogs lidocaine, 2–6 mg/kg slowed the rate of the tachycardia by an average of 36 beats/min. However, in a small percentage (Table III) a definite aggravation of the induced, sustained tachycardia was noted, i.e., a pro-

Table II. The incidence of sustained ventricular tachycardia in infarcted dog hearts 4 days after coronary artery ligation.

No. of dogs	Intervention	Sustained VT
11	MP, 30 mg/kg	9*
10	Untreated	2*

MP = Methylprednisolone, sodium succinate
VT = Ventricular Tachycardia
*p = 0.007, Fisher's test
*p = 0.016, corrected chi-square

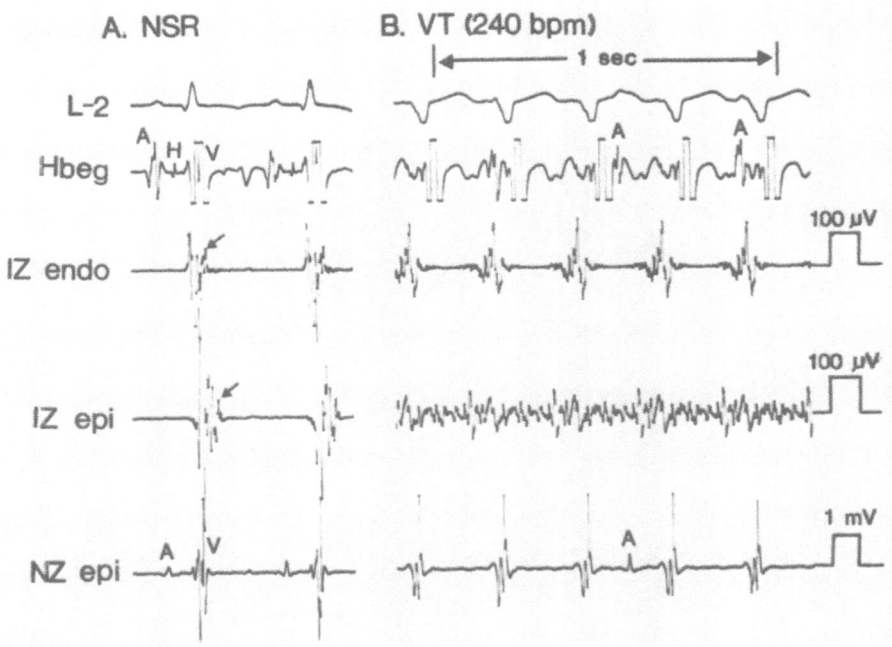

Figure 1. Electrical recordings from a dog with a 4-day old myocardial infarction. In panel A, during normal sinus rhythm (NSR) the following traces are shown: lead II (L-2) electrocardiogram; His bundle electrogram (Hbeg); electrode catheter recording from the left ventricular subendocardium near the infarct zone (IZ endo); composite electrogram from the sub-epicardium overlying the infarct zone (IZ epi) and normal zone (NZ epi). Sustained ventricular tachycardia was induced by a three beat burst of ventricular pacing at a rate of 240/minute delivered to the right ventricular outflow tract. Note the occurrence of continuous electrical activity on the IZ epi recording indicative of a single reentry circuit (see text). Atrial activity (A) is indicated on the Hbeg as well as on the composite electrogram in the normal zone which is close to the left atrium.

arrhythmic effect. An electrophysiological basis for this effect is seen in the following figures (2–6).

Figure 2 is an example of a multiple circuit, sustained ventricular tachycardia. In this case, 4 mg/kg of lidocaine was administered intravenously to the same dog in whom the single circuit reentrant sustained ventricular tachycardia was induced without the drug (figure 1). We have previously shown that therapeutic doses of lidocaine selectively act on abnormal potentials while normal electrical

Table III. Incidence of Pro-arrhythmic Effects of lidocaine as a Function of Increasing Dose.

Lidocaine dose	2 mg/kg	4 mg/kg	6 mg/kg	8 mg/kg
Incidence	1/9	1/9	3/9	2/3

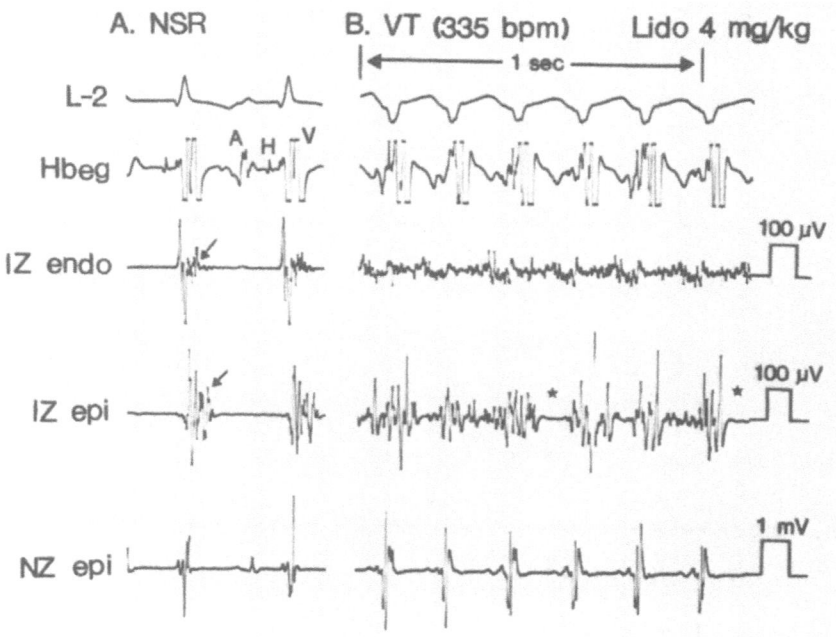

Figure 2. An example of multiple reentrant circuits during sustained ventricular tachycardia in the same dog as shown in Figure 1. (Tracings are the same as in Figure 1.) Prior to induction of this tachycardia, 4 mg/kg of lidocaine was administered causing a decrease in the amplitude and increase in the fractionation of the late potentials (arrows) recorded in the infarct zone electrograms. Sustained ventricular tachycardia is associated with the continuous electrical activity recorded on the sub-endocardial and sub-epicardial IZ recordings but with intermittent isoelectric periods on the latter (stars). See text for further discussion.

activity is unaffected [15]. During normal sinus rhythm (panel A) lidocaine caused a diminution of the amplitude and exacerbated the delay of the depressed potentials recorded both in the subendocardium, in or around, the infarct zone (arrows, compare with similar potentials in figure 1). Induction of sustained ventricular tachycardia was associated with continuous electrical activity which was regular and reproducible only in the endocardial electrogram but irregular and discontinuous in the epicardial recording. Moreover, the rate of the ventricular tachycardia was 335/min compared to 240/min seen in the control state with a single, epicardial reentry circuit (figure 1). The evidence that this was a multiple reentrant circuit, i.e., potential reentry going on at 2 sites, was deduced from the occurrence of continuous electrical activity from both endocardial and epicardial infarct zone recordings, albeit the activity from the epicardial recordings showed intermittent isoelectric periods. Another indication of the involvement of more than one reentrant circuit is seen in figure 3.

UNIFORM SUSTAINED VENTRICULAR TACHYCARDIA
WITH INTERACTIVE REENTRY LOOPS

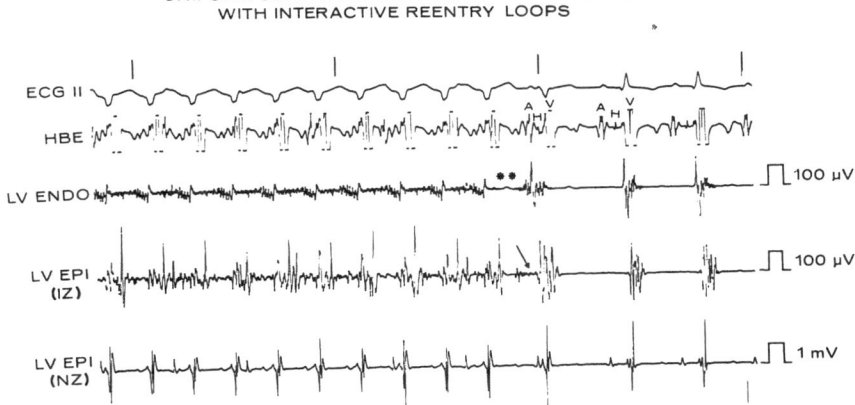

Figure 3. Evidence for concealed interaction between simultaneously operating reentrant circuits. Spontaneous termination of the sustained ventricular tachycardia shown in Figure 2 is associated with cessation of continuous electrical activity (asterisks) on the sub-endocardial recording in the infarct zone (LV endo). The last ventricular ectopic beat, similar in morphology to the tachycardia shown in Figure 1 is preceded by bridging electrical activity (arrow) on the sub-epicardial recording overlying the infarct (LV epi, IZ). See text for further discussion.

Spontaneous termination of the rapid, sustained ventricular tachycardia was associated with the abrupt loss of continuous electrical activity recorded from the sub-endocardial electrogram (asterisks, figure 3). However, the last ventricular ectopic beat not only is delayed, but also shows a slightly different QRS morphology than the previous ectopic tachycardia. Note the similarity of this morphology (last ectopic beat) and that of the sustained tachycardia in figure 1. Also note the fractionated electrogram (arrow) in the epicardial recording which precedes this last beat. Except for this last beat the subendocardial reentry circuit dominates the rhythm of the heart; the interaction of the subepicardial and subendocardial circuits is concealed, for the most part.

At a higher concentration of lidocaine, 6 mg/kg, evidence was found that these 2 simultaneously operative reentry circuits, which were showing only concealed interaction (figure 3, above), could now manifest interaction on the ECG. At the beginning of the ECG trace in figure 4 variable QRS morphologies are associated with continuous electrical activity at both subepicardial and subendocardial left ventricular sites in the infarction zones, LV endo, LV epi (IZ). The unstable ventricular tachycardia spontaneously converted to a stable but slower ventricular tachycardia at a rate of 208/min from the faster unstable ventricular tachycardia (330/min). Note that the reproducible interectopic activation patterns during the slower ventricular tachycardia shows fractionated electrical activity initially contributed by the epicardial electrogram and the terminal portion provided by the endocardial recording (arrows). We postulated that in this case the 2 shorter reentrant circuits, as a result of interaction, have merged into a single, longer circuit and thus a slower heart rate.

CONVERSION OF UNSTABLE VT TO STABLE VT

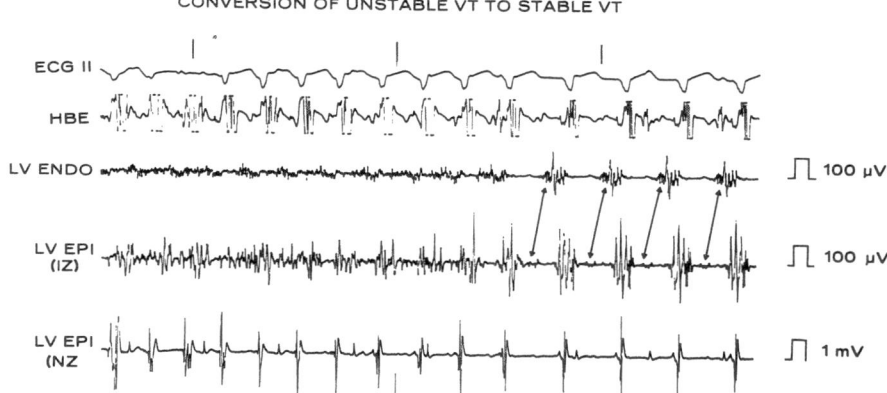

Figure 4. An example of multiple reentrant circuits showing interaction that manifests itself on the electrocardiogram. After 6 mg/kg of lidocaine, in the same dog as above, the continuous electrical activity seen in both sub-epicardial and sub-endocardial recordings were associated with intermittent alterations of the morphology and timing of the QRS complexes in the Lead II cardiogram. Termination of the continuous electrical activity in the endocardial recording gives way to a slower tachycardia with interectopic activation contributed from both sub-epicardial and sub-endocardial sites. See text for further discussion.

INITIATION OF MULTIFORM VENTRICULAR TACHYCARDIA
WITH 2 INTERACTIVE REENTRY LOOPS

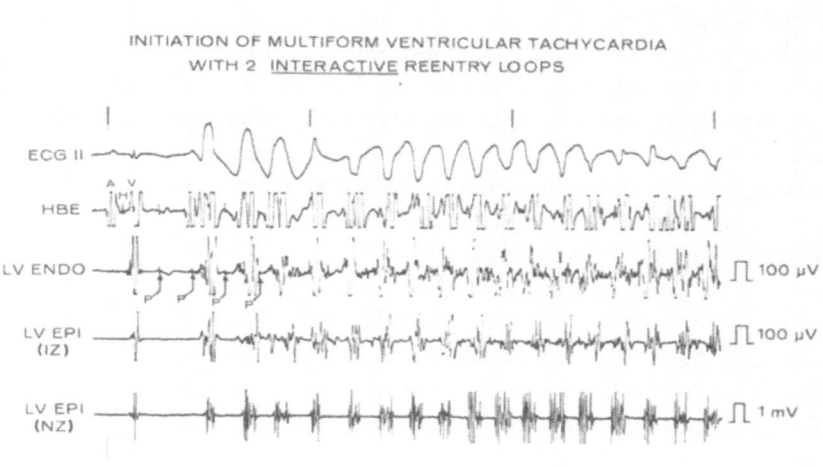

Figure 5. Induction of polymorphic ventricular tachycardia in another 4-day-old infarct caused by provocative ventricular pacing and a toxic dose of lidocaine, 8 mg/kg. Dual sites of continuous electrical activity were induced each showing intermittent isoelectric periods. Interaction in this instance was shown by the irregular, polymorphic nature of the QRS complexes. The rate of the ventricular tachycardia was 380/min. Note the clear isoelectric intervals recorded from the normal zone composite electrogram.

INTERACTION OF REENTRY LOOPS DURING MULTIFORM
VENTRICULAR TACHYCARDIA → VENTRICULAR FIBRILLATION

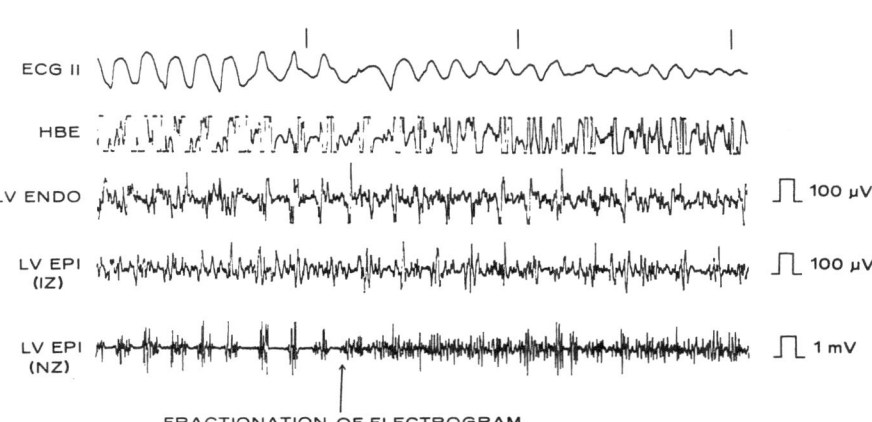

FRACTIONATION OF ELECTROGRAM
IN NORMAL LV EPICARDIUM

Figure 6. Further malignant degeneration of the rapid multiform tachycardia shown in Figure 5 is evidenced by an increase in the heart rate to 430/min which is associated with continuous electrical activity (no isoelectric intervals) shown on endo- and epi- recordings from the infarct zone. Deterioration of tachycardia to fibrillation is preceded by initiation of continuous electrical activity (arrow, bottom) at a new site, the normal zone.

Although the above example suggests a benign outcome of interaction of reentrant circuits, a malignant result may well be a more common consequence. In another 4 day infarcted dog heart a toxic dose of lidocaine, 8 mg/kg, in association with provocative ventricular pacing induced a polymorphic or multiform ventricular tachycardia. In figure 5, 3 ventricular paced beats induced a sustained ventricular tachycardia with variable QRS morphologies. This was associated with runs of continuous and discontinuous electrical activity in both endo and epicardial electrograms in the infarct zone; the heart rate averaged 390/min. Note the discreet isoelectric intervals during every interectopic interval in the normal zone electrogram during the induced tachycardia. However, in figure 6 progression of the degree of interaction of the subendo- and subepicardial reentry circuits increases, which is reflected in the increased rate of the polymorphic tachycardia (420/min) as well as the presence of continuous electrical activity in both endo- and epicardial electrograms in the infarct zones.

The degeneration of ventricular tachycardia to ventricular fibrillation (figure 6) was preceded by the appearance of continuous electrical activity in the normal zone electrogram (arrow, bottom) probably indicating another reentrant circuit which interacts with the other two causing disorganization of cardiac activation and manifesting as ventricular fibrillation.

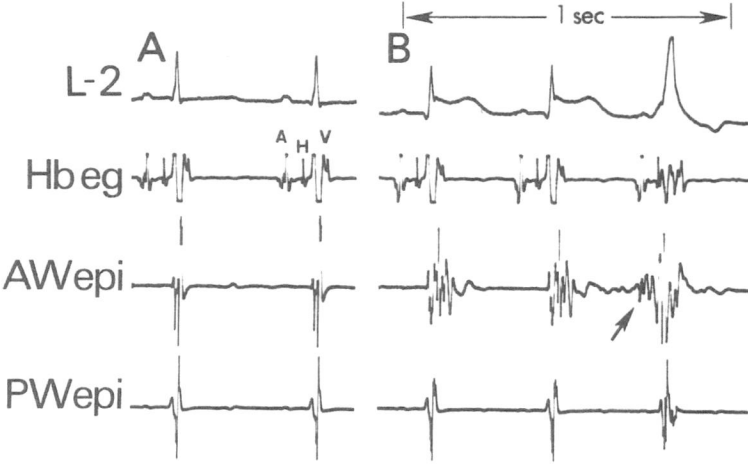

Figure 7. Effect of left circumflex coronary artery stenosis on regional epicardial electrograms. In each panel L-2 = lead II electrocardiogram; Hbeg = His bundle electrogram; AWepi and PWepi = epicardial composite recordings from anterior and posterior left ventricle, respectively. A, During sinus rhythm, prior to coronary artery stenosis, stable fractionation and delay are evident in the anterior wall epicardial recording (infarct zone). B, Sinus rhythm at 5 minutes after coronary artery stenosis. Note that fractionation and delay of the electrogram recorded from the anterior wall have increased with little change in the posterior wall electrogram. Also there is marked ST elevation in lead II and preectopic activity appears in the anterior wall electrogram (arrow), which precedes the ectopic beat. Reproduced by Permission: Kabell et al., American Heart J. (1984) 108: 447–462.

Destabilization of the reentrant substrate by transient myocardial ischemia

In a recent report from our laboratory Kabell et al. studied 15 anesthetized dogs with 4 day old anterior myocardial infarction [16]. Transient (5 minute) myocardial ischemia was induced by graded stenosis of the left circumflex coronary artery which provided the primary flow to the posterior left ventricular wall and collateral flow to the surviving anterior epicardial tissue overlying the infarct. In 12 dogs transient ischemia caused by left circumflex stenosis resulted in fractionation and delay of anterior wall electrograms leading to bridging electrical activity between sinus beats and spontaneously occurring ventricular ectopic beats (figure 7B) in 5 of the 12 dogs. Note the lack of fractionation and delay in the posterior wall in which epicardial flow, measured with the use of radioactive microspheres, diminished by only 10%. Average flow reduction in the anterior wall sub-epicardium was 41% of the flow prior to stenosis of the left circumflex coronary artery.

In 4 of 8 dogs provocative ventricular pacing could not induce sustained ventricular tachycardia prior to left circumflex stenosis. Figure 8 illustrates the induction of a non-sustained ventricular tachycardia in response to provocative ventricular pacing. Note the bridging electrical activity during the interectopic intervals of the non-sustained ventricular tachycardia. After left circumflex ste-

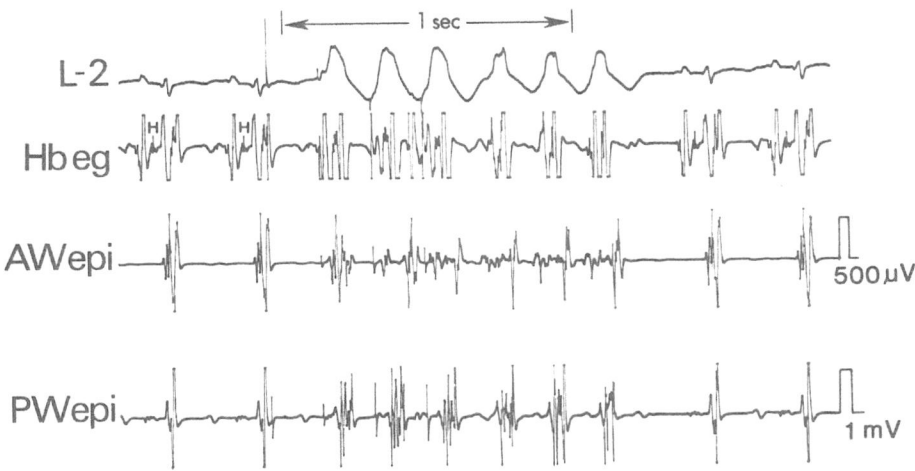

Figure 8. Response to ventricular pacing prior to left circumflex coronary artery stenosis. Tracings are the same as in figure 7. During sinus rhythm (first two beats) three ventricular paced beats are introduced which induce three ventricular ectopic beats. Note the fractionation of the anterior wall epicardial electrogram (A Wepi) during the stimulated and non-stimulated ectopic beats compared to the same electrogram seen in the sinus beats and in electrograms from the posterior wall in all beats. Reproduced by Permission: Kabell et al. American Heart J (1984) 108: 447–462.

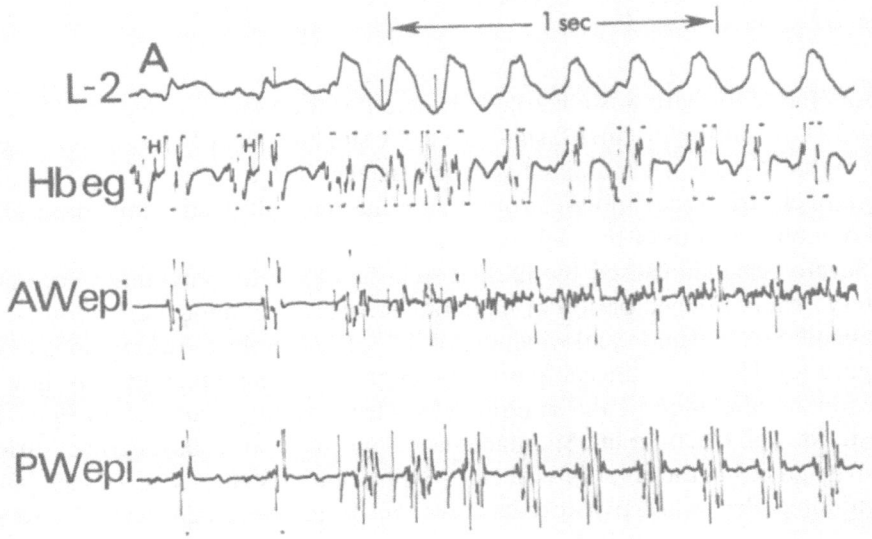

Figure 9. Response to ventricular pacing in the same dog as shown in Figure 8 after coronary artery stenosis. The sinus beats show a slight widening of the QRS complex and appreciable ST elevation in lead II (L-2). Three ventricular paced beats, as in Figure 8 now induced a sustained ventricular tachycardia. Note the greater degree of fractionation during the stimulated and ectopic beats. (Reproduced by Permission: Kabell et al. American Heart J. (1984) 108: 447–462.)

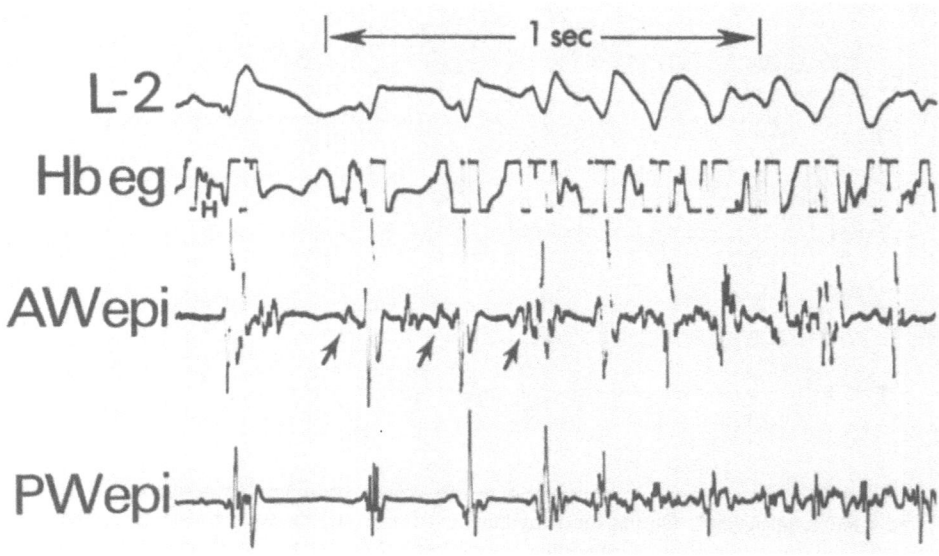

Figure 10. Onset of ventricular fibrillation 8 minutes after left circumflex coronary artery stenosis. There "s" is a widening of the QRS complex and marked ST elevation in the last sinus beat (first beat shown in the electrocardiogram [L-2]). Fractionation and delay in the anterior wall electrogram exceeded that observed in the posterior wall electrogram and ectopic beats are preceded by bridging activation in the anterior wall recording (arrows) but not in the posterior wall recording until ventricular fibrillation ensues.

nosis (figure 9) there was a marked elevation of the S–T segment in the lead II ECG (L-2) during the first 2 sinus beats. A similar 3 beat burst of ventricular pacing now induces a sustained ventricular tachycardia with reproducible patterns of electrical activation seen only in the anterior wall electrograms during the interectopic periods of the tachycardia.

Severe ischemia caused by marked stenosis of the left circumflex coronary artery or a prolonged period of moderate stenosis 6–10 minutes, both induced dramatic S–T elevation and widening of the QRS complexes during sinus beats (figure 10). However, the composite electrograms during this sinus beat showed greater fractionation of the anterior wall electrogram (infarct zone) than the posterior wall electrogram. Spontaneous ectopic beats also show early electrical activity arising in the anterior wall electrograms until the fifth beat at which point continuous electrical activity occurs at both recording sites. Ventricular tachycardia proceeds on to ventricular fibrillation. Note the similarity in the destabilization of the reentrant substrate and the recruitment of new circuits of reentry (indicated by bridging or continuous electric activity) induced by ischemia compared to the previous records (figures 2–6) in which the pro-arrhythmic agent was lidocaine. Of course, provocative ventricular pacing was an important, albeit artificial trigger, in these processes.

Discussion

On the basis of these studies and previous experience with recording of continuous electrical activity during various forms of sustained ventricular tachycardia, [14, & 17–19] we have postulated a classification system encompassing various types of reentrant circuits that may operate both in experimental preparations and under clinical circumstances:

1. Single circuit, sustained ventricular tachycardia
   a. monomorphic
   b. pleomorphic
2. Multiple circuit, sustained ventricular tachycardia
   a. non-interactive or concealed interaction
   b. interactive with intermittent manifestation in the ECG
   c. competitive; two or more circuits vying for domination of the heart's rhythm with concealed or manifest interaction

In the subacute stages of myocardial infarction in the dog (after anterior descending coronary artery occlusion) multiple sites for potential reentry circuits exist. The tissues most often involved in reentry circuits is the epicardium which overlies the necrotic or infarct zone that is ischemically damaged yet remains viable and electrophysiologically deranged [20, 21]. The demonstration of macro- as well as micro-reentry circuits has been reported using a number of recording techniques and devices from composite electrodes [20, 21], hand-held close bipolar recordings [22, 23], multiple close bipolar electrodes [24] and extensive mapping procedures [24, 25].

Several studies, have provided evidence either by showing continuous electrical activity arising from the epicardium overlying the infarct or by extensive epicardial mapping, that there is a circus movement or reentry going on during ventricular tachycardia. We have categorized these as single circuit reentrant rhythms (see classification above). The heterogenity of the reentry substrate even on the epicardial surface can be seen in the ability to induce many pleomorphic forms of ventricular tachycardia each with its associated form of continuous electrical activity only in epicardial recordings [17]. Although, different single circuits manifesting different QRS morphologies can be induced in one infarcted heart, i.e., pleomorphism [17] these circuits show little if any interaction.

The existence of this type of substrate consisting of viable but sick *epicardial* cells is not readily found in man probably due to: 1) The infarction process in Man is probably more severe since patients with complex arrhythmias are more likely to present with multiple vessel disease. Epicardial activation is much more depressed. 2) In the dog, with only one major coronary artery ligated and a greater potential for collateral development than in Man, survival of epicardial tissues is more likely [26].

Anti-arrhythmic drugs (figures 2–6) or new ischemic episodes (figures 7–10) can destabilize the substrate for single circuit reentry in the 4 day-old-infarcted hearts. After drugs or ischemia two reentry circuits involving both the subendo- and subepicardium can be shown to be operative simultaneously (figure 2) with only latent evidence of interaction (figure 3). Further destabilization, may lead to overt interaction between reentrant circuits manifesting as disturbances of QRS morphology and timing on the standard ECG. These ECG changes, are closely associated with changes in continuous electrical activity recorded from both subendo- and subepicardial infarct zones.

It might be interesting at this point to contemplate the basis of the recently reported but little understood proarrhythmic action of anti-arrhythmic agents [27]. From the data presented above it can be seen that lidocaine through its usual mode of action suppresses conduction in the single reentry circuit by changing the activity from continuous (figure 1) to discontinuous (figure 2). In most cases this results in slowing of the ventricular tachycardia. However, at the same time lidocaine can depress moderately sick tissue, e.g. on the subendocardial surface to the extent that these sites can now participate in a reentry circuit. But why should the new reentrant tachycardia be faster? Probably because it originates in tissues that were less depressed than the original circuit even with the added action of the depressant drug. Indeed, factors other than conduction depression, e.g. refractoriness and circuit length, may enter into the equation thus allowing new reentry circuits to be faster (figure 2) or even slower (figure 4) than pre- viously induced tachycardias. Figure 4 is an example suggesting manifest interac- tion of two circuits due to a proarrhythmic drug action. The interaction of multiple circuits in this case stabilizes and slows the tachycardia probably due to a lengthening of the circuit pathway so that the loop included both subepicardial and subendocardial activation sites.

Severe destabilization was shown with multiple reentry circuits which not only interacted but competed for dominance of the heart rhythm (figures 5 and 6). Such interaction particularly at fast rates can lead directly to ventricular fibrilla- tion or to severe decompensation of ventricular function. In the latter event ventricular fibrillation is a secondary consequence, but no less malignant.

Recording of continuous electrical activity

In the present study we have utilized the recording of continuous electrical activity as an indicator of a site of a reentry circuit. This contention has been questioned in previous clinical [28, 29] reports which has demonstrated the transient or intermittent nature of continuous electrical activity during sustained ventricular tachycardia. These reports suggest that the recording of continuous electrical activity may not necessarily be associated with the onset, perpetuation or termination of a ventricular tachyarrhythmia. Do these findings invalidate those presented herein or those reported in previous animal [17, 23] and clinical [30] reports? Just as continuous electrical activity may be unrelated or play an indeterminate role in certain sustained ventricular tachycardias [17, 28, 29] there are others in which there is a close cause-and-effect relationship between the functional properties of the continuous electrical activity and the behavior of the ventricular tachycardia [17]. Thus, the continuous electrical activity in the present study was not seen during sinus rhythm and started, on repeated occasions, with the start of the induced ventricular tachycardia. Also continuous electrical activity ended with the termination, induced or spontaneous, of the tachycardia (figure 3). Changes in the rate, morphology or type of tachyarrhythmia as indicated from the ECG were preceded or directly associated in time with changes in continuous electrical activity in one or more sites.

We do not believe that the recording of continuous electrical activity can be directly or easily used to interpret functional aspects of reentrant circuits unless several criteria such as those mentioned above are observed. Additional criteria and caveats in the relation between continuous electrical activity and reentrant ventricular tachycardia have been pointed out by others [31].

How useful the recording of continuous activity will be in discerning the functional aspects of reentrant circuits in the clinical setting will depend on the ability to localize such sites which have been postulated to be relatively small [30]. The use of close bipolar mapping techniques and appropriate amplification will probably facilitate recording of continuous electrical activity. Experimentally, recent reports using close bipolar recording electrodes have indicated that small areas of deranged myocardium can be the site of continuous electrical activity associated with sustained ventricular tachycardia [23, 32]. Within the confines of carefully delineated criteria, the recording of continuous activity remains a strong presumptive marker for reentry.

Acknowledgement

We thank LaVonna Blair for her surgical and technical expertise in the performance of these experiments; and we thank Melinda Lyon for her able assistance in the preparation of the manuscript.

References

1. Han J. 1969. Mechanisms of ventricular arrhythmias associated with myocardial infarction. Am J Cardiol 24: 800–812, 1969.
2. Scherlag BJ, Helfant RH, Haft JI, Damato AN. 1970. Electrophysiology underlying ventricular arrhythmias due to coronary ligation. Am J Physiology 219 (6): 1665–1617.
3. Boineau JF, Cox JL. 1973. Slow ventricular activation in acute myocardial infarction. A source of reentrant premature ventricular contraction. Circulation 48: 702–713.
4. Waldo AL, Kaisar GA. 1973. Study of ventricular arrhythmias associated with acute myocardial infarction in the canine heart. Circulation 47: 1222–1228.

40

5. Scherlag BJ, El-Sherif N, Hope R, Lazzara R. 1974. Characterization and localization of ventricular arrhythmias resulting from myocardial ischemia and infarction. Circ Res 35: 372–383.
6. Kaplinksy E, Ogawa S, Kmetzo J, Blake CM, Dreifus LS. 1980. Intramyocardial activation in early ventricular arrhythmias following coronary artery ligation. J Electrocardiol 13: 1–6.
7. Janse MJ, vanCapelle FJL, Morsink H, Kleber AG, Wilms-Schopman F, Cardinal R, d'Alnoncourt CN, Durrer D. 1980. Flow of 'injury' current and patterns of exictation during early ventricular arrhythmias in acute regional myocardial ischemia in isolated porcine and canine hearts. Circ Res 47: 151.
8. Wellens HJJ. 1971. Electrical stimulation of the heart in the study and treatment of tachycardias. Baltimore, University Park Press.
9. Josephson ME, Seides SF. 1971. Clinical cardiac electrophysiology. Techniques and Interpretations. Lea and Febiger, Philadelphia, 1979; chap. 12.
10. Ruskin JN, DiMarco JP, Garan H. 1980. Out-of-hospital cardiac arrest. Electrophysiologic observations and selection of long-term anti-arrhythmic therapy. New Engl J Med 303: 607–613.
11. Myerburg RJ, Conde CA, Sung RJ, Mayorga-Cortes A, Mallon S, Sheps DS, Appel RA, Castellanos A. 1980. Clinical, electrophysiological and hemodynamic profile of patients resuscitated from prehospital cardiac arrest. Am J Med 68: 568–576.
12. Scherlag BJ, Harrison LA, Kabell G, Brachmann J, Harrison LH, Lazzara R. 1908. Lidocaine unmasks ventricular arrhythmias in chronic myocardial infarction. Circulation 62: III–173.
13. Patterson E, Gibson JK, Lucchesi BR. 1982. Electrophysiologic actions of lidocaine in a canine model of chronic myocardial ischemic damage – Arrhythmogenic actions of lidocaine. J Cardiovasc Pharmacol 4: 927.
14. Scherlag BJ, Brachmann J, Harrison LA, Harrison L, Lazzara R. Mechanisms of ventricular arrhythmias in chronic myocardial infarction: The concept of latent ischemic damage. In proceedings of the International Symposium on Holter Monitoring. Eds. Hilger J and Hombach V. Schattaeuer, Cologne, In Press.
15. Lazzara R, Hope RR, El-Sherif N, Scherlag BJ. 1978. Effects of lidocaine on hypoxic and ischemic cardiac cells. Am J Cardiol 41: 872–879.
16. Kabell G, Brachmann J, Scherlag BJ, Harrison L, Lazzara R. 1984. Mechanism of ventricular arrhythmias in multi-vessel coronary disease: The effects of collateral zone ischemia. Amer Heart J. 108: 447–462.
17. Kabell G, Scherlag BJ, Hope RR, Lazzara R. 1982. Patterns of interectopic activation recorded during pleomorphic ventricular tachycardia after myocardial infarction in the dog. Am J Cardiol. 49: 56–62.
18. Brachmann J, Kabell G, Scherlag BJ, Harrison L, Lazzara R. 1983. Analysis of interectopic activation patterns during sustained ventricular tachycardia. Circulation 67: 449.
19. Scherlag BJ, Brachmann J, Kabell G, Harrison LA, Guse P. Lazzara R. 1985. Sustained ventricular tachycardia: Common functional properties of different anatomic substrates. In: Cardiac Electrophysiology and Arrhythmias. Eds. Zipes DP, Jalife J. Grune & Stratton, Orlando, Fl, 379–387.
20. Hope RR, Scherlag BJ, El-Sherif N, Lazzara R. 1977. Continuous concealed ventricular arrhythmias. Am J Cardiol. 40: 733–738.
21. El-Sherif N, Scherlag BJ, Lazzara R, Hope RR. 1977. Reentrant ventricular arrhythmias in the late myocardial infarction period. I. Conduction characteristics in the infarction zone. Circulation 55: 686–702.
22. Brachmann J, Scherlag BJ, Harrison LA. 1981. Localization of sites of slow conduction and unidirectional block in infarcted hearts. Circulation 64: IV–217.
23. Garan H, Ruskin JN. 1984. Localized reentry: Mechanism of induced sustained ventricular tachycardia in canine model of recent myocardial infarction. J Clin Invest. 74: 377–392.
24. Wit AL, Allessie MA, Bonke FIM, Lammers W, Smeets J, Fenoglio JJ Jr. 1982. Electrophysiologic mapping to determine the mechanism of experimental ventricular tachycardia

initiated by premature impulses. Experimental approach and initial results demonstrating re-entrant excitation. Am J Cardiol 49: 166–185.

25. El-Sherif N, Smith RA, Evans K. 1981. Canine ventricular arrhythmias in the late myocardial infarction period 8. Epicardal mapping of reentrant circuits. Circ Res 49: 255–265.

26. Bishop SP, White FC, Bloor C. 1976. Regional Myocardial blood flow during acute myocardial infarction in the conscious dog. Circ Res 38: 429.

27. Velebit V, Podrid P, Lown B, Cohen BH, Grayboys TB. 1982. Aggravation and provocation of ventricular arrhythmias by anti-arrhythmic drugs. Circulation 65: 886–894.

28. Waxman HL, Sung RJ. 1980. Significance of fragmented ventricular electrograms observed using intracardiac recording techniques in man. Circulation 62: 1349–1356.

29. Brugada P, Abdollah H, Wellens HJJ. 1985. Continuous electrical activity during sustained monomorphic ventricular tachycardia: Observations on its dynamic behavior during the arrhythmia. Am J Cardiol 55: 402–422.

30. Josephson ME, Horowitz LN, Farshidi A, Spielman SR, Michelson EL, Greenspan AM. 1978. Sustained ventricular tachycardia-evidence for protected localized reentry. Am J Cardiol 42: 416–424.

31. Wit AL, Josephson ME. 1985. Fractionated electrograms and continuous electrical activity: Fact or artifact. In: Cardiac Electrophysiology and Arrhythmias. Eds. Zipes DP, Jalife J. Grune & Stratton, Orlando Fl. pp. 343.

32. Gessman LJ, Endo T, Egan J, Gallagher JD, Hastie R, Maroko PR. 1983. Dissociation of the site of orgin from the site of cyro-termination of ventricular tachycardia. Pace 6: 1293–1305.

4. Parasympathetic effects on electrophysiological properties of mammalian ventricular tissues

JOHN C. BAILEY and ERIC N. PRYSTOWSKY

The heart is regulated by both limbs of the autonomic nervous system. In the sinoatrial node, the parasympathetic nervous system predominates over the sympathetic nervous system in control of heart rate (Jose and Taylor, 1969; Levy and Zieske, 1969; Prystowsky et al. 1981). In animals and human AV nodal function is under balanced influence of the parasympathetic and sympathetic nervous systems (Levy and Zieske, 1969; Prystowsky et al. 1981). The importance of resting parasympathetic tone on human ventricular refractoriness has only recently been postulated (see Reviews by Higgins, et al. 1973; Zipes et al. 1981; Rardon and Bailey, 1983).

The parasympathetic nervous system regulates cardiac function not only directly, but also by means of parasympathetic modulation of sympathetic effects on the heart (Levy, 1971). The importance of parasympathetic influence on the sinoatrial and AV nodes is well established. Parasympathetic effects on ventricular electrical function have also recently been recognized to be physiologically important, and may influence significantly the pathophysiological milieu responsible for the initiation or termination of certain ventricular arrhythmias.

Contrary to early histological studies that indicated an absence of parasympathetic innervation of the mammalian ventricle, more recent studies suggest the presence of parasympathetic nerve fibers distal to the AV node. The evidence includes histological demonstration of sparse numbers of cholinergic nerve endings in the ventricular myocardium, but a great abundance of cholinergic nerve terminals in ventricular conducting tissue of both canine and human hearts (Kent, et al. 1974). Histochemical studies have also localized choline acetyltransferase (Jacobowitz, et al. 1967; Roskoski, et al. 1975), the enzyme that catalyzes the synthesis of acetylcholine, within the ventricles, and have demonstrated the presence of acetylcholine in the ventricle myocardium (Brown, 1976). In addition to the evidence establishing the presence of cholinergic nerves in the ventricles, muscarinic cholinergic receptors on myocardial cells have been demonstrated directly with ligand-binding assays to label these receptors (Fields, et al. 1978). These receptors are located both on the ventricular myocardial cell and in the

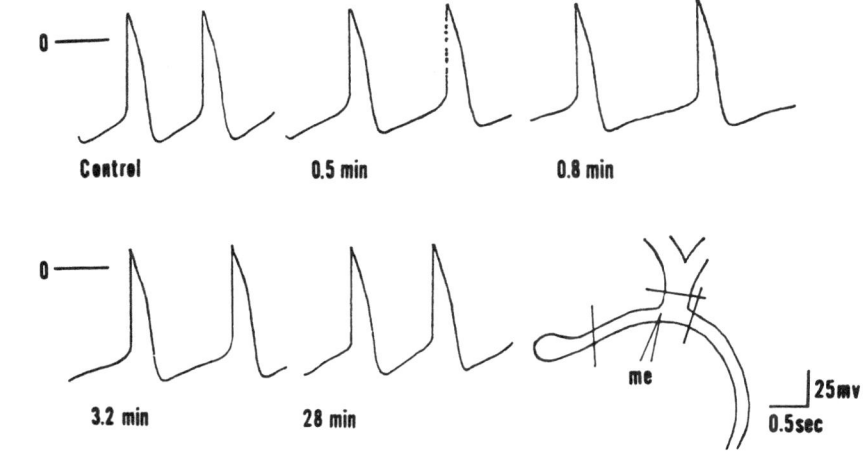

Figure 1. Spontaneous action potentials recorded from the bundle of His. The sketch indicates the proximal intraventricular conducting system and the location of the microelectrode (me). Acetylcholine (2×10^{-5} M) induced slowing of the rate of discharge and reduction of the slope of phase 4 depolarization at 0.5 and 0.8 min. Washout of acetylcholine (3.2 and 28 min) allowed return to control of the spontaneous rate and slope of phase four. Reproduced from ref. 13 by permission of the American Heart Association, Inc.

prejunctional sites on the sympathetic nerve terminals innervating the myocardium.

In this presentation, we review evidence from our laboratories that parasympathetic innervation in the mammalian ventricle is physiologically important and may have clinical implications in altering arrhythmogenesis. First we review the electrophysiological effects of muscarinic cholinergic stimulation. We then describe evidence indicating an indirect electrophysiological effect of muscarinic cholinergic stimulation in the ventricle. Third we present evidence demonstrating that acetylcholine exerts a direct electrophysiological effect in the ventricle.

Our first evidence for the effects of acetylcholine operating at muscarinic cholinergic receptors distal to the AV node was derived from studies of the isolated exposed canine bundle of His and proximal bundle branches (Bailey, et al. 1972). As seen in Figure 1, we recorded action potentials from the bundle of His that demonstrated spontaneous phase four depolarization. These preparations were exposed to acetylcholine and demonstrated time and concentration dependent slowing of spontaneous phase four depolarization, and this effect was reversed with washout or with the addition of atropine. Figure 2, a similar experiment, was recorded with a microelectrode recorded in the mid His bundle and a second microelectrode in the right bundle branch. These preparations were isolated from each other and discharged at their own inherent rates. The rate of discharge of the bundle of His was more rapid in the drug-free state than the rate of discharge of the right bundle branch. However note that there is a time-

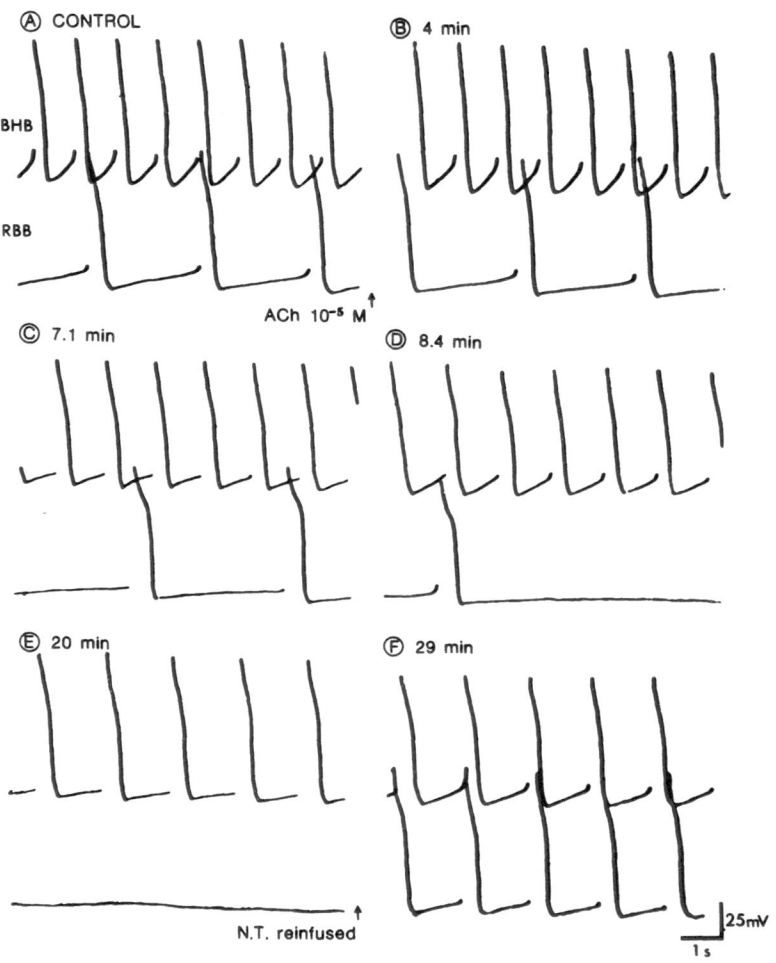

Figure 2. The time-dependent effects of acetylcholine (10^{-5} M) on spontaneous phase four depolarization of canine bundle of His and right bundle branch. Note that these two portions of the conducting system were isolated from each other. Drug-free normal Tyrode's solution (N.T.) reinfusion restored automaticity in both cells toward control state.

dependent slowing of spontaneous phase four depolarization in both portions of the specialized intraventricular conduction system in response to acetylcholine. Automaticity in the right bundle branch was eventually totally suppressed with acetylcholine, an effect that was reversed in both portions with washout of the choline ester. These data demonstrate that acetylcholine can affect electrophysiological properties of the intraventricular specialized conducting system by reducing the rate of spontaneous phase four depolarization and by reducing the rate of spontaneous discharge of these cells.

We then performed a study to determine the extent to which acetylcholine

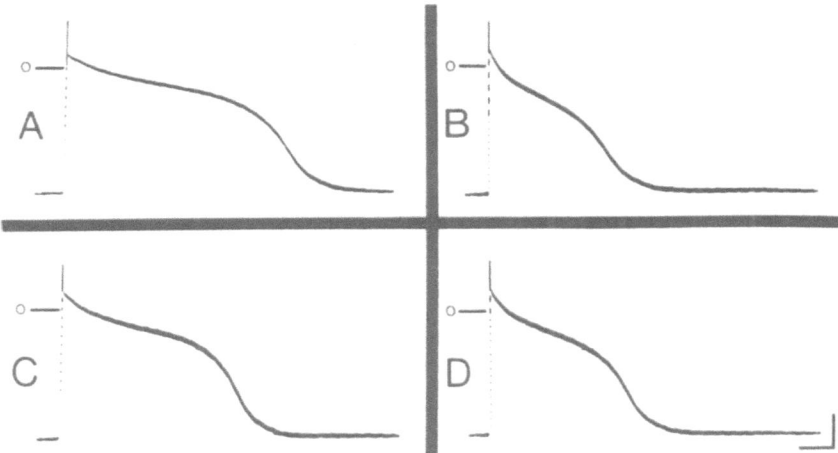

Figure 3. The effects of acetylcholine on the shortening of action potential duration effected by isoproterenol. A: A control cardiac Purkinje fiber action potential. B: Action potential duration shortening produced by isoproterenol (10^{-7}M). C: The addition of acetylcholine (10^{-6}M) partially reversed the shortening of action potential duration effected by isoproterenol. D: Atropine (10^{-6}M) attenuated the effects of acetylcholine, resulting in an action potential duration resembling that produced by the superfusion of isoproterenol alone. Zero potential indicated in each panel. Calibrations: horizontal bat = 50 msec; vertical bar = 25 mV. Reproduced from ref. 14 by permission of the American Heart Association, Inc.

might antagonize the electrophysiological effects of simultaneous beta adrenergic stimulation of ventricular tissue (Bailey, et al. 1979). A typical experiment is depicted in Figure 3. Transmembrane action potentials were recorded from normal canine cardiac Purkinje fibers, panel A. In panel B the fiber was exposed to isoproterenol 10^{-7}M, and action potential duration shortened as expected. In panel C isoproterenol was continued but acetylcholine 10^{-6}M was added, and the choline ester attenuated the effects of isoproterenol on action potential duration. As can been seen from panel D, the attenuating effects of acetylcholine were abolished by addition of atropine to the superfusate. To demonstrate that the antagonistic effects of acetylcholine were specific for beta adrenergic mediated action potential duration shortening, we exposed canine cardiac Purkinje fibers to acetylstrophanthidin, Figure 4, that also produced shortening of action potential duration. Concomitant superfusion of acetylcholine, 10^{-5}M, did not reverse the action potential duration shortening produced by acetylstrophanthidin. In another set of experiments we paced canine cardiac Purkinje fibers at a constant cycle length but introduced premature beats every tenth stimulus. The premature beats demonstrated shortened action potential duration. Addition of acetylcholine did not shorten further the action potential duration of the premature beats. These experiments suggest to us that the antagonistic effects of acetylcholine were specific for action potential duration shortening produced by isoproterenol.

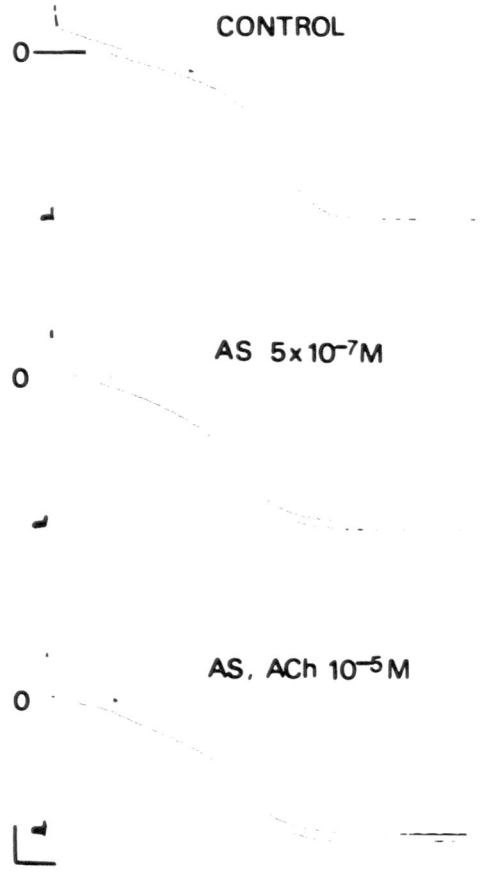

CONTROL

AS 5×10⁻⁷M

AS, ACh 10⁻⁵M

Figure 4. The effects of acetylcholine on action potential shortening effected by the superfusion of acetylstrophanthidin, 5×10^{-7} M. A: Control Purkinje fiber action potential. B: Action potential duration shortened by superfusion with acetylstrophanthidin. C: Addition of acetylcholine (10^{-5} M) produced no effect on action potential duration shortening due to acetylstrophanthidin. Administration of acetylstrophanthidin was continued during superfusion of acetylcholine. Zero potential lines and calibrations as in Figure 3. Reproduced from ref. 14 by permission of the American Heart Association, Inc.

We examined the antagonistic effects of acetylcholine on another well recognized isproterenol-induced electrophysiological phenomenon (Bailey, et al. 1979). Figure 5 depicts the effects of acetylcholine on an isoproterenol-restored slow response. Panel A depicts a normal, polarized, canine cardiac Purkinje fiber superfused with 4 mM potassium. We then increased the potassium concentration, panel B, to 22 mM, and this resulted in depolarization of the membrane and inexcitability. In panel C the elevated potassium solution was superfused while isoproterenol, 10^{-7} M, was added. This resulted in return of excitability in the form of a low amplitude, slowly rising, so-called slow response action potential.

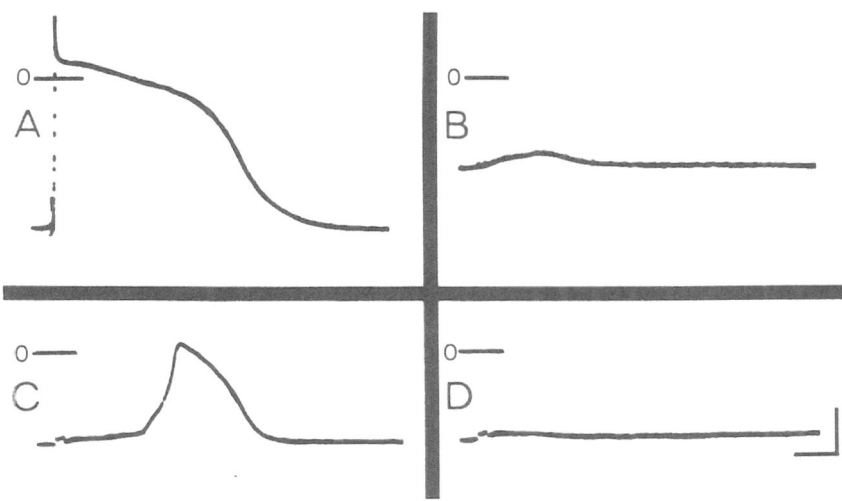

Figure 5. The effects of acetylcholine on an isoproterenol-dependent 'slow response.' A: Control Purkinje fiber action potential in 4 mM potassium. B: Generalized depolarization and loss of excitability produced by superfusion of Tyrode's solution containing 22 mM potassium. C: Restoration of excitability by the addition of 10^{-7} M isoproterenol. D: The addition of acetylcholine (10^{-5} M) abolishes the 'slow response' generated by the addition of isoproterenol. Zero potential lines and calibrations as in Figure 3. Reproduced from ref. 14 by permission of the American Heart Association, Inc.

This slow response, panel D, was abolished by the addition of acetylcholine to the solution containing elevated potassium and isoproterenol. To demonstrate again that acetylcholine antagonism was directed specifically toward isoproterenol mediated events, we looked at the effects of acetylcholine on another model of slow response electrical activity. Figure 6, Panel A depicts a normally polarized canine cardiac Purkinje fiber. Panel B depicts a so-called slow response generated in nominally zero sodium, 20 mM calcium Tyrode solution. Panel C depicts the fact the acetylcholine, 10^{-5} M, did not abolish the slow response generated in this beta adrenergic receptor-independent model of slow response electrical activity.

In the very first series of experiments we have described so far, we demonstrate that acetylcholine can affect automaticity in the intraventricular specialized conducting system. The last series of experiments demonstrate that acetylcholine is capable of antagonizing the effects of prior beta adrenergic stimulation of canine Purkinje fibers in the ventricle. Neither of these two studies addressed the issue of whether or not acetylcholine might exert an effect in the ventricle independent of the presence of concomitant beta adrenergic tone. Therefore we undertook a series of experiments in guinea pigs to determine whether acetylcholine might affect automaticity in guinea pig Purkinje fibers (Rardon and Bailey, 1983). In these experiments the guinea pigs were pretreated with reserpine to deplete

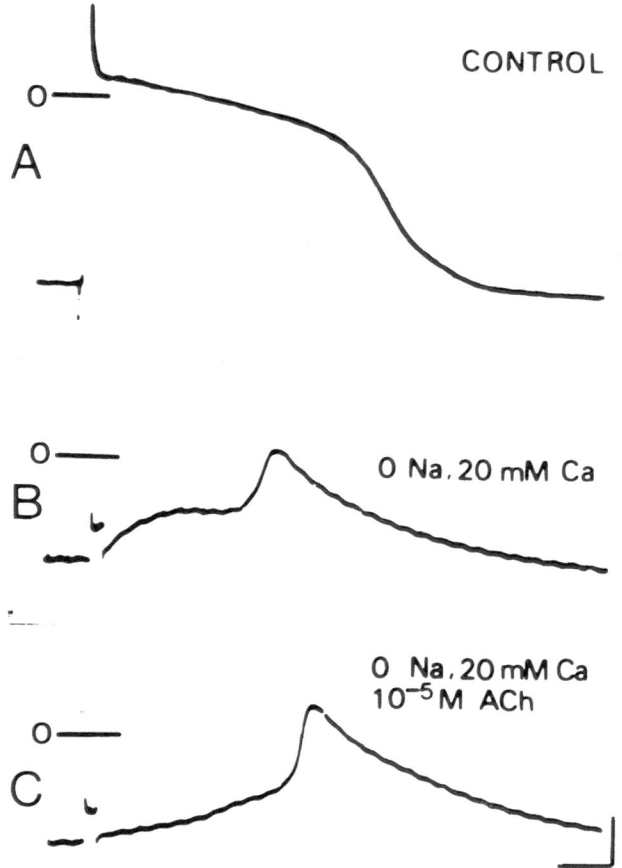

Figure 6. The effects of acetylcholine on a 'slow response' that is not isoproterenol-dependent. A: A control canine cardiac Purkinje fiber action potential. B: 'Slow response' generated in a sodium-free, 20 mM calcium solution. C: Addition of acetylcholine (10^{-5} M) did not affect excitability. Zero potential lines and calibrations as in Figure 3. Reproduced from ref. 14 by permission of the American Heart Association, Inc.

myocardial norepinephrine stores. The results of one such experiment are depicted in Figure 7. The top panel depicts a tachometer tracing recording beat to beat changes in spontaneous cycle-length of a guinea pig Purkinje fiber. Please recall that these fibers are from animals pretreated with reserpine. The first portion of the record demonstrates the control spontaneous cycle-length. Note that tyramine, 10^{-4} M, does not alter the rate of discharge of these Purkinje fibers. In a normal Purkinje fiber from guinea pig, tyramine would decrease significantly the spontaneous cycle-length of these fibers. Physostigmine produces a significant time-dependent decrease in the cycle-length of these reserpine pretreated fibers, an effect that is reversed with atropine. The same observations are noted in the bottom panel. Tyramine does not alter the cycle-length of these reserpine

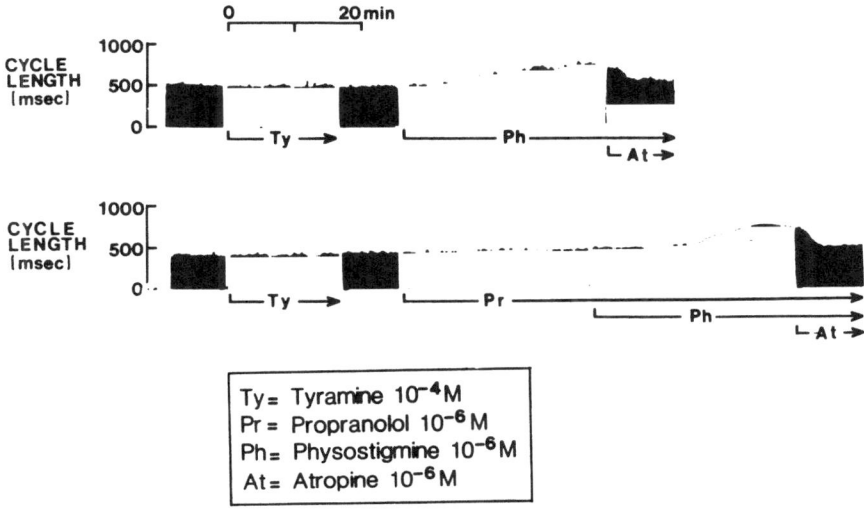

Ty = Tyramine 10^{-4}M
Pr = Propranolol 10^{-6}M
Ph = Physostigmine 10^{-6}M
At = Atropine 10^{-6}M

Figure 7. Effects of tyramine, propranolol, physostigmine, and atropine on spontaneous ventricular rate in reserpine-pretreated guinea pigs. Cycle length (msec) is plotted on the vertical axis, and time (minutes) is plotted on the horizontal axis. The initial portion of each tachometer recording represents the last 5 minutes of the 20-minute control period. Each ventricular strip was superfused with tyramine 1×10^{-4}M (Ty) which was washed out of the tissue bath prior to superfusion of physostigmine 1×10^{-6}M (Ph), propranolol 1×10^{-6}M (Pr), atropine 1×10^{-6}M (At), or a combination of drugs as noted. Reproduced from ref. 15 by permission of the American Heart Association, Inc.

pretreated fibers. Propranolol also has no effect on the spontaneous cycle-length. Note that physostigmine still produces a significant slowing of the rate of discharge of these fibers despite the propranolol. The effects of physostigmine in the lower panel are also reversed with atropine. The response in the normal guinea pigs was clearly different from that seen in reserpine pretreated animals as depicted in Table I. In normal animals tyramine, as expected, increased the rate of spontaneous discharge of ventricular pacemakers. Both physostigmine and propranolol induced time-dependent slowing of these normal fibers. However, as shown in Table II, in the reserpine pretreated animals tyramine did not alter the

Table 1. Chronotropic response to physostigmine, propranolol, and tyramine in the control group.

	n	Control	10 min	20 min	30 min
Physostigmine (10^{-6}M)	12	97 ± 36	79 ± 35‡	60 ± 34‡	53 ± 24‡
Propranolol (10^{-6}M)	7	141 ± 30	128 ± 38	118 ± 40	108 ± 35†
Tyramine (10^{-5}M)	7	87 ± 42		109 ± 29*	

Spontaneous ventricular discharge rate per minute, mean $\pm$ SD, at 10, 20, and 30 minutes of superfusion. * $P<0.05$, † $P<0.01$, ‡ $P<0.001$ compared to control.

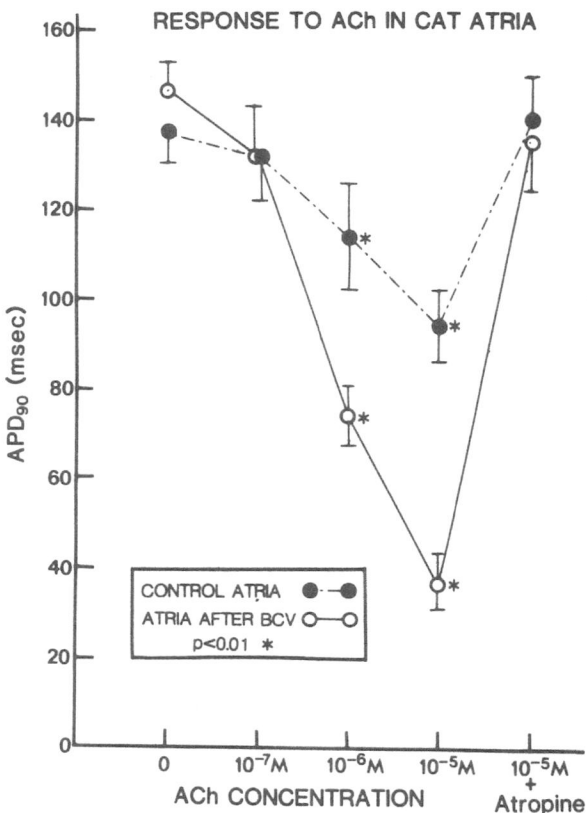

Figure 8. Comparison of action potential duration shortening at 90% repolarization (ADP$_{90}$) atria from cats with intact vagi (●) and cats following bilateral cervical vagotomy (○). APD$_{90}$ is plotted as a function of acetylcholine concentration. An (*) indicates a significant (P<0.01) difference from the value for APD at 0 concentration of ACh within that group. Differences in the response to ACh between the two groups were analyzed by two-way ANOVA with repeated measures. There is a significant difference in APD response to ACh between cats with intact vagi and cats after BCV when measured at 90% repolarization (interaction F = 7.88 P<0.001). This exaggerated effect of ACh is graphically illustrated by the increased steepness of the curve for animals after BCV. Reproduced from ref. 16 by permission of the American Heart Association, Inc.

Table 2. Chronotropic response to physostigmine, propranolol, and tyramine in the reserpine-pretreated group.

	n	Control	10 min	20 min	30 min
Physostigmine (10^{-6}M)	12	94 ± 53	73 ± 40*	55 ± 42*	48 ± 45*
Propranolol (10^{-6}M)	5	98 ± 26	99 ± 23	92 ± 23	90 ± 21
Tyramine (10^{-4}M)	19	94 ± 44		92 ± 45	

Spontaneous ventricular discharge rate per minute, mean ± SD, at 10, 20, and 30 minutes of superfusion. * P<0.001 compared to control.

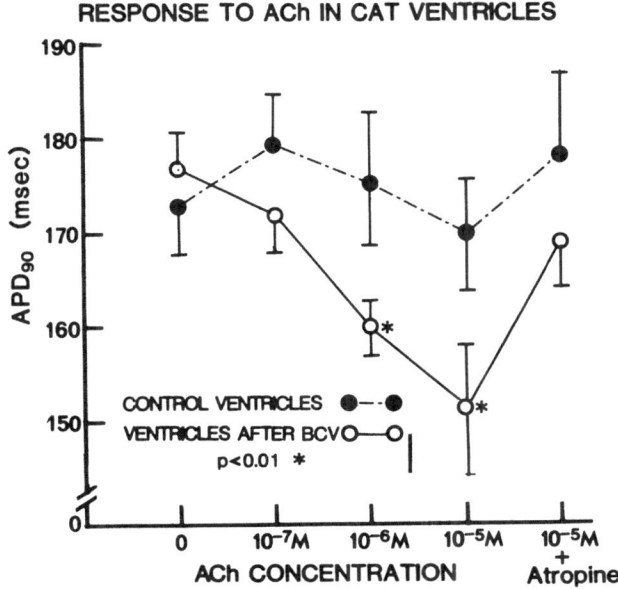

Figure 9. Comparison of effects of acetylcholine ($10^{-7} - 10^{-5}$ M) on APD_{90} in ventricles from cats with intact vagi (●) and cats following bilateral cervical vagotomy (○). In normally innervated ventricles, acetylcholine did not alter APD_{90} at any concentration. However the choline ester produced a significant concentration-dependent shortening of APD_{90} in ventricles following bilateral cervical vagotomy. Reproduced from ref. 16 by permission of the American Heart Association, Inc.

spontaneous rate of discharge. Furthermore, propranolol had no effect on the rate of spontaneous discharge although physostigmine continued to induce a time-dependent slowing in the rate of ventricular discharge of these guinea pig fibers pretreated with reserpine. We interpreted these data to indicate that acetylcholine was capable of producing negative chronotropic effects in the ventricle even in the absence of basal beta adrenergic tone. These data, therefore, indicate a direct, that is an adrenergic independent, role for vagal modulation of the electrophysiological effects on mammalian ventricular specialized conducting tissue.

The previous data indicate that acetylcholine can alter electrophysiological parameters in the ventricle during elevated or absent beta adrenergic tone. We then undertook a series of experiments to determine whether the chronic removal of muscarinic cholinergic tone might result in alterations in the electrophysiological response to acetylcholine and beta adrenergic stimulation (Kovacs and Bailey, 1985). We subjected cats to bilateral cervical vagotomy, and three days later sacrificed the cats and mounted the atria in muscle chambers exposed to increasing concentrations of acetylcholine. Figure 8 demonstrates the response to acetylcholine in both the experimentally denervated atria as well as on a control group with normal innervation. Note that acetylcholine produced, as expected, a dose-dependent decrease of action potential duration of normally innervated cat atrium. However following bilateral cervical vagotomy there was an exaggerated decrease in action potential duration in response to this choline ester. The response to acetylcholine in cat ventricles is illustrated in Figure 9. In normally innervated ventricles there was no dose-dependent alteration in cat ventricular muscle action potential duration in response to acetylcholine. However in those animals subjected to bilateral cervical vagotomy there was a significant dose-dependent decrease in the action potential duration in response to acetylcholine, effects that were reversed with atropine. Thus, following bilateral cervical vagotomy, cat ventricular myocardium behaved much like normally innervated cat atrium in response to acetylcholine. Therefore these studies demonstrate that, following vagotomy in cat, the atria become supersensitive to the effects of acetylcholine, whereas the ventricles, in the normally innervated preparations unresponsive to this neurotransmitter, become sensitive to the effects of acetylcholine.

What are the clinical implications of these animal findings? In the first place it would appear that data derived from numerous animal species might also apply to man. In this regard Prystowsky, et al. (1981) demonstrated in conscious man that, although beta adrenergic blockade did not alter ventricular effective refractory periods significantly, the administration of atropine produced significant shortening of the effective refractory periods ($238 \neq 23$ to $218 \neq 19$ msec., $p<0.05$) in ventricles subjected to prior beta adrenergic blockade. Waxman and Wald (1977) have also reported termination of ventricular tachycardia in man by elevating vagal tone.

In conclusion, we have demonstrated that mascarinic cholinergic stimulation with acetylcholine exerts potent effects on the ventricle, regardless of the state of adrenergic tone. The extent to which these potent effects are relevant to the offset or onset of clinically relevant arrhythmias remains to be determined.

References

1. Jose AD, Taylor RR. 1969. Autonomic blockade by propranolol and atropine to study intrinsic myocardial function in man. J Clin Invest 48: 2019–2031.
2. Levy MN, Zieske H. 1969. Autonomic control of cardiac pacemaker activity and atrioventricular transmission. J Appl Physiol 27: 465–470.
3. Prystowsky EN, Jackman WM, Rinkenberger RL, Heger JJ, Zipes DP. 1981. Effect of autonomic blockade on ventricular refractoriness and atrioventricular nodal conduction in humans. Circ Res 49: 511–518.
4. Higgins CB, Vatner SF, Braunwald E. 1973. Parasympathetic control of the heart. Pharmacol Rev 25: 119–155.
5. Zipes DP, Martins JB, Ruffy R, Prystowsky EN, Elharrar V, Gilmour RF. 1981. Roles of autonomic innervation in the genesis of ventricular arrhythmias. In: FM Abboud, HA Fozzard, JP Gilmore, DJ Reis, eds. Disturbances in Neurogenic Control of the Circulation, pp 225–250. Bethesda, MD: American Physiological Society.

6. Rardon DP, Bailey JC. 1983. Parasympathetic effects on electrophysiological properties of cardiac ventricular tissue. J Amer Coll Cardiol 2: 1200–1215.

7. Levy MN. 1971. Sympathetic-parasympathetic interactions in the heart. Circ Res 29: 437–445.

8. Kent KM, Epstein SE, Cooper T, Jacobowitz DM (1974) Cholinergic innervation of the canine and human ventricular conducting system: Anatomical an electrophysiological consideration. Circulation 50: 948–955.

9. Jacobowitz DM, Cooper T, Barner HB. 1967. Histochemical and chemical studies of the localization of adrenergic and cholinergic nerves in normal and denervated cat hearts. Circ Res 20: 289–298.

10. Roskoski R, Schmid PG, Mayer HE, Abboud FA. 1975. In vitro acetylcholine biosynthesis in normal and failing guinea pig hearts. Circ Res 36: 547–552.

11. Brown OM. 1976. Cat heart acetylcholine: structural proof and distribution. Am J Physiol 231: 781–785.

12. Fields JZ, Roeske WR, Morkin E, Yamamura HI. 1978. Cardiac muscarinic cholinergic receptors. Biochemical identification and characterization. J Biol Chem 253: 3251–3258.

13. Bailey JC, Greenspan K, Elizari MV, Anderson GJ, Fisch C. 1972. Effects of acetylcholine on automaticity and conduction in the proximal portion of the His-Purkinje specialized conduction system of the dog. Circ Res 30: 210–216.

14. Bailey JC, Watanabe AM, Besch HR Jr, Lanthrop DA. 1979. Acetylcholine antagonism of the electrical effects of isoproterenol on canine cardiac Purkinje fibers. Circ Res 44: 378–383.

15. Rardon DP, and Bailey JC. 1983. Direct effects of cholinergic stimulation on ventricular automaticity in guinea pig myocardium. Circ. Res. 52: 105–110.

16. Kovacs RJ, and Bailey JC. 1985. Effects of acetylcholine on action potential characteristics of atrial and ventricular myocardium after bilateral cervical vagotomy in the cat. Circ Res 56: 613–620.

17. Waxman MB, and Weld RW. 1977. Termination of ventricular tachycardia by an increase in cardiac vagal drive. Circulation 56: 385–391.

5. Clinical evaluation of the role of the autonomic nervous system in ventricular arrhythmias

PHILIPPE COUMEL, JEAN-FRANÇOIS LECLERCQ, JEAN-SYLVAIN HERMIDA and MARC ZIMMERMAN
Hôpital Lariboisière, 2 rue Ambroise-Paré, 75010 – Paris, France

The role of the autonomic nervous system (ANS) in ventricular arrhythmias is a very wide topic which may be evaluated clinically from many different aspects. The present chapter does not pretend to cover in depth all of them, but simply to remind the clinician what evidences he has of the importance of this role, what tools he has at his disposal to explore it, and what difficulties he will meet when using them.

The role of the ANS in the genesis of cardiac arrhythmias has been suspected for a long time [1], especially in relation to the role of the sympathetics in experimental ventricular arrhythmias. However, the problem has not been systematically explored in humans, except for ventricular arrhythmias in patients with coronary heart disease, and for those with the long QT-sudden death syndromes and their variants [2–4]. An important reason for this lack of knowledge is that invasive and non-invasive electrophysiological (EP) methods are not well-adapted to explore the problem, or at least not oriented towards its exploration [5].

The methods of exploration

Invasive EP evaluation

Evaluating ventricular arrhythmias and their sensitivity to the ANS is rarely done using beta-adrenergic agonists and antagonists during programmed stimulation. At best in some publications, the stimulation protocol includes isoprenaline infusion in case of non-inducibility of the arrhythmia which was looked for. Theoretically, isoprenaline should decrease false negatives of the tests (patients with a non-inducible but spontaneously relapsing arrhythmia) with the risk of increasing false positives (induction of non-clinical arrhythmias). Protocols of isoprenaline administration can be based on the level of sinus rhythm attained, or on the amount of drug and infusion rate. This might be the right way to bridge the gap between the 33% exercise-related and the 75% not-exercise-related induci-ble idiopathic VTs [6], rather than refining the stimulation protocols. Performing them during standardized isoprenaline or exercise tests would evidence and quantify common though rarely referred to findings about the much easier induction of any arrhythmia: the smaller the necessary adrenergic stimulation, the greater the arrhythmia sensitivity. On the other hand, using beta-blockers should decrease false positives of EP testing, the risk being to increase false negatives thus decreasing sensitivity. Continuing oral beta-blocking therapy after EP testing may be the best way to improve its reliability.

One should not forget however, that administration of beta-adrenergic ago-nists or antagonists may fail to reproduce the complex interactions of the 2 limbs of the ANS, and may fail to recognize possible differences between beta 1 and beta 2 receptors as far as the sinus node on the one hand, and ventricular arrhythmias on the other hand are concerned. Figure 1 is illustrative of this situation. In a patient with documented, idiopathic paroxysmal attacks of ven-tricular tachycardia (VT), all attemps for inducing them in the laboratory failed, even when isoproterenol was administered. A non-clinical atrial fibrillation was then artificial induced, and lasted during 10 minutes: panel 2 of the figure shows its spontaneous termination followed by 17 sinus beats after which the clinical VT starts spontaneously. Then the VT became inducible and could be terminated at will during the rest of the study. It is likely that the hemodynamic consequences of the attack of atrial fibrillation had modified the vago-sympathetic balance in a way which was indeed more effective than, and probably different from the isoprenaline administration. We are possibly facing such a situation any time we cannot reproduce a clinical VT in the laboratory, and many false negatives or false positives of this technique may be related to ANS.

Non-invasive EP evaluation

The technique of ambulatory monitoring seems much better adapted to evidenc-ing the role of the ANS than invasive electrophysiology, because it deals with the natural behavior of arrhythmias. This technique does have its limitations: explor-ing the role of the ANS first supposes that the arrhythmias are recorded, which may be difficult when they are paroxysmal and very occasional. This condition can be met with some luck and patience, but the real problem is to define the right parameters related to ANS. The heart rate reflects the balance between sympa-thetic and vagal drive. Sinus function constitutes a useful though global indica-tion, and should be studied systematically at the beginning of the arrhythmia in an effort to define the autonomic tone at that time. This marker of the ANS balance reflects what happens in the sinus node, which does not necessarily parallel the ventricle: at this level, monitoring the QT interval despite the considerable practical difficulty [7] theoretically is more appropriate. Overall, our experience

56

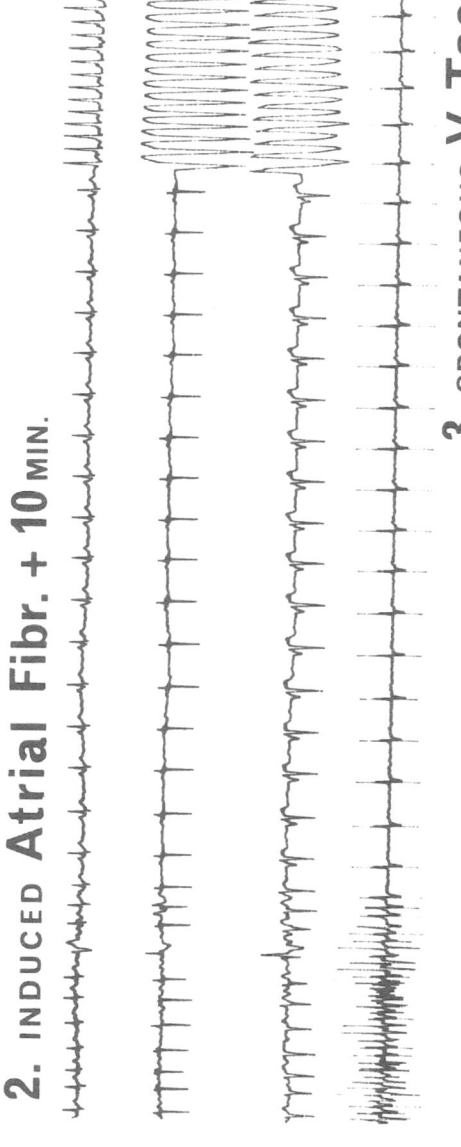

1. NON-INDUCIBLE **V. Tach.**

2. INDUCED **Atrial Fibr. + 10**MIN.

I

III

V1

A

3. SPONTANEOUS **V. Tach.**

4. INDUCIBLE **V. Tach.**

Figure 1. False negative of an EP study. A known, clinical ventricular tachycardia could not be obtained by programmed stimulation, even after isoproterenol infusion, as it frequently happens in undiseased hearts (1). Then an atrial fibrillation was artificially provoked (2). Sinus rhythm resumed after 10 minutes. A few seconds later the clinical VT spontaneously occured (3) and then became quite easy to start again and to terminate artificially (4).

in using the sinus frequency shows a serious limitation of this marker that is at the same time very logical and paradoxical: one must realize that the greater the arrhythmia dependency on the sympathetic drive, the smaller the necessary adrenergic stimulation, hence the less apparent the sinus rate changes. We shall give illustrative examples of this situation, which unsurprisingly also applies to the QT evaluation [8].

The role of the ANS in non-sustained ventricular tachycardias
In two recent studies [9, 10] we analyzed the determinants of non-sustained VT (NSVT) in various categories of patients according to the clinical and ECG pattern of the arrhythmia. Three determinants could be individualized: the cycle length of the last sinus beat immediately preceding the NSVT, the coupling interval of the extrasystole (ES) forming the first beat of the arrhythmia, and the mean heart rate during the 3 minutes that precede it. This was done in different categories of patients forming 2 groups of 30 (fig. 2). Group A included 30 patients (16 males, 14 females, aged 42 ± 17 years – mean $\pm$ SD) with recurrent monomorphic NSVT (86% with a left bundle branch block pattern and a normal or right axis deviation) without any evidence of heart disease (Fig. 2A). Group B also included 30 patients (25 males, 5 females, aged 57 ± 12 years) with an identified heart disease (18 coronary heart disease, 11 cardiomyopathies, 1 aortic stenosis) and various degrees of left ventricular function impairment (mean ejection fraction = 41%). This group was subdivided according to the ECG pattern: a B′ subgroup of 18 patients with a monomorphic VT (right bundle branch block pattern in 78% of the cases, fig. 2 B′), and a B″ subgroup of 12 patients with polymorphic NSVTs (Fig. 2 B″). The number of the analyzed events were equivalent in groups A en B, and for the purpose of the present chapter we do not consider the role of 2 determinants which can be briefly summarized as follows: the longer the last sinus cycle length, and the longer the coupling interval, the longer the duration of the repetitive activity from couplets to salvos of NSVT. The role of the third determinant will be more detailed.

The different types of arrhythmia were classified as isolated ES (type 1), couplets (type 2), triplets (type 3), salvos of 4, 5, 6 to 10 and more than 10 beats of VT. For each of the events (with a total of several thousands per patient per 24 hours) the computer we use in the ATREC II system [11] calculated the mean RR interval during the 3 preceding minutes, and the global results are displayed in figure 3. In group A the correlation between the heart rate and the type of events is highly significant ($r = 0.98$, P<0.001) and indicates the strong relationship between the arrhythmia and the level of the sympathetic tone reflected by the 3-min heart rate. In subgroup B′ patients the relationship is still present but less marked ($r = 0.67$, P = 0.09), and in subgroup B″ patients only a trend is visible ($r = 0.51$, p = 0.29).

At this point, the progressively decreasing apparent ANS-to-NSVT relation-ship as the severity of ECG and clinical pattern of NSVT increases have only two

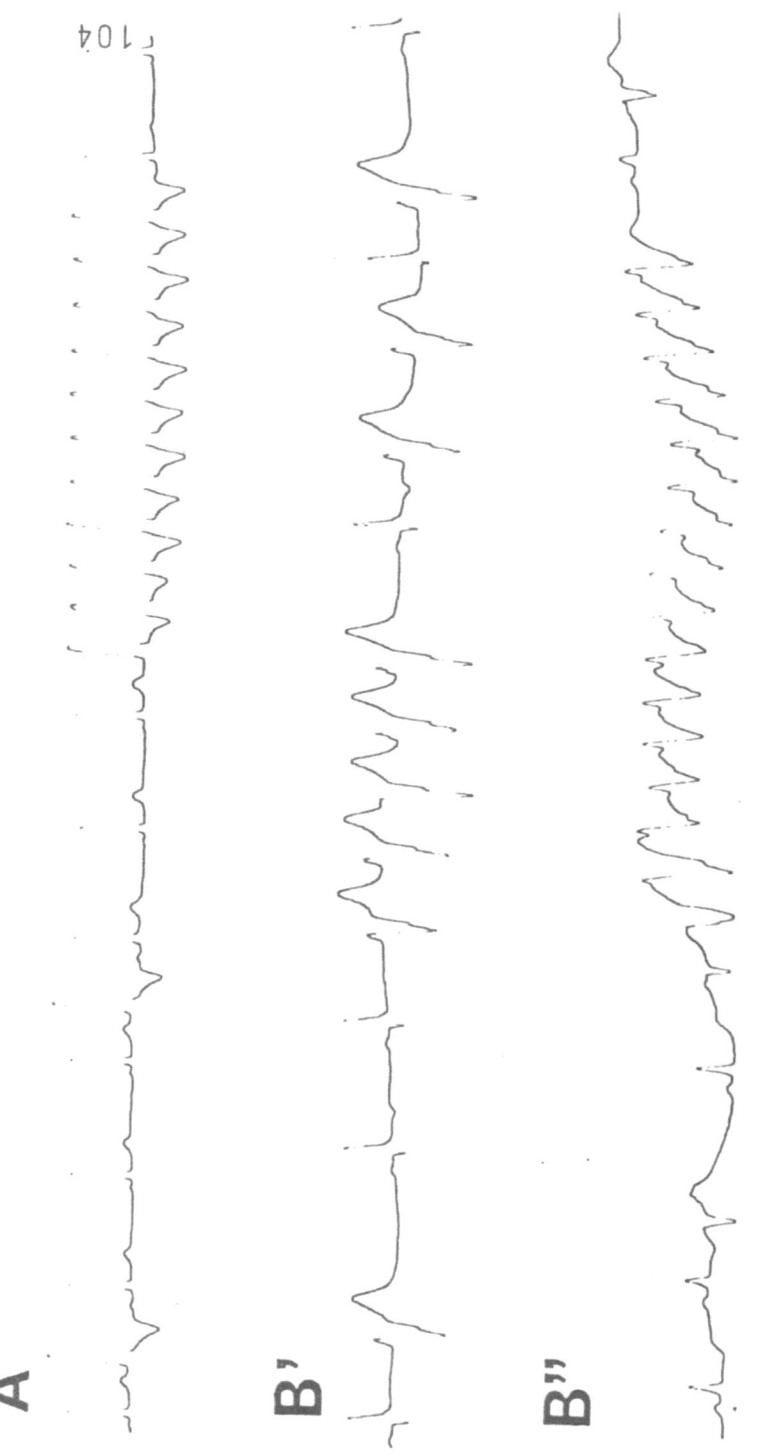

Figure 2. Various forms of non-sustained ventricular tachycardias. In group A patients (n = 30) the NSVT was monomorphic (left bundle branch block pattern and right axis deviation) and idiopathic. Group B' patients (n = 18) had a known left heart disease and a monomorphic NSVT (right bundle branch block pattern). Group B" patients (n = 12) had polymorphic NSVTs and a more severely diseased left ventricle (see also figure 3).

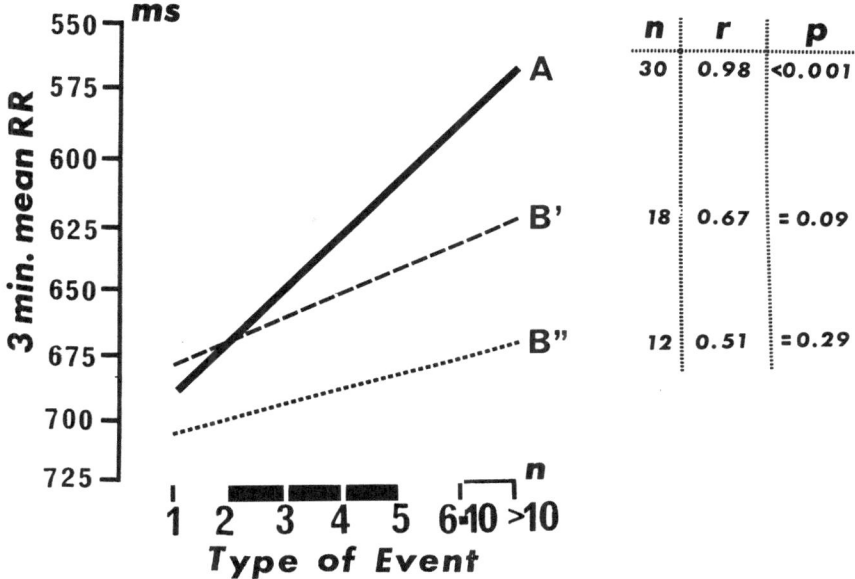

Figure 3. Preceding heart rate and NSVT relationships. The mean RR interval during the 3 minutes before each arrhythmia is plotted with the type of this arrhythmia: isolated ES (1), couplets (2), triplets (3), runs of 4 or 5, 6-to-10 (6–10) and longer than 10 salvos (>10) of NSVT. The number of patients (n) in groups A, B' and B" is indicated on the right, with the correlation coefficient (r) of the regression line and the corresponding p value.

possible explanations: an actual loss of adrenergic dependency of the arrhythmia, or on the contrary an increased sensitivity to smaller, hence less visible and detectable changes in the sympathetic drive, according to the 'adrenergic paradox' concept.

Patent and latent adrenergic dependency of sustained VTs

The same rules apply to sustained VT as to NSVT. The former does not fundamentally differ from the latter. Their definitions are purely arbitrary: there are no criteria except conventions to decide whether the cutting point between the two forms should be their duration for 3, 5, 10, 15 beats or 30 seconds, 1 or 3 minutes. Whether spontaneous or induced, non-sustained and sustained VTs obviously correspond to the same phenomenon [12] and they are observed in the setting of the same diseases (or their absence). After all, the reasons for a VT to be sustained or not reside in the termination of the repetitive activity rather than in its initiation. However, a major practical difference between the two forms is that the computerized analysis cannot be used in the same way, for the simple reason that not the same, and not as many events are available. At best in sustained VTs, one can study the 2 extremes of the continuous spectrum formed by the NSVTs: logically the ANS influence should increase from ES to VT, but here the intermediate forms are lacking to validate the hypothesis. Even if available, ESs and VTs do not necessarily have the same EP mechanism, the same meaning and the same relationships with the ANS. The VT corresponds to the existence of a substrate, the activity of which obviously has to be triggered by some initiating factor, usually an ES [5]: if this condition were not present the VT would be permanent, and invasive EP studies are but a means to artificially provide an initiating factor. We shall give 2 examples which illustrate for sustained VTs situations analogous to what we observed in NSVTs.

The patient of figure 4 had a common history of post-infarct paroxysmal VTs, with the particularity of their preferable occurrence at daytime, and more precisely during physical activity. There was no evidence of clinical heart failure or ECG ischemia since the infarction 3 years before the first attack of VT. During a 24-hour ambulatory monitoring, various forms of ES were recorded, which could be classified into 2 clearly separated groups (Fig. 5): a total of 162 ES distributed into 3 morphologic types (A, B and C) always occurred in the setting of a sinus tachycardia corresponding to physical activity, whereas a total of 2347 ESs distributed into 3 other types (D, E and F) always occurred in the setting of a slower heart rate. Focusing on the former 3 types, the systematic computerized analysis showed that the 119 type C ESs were always preceded by a 2-minute dramatic acceleration of sinus frequency (fig. 6). The 12 type B ESs had the slightly different pattern of a sinus acceleration occuring during the 4 to 7 preceding minutes but slightly decreasing secondarily. The 28 type A ESs, in addition to the same behavior, had the important characteristic of having the same morphology as 3 runs of 7-beat to 2-minute VTs reproducing the clinical sustained VT. Focusing on these type A ESs and VTs in figure 7 shows that indeed a sinus acceleration followed by a deceleration always precedes the ESs by 5 to 8 minutes, and that runs of VT precisely follow a more important and prolonged previous sinus acceleration. Thus, the adrenergic origin of the VT was clear in this patient, and further confirmed by an easy control of the arrhythmia by acebutolol. Occasionally, one should note that types D-to-F ESs were not affected by this treatment: this illustrates how misleading it may be to take indifferently any type of ES as the marker for treatment efficacy if a VT is indeed the real clinical target. Finally, one should note how arrhythmias that do have in common their ANS-dependency in this patient may well have a different behavior vis-à-vis the marker, i.e. the sinus rate: type C ESs reacted immediately to sinus acceleration whereas a lag time was observed for ESs types A and B.

The example given in figure 8 illustrates a quite opposite situation. An infarcted patient with a clinical heart failure (NYHA class III) and a 28% ejection fraction had attacks of sustained VT which proved resistant to amiodarone and quinidine combined therapy. They occured preferably in the morning though apparently not related to the limited physical activity. An episode was recorded, and no visible heart rate change could be detected by a precise, minute-by-minute and even beat-to-beat analysis. Still, an indication was given by studying the

61

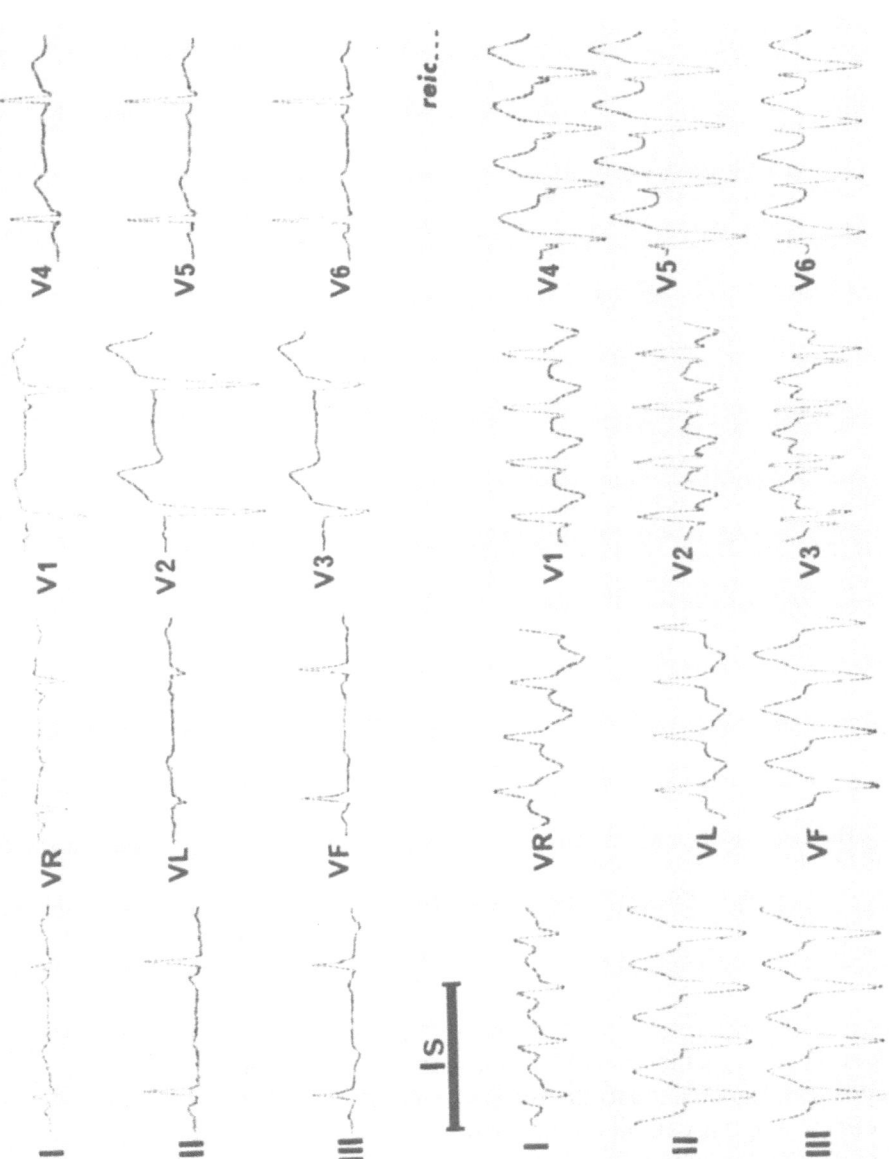

reic...

Figure 4. Post-myocardial infarction ventricular tachycardia. Basic tracings show the healed anterior myocardial infarction during sinus rhythm. The VT with a left axis deviation and a right bundle branch block pattern also shows Q waves in leads V1–V4 (see also figures 5–7).

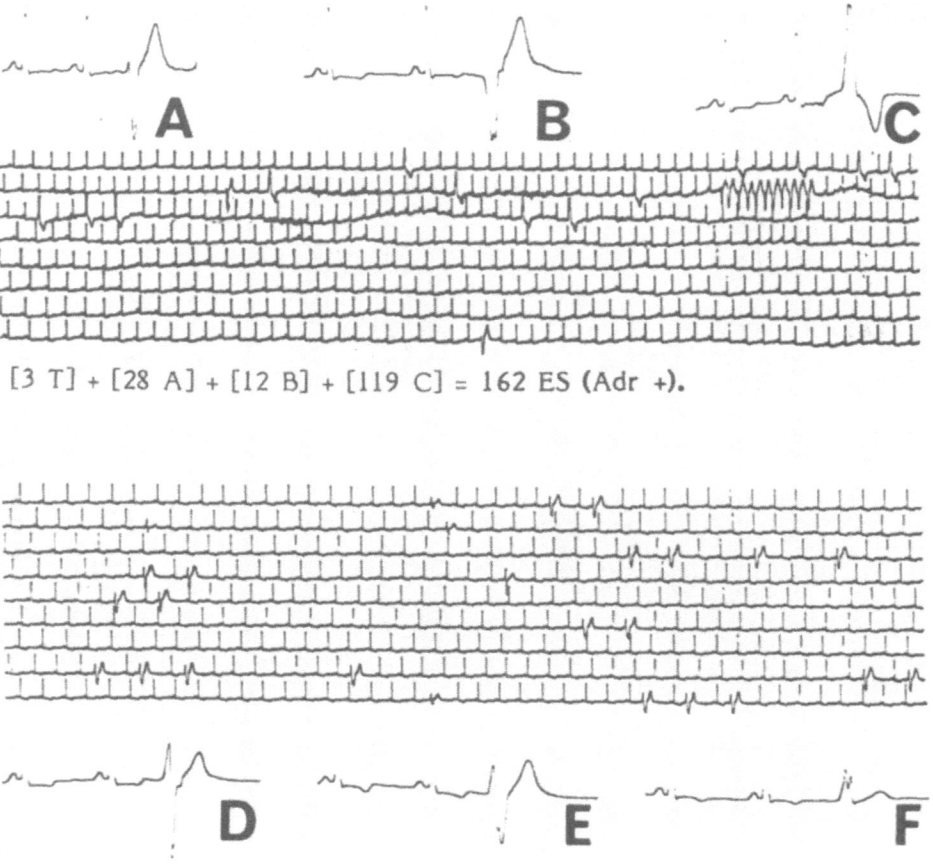

[3 T] + [28 A] + [12 B] + [119 C] = 162 ES (Adr +).

Figure 5. Holter monitoring in a post-infarc paroxysmal VT. Seven types of events observed during the 24-hour ambulatory recording could be grouped in 2 sets. The upper panel displays the events occuring in the setting of a sinus tachycardia: a total of 162 'Adr +'; extrasystole of type A (n = 28), B (n = 12) or C (n = 119), and runs of VT (T, n = 3) with a type A configuration. In contrast, the lower panel displays 3 other types of extrasystoles (types D, E, F, n = 2347) occuring only with a slower sinus rate.

extrasystolic rate as a function of the heart rate (right upper diagram of figure 8), and a positive, significant correlation was found. A beta-blocking treatment was quite effective in this patient on the condition to be combined with a previously ineffective type I anti-arrhythmic drug.

At this point, again the same problem of interpretation applies to VTs and to NSVTs: in our first case the dependency on the sympathetic drive was obvious. In the second case however, the clinical and ECG pattern of the arrhythmia could be interpreted in two opposite ways: a lesser dependency on, or an increased sensitivity to the sympathetic drive. Yet this time the beta-blockers effectiveness

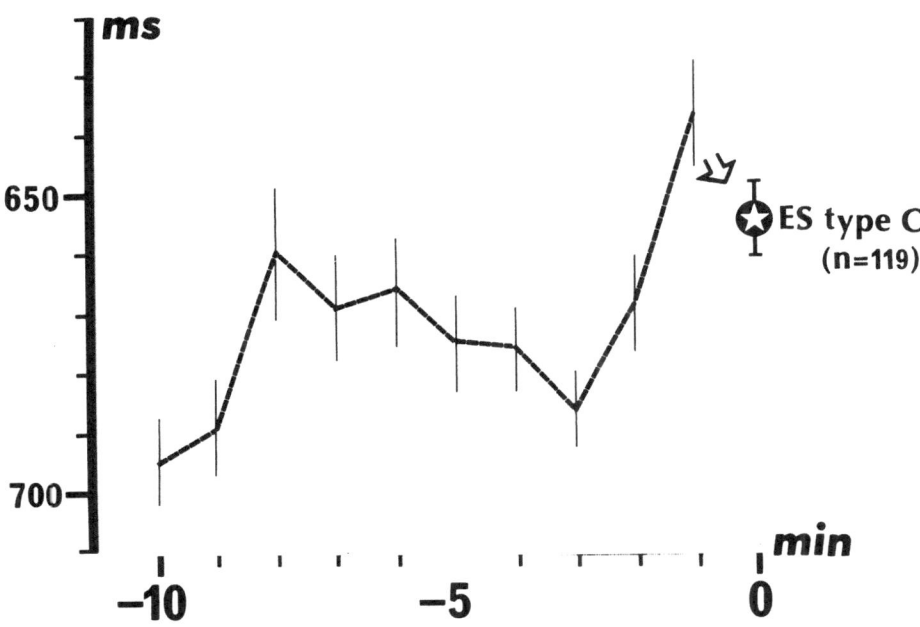

Figure 6. Extrasystoles and the preceding heart rate. Type C extrasystoles of the patient of figures 4 and 5 were studied individually in terms of heart rate during each of the 10 preceding minutes. The mean cycle length/min is represented (±SEM). Significant heart rate changes occur as early as 5 to 10 minutes before the extrasystoles, but the most significant phenomenon is a dramatic acceleration in the last 2 minutes. The star figures the mean sinus cycle length of the 10 beats immediately preceding the 119 extrasystoles, which is slightly longer than the last minute mean cycle length.

clearly indicated on an a posteriori basis that the latter interpretation was correct and that the 'adrenergic paradox' was a reality rather than an attractive and logical concept: a highly sensitive arrhythmia only needs tiny changes of the sympathetic drive at the ventricular level, and they are not necessarily detectable by monitoring the sinus node frequency. Arguments provided by the effect of beta-blocking therapy will be now further developed.

The effect of beta-blockers in ventricular arrhythmias

The adrenergic paradox implies therapeutic corollaries. One should expect that arrhythmias clearly preceded by a 'warning' sinus tachycardia would be theoretically amenable to beta-blocking therapy without forgetting, however, that if the arrhythmia is indeed sensitive to a strong adrenergic stimulation, it means that the adenergic component is possibly neither the only nor even the predominant mechanism of the arrhythmia. Therefore, the beta-blocking treatment would be of interest, but probably not on its own. In addition, as the aim of the treatment

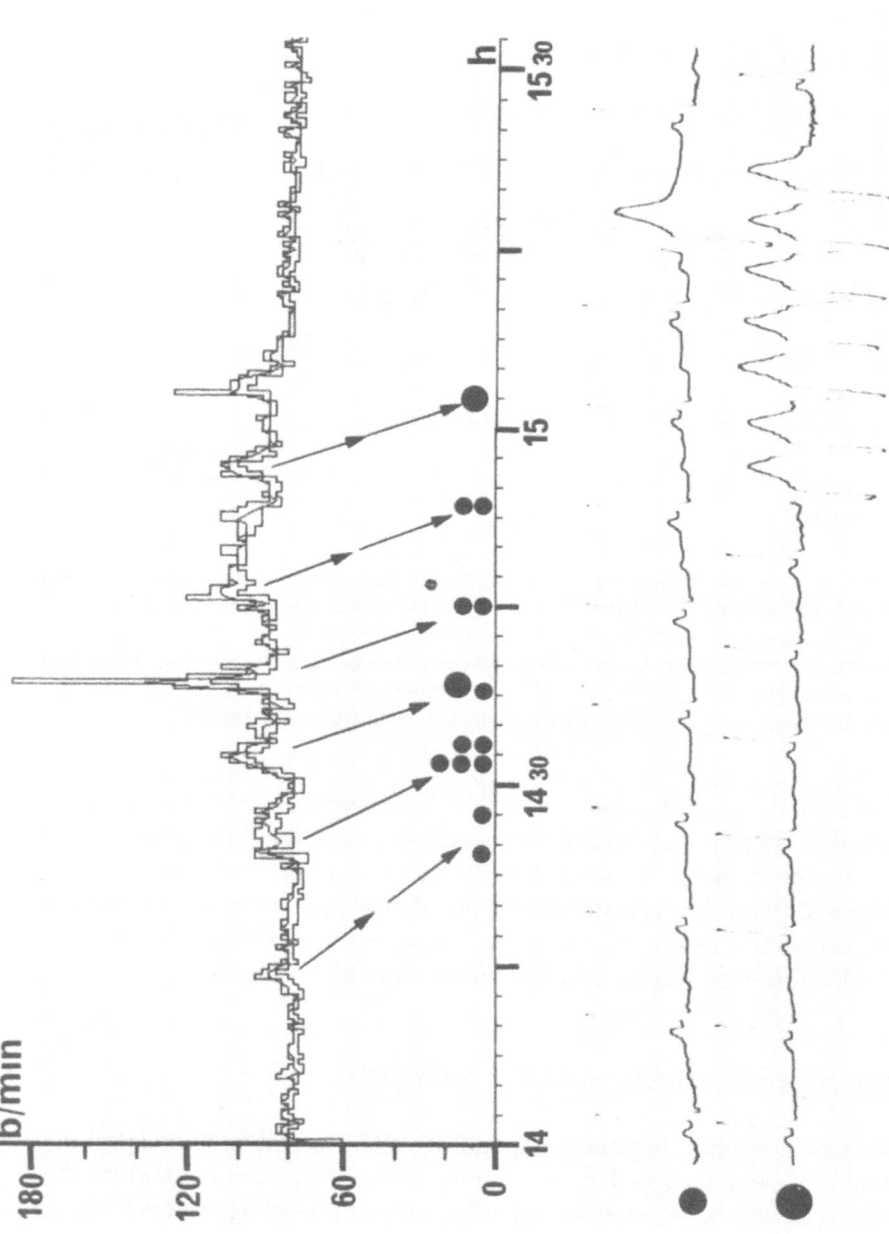

Figure 7. Type A extrasystoles and ventricular tachycardias. The computerized analysis of a 1-and-a-half-hour ambulatory recording is displayed (the 3 curves refer to the mean, maximal and minimal heart rates for each 25-second studied block). It includes the exact timing of 12 type A extrasystoles (small solid circles) and 2 runs of ventricular tachycardia (large solid circles) lasting 11 and 7 beats respectively. The arrhythmias are not randomly distributed: they systematically occur several minutes after a sinus acceleration had occured, and this lag time tends to shorten (arrows) as the heart rate becomes higher.

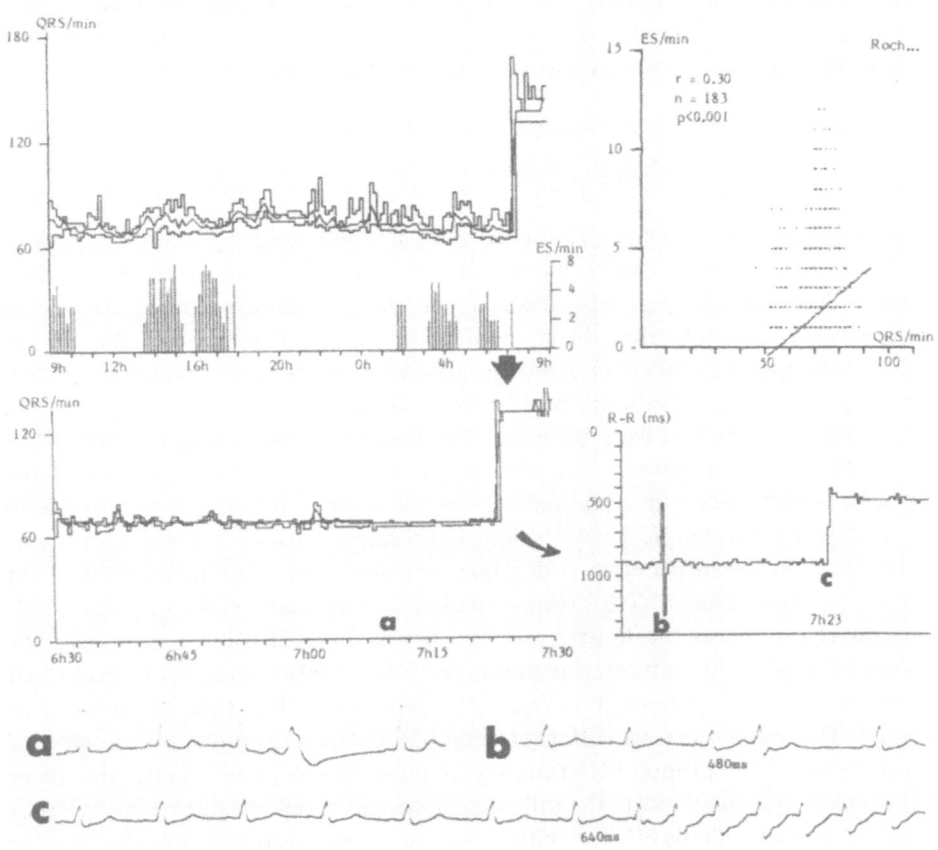

Figure 8. Behavior of extrasystoles and paroxysmal ventricular tachycardia. The left upper panel shows the computerized analysis of a 24-hour recording. A paroxysmal VT starts at 7h.23 am (left lower diagram) without any previous heart rate change, even when a beat-to-beat analysis is carried out (right lower diagram and bottom strip C). The only indication about the possible adrenergic dependency of the arrhythmia is suggested by the positive relationship between the extrasystolic rate (ES/min) and the heart rate (QRS/min) in the right upper panel. The resistant VT could be controlled only when nadolol was added to the antiarrhythmic treatment.

will be to prevent mainly strong adrenergic stimulations, one may in principle use moderate dosages of this type of drugs, and does not have to use the strongest ones.

If the adrenergic paradox concept is valid, a second corollary is that arrhythmias which are very sensitive to catecholamines, i.e. preceded by tiny changes or even no apparent changes of sinus rate, should be indeed protected against small modifications of the adrenergic drive in order to have a good clinical outcome: this implies using larger dosages of powerful beta-blockers. Clinicians are not used to making distinctions between the various presentations of the class II drugs, and in any case they are concerned by indicating these drugs precisely in the context of an impaired contractile myocardial function.

Beta-blockers in ventricular arrhythmias without heart failure

We compared the effects of 2 beta-blockers, nadolol and propranolol, in patients without heart failure, and with non-ischemic ventricular arrhythmias [13]. They were distributed in 2 groups according to the precipitating factors of the arrhythmia and its tolerance during activity. Ten patients with idiopathic ES and NSVT disappearing at exercise were allocated to the 'non-adrenergic' group. Nine patients with disabling, polymorphic, irregular arrhythmias occuring particularly at stress and exercise were allocated to the 'adrenergic' group which included 3 cases of mitral valve prolapse, 1 case of obstructive cardiomyopathy, and 5 cases of more or less idiopathic catecholamine-induced severe arrhythmias.

In the non-adrenergic group the hourly ES rate was 478 ± 439 and there was no significant difference between daytime and nighttime. The mean cardiac rate over 24 hours was 74.7 ± 8.6 bpm, with a day-to-night ratio of 1.26. In the adrenergic patients the hourly rate of ES was 201 ± 267 and a significant difference was found between day and night (252 ± 390 vs. 84 ± 78, $p < 0.05$). The cardiac rate over 24 hours was 78.5 ± 9.3 bpm with a day-to-night ratio of 1.35. All these parameters were different ($p < 0.05$) when the 2 groups were compared. The results of propranolol (160 mg/day) and nadolol (160 mg/day) treatments are presented in figure 9 where the following messages should be drawn from: 1/ there was no antiarrhythmic effect of either drug in the non-adrenergic group, whereas in the adrenergic group nadolol had a stronger effect than propranolol and 2/ both nadolol and propranolol significantly reduced the 24-hour heart rate in the adrenergic group, whereas only nadolol did so in the non-adrenergic group.

These results suggested that 1/ the antiarrhythmic effects of beta-blockers depend on the arrhythmia mechanism, 2/ in patients with adrenergic arrhythmias but without heart failure the 24-hour heart rate may be a marker of this mechanism which can be further explicited by beta-blocking therapy, and 3/ nadolol had a stronger effect than propranolol on both parameters, at least at the dosages used.

The differences between beta-blockers according to drugs and patient's condition

Recently we investigated further the effect of various beta-blockers on sinus frequency in 42 patients using 4 beta-blockers at different dosages [14]. We confirmed the differences between acebutolol and the drugs without intrinsic sympathetic activity [15], but differences were also found between the latter given

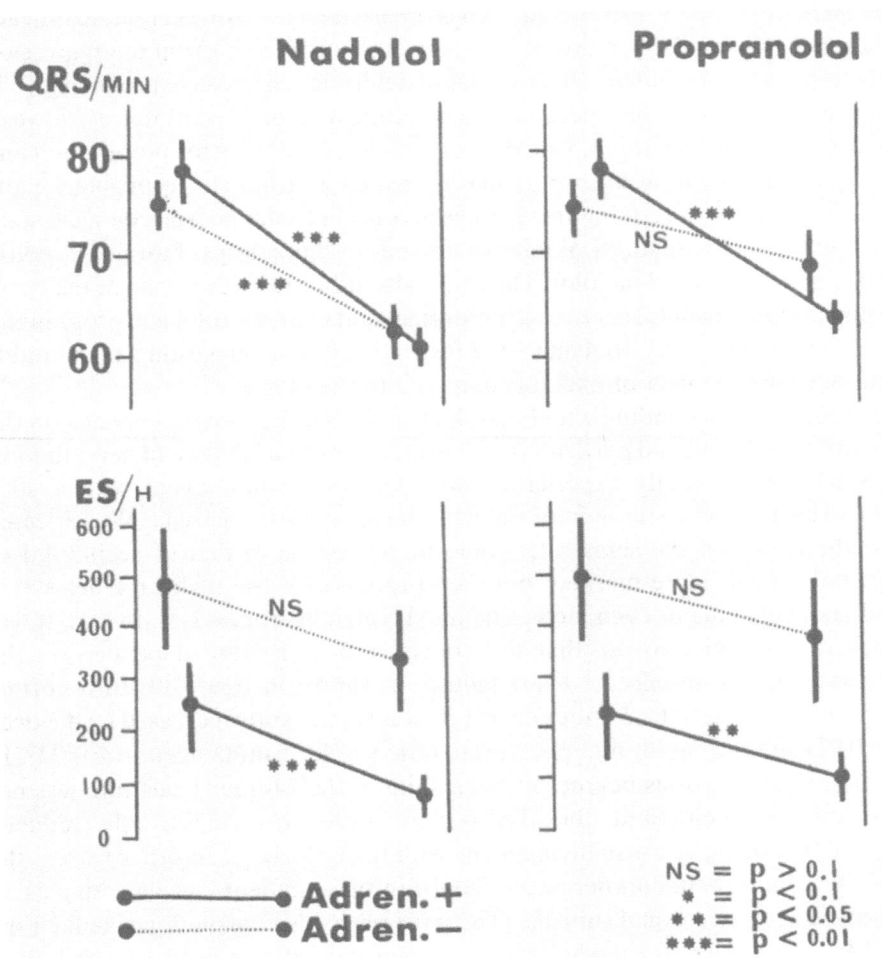

Figure 9. Effects of nadolol and propranolol in 'non-adrenergic' and 'adrenergic' patients with ventricular arrhythmias and no heart failure. The 24-hour heart rate (in QRS/min) and the 24-hour extrasystolic rate (in ES/hour) are represented for the adrenergic (circles ± SEM, n = 9) and the non-adrenergic (n = 10) group of patients. The control values are on the left and values during nadolol and propranolol treatments on the right of each panel. The drugs have no effect on non-adrenergic arrhythmias, and nadolol is more effective than propranolol on adrenergic arrhythmias. The mean heart rate is higher in patients with adrenergic arrhythmias, and it is significantly decreased by either drug. In patients with non-adrenergic arrhythmias, the mean heart rate is slower, and less influenced by propranolol than nadolol.

at different dosages: propranolol (80, 160 and 320 mg/day), metoprolol (200, 400 and 800 mg/day) and nadolol (40, 80 and 160 mg/day). Just considering the 24-hour mean heart rate in this study, it appears dose-dependently reduced in all patients, but the 3 drugs differed by the intensity of the effect. The maximal effect was similar (−26%, −25% and −26% respectively). However, a significant difference appeared when lower dosages were considered. From the regression line of the dose-dependent effect we could determine the dosage producing 50% of the maximal effect, thus permitting a quantification of the differences between the drugs: this dosage was 0.3 mg/day for nadolol, 47 mg/day for propranolol and 120 mg/day for metoprolol, a relationship which is strikingly surprising for the clinician used to prescribing these drugs according to the pharmacological standards based on the theoretical relative potency of these drugs: 1 for propranolol, 0.5 for metoprolol and nadolol. The drugs also differed by the slope of the dose-response curve: nadolol curve was flatter than that of metoprolol and propranolol (the slope being −2.0, −6.4 and −6.7 respectively) thus suggesting a qualitative difference in the effect of nadolol compared to the others.

Another curious finding with beta-blockers is that their effect depends on the patient's condition, and particularly the presence of some degree of heart failure. It is what we recently experienced with Corwin, a new agent with a 40% betaadrenergic agonistic activity and a partial antagonistic activity. We expected that the effect on the sinus rate would be analogous to that of acebutolol or pindolol though more marked: both tend to increase the nighttime heart rate while not changing or even increasing the daytime heart rate [15]. In fact, it was much of a surprise to see that the effect on sinus rhythm depended on the existence or the absence of heart failure, as shown in figure 10. In 6 normal subjects (left panel) the 24-hour heart rate was significantly increased by the drug ($p < 0.01$) and the day-to-night heart rate ratio was little influenced ($p = 0.22$). In 6 patients with various degrees of heart failure, the 24-hour heart rate was not changed ($p = 0.60$), but the day-to-night ratio was significantly reduced ($p < 0.02$), exactly as it usually happens with beta-blockers. In other words, the drug acted as a beta-adrenergic antagonist in these patients, while acting as an agonistic agent in normal subjects. The most probable explanation is indeed the well-known increased catecholamines plasma level in congestive heart failure [16]. A consequence is that one can expect a different effect of any beta-blocker according to the patient's hemodynamic condition.

This does not imply that the effect on arrhythmias and on sinus rate should be parallel in the same patient. Figure 11 shows that if the agonistic effect of Corwin was not detectable on the sinus rhythm in a patient with heart failure, this was indeed the case for the arrhythmia: salvos of NSVT increased in number and rate, and trigeminated ESs also augmented, with a shorter coupling interval.

Beta-blockers and ventricular arrhythmias with heart failure

In the light of the preceding experiences, in the past several years we used beta-blockers in cases of resistant ventricular arrhythmias, notwithstanding the existence or the absence of arguments in favor of their adrenergic dependency. We

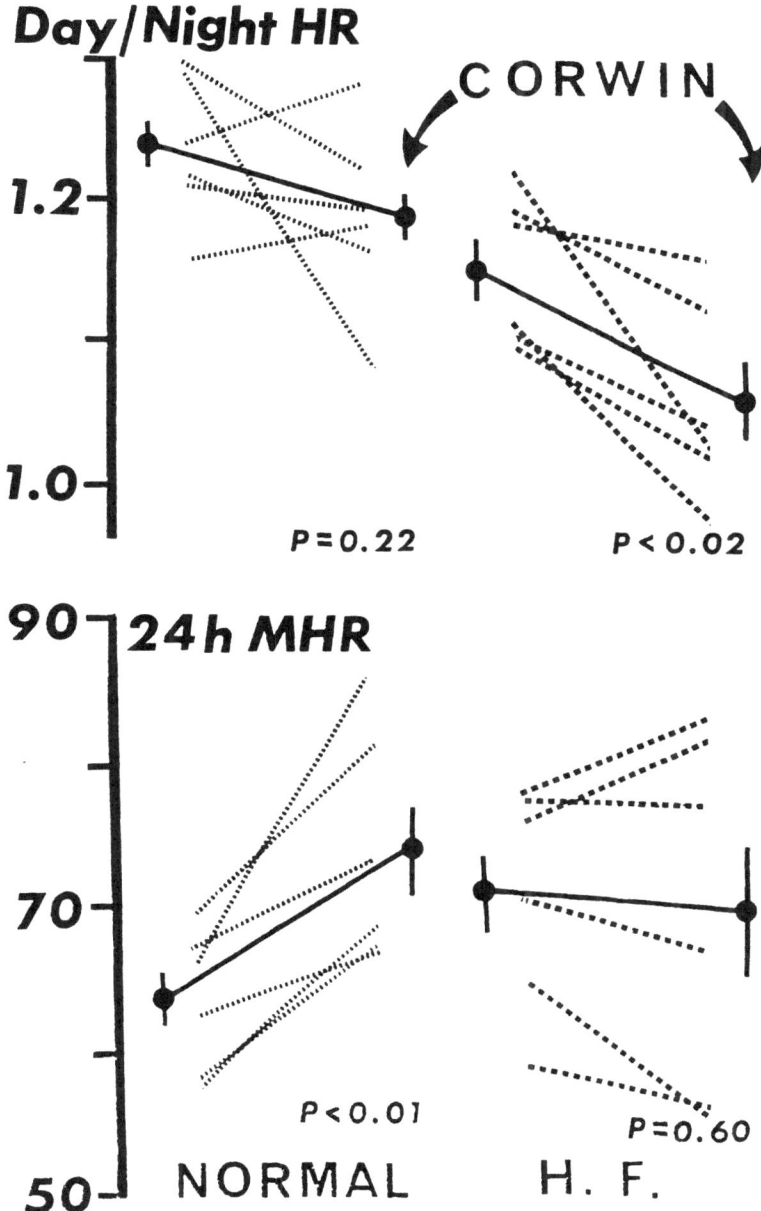

Figure 10. Heart failure and the effect of a beta-adrenergic agonist. The effect of corwin, a partially beta-adrenergic antagonist with a 40% intrinsic adrenergic activity, was studied on the 24-hour mean heart rate (24 h MHR) and the day-to-night ratio (8-hour daytime vs. 4-hour nighttime) in 6 patients without (normal) and 6 patients with heart failure. Individual values and average values (±SEM) are displayed in the control conditions in the left part of each panel) and during treatment (right part). The beta-adrenergic effect is manifest on the 24 h MHR in patients without heart failure, and the beta-blocking effect is better evidenced by the day-to-night ratio in patients with heart failure.

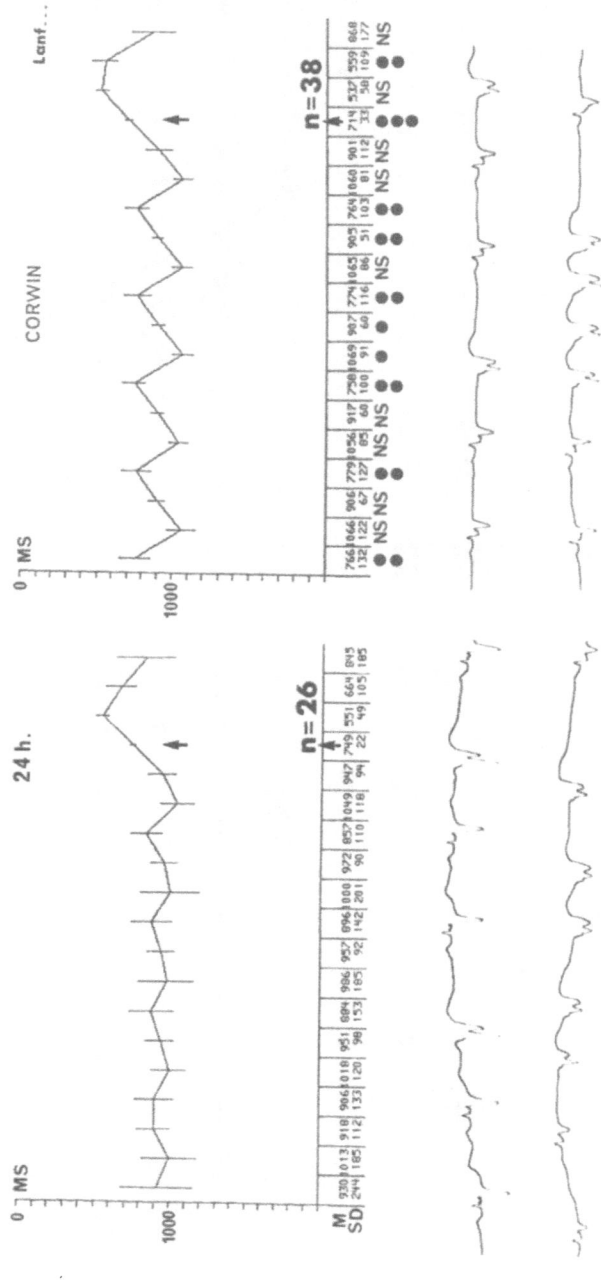

Figure 11. Arrhythmia sensitivity to beta-adrenergic stimulation. Short salvos of ventricular tachycardia occuring in a patient with heart failure (NYHA class IV) were studied in control conditions (left diagram) and during treatment by corwin. The total number of salvos collected by the computer during the 24-hour period was not significantly modified (38 *vs* 26). However, the coupling interval and the proper cycle length of the runs were dramatically shortened. Their mean value (±SD) is displayed in the bottom line where the arrows points to the first coupling interval (714 ± 33 ms *vs.* 749 ± 22, p<0.001). The 15 cycles preceding each salvo were also collected and show the pattern of a frequent trigeminy: significant differences (2 solid circles = P<0.01, 1 solid circle = p<0.05) reflect an increased number of more shortly coupled isolated extrasystoles.

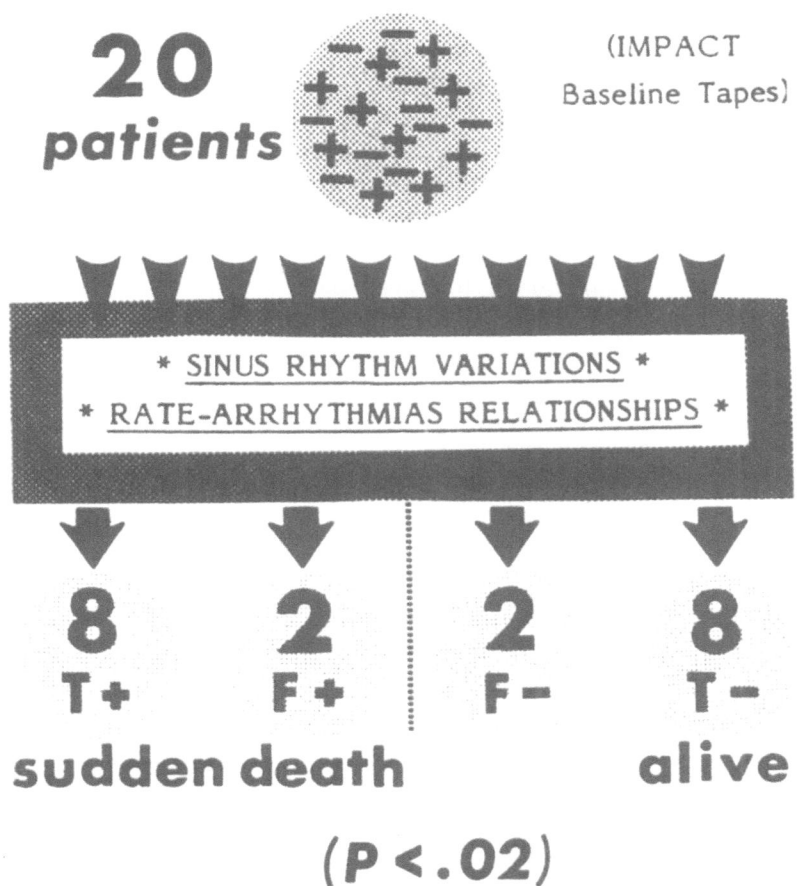

Figure 12. Sudden death prognosis from baseline 24-hour ambulatory recording in patients with healed myocardial infarction and no heart failure. Twenty baseline tapes from IMPACT study were blindly analyzed in terms of sinus rhythm frequency and variability, and rate-arrhythmias (atrial and ventricular) relationships. Using these parameters allowed to predict 8 out of the 10 patients who died suddenly during the 1-year follow-up ('T+' = true positives), and 8 of the 10 who survived ('T+' = true negatives), a result which was significant at p<0.02 (exact test).

have just collected [17] our experience with 20 patients (19 males, 1 female, aged 55 ± 12 years) with particularly severe ventricular arrhythmias. All had a heart failure (NYHA functional class II–IV, ejection fraction 29.7% ± 7.8) due to advanced, chronic coronary heart disease (18 cases) or dilated cardiomyopathy (2 cases), and a history of 12.4 ± 18 months of arhythmias definitely proved resistant to amiodarone and/or a class 1A (19 cases) or class IC (16 cases) agents. The VTs were monomorphic in 8 cases, polymorphic in 12, and generally both non-sustained (18 cases) and sustained (19 cases with 8 ± 6 episodes/patient). Nine cases had necessitated resuscitation.

The results were surprisingly good in this cohort of particularly severe patients. On a short-term basis, these resistant NSVTs and VTs were controlled in 17 cases. There were 2 failures which underwent surgery, and one death was due to an acute, nadolol-induced low cardiac output a few hours after incessant attacks of VT and ventricular fibrillation had been controlled. Two of the controlled patients were operated on, so that the long-term follow-up concerned only 15 patients during 14 ± 7 months. Heart failure was not aggravated: NYHA functional classes and ejection fractions remained unchanged. We observed 1 secondary failure leading to surgery, and 1 sudden death which, interestingly, occurred at night in the patient of figures 4–7 whose adrenergic arrhythmias were indeed controlled by acebutolol but who was left with polymorphic ESs. The other 13 patients are alive and controlled: in 1 nadolol is given alone, in 2 it is combined with a class I antiarrhythmic, in 9 with amiodarone, and 1 patient receives a combination of nadolol, amiodarone and a class I agent. In short, in this high-risk cohort with an expected 1-year mortality of about 30 to 50%, we had a total of 2 deaths which can be considered as very encouraging. It should be noted also that all failures but one were observed with beta-blockers other than nadolol, thus suggesting that one of the proposed corollaries of the 'adrenergic paradox' might be correct: the more resistant the arrhythmia in the setting of heart failure, the more adrenergic-dependent it is, and the stronger the beta-blocking treatment should be.

Mechanism, prevention and prediction of sudden death

In another chapter of this book, we report our observations on the mechanisms of sudden death in the light of a cooperative study including 74 cases recorded during ambulatory monitoring. With regard to the present chapter, of particular interest was the finding that in the 45 patients dying from primary ventricular fibrillation or VT degenerating into ventricular fibrillation, a common denominator in terms of 'warning arrhythmia' was a sinus rate acceleration in the hour preceding death: from 92 ± 19 bpm to 89.8 ± 25 ($p<0.001$). This indicates that an increased sympathetic drive is indeed present as a component of lethal tachyarrhythmias: it should be looked for systematically because an average increase of 7 bpm over a 1-hour period is not necessarily evident, and many studies dealing with the sudden death mechanisms tend to mix these ventricular tachyarrhythmias with others like torsades de pointes and cardiac standstill in which we did not find this criterion.

It is now largely admitted that beta-blocking therapy is capable of reducing the sudden death rate in high-risk patients by as much as 15 to 30% [18], and if one considers our experience with resistant VTs and recorded sudden death, the mechanism of the treatment efficacy clearly implies the direct antiarrhythmic effect of beta-blockade. That such an effect can be combined with others, like prevention of ischemia is probable, but our experience is that the evidence of ischemia is much more frequent in cardiac standstill and electromechanical dissociation than in tachyarrhythmias as the mechanism of sudden death.

An important remark concerns the results of sudden death intervention trials with beta-blockers: though it is difficult and somewhat questionable to pool studies with various protocols, drugs, cohorts of patients, there seems to exist a direct correlation between the mortality rate reduction and the percentage of reduction of the sinus rate during beta-blockade [19]. If this correlation is not coincidental, the various findings we reported suggest 3 possible explanations, which may be combined:

– the stronger the beta-blockade, the greater the heart rate reduction and the better the prevention of adrenergic tachyarrhythmias;
– the more frequent the heart failure in the studies, the greater the proportion of adrenergic dependent tachyarrhythmias, and the more the bradycardic effect of beta-blockers on the sinus rate;
– in the absence of heart failure, adrenergic related tachyarrhythmias are observed in the context of a generally increased mean heart rate which suggests a basically augmented sympathetic drive in these patients.

The last statement is not purely theoretical. Not only our experience with sinus rhythm in 2 groups of patients with adrenergic and non-adrenergic ventricular arrhythmias [13] was very suggestive, but also a more recent one which will be briefly reported (fig. 12). We analyzed baseline 24-hour tapes of 20 patients belonging to the data bank of the IMPACT study [20]. Two sets of 10 tapes had been matched in such a way that the number of classically evaluated arrhythmic events ('simple' and 'complex' arrhythmias . . .) were equivalent. Our analysis was conducted blindly (clinical and ECG data), and its aim was to detect, from this baseline tape, which 10 patients died or survived during the 1-year follow-up of this intervention trial using mexiletine. Just taking into account an increased sinus rhythm frequency and variability, and the occurrence of any arrhythmias (atrial as well as ventricular) in the context of a sinus tachycardia, we were able to find out 8 of the ultimately dead patients (true positives), 8 of the surviving patients (true negatives), with only 2 false positives and 2 false negatives. The probability of obtaining such a result by chance was less than 2% (exact test). Though such a result suggests how important it may be to consider such parameters in studies dealing with sudden death predictivity, it is important to underline that the absence of heart failure was a required criterion for inclusion in the IMPACT study.

Conclusion

The evidence of the role of the ANS in ventricular tachyarrhythmias cannot be circumvented. This should not be astonishing, as most experimental arrhythmias do include this paramater. The problem is that the clinician only has a few ways for evaluating the importance of this factor in human tachyarrhythmias. They must be developed in the two major methods of investigation we routinely use: invasive and non-invasive EP evaluation [5]. Then it appears that not only do we not have so many possible approaches, but they have serious limitations which are probably due to a common denominator: the biological consequence of heart failure is the development of an increased sympathetic drive which makes much less reliable the most convenient parameter we can use, i.e. the sinus rate. The phenomenon of the adrenergic paradox may well explain our difficulties but it does not provide any way for solving them. Finally, in extreme cases the only way to evidence the ANS role is first to block its eventual role by the appropriate drugs. Then comes the problem of finding some consistency between the effect of drugs and the mechanism of this effect according to the many different possible combinations of arrhythmia EP mechanisms, mechanisms of occurrence of clinical arrhythmias in the presence or in the absence of heart failure, and finally the multifactorial antiarrhythmic action of beta-blockers: direct competition with beta-adrenoceptors, class I action of some of them, prolongation of action potential which may constitute a class III effect [21], reduction of catecholamine release by a pre-synaptic action, just to speak of arrhythmias without taking into account the anti-ischemic and metabolic properties.

References

1. Randall WC, Euler DE, Jacobs HK, Wehrmacher W, Kaye MP, Hageman GR. 1976. Autonomic neural control of cardiac rhythm: the role of autonomic imbalance in the genesis of cardiac dysrhythmias. Cardiology 61: 20.
2. Verrier RL. 1980. Neural factors in ventricular electrical instability. In 'Sudden Death', HE Kulbertus & HJJ Wellens edit, Martinus Nijhoff Publ, The Hague/Boston/London, p. 137–155.
3. Schwartz PJ, Periti M, Malliani A. 1975. The long Q-T syndrome. Am Heart J 89: 378.
4. Coumel Ph, Leclercq JF, Lucet V. 1985. Possible mechanisms of the arrhythmias in the long QT syndrome. In 'Prolonged ventricular repolarization. Benefits and drawbacks', P Amlie Ed. Eur Heart J 6D: 115–29.
5. Coumel Ph. 1987. The management of clinical arrhythmias. An overview on invasive versus non-invasive electrophysiology. Eur Heart J 8: 92.
6. Brugada P, Wellens HJJ. 1984. Standard diagnostic programmed electrical stimulation protocols in patients with paroxysmal recurrent tachycardias. Pace 7: 1121–8.
7. Campbell RWF, Gardiner P, Amos PA, Chadwick D, Jordan RS. 1985. Measurement of the QT interval. Eur Heart J 6D: 81–4.
8. Romano M, Di Maro T, Garella G, Cotecchia MR, Ferro G, Chiariello M. 1985. Relation between heart rate and QT interval in exercise-induced myocardial ischemia. Am J Cardiol 56: 861–2.
9. Zimmerman M, Maisonblanche P, Cauchemez B, Leclercq JF, Coumel Ph. 1986. Déterminants de l'activité répétitive dans les tachycardies ventriculaires en salves. Arch mal Coeur 79: 1420.
10. Zimmermann M, Maisonblanche P, Cauchemez B, Leclercq JR, Coumel Ph. 1986. Déterminants of the repetitive activity in benign incessant monomorphic ventricular tachycardia. JACC 7: 1219.

11. Coumel Ph, Leclercq JF, Maisonblanche P, Attuel P, Cauchemez B. 1985. Computerized analysis of dynamic electrocardiograms: a tool for comprehensive electrophysiology. A description of the ATREC II system. Clin Progress 3: 181–201.
12. Platia EV, Reid PR. 1985. Nonsustained ventricular tachycardia during programmed ventricular stimulation: criteria for a positive test. Am J Cardiol 56: 79–83.
13. Coumel Ph, Rosengarten MD, Leclercq JF, Attuel P. 1982. Role of sympathetic nervous system in non-ischaemic ventricular arrhythmias. Br Heart J 47: 137–43.
14. Escoubet B, Leclercq JF, Maisonblanche P, Poirier JM, Gourmel B, Delhotal-Landes B, Coumel Ph. 1986. Dose-related effect of four beta-blockers on heart rate assessed by 24-hour recordings. Clin Pharmacol Ther 39: 361.
15. Leclercq JF, Rosengarten MD, Kural S, Attuel P, Coumel Ph. 1981. Effects of betablocker's intrinsic sympathetic activity on SA and AV nodes in man. Europ J Cardiol 12: 367–75.
16. Bristow MR, Laser JA, Minöbe W, Ginsburg R, Fowler MB, Rassmussen R. 1984. Selective down regulation of beta 1 adrenergic receptors in failing human heart. Circulation 70: suppl. II, 117.
17. Hermida JJ, Coumel Ph, Leclercq JF, Cauchemez B, Maison Blanche P, Leenhardt A, Slama R. 1987. Apport des bêta-bloquants dans le traitement des tachycardies ventriculaires résistantes chez l'insuffisant cardiaque. Arch Mal Coeur 80: 290.
18. Yussuf S, Peto R, Lewis J, Collins R, Sleight P. 1985. Beta-blockade during and after myocardial infarction. An overview of the randomized trials. Prog Cardiovasc Dis 77: 335.
19. Kjekshus J. 1985. Beta-blockers: heart rate reduction, a mechanism of benefit. Eur Heart J 6 (suppl. A): 29–30.
20. IMPACT RESEARCH GROUP. 1984. International Mexiletine and Placebo Antiarrhythmic Coronary Trial: I. Report on arrhythmia and other findings. JACC 4: 1148–63.
21. Vaugham-Williams EM. 1982. Beta-blockers in the control of arrhythmias. In 'Advances in beta-blocker therapy II', A Zanchetti ed, Excepta Medica, Amsterdam-Oxford-Princeton publ. p. 110–6.

6. Sustained ventricular tachycardia in the acute phase of myocardial infarction

Ch. DUBOIS, J.P. SMEETS, L. PIERARD and H.E. KULBERTUS

Service de Cardiologie, CHU de Liège, Hôpital de Bavière, 66 Bvd de la Constitution, 4020 Liège, Belgium

Introduction

Ventricular arrhythmias seen on predischarge 24 hour electrocardiographic recordings after acute myocardial infarction (MI) carry a guarded prognosis [1–4].

The correlation, however, between these predischarge arrhythmias and the ventricular arrhythmias – especially ventricular tachycardia – which occur in the coronary care unit is a matter of controversy [5, 6].

We decided to undertake a prospective study in a large population of patients with acute MI to delineate the incidence, clinical significance and prognosis of sustained ventricular tachycardia during hospitalization.

Patients and methods

From December 1, 1977 to April 30, 1980, 1013 patients were admitted consecutively to our CCU with a diagnosis of acute MI. There were 182 women and 831 men, with a mean age of 58.8 ± 9.9 years. The diagnosis of MI was based either on a history of typical prolonged chest pain accompanied by pathognomonic ECG changes with the development of new Q waves, or by ST-T wave changes suggestive of an acute MI associated with an elevation of serum creatine kinase (CK). The mean delay between the onset of chest pain and admission to CCU was 12.9 ± 28.4 hours. None of the 1013 patients received prophylactic antiarrhythmics.

A series of parameters were coded, stored and studied in a prospective manner. They included:
1. Demographic and past medical history: age, sex, prior MI, history of angina, of hypertension, tobacco abuse, cardiac treatment before admission (beta-blockers, diuretics, digitalis, class I antiarrhythmics)
2. Characteristics of the infarction: delay of admission to CCU, type and location of infarct, serum CK peak (measurements made every 4th hour)

3. In hospital complications (within two weeks): recurrence of MI, development of angina pectoris (typical chest-pain at least 72 hours after admission); left ventricular failure (LVF) coded from 0 to 4 (0: no rales; 1: basilar rales; 2: rales up to scapular level; 3: acute pulmonary oedema; 4: cardiogenic shock); development of a pericardial friction rub, of frequent premature ventricular contractions (VPC's >30/hours, diagnosed by well trained doctors or nurses using conventional oscilloscope and direct write-out recordings), of unusual bradycardia (<50/min), of atrial fibrillation or flutter, of ventricular fibrillation (VF), of 2nd or 3rd degree atrio-ventricular block (AVB), of right or left complete bundle branch block (BBB); cardiothoracic ratio measured on the pre-discharge chest X-ray.

We considered ventricular tachycardia (VT) as sustained if, for its termination, it required either a DC shock or the intravenous administration of a drug. All episodes of VT occurring later than 24 hours after an initial episode were considered as recurrences.

The quantitative variables were statistically analysed by a Student T-test and the nominative variables by a chi-square test.

Results

Among the 1013 patients admitted for acute MI, 66 (6.5%) developed a sustained VT. This complication occurred in 39 (59.8%) within the 24 hours of admission, in 8 (12.1%) between 24 and 72 hours after admission, in 8 (12.1%) between the 4th and the 7th day and in 11 (16.7%) during the second week.

The characteristics of these 66 patients with VT are shown in Table 1. The incidence of VT did not vary with age, sex, past cardiac history or treatment, or MI location. In comparing the 66 patients with sustained VT to the 947 patients without, we noted that the former group had more extensive MI (CK peak: 1898 ± 1717 UI/1, vs 1350 ± 1040 UI/1; p<0.02), more frequently complicated by LVF (62.1% vs 39.4%, p<0.001), frequent VPC's (68.2%, vs 43.1%, p<0.001), VF (37.9% vs 7.7%, p<0.001), AVB (24.2% vs 11.5%; p<0.01).

The hospital course of the 66 patients with VT was poor. Nine (13.6%) had a recurrence of sustained VT. Twenty-five (37%) developed a VF, 13 on the same day as the VT. Twenty patients (30.3%) died in hospital, during the first two weeks. This figure was considerably higher than the in-hospital mortality of the patients without VT (10.6%, p<0.001).

Among the 20 patients who died, 16 died from cardiogenic shock, 4 from untractable primary VF (LVF ≤1 on the day of the arrhythmia). The mean delay of death was 7.2 ± 6.5 days.

To be noted that 7 patients died on the same day as the VT and that 6 of the 20 dead had had their VT more than 72 hours after admission.

A comparison of survivors with non survivors within the group of 66 patients with VT (Table 2, column 1 and 2) showed that those who died were older (62.8 ± 8.2 years, vs 55.3 ± 9.2 years, p<0.01), had a higher incidence of prior MI (65% vs 26.1%, p<0.01), LVF (95% vs 47.8%, p<0.001), VF (60% vs 28.3%, p<0.05) and BBB (30% vs 6.5%, p<0.05).

If we compare, among the 120 in-hospital deaths, the 20 patients who developed a sustained VT with the 100 patients who did not (Table 2, columns 2 and 3), the groups were similar except that the VT patients had a higher incidence of

Table 1. Comparison of patients with and without sustained ventricular tachycardia.

	947 patients without VT	66 patients with VT
Admission delay (hours)	13.2 ± 29.0	7.31 ± 16.1*
Age (years)	58.8 ± 9.9	57.6 ± 9.6
Sex (% female)	18.2	15.2
Past history infarction (%)	27	37.9
angina (%)	66.5	74.2
tobacco abuse (%)	81.9	80.3
hypertension (%)	33.9	25.8
Therapy on admission		
beta-blockers (%)	14.5	13.6
diuretics (%)	10.9	12.1
digitalis (%)	8.2	15.2
class I antiarrhythmics (%)	5.4	3.0
Infarct		
inferior (%)	44.7	36.4
anterior (%)	38.5	47.0
non-q-wave (%)	14.0	13.6
other (%)	2.7	3.0
Creatine-kinase peak (UI/1)	1350 ± 1040	1898 ± 1717*
Grade of LVF	1.1 ± 1.2	1.7 ± 1.3***
Grade of LVF >1 (%)	39.4	62.1***
Recurrence of infarct (%)	3.0	4.5
Development of angina (%)	17.4	15.2
Pericarditis (%)	24.2	40.9**
Bradycardia (%)	15.2	21.2
Atrial fibrillation of flutter (%)	13	19.7
Frequent PVC's (%)	43.1	68.2***
Ventricular fibrillation (%)	7.7	37.9***
Atrio-ventricular block (%)	11.5	24.2**
Bundle branch block (%)	10	13.6
Cardio-thoracic ratio (%) on discharge	46.3 ± 5.6	45.8 ± 6.3
In-hospital mortality (%)	10.6	30.3***

VT: ventricular tachycardia.
LVF: left ventricular failure.
PVC's: premature ventricular complexes.
* p<0.02; ** p<0.01; *** p<0.001.

prior MI (65% vs 39%, p<0.05), of pericarditis (45% vs 21%, p<0.05), and VF (60% vs 30%, p<0.05).

The 3 years follow-up of the hospital survivors showed that, of the 46 patients who had survived in the VT group, 12 died (26.1%). This figure was not significantly different from the mortality (19.4%) seen among the 847 survivors who had had no VT. To be noted however that, in the VT groups, the 7 patients who died within the first 18 months met a sudden death.

We also noted that only 2 patients who had developed VT during their hospital stay, developed an episode of sustained VT during the 3-years follow-up: one at 2 months and the other at 3 months; the latter died suddenly at 7 months.

*Table 2.*Sustained ventricular tachycardia and in-hospital mortality.

	Sustained ventricular tachycardia		Dead without VT
	Survivors	Dead	
No. of patients	46	20	100
Admission delay (hours)	7.4 ± 15.9	9.2 ± 17.5	14.9 ± 22.9
Age (years)	55.3 ± 9.2**	62.8 ± 8.2	64.2 ± 8.7
Sex (% female)	10.9	25	24
Past history			
infarction (%)	26.1**	65	39*
angina pectoris (%)	76.1	70	71
Infarct			
inferior (%)	41.3	25	31
anterior (%)	41.3	60	57
non-q-wave (%)	17.4	5	8
others (%)	0	10	4
Creatine-kinase peak (UI/1)	1771 ± 1612	2254 ± 1890	1808 ± 1179
Grade of LVF (mean)	1.3 ± 1.2***	2.8 ± 0.9	2.4 ± 1.4
Grade of LVF >1 (%)	47.8***	95	78
Recurrence of infarct (%)	0	15	11
Development of angina pectoris (%)	17.4	10	10
Pericarditis (%)	39.1	45	21*
Bradycardia (%)	21.7	20	19
Atrial fibrillation or flutter (%)	17.4	25	18
Frequent PVC's (%)	71.7	60	44
Ventricular fibrillation (%)	28.3*	60	30*
Atrio-ventricular block (%)	10.6	35	30
Bundle branch block (%)	6.5*	30	27

VT: ventricular tachycardia.
LVF: left ventricular failure.
PVC's: premature ventricularcomplexes.
* p<0.05; ** p<0.01; *** p<0.001.

Discussion

In the literature, the incidence of VT during the acute MI phase varies from 6 to 40%; this is due to differences in definition and detection techniques [5–10]. Our low incidence (6.5%) of VT is explained by the choice of very stringent criteria for sustained VT.

As Marchlinski [11], we observed that patients at risk of VT are best identified by the presence of an extensive necrosis (assessed by CK-peak), associated with LVF. In our study, as was the case in the report by Nordrehaug et al. who studied non sustained VT [12], the VT incidence did not vary with age, sex, past cardiac history or treatment, or MI location. Nordrehaug et al. [12] had noted that the patients with VT had a more frequent history of systemic hypertension and, in accordance with Julian et al. [7], but in contrast with our and Mogensen's results, that these patients were older. One must also underline that Marchlinski et al. [14] observed an unusually high frequency of BBB among patients with sustained VT. We could not confirm this, but instead observed a higher incidence of AV block.

The poor in-hospital prognosis of patients with VT, especially associated with LVF, is well known [10, 15]. Among our 66 patients with VT, 20 died during the hospital phase. Their characteristics were very similar to those of the 100 patients without VT who also died in-hospital. The only exception is a higher incidence of VF and prior MI among the VT patients.

If the VT patients have a high in-hospital mortality, their long-term prognosis is better: the 3-years mortality was 26% among the patients with VT and 19% among those without VT. These findings confirm the study of Wong et al. [6] who showed that VT in the CCU is correlated with an increase in ventricular arrhythmias on predischarge Holter, but does not predict late mortality of sudden death. We must underline however that during the 3-year follow-up, the 7 deaths which occurred during the first 18 months were all sudden. Two patients also developed an episode of sustained VT at a later stage.

In conclusion: we observed a low incidence of sustained VT (6.5%) during the hospital phase of acute MI. The patients with this arrhythmia are best identified by the presence of an extensive cardiac necrosis associated with LVF. They have a high in-hospital mortality (30%) but once they have survived the acute phase, their long term prognosis is similar to that of the MI patients who did not suffer an episode of VT.

References

1. Bigger JT Jr, Fleiss JL, Kleiger R, Miller JP, Rolnitzky LM and The Multi-Center Post-Infarction Group. 1984. The relationship between ventricular arrhythmias, left ventricular dysfunction and mortality in the 2 years after myocardial infarction. Circulation 69: 250–258.

2. Mukharji J, Rude RE, Poole WK, Croft C, Thomas LJ Jr, Braunwald E, Willerson JT and Cooperating investigators. Multicenter Investigation of the Limitation of Infarct Size (MILIS). 1982. Late sudden death following acute myocardial infarction, importance of combined presence of repetitive ventricular ectopy and left ventricular dysfunction (abstr). Clin Res 30: 108A.

3. Mukharji J, Rude RE, Poole WK, Gustafson N, Thomas LJ Jr, Strauss HW, Jaffe AS, Muller JE, Roberts R, Raabe DS Jr, Croft CH, Passamani E, Braunwald E, Willerson JT and The MILIS Study Group. 1984. Risk factors for sudden death after acute myocardial infarction: two- year follow-up. Am J Cardiol 54: 31–36.

4. Bigger JT Jr, Weld FM, Coromilas J, Rolnitzky LM, De Turk WE. 1983. Prevalence and significance of arrhythmias in 24-hour ECG recordings made within one month of acute myocardial infarction. In: Kulbertus HE, Wellens HJJ (eds) The First Year after a Myocardial Infarction. The Hague: Martinus Nijhoff, 161–175.

5. Bigger JT Jr, Coromilas J. 1984. Ventricular tachyarrhythmias in the various stages of ischemic heart disease. In: Surawicz RCP, Prystowsky EN (eds) Tachycardias. Boston: Martinus Nijhoff, 355–371.

6. Wong P, Radwaner BA, Case RB, Hochman JS. 1985. Prognosis of ventricular tachycardia in survivors of myocardial infarction (Abstr). Circulation 72: III-360.

7. Julian DG, Valentine PA, Millet GG. 1964. Disturbances of rate, rhythm and conduction in acute myocardial infarction. A prospective study of 100 consecutive unselected patients with the aid of electrocardiographic monitoring. Am J Med 37: 915–927.

8. De Sanctis RW, Block P, Hutter AM Jr. 1972. Tachyarrhythmias in myocardial infarction. Circulation 45: 681–702.

9. Meltzer LE, Kitchell JB. 1966. The incidence of arrhythmias associated with acute myocardial infarction. Progress Cardiovasc Diseases 9: 50–63.

10. Meltzer LE, Cohen HE. 1972. The incidence of arrhythmias associated with acute myocardial infarction. In: Meltzer LE, Dunning AJ (eds) Textbook of Coronary Care. Philadelphia. Charles Press.

11. Marchlinski FE. 1984. Ventricular tachycardia soon after myocardial infarction: risk and management. Intern J Cardiol 5: 761–766.

12. Nordrehaug JE, Johannessen KA, Von der Lippe G. 1985. Serum potassium concentration as a risk factor of ventricular arrhythmias early in acute myocardial infarction. Circulation 71: 645–649.

13. Mogensen L. 1970. Ventricular tachyarrhythmias and lignocaïne prophylaxis in acute myocardial infarction. Acta Med Scand 513 (suppl): 1.

14. Marchlinski FE, Waxman HL, Buxton AE, Josephson ME. 1983. Sustained ventricular tachyarrhythmias during the early postinfarction period: electrophysiologic findings and prognosis for survival. JACC 2: 240–250.

15. Kitchin AH, Pocock SJ. 1977. Prognosis of patients with acute myocardial infarction admitted to a coronary care unit. 1. Survival in hospital. Br Heart 39: 1163–1166.

7. Ventricular tachycardias in non ischemic disease

BÉATRICE BREMBILLA-PERROT*, ETIENNE ALIOT* *, ARNAUD
TERRIER DE LA CHAISE*, JOEL DONETTI*, KHALIFE KHALIFE* *
* Services de Cardiologie A-B (Pr Pernot, Pr Cherrier) Chr de Brabois,
54500 Vandoeuvre Les Nancy, France
* * Service de Cardiologie, (Pr Gilgenkrantz) Chr Hopital Central, 54000 Nancy,
France

The association of ventricular tachycardia and underlying heart disease is known as a predictor of sudden death. However, the risk of sudden death is dependent on the type of heart disease.

In this review we comment upon the incidence and the significance of ventricular tachycardia in some non-ischemic diseases. The review has been restricted to three frequent non-ischemic diseases which are known to be associated with increased risk of sudden death: mitral valve prolapse, hypertrophic cardiomyopathy, and dilated cardiomyopathy.

Mitral valve prolapse

Patients with mitral valve prolapse (MVP) frequently are found to have ventricular arrhythmias and sudden death in patients with this entity have been described.

However, mitral valve prolapse may be associated with other conditions which in their own right may be important determinants of prognosis. Also the study will be limited to the isolated MVP without enlargement of left ventricle nor coexisting heart disease.

The diagnostic of MVP should be generally based on the presence of two of the following three criteria:
– suggestive clinical signs, i.e. mid-late systolic click ± a mid-late or pansystolic mitral murmur.
– echocardiographic mitral valve prolapse, i.e. posterior excursion of the leaflet >2 mm during systole, lasting more than 0.05s.
– angiographic mitral prolapse, i.e. systolic protrusion of a portion of the base of the left ventricular contrast shadow across the atrioventricular ring into the left atrium during selective left ventricular cinéangiography.

This diagnosis of MVP could be made in 5 percent of general population [1].
The complications related to MVP are discussed.

Frequency of ventricular tachycardia in MVP

Patients with MVP frequently are found to have ventricular arrhythmias. However the incidence of complex ventricular arrhythmias is very variable and dependent on the effect of patient selection. A high incidence of ventricular tachycardia (VT) has been found in studies which included patients with MVP and other structural disease [2]. In patients with MVP and without other structural disease, repetitive ventricular premature beats ($\geqslant$3) have been found in 5 to 15 percent of subjects [3, 4]. The reported ventricular tachycardias are nonsustained, polymorphic and noted during the daily period.

VT is rarely the cause of tachycardia-feeling in patients with MVP. In a personal study [5] the mechanism of tachycardia in 22 patients with MVP, admitted for this problem of tachycardia , has been related to a supraventricular tachycardia in 20 patients and a ventricular tachycardia in 2 patients.

Moreover, a sustained VT is very rare and should lead to a search for another cause. In particularly the association MVP-right ventricular dysplasia [5], left ventricular myopathy, coronary heart disease or prolongation of QT interval should be excluded.

Mechanism of ventricular tachycardia in MVP

The cause of the dysrhythmias in subjects with MVP remains an enigma. Some mechanisms are discussed [6].

Endocardial friction lesions have been frequently found in patients who had presented a sudden death. These lesions are the results of friction between chordae and the left ventricular mural endocardium which may lead to a fibrosis of the mural endocardium. Mechanical stimulation of the endocardium by the thickened chordae could be responsible for the ventricular dysrythmias. Aggregates of platelet and fibrin found in the angle between the posterior leaflet of the mitral valve and the left atrial wall could be responsible for small coronary emboli, the latter causing dysrythmias. Prolongation of QT interval has been reported in MVP. Abnormalities of conduction system has been noted in MVP and would explain reentrant mechanisms as a potential cause of ventricular ectopy.

However these findings in the pathogenesis of tachy-arrhythmias are uncertain since their frequency in hearts without myxomatous mitral valves is unknown. Only one factor has been proved in MVP. That is, an autonomic dysfunction in MVP [7, 8] with a decreased parasympathetic, increased α and normal β adrenergic tone and responsiveness.

Methods of study

a) Holter monitoring

Although the incidence of ventricular premature beats (VPB) (50 to 75%) and of pairs or runs (5 to 15%) [3, 4, 8] seems high, the comparison with Holter monitoring of patients without MVP shows that this excess of VPBs in those with MVP does not reach statistical significance. These contrasts with the findings of other studies [9], which indicated a significantly higher prevalence of complex VPBs in subjects with MVP than in normal subjects, are probably related to the effect of selection bias [3]: the problem is to identify a control population and to study only patients with MVP and without other cardiac disease.

The interest of Holter monitoring is to assess the relationship with autonomic function [8]: the ventricular arrhythmias occur generally in day-time, suggesting an increased adrenergic tone.

b) Exercise testing

The interest of Holter monitoring is also to assess the relationship between the ventricular arrhythmias and the exercise: 10% of the Framingham subjects [4] have complex or frequent VPBs. A similar incidence was found by Demaria [9] during treadmill testing. This higher incidence of ventricular arrhythmias than in non-MVP population may be related to the increased adrenergic responsiveness.

c) Programmed electrical stimulation (PES)

Two studies in patients with MVP and ventricular arrhythmias (VPB's, non-sustained ventricular tachycardia and ventricular fibrillation) have demonstrated a high incidence of inducible polymorphic VT (65%) by triple ventricular extra-stimuli [10, 11]. Only one patient had sustained VT, and that VT was induced by stimulation [10]. The patients with MVP were more susceptible to inducible ventricular tachyarrhythmias than patients without structural heart disease, but no relationships between the response to PES and subsequent prognosis in the MVP group could be demonstrated. This high incidence of inducible polymorphic VT may be also related to the method of stimulation using three extrastimuli. In a personal study in 20 patients withMVP and without ventricular arrhythmia, only one nonsustained VT was induced by the method of 2 extrastimuli delivered on sinus rhythm and paced rhythm. Only one patient had sustained VT and the VT was reproduced by stimulation.

The sensitivity of PES is difficult to etablish, while few sustained VT have been found in MVP. Usually the patients with MVP have nonsustained VT and it is known that patients with nonsustained VT have rarely inducible sustained VT.

In our experience, and with the method of double ventricular extrastimuli, the specificity of ventricular stimulation is excellent (95%).

Prognostic: what is the significance of VPB's runs?

Although MVP is frequent in the general population (5%) [1], only 60 cases of sudden death have been reported [6, 12, 13]. Two factors could favour sudden death: the development of a complication (ruptured chordae tendinae, progression of mitral regurgitation, infective endocarditis) and the usage of antiarrhythmic drugs [14]: the discontinuation of antiarrhythmic measures results often in an abrupt cessation of seemingly malignant arrhythmias in patients with MVP.

Jeresaty [12] identified the potential victim as having the following features: a young women with a history of syncope who has a late systolic murmur preceded by a click, and whose ECG shows abnormal repolarization and ventricular premature beats. Patients with 'silent' mitral valve prolapse or an isolated click do not appear to be susceptible. A family history of sudden death is an added risk factor.

Also, the prognosis in mitral valve prolapse should be considered as benign and a permissive attitude would seem warranted [13] except in the presence of disabling chest pain, syncope, prolonged QT interval, complex ventricular arrhythmias, or significant mitral regurgitation. In these latter patients a complete study is required, with Holter monitoring, exercise testing and programmed electrical stimulation. The PES should be completed by an isoproterenol test to detect the high adrenergic tone associated with MVP.

In summary, an isolated mitral valve prolapse should be considered as benign. Sustained VT in MVP have rarely been documented, have rarely been induced, are rarely the cause of tachycardia and syncopes, and should lead to a search for an associated heart disease.

Hypertrophic cardiomyopathy

Hypertrophic cardiomyopathy is defined as a heart muscle disorder of unknown etiology which is characterized by a hypertrophied and non-dilated left ventricle. The natural history of the patient with hypertrophic cardiomyopathy (HCM) is a slow progression of symptoms and a high risk of death, which is generally sudden and occurs irrespective of the functional status of the patient.

Frequency of VT in HCM

If the ventricular arrhythmias are common in HCM, (60 to 90%), the VT are less frequent: an incidence of 7 to 28% has been reported [15–16]. Generally the VT are nonsustained.

VT are not the only cause of tachycardia in HCM. A high incidence of supraventricular tachycardias, including paroxysmal junctional tachycardia and atrial tachycardia, has been reported [15]. In 11 of our patients with HCM and admitted for tachycardias, the mechanism of tachycardia could be related to a VT in 2 patients and a supraventricular tachycardia in 9 patients (paroxysmal junctional tachycardias 4, atrial tachycardias 5).

Mechanism of VT

There are several factors peculiar to hypertrophic cardiomyopathy which are potential causes for arrhythmias [16]. Myocardial disorganization responsible for structural and metabolic abnormalities could provide the substrate for either automatic or reentrant initiation of arrhythmia. Cellular disorganization also provides the substrate for the propagation of arrhythmias. Necropsy changes of subendocardial ischemia are common and would be responsible for the initiation of arrhythmias. However, the fact that episodes of VT occur following periods of normal or slow heart rate, and often during periods of high vagal tone, would favor reentry and make ischemia due to increased metabolic demand unlikely to be important.

Some relations between the echocardiographic patterns of HCM and the occurrence of ventricular arrhythmias have been reported but are not proved [17]. VT would be more frequent when the septal movement is severely pathological [18] with a systolic anterior valve motion of mitral valve more important. VT would be also correlated with a septal hypertrophy exceeding 20 mm [19, 20].

The study of hemodynamic characteristics of HCM [21] would show that indexes of ventricular function contribute to the identification of patients at particular risk of sudden death.

The combination of increased end-diastolic volume, small end-systolic volume and low peak filling rate has the best predictive value of sudden death. However its predictive power is poor (predictive accuracy 32%).

Methods of study

a) Holter monitoring
Ventricular arrhythmias of grade 3 and above is noted in 60 to 95% of patients [22, 23, 24]. Ventricular tachycardia could be identified in 15 [22] to 19% [23] of asymptomatic patients with HCM. However, the incidence of VT is higher if a more prolonged period of 72 hours of Holter monitoring is performed [24]: 24 of 86 unselected patients have ventricular tachycardia.

The ventricular tachycardias are nonsustained; their morphology is variable and most of the episodes occur between midnight and 8.00 am and most follow periods of relative bradycardia. The variability of ventricular arrhythmia is marked and it seems that a period 48 of 72 hours of electrocardiographic monitoring should be performed at least annually to detect épisodes of VT.

b) Exercise testing

Exercise testing is less sensitive than Holter monitoring in detecting VT [19]. Although ventricular premature beats are frequently induced by exercise testing, VT are generally not induced in different studies that compare Holter monitoring and exercise testing [19, 22, 25].

c) Programmed electrical stimulation

Patients with HCM have a high incidence of inducible polymorphic ventricular tachycardia [26, 27]. Ventricular fibrillation was induced in 8/17 patients of Watson [27] who had history of ventricular arrhythmias and 14/16 patients of Anderson [26] who were undergoing myomectomy. The protocol of stimulation of both studies used 3 extrastimuli. These authors suggested that this high vulnerability to ventricular arrhythmia could be a primary cause of sudden death in HCM. However, inducible ventricular fibrillation is generally considered as a nonspecific finding. Moreover the follow-up of patients with inducible ventricular fibrillation and without inducible arrhythmias shows that, for identifying patients with HCM at risk for sudden death, sensitivity of programmed electrical stimulation is markedly lower than Holter monitoring [28]. Comparing programmed electrical stimulation and Holter monitoring the sensitivity was 22% and 67% respectively. However, the specificity of programmed stimulation was higher than the specificity of Holter monitoring (85% vs 53%).

In a personal study, similar results were found with a high incidence of inducible polymorphic VT in patients with and without ventricular arrhythmias. In 10 patients without ventricular arrhythmias on Holter monitoring, 3 nonsustained polymorphic VT and 1 ventricular fibrillation were induced by 2 ventricular extrastimuli. In 4 patients without VT on Holter monitoring, 1 ventricular fibrillation was induced.

The rarity of spontaneous sustained VT in patients with HCM should be noted and could explain the weak sensitivity of programmed stimulation in these patients. Generally, patients with spontaneous nonsustained VT have rarely inducible sustained VT.

Prognostic

Patients with HCM have a high risk of sudden death [15, 16]. In the study by McKenna [29], two hundred fifty-four patients with HCM were followed-up from 1 to 23 years (mean 6). The study disclosed 58 deaths, 32 of them sudden.

However many mechanisms have been suggested to explain sudden death in HCM [16].

– Complete heart block has been reported but is rare. One case could be recorded

in Nancy on a Holter monitoring but was related to verapamil therapy [30].
– Rapid atrial arrhythmias through an accessory pathway may occur but this is no likely to be a common cause of sudden death in HCM.
– The role of myocardial ischemia or infarction as a cause of sudden death may have been overlooked because of the absence of the typical markers, or the inability of the pathologist to assess myocardial ischemia or the early changes of myocardial infarction.
– Tract spasm has been speculated but not proved.
Acute changes in filling may cause sudden death and this mechanism would be important in older patients; impaired diastolic filling may occur because of decreased venous return following peripheral vasodilation, increased heart rate with decreased time for filling or increased myocardial stiffness after ischemia or catecholamine stimulation.
– However, it seems that, although it is unproven, ventricular arrhythmias are the antecedent of most sudden deaths. The comparison of patients with HCM who had presented a sudden death with those who were alive, shows that ventricular tachycardia was significantly more common in those patients who died suddenly (p <0.001) [16]. However, some survivors also had VT and indicate that this arrhythmia is not a highly specific marker for sudden death and that yet undefined factors must determine ventricular fibrillation.

The combination of a young age (≤14 years), syncope at diagnosis, severe dyspnea at last follow-up a family history of HCM and sudden death best predicted the possibility of sudden death [15], although in adults the indexes of ventricular function are a more important determinant [21]. The most extensive disorganization of myocardial cellules was found in young asymptomatic patients who died suddenly [31], supporting the probability that sudden death was most likely due to a primary arrhythmia.

VT in HCM is of prognostic rather than symptomatic importance. The factors that determine whether or not the VT will degenerate to fibrillation are unknown. The use of programmed electrical stimulation in detecting these patients at risk of ventricular fibrillation has not been proved.

In summary, runs of ventricular tachycardia are frequent in asymptomatic hypertrophic cardiomyopathy. 72-hour Holter monitoring is the most sensitive method of detecting VT, while programmed stimulation seems poorly sensitive. VT are associated with a high risk of sudden death.

Dilated cardiomyopathy

Dilated cardiomyopathy is defined as a heart muscle disorder of unknown etiology in which there is impaired contractile function and dilatation of one or both ventricles. The natural history of dilated cardiomyopathy (DCM) is unknown because the majority of patients are not diagnosed until they develop symptoms of left ventricular impairment. Once clinical evidence of impaired ventricular performance is apparent the prognosis is poor and is related to the degree of left ventricular impairment.

Frequency of VT in DCM

The incidence of ventricular arrhythmias is very high and reported in 43 to 93% of patients [15, 16]. Nonsustained VT also are common and have been noted in 43 to 93% of patients. Generally these VT are asymptomatic.

Mechanisms of VT [32]

Arrhythmias in dilated cardiomyopathy are presumably due to myocardial cellular abnormalities as well as the secondary chamber dilatation. Ventricular tachycardia and sudden death are more common when the left ventricular function is severely compromised [33]. However, the relationship of incidence of VT to severe impairment of left ventricular function is uncertain and not proved [34]. The mechanism of VT initiation remains uncertain.

Although some reports have validly emphasized the importance of structural and hemodynamic factors (such as myocardial fibrosis and ventricular wall stress) in predisposing to the reentry phenomena, recent evidence points to three potentially reversible arrhythmogenic factors in patients with congestive failure [32].

– Electrolyte depletion: patients with congestive heart failure have maked deficits of total body and intracellular potassium and a magnesium depletion.

– Activation of neurohormonal mechanisms: the sympathetic nervous system and the renin-angiotensin are activated in patients with congestive heart failure. Circulating levels of catecholamines may be directly arrhythmogenic or may contribute to potentiating the arrhythmogenic effects of hypokaliemia. Angiotensin II may exacerbate ventricular arrhythmias.

– Therapy with drugs used to heart failure: diuretic drugs may prove to be the most arrhythmogenic, activating both the sympathetic nervous and renin-angiotensin systems and promoting the renal loss of potassium and magnesium. Digitalis may produce serious ventricular arrhythmias. Recently developed potent inotropic agents such amrinone, milrinone, enoximone enhance cardiac contractility by increasing intramyocellular levels of cyclic AMP either by promoting its synthesis (catecholamines) or by retarding its degradation (phosphodiesterase inhibition); both mechanisms are potentially arrhythmogenic.

– Antiarrhythmic therapy is often responsible for a proarrhythmic effects in patients with heart failure.

Methods of study

a) Holter monitoring
In recent years a number of studies have emerged documenting the high incidence of serious ventricular arrhythmias; most of the patients have multifocal ectopic beats [35, 36]; 43 to 77% of patients with DCM have ventricular tachycardias [16, 35, 36, 37]. The VT are often nonsustained, polymorphic and daily related [38].

b) Exercise testing
In favor of the proarrhythmic effect of catecholamines is the increase of ventricular arrhythmias during exercise testing in 28% of patients [37]. Repetitive ventricular premature beats are noted in 21% of patients.

c) Programmed electrical stimulation
The diagnosis value of programmed electrical stimulation is discussed because of the differences between the studied population. In patients with sustained VT, the sustained VT could be induced by programmed electrical stimulation in all patients [39]. This induction of sustained VT was associated with a high risk of sudden death and recurrence of VT. In patients with various ventricular arrhythmias on Holter monitoring, but without spontaneous sustained VT, a monomorphic VT was not induced by 1 and 2 ventricular extrastimuli. A high incidence (86%) of inducible polymorphic ventricular arrhythmias was found [40], but only 4.8% of polymorphic sustained VT and 2.4% of VF were induced and were not correlated with the occurrence of sudden death. A mean sensitivity was found in a population including patients with sustained VT or nonsustained VT, or ventricular fibrillation [41]: Electrophysiologic testing reproduced the clinical arrhythmia in approximately 50% of patients. However, inducibility did not predict the outcome.

In our experienc simular results were found. In 4 patients with sustained VT, a sustained VT was reproducibly induced; in 8 patients with nonsustained VT, only 1 sustained VT and 2 nonsustained VT were induced and the significance of this arrhythmia is unknown. The sensitivity of PES to reproduce sustained VT is excellent but its specificity seems weaker.

d) Signal averaged electrograms
The signal averaged electrogram could identify patients with non-ischemic congestive cardiomyopathy and sustained ventricular arrhythymias [42]. The filtered QRS duration was longest and the voltage in the last 40 msec of the filtered QRS was lower, in patients with sustained ventricular arrhythmias. Similar results have been assessed in Nancy: abnormal late potentials have been registered in 3 patients, 2 of them with sustained VT; 7 patients with nonsustained VT did not have abnormal late potentials. In patients with inducible polymorphic VT [40] an abnormal late potential had been detected in only 1 of the 30 patients. Also,

abnormal late potential could be a marker for the risk of monomorphic sustained VT.

Prognostic of VT in DCM

VT are associated with a high mortality [32, 43]. Some investigators have suggested that the finding of complex ventricular rhythm disturbances predicts future fatal arrhythmias, but such malignant ventricular ectopy is usually a reflection of the severity of hemodynamic and therefore predicts total mortality rather than the occurrence of sudden unexpected death [32].

The high incidence of mortality (about 20% per year) in patients with ventricular arrhythmias could be related either to sudden death (50%) or to cardiac heart failure (50%) [33, 43].

However, some authors [44, 45, 46] have proposed that the finding of sustained VT is associated with a substantial risk of sudden death: the comparison of patients with and without VT would have assessed a higher incidence of sudden death in patients with VT.

Different results have been found by other observers; the incidence of ventricular arrhythmias is very high in DCM; the mortality is important but most of the deaths would be secondary to worsening cardiac heart failure and VT did not appear to be a predictor of prognosis [35, 36, 41]. In our experience, 13 patients with VT have been followed up: 7 patients with nonsustained VT are alive, 6 patients had sustained VT: 3 died, one from heart failure, one from VT, one from unknown causes.

Also, some patients with VT and DCM are at high risk of sudden death. However, at present there is no validated means of identifying these patients, although some investigators have suggested that the finding of sustained VT during programmed electrical stimulation or late potentials on signal averaged electrograms could distinguish these paients with heart failure predisposed to potentially lethal arrhythmias [42].

In summary, there is a high incidence of VT in DCM. VT are more common when the left ventricular function is severely compromised. This association explains the high mortality which has been correlated with VT. But the deaths have differents causes, and could be related either to a sudden death or to worsening of heart failure. The antiarrhyhmic drugs may precipitate the cardiac heart failure. There is no validated means of identifying the patients at high risk of sudden death.

In conclusion, the frequency and the significance of ventricular tachycardia in non-ischemic diseases are dependent on the underlying heart disease.
– In mitral valve prolapse sustained ventricular tachycardia are very rare when mitral valve prolapse is not associated with cardiac enlargement or another heart disease, and are difficult to induce. The ventricular tachycardias could rarely lead

to sudden death. Only young patients with syncopes should be controlled.

– In hypertrophic cardiomyopathy nonsustained polymorphic ventricular tachycardia are frequent, are difficult to induce but are detected by a 72 hour holter monitoring. Ventricular tachycardia are associated with a high risk of sudden death and should be treated.

– In dilated cardiomyopathy nonsustained or sustained ventricular tachycardia are very frequent, are easy to induce when sustained and are often facilitated by an enhanced sympathetic activity. Ventricular tachycardias are associated with a high mortality from sudden and nonsudden cardiac death. Antiarrhythmic therapy is difficult to use and often dangerous or inefficacious; adrenergic activation may be present and lead to indicate β blocker therapy. The means of identifying the patients at high risk of sudden death are unknown.

References

1. Savage DD, Garrison RJ, Devereux RB, Castelli WP, Anderson SJ, Levy D, Mc Namara P, Stokes J, Kannel WB, Feinleib M. 1983. Mitral valve prolapse in the general population. I – Epidemiologic features: the Framingham study. Am Heart J 106: 571–576.
2. Fauchier JP, Neel CH, Charbonnier B, Brochier M. 1980. Les troubles du rhythme du prolapsus mitral. Etude de 59 cas. Ann Cardiol Angéiol 29: 281–290.
3. Kramer HM, Kligfield P, Devereux RB, Savage D, Kramer-Fox R. 1984. Arrhythmias in mitral valve prolapse. Effect of selection bias. Arch Intern Méd 144: 2360–2364.
4. Savage DD, Levy D, Garrisson RJ, Castelli WP, Kligfield P, Devereux RB, Anderson SJ, Kannel WB, Feinleib M. 983. Mitral valve prolapse in the general population. 3 dysrhythmias: the Fragmingham study. Am Heart J 106: 582–586.
5. Perrot B, Danchin N, Preiss MA, Bara P, Cherrier F, Faivre G. 1985. Prolapsus de la valve mitrale. Résultats des études électrophysiologiques. Arch Mal Coeur 78: 1001–1008.
6. Chesler E, King RA, Edwards JE. 1983. The myxomatous mitral valve and sudden death. Circulation 67: 632–639.
7. Gaffney FA, Karlsson ES, Campbell W, Schutte JE, Nixon JV, Willerson JT, Blomqvist CG. 1979. Autonomic dysfunction in women with mitral valve prolapse syndrome. Circulation 59: 894–901.
8. Leclercq JF, Malergue MC, Milosevic D, Rosengarten MD, Attuel P, Coumel PH. 1980. Troubles du rhythme ventriculaire et prolapsus mitral. A propos de 35 observations. Arch Mal Coeur 73: 276–287.
9. Demaria AN, Amsterdam EA, Vismara LA, Neumann A, Mason DT. 1976. Arrhythmias in the mitral valve prolapse syndrome: prevalence, nature and frequency. Ann Intern Med 84: 656–.
10. Morady F, Shen E, Bhandari A, Schwartz A, Scheinman HM. 1984. Programmed ventricular stimulation in mitral valve prolapse: analysis of 36 patients. Am J Cardiol 53: 135–138.
11. Rosenthal ME, Halmer A, Gang ES, Oseran DS, Mandel WJ, Peter T. 1985. The yield of programmed ventricular stimulation in mitral valve prolapse patients with ventricular arrhythmias. Am Heart J 110: 970–976.
12. Jeresaty RM. 1979. Mitral valve prolapse. New York, Roven Presss,219.
13. Jeresaty RM. 1986. Mitral valve prolapse: definition and implications in athletes. J Am Coll Cardiol 7: 231–236.
14. Lown B. 1982. Management of patients at high risk of sudden death. Am Heart J 101: 689–697.
15. Brandenburg RO. 1985. Cardiomyopathy and their role in sudden death. J Am Coll Cardiol 5: 185B–189B.

16. McKenna WJ, Krikler DM, Goodwin JF. 1984. Arrhythmias in dilated and hypertrophic cardiomyopathy. Symposium on cardiac arrhythmias. Medical clinics of north america 68: 983–1000.

17. Maron B, Roberts W, Epstein S. 1982. Sudden death in hypertrophic cardiomyopathy. A profile of 78 patients. Circulation 65: 1388–1394.

18. Doy Y, Mc Kenna WJ, Chetty S, Dakley C, Goodwin J. 1980. Prediction of mortality and serious ventricular arrhythmias in hypertrophic cardiomyopathy. An echocardiographic study. Brit Heart J 44: 150–157.

19. Savage DD, Seides SF, Maron BJ, Myers DJ, Epstein SE. 1979. Prevalence of arrhythmias during 24 hour electrocardiographic monitoring and exercise testing in patients with obstructive and non obstructive hypertrophic cardiomyopathy. Circulation 59: 866–875.

20. Bjarnason I, Hardarson T, Jousson S. 1982. Cardiac arrhythmias in hypertrophic cardiomyopathy. Br Heart J 48: 198–203.

21. Newman H, Sugrue D, Oakley CM, Goodwin JF, Mc Kenna WJ. 1985. Relation of left ventricularfunction and prognosis in hypertrophic cardiomyopathy: an angiographic study. J Am Coll Cardiol 5: 1064–1074.

22. Baille N, Aliot E, Perrot B, Ethevenot G, Neimann JL, Godenir JP, Gilgenkrantz JM, Faivre G. 1984. Enregistrements électrocardiographiques de longue durée chez 33 patients atteints de cardiomyopathie obstructive. Arch Mal Coeur 77: 730–737.

23. Maron BJ, Savage DD, Wolfson JK, Epstein SE. 1981. Prognostic significance of 24 hour ambulatory electrocardiographic monitoring in patients with hypertrophic cardiomyopathy: a prospective study. Am J Cardiol 48: 252–257.

24. Mc Kenna WJ, England D, Doi YL, Deanfield JE, Oakley C, Goodwin JF. 1981. Arrhythmia in hypertrophic cardiomyopathy. I influence on prognosis. Br Heart J 46: 168–172.

25. Mc Kenna WJ, Chetty S, Oakley CM, Goodwin JF. 1980. Arrhythmia in hypertrophic cardiomyopathy: exercise and 48 hour ambularoty electrocardiographic assessment with and without beta adrenergic blocking therapy. Am J Cardiol 45: 1–5.

26. Anderson KP, Stinson EB, Derby GC, Oyer PE, Mason JW. 1982. Vulnerability to ventricular arrhythmia induction in patients with hypertrophic obstructive cardiomyopathy. Circulation 66 (suppl. II): 146.

27. Watson R, Liberati JM, Tucker E, Cannon RO, Rosing DR, Epstein SE, Josephson ME. 1985. Inducible ventricular fibrillation in patients with hypertrophic cardiomyopathy. J Am Coll Cardiol 5: 395.

28. Kuck KH, Kunze KP, Bernedde J. 1985. Value and limitations of programmed electrical stimulation in hypertrophic cardiomyopathy. Circulation 72 (suppl. III): 158.

29. Mc Kenna WJ, Deanfield J, Faruqui A, England D, Oakley C, Goodwin JF. 1981. Prognosis in hypertrophic cardiomyopathy: role of age and clinical electrocardiographic and hemodynamic features. Am J Cardiol 47: 532–538.

30. Perrot B, Danchin N, Terrier De La Chaise A, Cherrier F, Faivre G. 1984. Vérapamil cause of sudden death in a patient with hypertrophic cardiomyopathy. Brit Heart J 51: 352–354.

31. Maron BJ, Roberts WC, Edwards JE, Mc Allister HA, Foley DO, Epstein SE. 1978. Sudden death in patients with hypertrophic cardiomyopathy: characterization of 26 patients without functional limitation. Am J Cardiol 4: 803–810.

32. Packer M. 1985. Sudden unexpected death in patients with congestive heart failure: a second frontier. Circulation 72: 681–685.

33. Chakko CS, Gheorghiade M. 1985. Ventricular arrhythmias in severe heart failure: incidence, significance and effectiveness of antiarrhythmic therapy. Am Heart J 109: 497–504.

34. Constanza-Nordin MR, O'Connel JB, Engelmeier RS, Moran JF, Scanlon PJ. 1984. Ventricular tachycardia in dilated cardiomyopathy: a variable independent of hemodynamics, morphology and prognosis (Abstr.). J Am Coll Cardiol 3: 594.

35. Maskin CS, Siskind SJ, Le Jemtel TH. 1984. High prevalence of nonsustained ventricular tachycardia in severe congestive heart failure. Am Heart J 107: 896–901.

36. Huang SK, Messer JV, Denes P. 1983. Significance of ventricular tachycardia in idiopathic dilated cardiomyopathy: observations in 35 patients. Am J Cardiol 51: 507–512.
37. Haissaguerre M, Bonnet J, Le Goff G, Gueguen A, Broustet JP, Choussat A, Dallochio M, Besse P, Bricaud H. 1986. Prevalence, signification et pronostic des troubles du rhythme ventriculaire dans 236 myocardiopathies dilatées. Arch Mal Coeur 79: 32–38.
38. Leclercq JF, Maisonblanche P, Cauchemez B, Attuel P, Coumel Ph. 1984. Les troubles du rhythme ventriculaire des myocardiopathies congestives. Arch Mal Coeur 77: 937–945.
39. Poll DS, Marchlinski FE, Buxton AF, Doherty JU, Waxman HL, Josephson ME. 1984. Sustained ventricular tachycardia in patients with idiopathic dilated cardiomyopathy: electrophysiologic testing and lack of response to antiarrythmic drug therapy. Circulation 70: 451–456.
40. Meinertz T, Treese N, Kasper W, Geibel A, Hofmann T, Zehender M, Bohn D, Pop T, Just H. 1985. Determinants of prognosis in idiopathic dilated cardiomyopathy as determined by programmed electrical stimulation. Am J Cardiol 56: 337–341.
41. Milner PG, Lerman RB, Dimarco JP. 1986. Role of electrophysiological testing in patients with idiopathic dilated cardiomyopathy and ventricular arrhythmias. J Am Coll Cardiol 7: 159 (Abstr.).
42. Poll DS, Marchlinski FE, Falcone RA, Josephson ME, Simson MB. 1985. Abnormal signal averaged electrocardiograms in patients with nonischemic congestive cardiomyopathy: relationship to sustained ventricular tachyarrhythmias. Circulation 72: 1308–1313.
43. Wilson J, Schwartz S, St John-Sutton M, Ferraro N, Horowitz L, Reicheck N, Josephson M. 1983. Prognosis in severe heart failure: relation to hemodynamic measurements and ventricular ectopic activity. J Am Coll Cardiol 2: 403–410.
44. Kafka W, Petri H, Hansen W, Rudolph W. 1983. Prognostic implications on ventricular arrhythmias in patients with dilated cardiomyopathy. Eur Heart J 4: 71 (Abstr.).
45. Hofmann T, Kasper W, Treese N, Hartmuller E, Pop TL, Meinertz T. 1983. Prognostic significance of ventricular arrhythmias (VA) and cardiac function in dilative cardiomyopathy (DCM). Eur Heart J 4: 97 (Abstr.).
46. Holmes J, Kubo S, Cody R, Kligfield P. 1985. Arrhythmias in ischemic and non ischemic dilated cardiomyopathy: prediction of mortality by ambulatory electrocardiography. Am J Cardiol 55: 146–151.
47. Von Olshausen K, Schafer A, Mehmel MC, Schwartz F, Senges J, Kubler W. 1984. Ventricular arrhythmias in idiopathic dilated cardiomyopathy. Br Heart J 51: 195–201.

8. Ventricular tachycardias in individuals with apparently normal heart

E. ALIOT, B. BREMBILLA-PERROT, K. KHALIFE, A. TERRIER DE LA CHAISE, M. BIANCHI, J.M. GILGENKRANTZ
Département de Cardiologie, C.H.R.U. de Nancy, Hôpital Central, 543037 Nancy Cedex, France

Ventricular tachycardia (VT) is usually associated with heart disease. However, it may occur without clinically evident cardiac abnormalities, and, in this case, the benign character of this arrhythmia has been stressed, compared to VT associated with heart disease. Although clinically well known [1, 2] its pathophysiology is still not well defined. In this chapter, we'll envisage the clinical pattern of this particular kind of VT.

We based this study upon both current data from the literature and our own experience of 35 consecutive patients (22 male, 13 female), with a mean age of 35.1 years (range 8 to 59) with VT and apparently normal heart as judged by non invasive cardiac examination and referred to our department out of 210 VT's (Table 1).

Table 1. Patients evaluation (n = 35). Diagnosis of apparently normal heart was based upon results of non invasive evaluation.

Non-invasive	
Clinical	35
Chest x Ray	35
12 leads ECG	35
24 hours ECG	30
Exercise testing	29
Echocardiography (TM, 2D)	35
Signal averaging	18
Stress 201 T1, 99 mTc	17
Invasive	
Electrophysiological study	24
Right angiography	19
Left angiography + Coronarography	19
(RV endomyocardial biopsy)	3

Incidence, clinical features

The definition of 'apparently normal heart' is the crucial point from many of the studies dealing with the subject, and is the most important factor responsible for the inconsistent data in the literature. The way to ensure an apparently normal condition of the heart differs markedly between the studies. Although idiopathic VT's may produce no symptoms and are often identified during routine examination, incidence of idiopathic VT's, defined as more 3 premature ventricular complexes (PVCs), with a rate higher than 100 beats/min is about 1 to 2% [1, 3, 4, 5, 6] with range from 0% [7] to 6% [8] when studied by Holter recordings or exercise testing. Among chronic VT's, it represents 7 to 38% of the patients 16.6% in our series [2, 9–16]. As confirmed by our data, idiopathic VT's can be present in children [17–19], is frequent in young adults [14, 20], and, is rarely found in older patients either because the arrhythmia disappears with time as myocardial changes occur, or, in older patients the heart is more often abnormal or as suggested by some, patients may die at an early age, a possibility which seems unlikely given the good prognosis of these arrhythmias.

Of our 35 cases, 6 patients reported syncope (correlated with paroxysmal sustained VT (PSVT), 19 complained of dizziness, light-headeness, pre-syncope or palpitations: 10 were totally asymptomatic. No patient had history of cardiac arrest, or ventricular fibrillation. In contrast to VT associated with heart disease, the clinical tolerance is always almost good [14, 21–24] even when ventricular rate exceeds 200 beats/min [10]. Therefore the initial diagnosis in young patients may sometimes be mistaken for paroxysmal supraventricular tachycardia.

Electrocardiography

Schematically, two kinds of VT can be observed in subjects with apparently normal heart: repetitive monomorphic ventricular tachycardia (RMVT) and paroxysmal monomorphic sustained ventricular tachycardia (PMSVT).

In our series, 23 patients demonstrated RMVT defined as follows [20, 25] (Fig. 1): a) single PVCs coexisting with couplets, triplets and frequent runs of non sustained VT (from 5 beats to 30″, and terminated spontaneously); b) identical morphologic pattern of all premature PVCs; c) and normal intervening sinus conducted complexes, i.e., without axis deviation, intraventricular conduction disturbances, pathological Q waves, or abnormalities of the ST segment or T wave. The mean cycle length of the VT's was 443 ± 72.7 ms (range 280 to 520 ms), and, runs of VT occurred predominantly or exclusively during the activity period in ten of 23 patients. These cases look like the classical form of incessant VT described by Gallavardin [26] as 'extrasystolie ventriculaire à paroxysmes tachycardiques prolongés' and, later by Parkinson and Papp [27] as 'repetitive paroxysmal ventricular tachycardia'. Later reports described benign paroxys-

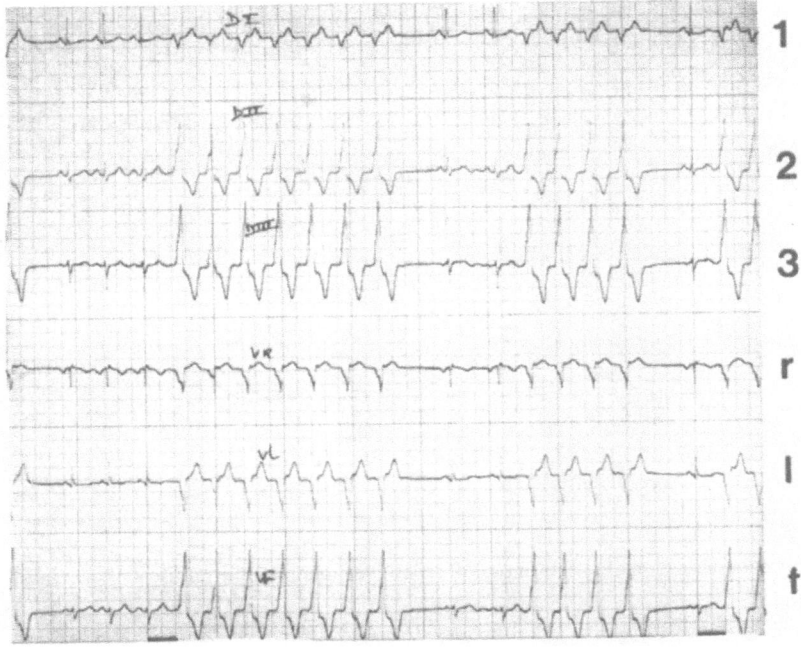

Figure 1. Peripheral leads: uncessant runs of repetitive monomorphic VT. The configuration of the ectopic complex is uniform and the sinus conducted complexes are normal.

mal VT [28], type II paroxysmal VT [11], tachycardies ventriculaires en salves [20], chronic recurrent right ventricular tachycardia [22, 23, 29] and repetitive monomorphic VT [14, 21]. The usual succession of events is as observed by Slama [10]: 'the coupling interval of the first beat of the tachycardia is relatively long (RV1), the first cycle of the tachycardia is the shortest (V1V2), the successive cycle length increases progressively and, VT stops after 5 to 10 complexes with a last cycle longer than all the preceding ones' (Fig. 2).

The 12 other patients demonstrated PMSVT (that lasted more than 30 seconds) with complete absence of any significant arrhythmias between the VT episodes (or very few PVCs on Holter recordings), and normal intercritic ECG. Normal QRS complexes of sinus origin between the VT were observed in all patients, and by definition, all PVCs had uniform QRS morphology. This type of VT may be mistaken for paroxysmal supraventricular tachycardia, with aberrant conduction [2, 10, 19, 22, 23, 30–35] in young patients with absence of severe symptoms. The mean cycle length of the VT was 316 ± 103 ms (range 250 to 500 ms).

The regular monomorphisms is one of the major criteria of this kind of arrhythmia [10, 20, 22–24] and, in contrast, this pattern is different from the polymorphism or the pleomorphism of VT's due to coronary artery disease, congestive cardiomyopathiy, or arrhythmogenic right ventricular dysplasia [10,

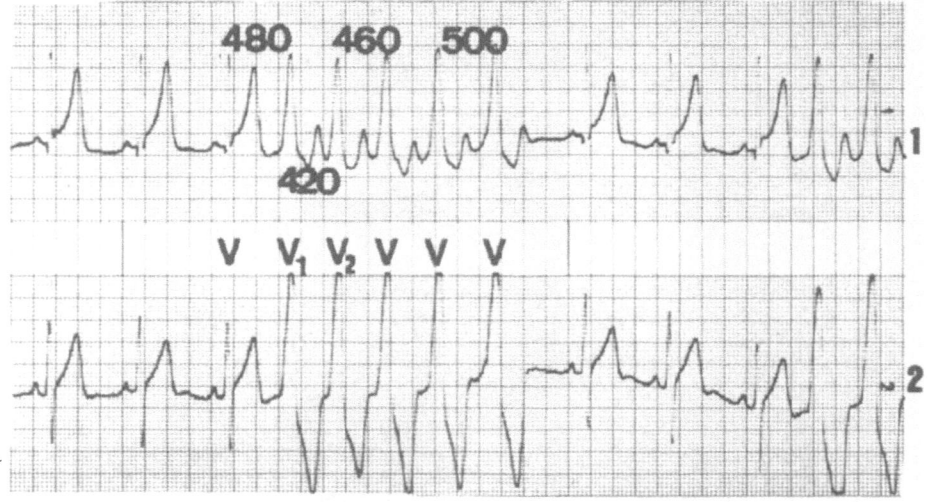

Figure 2. Usual succession of events in runs of repetitive monomorphic ventricular tachycardias (see text).

36]. The most frequent morphologic pattern of VT's was a left bundle branch block (LBBB) pattern, in 27 out of 35 patients (77%) (Fig. 3). In our group of idiopathic RMVT (n = 23) 16 patients had a LBBB morphologic pattern with a normal or right frontal plane axis, and 1 LBBB pattern with left axis; 6 patients had a right bundle branch block (RBBB) pattern with either right axis (n = 3), left axis (n = 1) or superior axis (n = 2). These findings of predominance of the LBBB morphologic pattern are in total agreement with most of the studies. In a recent paper, comparing morphology of 100 post myocardial infarction VT's, and 70 benign incessant idiopathic VT's, Coumel [37], considering only 2 parameters, QRS axis and morphology of VT in the precordial leads, found 4 major groups: inferior axis and LBBB pattern characterized 51% of idiopathic RMVT's; RBBB pattern with inferior axis (and exclusive R in V6) 24%; LBBB pattern with left axis deviation 7% and RBBB pattern in V1 (with rS in V6) with right or left deviation, 18%. Compared to post myocardial infarction VT, idiopathic RMVTs had a greater amplitude in peripheral leads, a smaller width, and most often a normal axis. The same applies to VT's due to congestive cardiomyopathy, but not to VT's with arrhythmogenic right ventricular dysplasia [10]. QR pattern in leads other then VR, and QS pattern in V5-V6 were constantly absent in RMVTs, and present in the majority of myocardial infarction VT's. The QRS morphology of RMVT with LBBB pattern and normal axis is related to its origin, first suggested by Rosenbaum [38], and recently proved to be the right ventricular outflow tract near the septum rather than the free wall surface [14, 22–24]. If the validity of prediction of the VT's origin based on the QRS morphology during VT has been questioned by endocardial mapping in patients with chronic ischemic heart disease, this phenomenon has not been demonstrated in patients without apparent heart disease [22, 30, 36, 39].

In the group of idiopathic PMSVT, LBBB morphologic pattern with normal or right axis, similar to RMVT, is also frequent, but LBBB pattern with left axis seems to be less common (respectively 6 and 4 of our 12 patients) [10, 22, 23, 30]. The 2 last patients had a particular kind of VT with RBBB pattern and left axis deviation, recently described as a possible unique ECG-electrophysiologic entity. This particularly interesting VT will be analysed below.

Exercise test

Response of these arrhythmias to exercise is variable [14, 17, 19, 22–24] as reported by others, and as shown by symptom limited exercise testing, performed in 29 of our patients. None of them had symptomatic or clinical evidence of ischemia during exercise. Patients with RMVT usually exhibited a marked decrease or total suppression of VT's salvos or PVC's (17 out of 19). For Coumel [21], this is due to a rate dependency and related to an 'upper threshold' of sinus rate. VT salvos may decrease or increase during exercise and of our two last patients with RMVT, one experienced a marked increase in spontaneous non sustained VT, and one no evident change. However, some studies insist on the higher frequency of exercise, provocable right VT [23,, 30], and for Buxton [23], this group of patients represent 75% of the non ischemic related exercise induced VT's observed in his institution. In patients with PMSVT, exercise induced VT seem to be more frequent (7 out of 10 patients in our group) [2, 23, 30]. In addition, exercise provocable right VT may represent a special group sharing different characteristics [23, 30, 40].

Signal averaging

Signal averaging system has recently been introduced as a method for non invasive detection of ventricular late potentials on the body surface [43]. The presence of low amplitude fragmented electrical activity ocuring at the end of QRS or during ST segment, originating from areas of slow conduction, seems to be closely corrected with the propensity to VT [41, 42]. Signal averaged ECG may permit non invasive identification of patients with spontaneous NSVT to develop sustained VT [44], but, to our knowledge, late potentials have not been recorded in patients with VT and apparently normal heart [23,, 45].

Signal averaged surface ECG was recorded in 18 of our patients with a previously described technique [46]. Four patients displayed an abnormally wide QRS (120 ± 11.8 msec, range 112 to 139 msec). The signal amplitude of the last

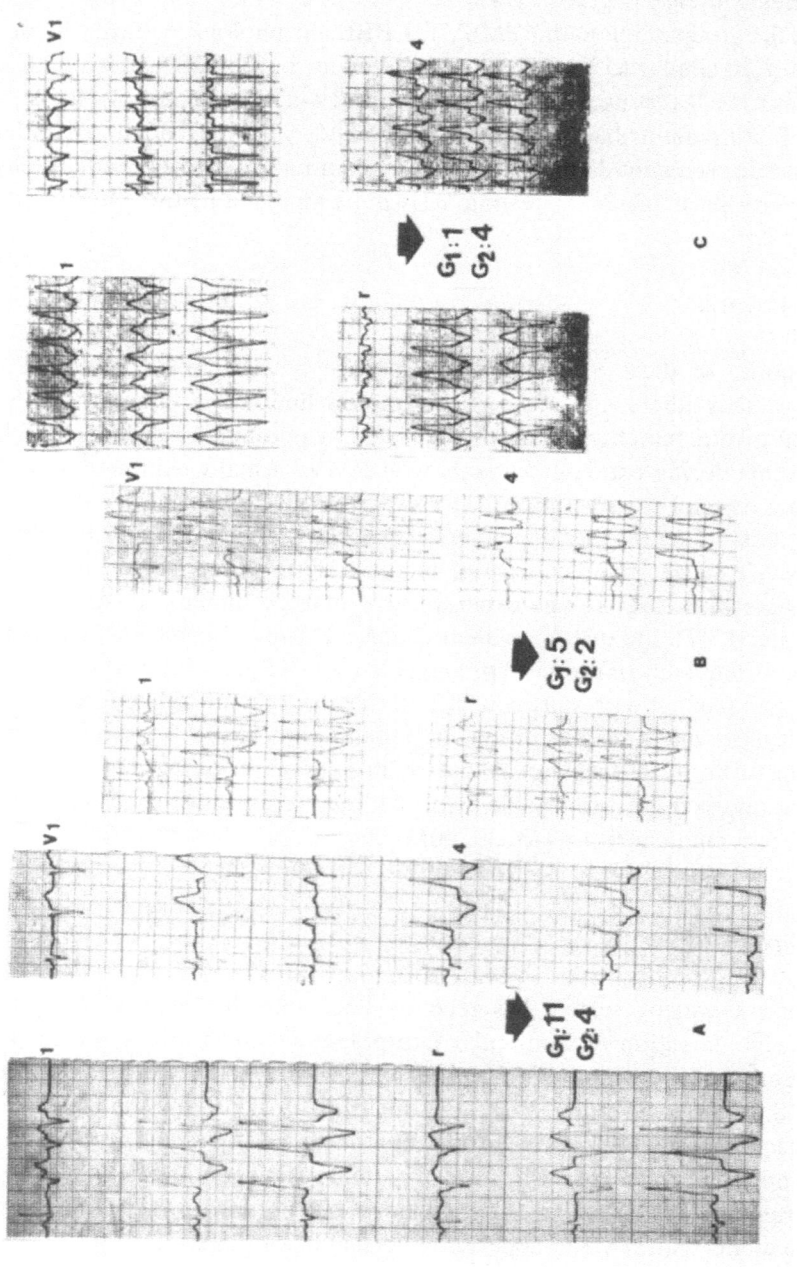

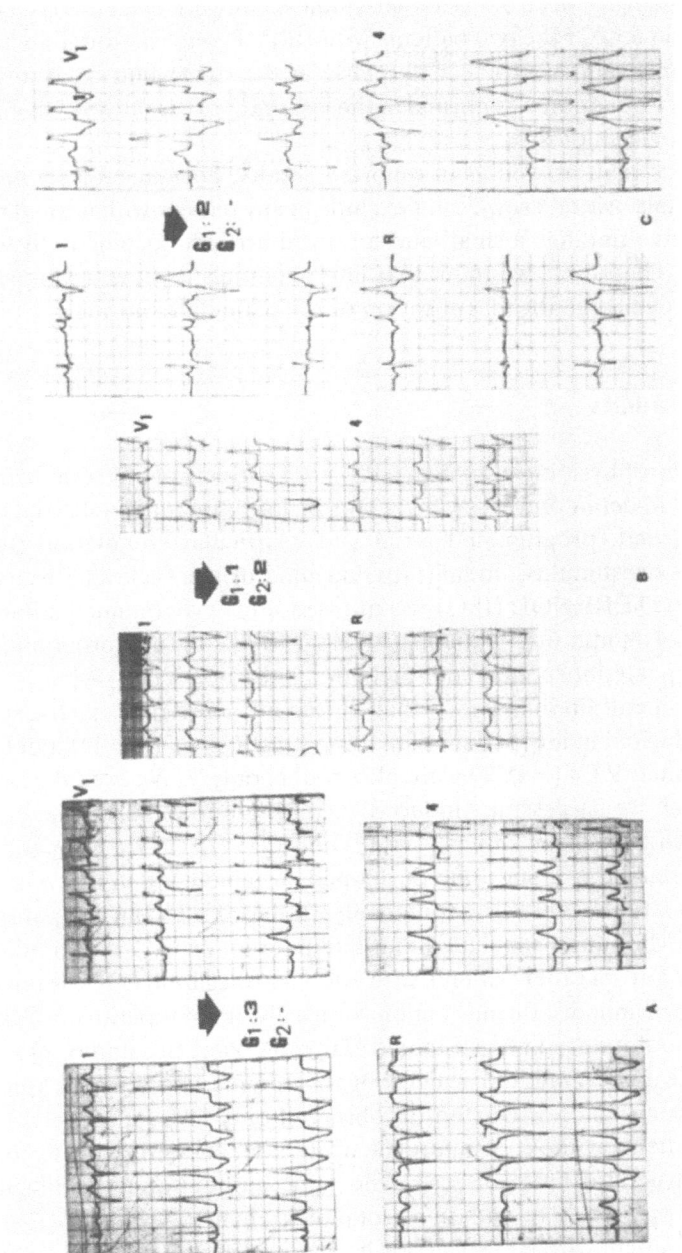

Figure 3. Morphologic types of VT in subjects with apparently normal heart: Gr 1: RMVT, Gr 2: PSVT; 3A: LBBB morphologic pattern (the most frequent: 77%) with right or normal axis (A, B) or left axis (C); 3B: RBBB morphologic pattern with right (A), left (B) or superior (C) axis.

40 msec of the filtered QRS was 10 ± 5.46 uv (range 2.34 to 14.88 uv), and duration of late potentials was 49 ± 4.7 msec. Of these 4 patients, two with PSVT had inducible SVT during electrophysiologic studies, but were evaluated only by non invasive techniques. Of the two patients with RMVT, one was found to have local arrhythmogenic right ventricular dysplasia at the right ventricular angiogram, and invasive evaluation was normal in the last one, with inducible NSVT at the electrophysiologic studies.

In our experience [46], as well as in reported results, normal subjects never display late potentials. Morever, we can't exclude in any patient with normal non invasive and invasive findings a small and localized arrhythmogenic right ventricular dysplasia. Therefore, we think that late potentials represent abnormal findings and must challenge the classification of the patients as normal.

Electrophysiologic studies

We performed electrophysiologic studies (EPS) in 24 patients of our series with a protocol described in detail previously [47]. This included incremental atrial and ventricular pacing and, programmed atrial and ventricular stimulation (with single and double extrastimulus), in sinus rhythm and 2 driven cycle lengths (600, 400 msec). ISOPROTERENOL (ISO) was infused after programmed stimulation at rate of 1 to 4 ug/min in 14 patients (9RMVT, 5PSVT), and programmed stimulation was repeated if spontaneous arrhythmia did not occur [48].

Our most prominent findings were that sustained ventricular tachycardia (SVT) was not inducible in any patient with idiopathic RMVT (n = 14) and that induced non sustained VT's (NSVT) were observed in only 2. We used the same protocol with which we successfully induced VT in more than 80% of patients with SVT and ischemic heart disease [47]. During ISO, (n = 9) 2 patients developed non sustained VT and, one developed sustained VT in response to programmed stimulation. Rahilly [14] found only 2 induced VT's out of 7 patients with 'idiopathic' RMVT, and concluded that failure to induce VT differentiates this group of RMVT from other patients with RMVT. Naccarelli [13] was unsuccessful in inducing sustained VT in any patient with a history of repetitive VT, and observed only 32% of induced non sustained VT; moreover, this author did not recommend routine electrophysiological testing for patients who have this kind of arrhythmia. In several studies, Buxton [9] observed only 29% of induced non sustained VT in patients without structural heart disease, and induced SVT only in patients with structural heart disease. The same author found 7 inducible RMVT's out of 22 patients [24], and, in a group of 30 right VT's, ten VT's were induced (only one patient with RMVT at rest had SVT induced), most frequently by atrial or ventricular rapid pacing [23]. The same kind of results have been noted by others, and demonstrate that this type of VT is generally non inducible by stimulation [10, 12, 30, 49]. ISO may either suppress the VT salves, or PVC's,

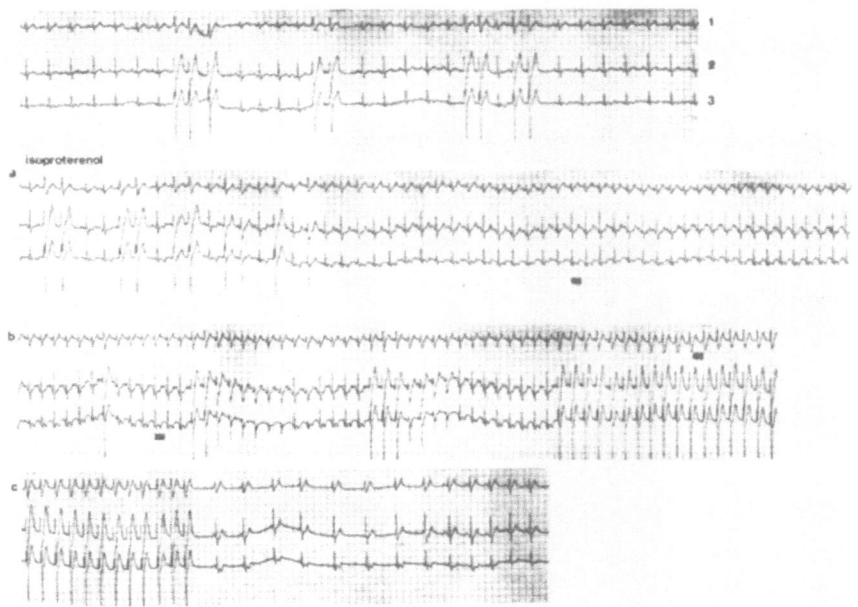

Figure 4. Induced isoproterenol .PSVT in an apparently normal subject. 4A: Infusion of cate-cholamines suppresses the VT when the sinus rate reaches a threshold value of 125/ms. 4B: When the adrenergic stimulation is adequate, VT starts spontaneously (sinus rate: 160). 4C: When the adre-nergic stimulation decreases (ISO stopped at the onset of the VT), VT stops spontaneously followed by a short period of junctional escape and sinus bradycardia (vagal response). (A and B in continuity; 90 seconds between B and C).

by increasing sinus rate to a threshold value [10], or induce VT (Fig. 4). In a group of 23 RVT, ISO infusion facilitated tachycardia induction in 13 cases (11 spontaneously, 12 with pacing), and stopped the arrhythmia in one patient [23]. As stressed by Coumel, ISO (or exercise) is not constantly effective and effects may be observed only after ISO infusion (or exercise) [20, 21]. Moreover, spontaneous changes and spontaneous termination of RMVT explain the difficulty of a systematic study and the impossibility to obtain reproducible results [14, 21, 23].

Idiopathic PSVT are normally easier to induce (or to stop) by pacing or programmed stimulation. In ten of our group of PMSVT, premature ventricular stimulation induced VT in 6 cases, but atrial pacing or programmed stimulation was unsuccessful, in contrast with some reports [23]. Brugada [45] and Prystowsky [12] successfully induced VT respectively in 88% and 83% of idiopathic SVT. ISO may be necessary for VT induction. Palileo [30] was able to induce VT only in one out of 6 patients with exercise provocable right ventricular tachycardia while ISO reproduced VT in 100% of cases, confirming the impression of Wellens that exercise induced VTs are not replicable by provocative techniques [50]. ISO

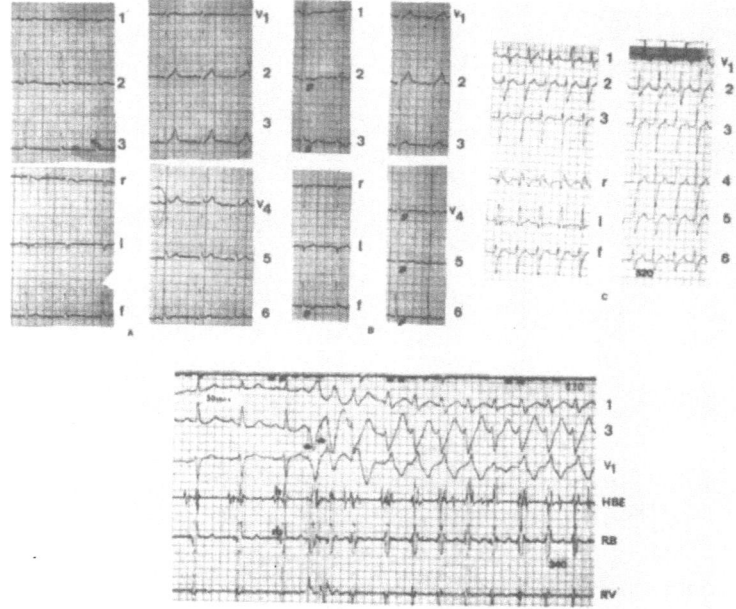

Figure 5. Idiopathic paroxysmal VT with a QRS pattern of RBBB and left axis deviation: – top left: ECG's in sinus rhythm, one week (A) (normal) then shortly after VT (B) (negative T waves in inferior and lateral precordial leads); – top right: spontaneous VT (C); – bottom: VT induced by 2 programmed ventricular stimulation.

induced SVT's were observed in 3 of 5 patients in our series of PSVT (1 spontaneously, 2 with programmed stimulation), and were similar to exercise induced VT.

These data confirm the point that inducibility of VT is related to heart disease. Programmed electrical stimulation induced VT less often in patients with a history of non sustained VT versus sustained VT, and less often in patients whom tachycardia is not due to coronary artery disease than in related to heart disease [9, 12, 24].

Idiopathic recurrent sustained VT with a RBBB QRS pattern and left axis deviation

One kind of idiopathic VT has been recently emphasized, first described by Belhassen [31] as a possible unique entity, then by German, Lin and Klein [32, 33, 34], following observations by several authors [39, 50, 51, 52] (Fig. 5). This type of tachycardia has been described in young patients with apparently normal heart. During sinus rhythm ECG shows ST depression and T waves inversion in the inferior and lateral leads. This has been related by some as a 'post tachycardia syndrome' due to the changes of ventricular repolarization following the altered depolarization [10]. QRS morphologic characteristics during episodes of VT showed a pattern of RBBB and left axis deviation. As VT's induction may be obtained by atrial (atrial pacing or extrastimulus) or ventricular stimulation, the tachycardia may be misdiagnosed as being supraventricular tachycardia with aberrant conduction. Finally, termination of tachycardia may be obtain by Verapamil. Earliest activity has been recorded usually from the left mid septum (or the LV apex). These features suggest that the tachycardia in these patients may be possibly due to a reentrant mechanism located in the proximal part of the left posterior fascicle, resulting in relatively narrow QRS, and early retrograde His deflection during VT, and possible induction by atrial beats. The abnormal conduction may be slow channel mediated, thus explaining the high efectiveness of Verapamil, which suggests involvement of the slow response in a reentry or a triggered automaticity mechanism.

Mechanism

If reentry, the most commonly advanced mechanism for SVT, is probaby involved in the mechanism of idiopathic PMSVT, their characteristics do not fulfill the normally admitted criteria and some features suggest other possible mechanisms. The ability of catecholamines to reproducibly induce tachycardias, even not replicable by stimulation [12, 23, 30, 50] suggests either enhanced normal activity, abnormal automatic rhythm or slow response reentrant rhythm, or triggered activity as a mechanism. Moreover, after-depolarizations giving rise to tachyarrhythmias may be due to catecholamines, or be triggered by pacing or premature stimulation, and triggered activity is abolished by Verapamil similarly to observations in the clinical setting [54, 55].

Data from the literature suggest that idiopathic RMVT's are probably due to automaticity abnormality and triggered activity may be responsible for the repetitive activity rather than reentry, although clinical findings are not really helpful in establishing what is the underlying mechanism. However the absence of structural disease, the absence of late potentials, the low frequency of induction by programmed ventricular stimulation, the effects of exercise or Isoproterenol (although they are inconstantly effective), the efficacy of calcium channel blockers in contrast with what is observed in reentrant VT, suggest a mechanism other than reentry such as triggered activity. Most of the authors are in agreement with that point [10, 13, 14, 20, 21, 23–25]. In idiopathic RMVT, Coumel [21] showed a dissociation between 'the triggering phenomenon' (the initial extrasystole) and 'the triggered phenomenon' (the repetitive activity) and found 3 major determinants of spontaneous activity:
1) the preceding mean heart rate, the length of runs increasing with increasing

preceding heart rate (adrenergic dependence),

2) the length of the RR cycle preceding the initial PVC, the length of runs correlating positively with the duration of the long preceding diastole (rate dependence), and

3) the coupling interval of the first PVC usually longer for runs than for single PVC [25].

Again, a mechanism of triggered activity responsible of idiopathic RMVT was suggered by these observations and the initial extrasystole showed the same characteristics as observed in uniform idiopathic isolated premature ventricular complexes, for which a modulated parasystole has been proposed as mechanism [56].

Morphologic findings

The term itself, 'apparently normal' heart, suggests a difficulty in conceiving that these hearts are completely normal. Although the majority of patients had non clinical evidence of structural heart disease, subtle histopathologic changes may have been present to account for the presence of VT. To investigate the anatomic substrate of idiopathic VT, 19 patients (out of our group of 35) underwent right and left ventriculography, and coronary angiography with RV endomyocardial biopsy in 3 cases. All patients had angiographically normal coronary arteries, and normal left ventricle (LV) with normal LV ejection fraction and end diastolic pressure. Six of them (32%) exhibited localized right ventricular wall abnormalities, similar to those described by Fontaine in patients with arrhythmogenic right ventricular dysplasia [57, 58]. All of them had VT with LBBB pattern and right or normal axis, and RV biopsy showed adipose tissue and thickening of endocardium compatible with ARVD in one patient.

Coronary artery disease, mitral valve prolapse and cardiomyopathy

As said before, features of idiopathic VT usually differ from VT in coronary artery disease, cardiomyopathy and mitral valve prolapse, in which pleomorphism and/or polymorphism of tachycardias, although inconstant, are a frequent observation, and exclude these kinds of arrhythmia from our study. The authors who performed coronary angiography, in patients without apparent heart disease, didn't find any significant abnormality, and we think it unnecessary to perform coronary arteriography in patients without clinical evidence or suspicion of coronary disease [9, 10, 13–15, 18, 23, 39, 63].

As far as TM and 2D echocardiography is probably the 'gold standard' to diagnose mitral valve prolapse (MVP), invasive tehniques are unnecessary to confirm this abnormality, and we excluded MVP from this study. However, considering the frequency of MVP, some studies included mild degree of MVP in the group of VT with apparently normal heart [10, 21, 23, 30, 35].

The diagnosis of cardiomyopathy is generally easy to make with non invasive techniques, but as VT may represent the first clinical sign of cardiomyopathy, it may be difficult to prove or to exclude [2, 10]. Subclinical evidence of myocardial dysfunction can be present in some patients without apparent disease and VT: subtle abnormalities as abnormal LV pressure and/or angiographics findings, increased LV volumes, and diastolic pressures, or decreased mean velocity of myocardial circumferential fibers shortening, or ejection fraction [57, 60, 61].

Arrhythmogenic right ventricular dysplasia (ARVD)

As foresaid, several distinctions between the group of patients with idiopathic VT and those with ARVD are apparent. In ARVD, VT may be pleomorphic with half of them having a left superior axis, and signal averaged surface ECG shows usually characteristic delayed activation [23]. ARVD, easy to recognize when must of the right ventricle is involved, may be difficult to diagnose unless the patients are carefully evaluated by 2D echocardiography or RV angiography or both [58]. However, this abnormality has been found as often as 70% in idiopathic ventricular arrhythmias [35]. This frequency appears overestimated, and, a rate nearly 30% seems us more likely [65]. In fact, Pietras [22], in a group of right ventricular tachycardias, observed 45% of 'RV disease' characterised by slight to moderate increase in RV volumes, associated in 18% with obvious left ventricular disease.

If very localized lesions of the RV wall (the LV wall as well) may be undetectable for usual means of investigations, it remains a group of patients with so called 'primary electrical disease' or 'VT with apparently normal heart' even in studies with complete cardiac evaluation. Recently, several studies have reported results of right and left biopsy in this group of patients [49, 61–64]. Indeed, majority of patients with idiopathic VT have histologic abnormalities bringing into question this concept. An interesting finding was that myocarditis may be more common than previously suspected. Recognition of this is important because of the serious nature of the disease, and the potential for treatment. Moreover a majority of patients had abnormal non specific biopsy findings such as myocardial cellular hypertrophy, interstitial or perivascular fibrosis, suggested to be compatible with early dilated cardiomyopathy. Findings compatible with ARVD were found respectively in 3 out of 10, 2 out of 18 and 1 out 15 patients [61, 63, 64].

We may insist on the fact that most reported studies may be considered biased by either the polymorphous aspect of VT, or the existence of patent abnormalities before invasive studies. However, the significance of these findings is unclear for the present. Utility of biopsy in majority of patients with otherwise normal ventricular function remains uncertain, as long as long term follow up don't show any prognostic implications.

Follow-up and therapy

With the exception of some reported sudden deaths [10, 66], a benign clinical course is reported in the majority of patients with idiopathic VT [8, 10, 13–15, 18, 21–24, 30, 67] even in patients with microscopic or macroscopic ventricular abnormalities [61] whatever the kind of VT, RMVT or PSVT.

The mean follow-up of our patients was 3.32 years (0.25 to 15 years) after the first documented VT and, in agreement with literature, during that period no patient had died suddenly, had cardiac arrest, symptomatic VT or progression of symptoms. More than that, some patients appear to have spontaneous resolution of RMVT [10, 14], PSVT as well. Conversely, frontier forms may exist, with either increase of the VT's salvos frequency and episodes of sustained VT, or decrease of VT's salvos and conversion to sinus rhythm [10, 20]. Only symptomatic patients have to be treated (40% of our patients are not on therapy). In that case, idiopathic VT are responsive to a wide variety of antiarrhythmic drugs, including type I agents, β-blockers and calcium blockers. All patients on drugs had no VT on 24 hours ambulatory ECG, and the recordings revealed only PVC's in 6 patients (Table 2). Special interest has been given to β-blockers in exercise or ISO induced VT [20, 21, 23, 24, 30]. The efficacy of calcium blockers in suppressing runs of RMVT has been stressed [14, 20, 21, 25] (as well as effectiveness on PSVT with RBBB pattern and left axis deviation, which has been mentioned), and give one more reason to think that slow channels are involved in the mechanism of these arrhythmias, as we mentioned previously. Other types of therapy, such as surgery or fulguration, may remain exceptional [10].

Table 2. Treatment of 35 idiopathic ventricular tachycardias. No recurrence of ventricular tachycardia in any patient.

	Group I (RMVT) n = 23	Group II (PSVT) n = 12	Total n = 35
No drug	12	2	14 (40%)
Amiodarone	2 (2)	4 (1)	6
Quinidine	2 (2)	2	4
Flecaïnide	–	3	3
Aprindine	2	1 (1)	3
Verapamil	1	–	1
β-blockers	1	3	4

( ) patients with persistent PVC's.

Conclusion

What usually makes the RV site of VT in patients without apparent heart disease? This remains unclear, although the fact that RV is a more anatomically complex chamber, prone to a selective degeneration process, has been advanced [22]. Whatever the mechanisms of VT or the possibility of histologic abnormalities, patients appear to have a benign course and need treatment only when smptomatic.

References

1. Clarke JM, Hamer J, Shelton JR, Taylor S, Venning GR. 1976. The rhythm of the normal human heart. Lancet 2: 508–522.
2. Sebastien P, Waynberger M, Beaufils P, Motte G, Slama R, Bouvrain Y. 1976. Les tachycardies ventriculaires isolées sans cardiopathie patente. Arch Mal Coeur 69: 919–928.
3. Bethge KP, Bethge D, Meiners G, Lichtlen PR. 1983. Incidence and prognostic significance of ventricular arrhythmias in individuals without detectable heart disease. Eur Heart J 4: 338–346.
4. Bjerregard P. 1982. Premature beats in healthy subjects 40–79 years of age. Eur Heart J 3: 493–503.
5. Brodsky M, Wu D, Denes P, Kanakis C, Rosen K. 1977. Arrhythmias documented by 24 hour continuous electrocardiographic monitoring in 50 male medical students without apparent heart disease. Am J Cardiol 39: 390–395.
6. Fleg JL, Lakatta EG. 1984. Prevalence and prognosis of exercise induced non sustained ventricular tachycardia in apparently healthy volunteers. Am J Cardiol 54: 762–764.
7. Kostis JB, Mc Crone K, Moreyra AE, Gotzoyannis S, Aglitz N, Natarajan N, Kuo PT. 1981. Premature ventricular complexes in the absence of identifiable heart disease. Circulation 63: 1351–1355.
8. Montague TJ, Mc Pherson D, Mc Kenzie BR, Spencer CA, Nanton MA, Horacek BM. 1983. Frequent ventricular ectopic activity without underlying cardiac disease: analysis of 45 subjects. Am J Cardiol 52: 980–984.
9. Buxton AE, Waxman HL, Marchlinski FE, Josephson ME. 1983. Electrophysiologic studies in non sustained ventricular tachycardia: relation to underlying heart disease. Am J Cardiol 52: 985–991.
10. Slama R, Leclercq JF, Coumel P. 1985. Paroxysmal ventricular tachycardia in patients with apparently normal heart. In: Cardiac electrophysiology and arrhythmias, D.P. Zipes and J. Jalife Ed., Grune and Stratton, Orlando: 545–552.
11. Froment R, Gallavardin L, Cahen P. 1953. Paroxysmal ventricular tachycardia. A clinical classification. Br Heart J 15: 172–178.
12. Prystowsky EN, Zipes DP. 1984. Electrophysiologic testing in ventricular tachycardia. In: Tachycardias, B. Sorawicz, C. Pratap Reddy, E.N. Prystowsky Ed., Martinus Nijhoff Publishers, Boston: 293–309.
13. Naccarelli GV, Prystowsky EN, Jackman WM, Heger JJ, Rahilly GT, Zipes DP. 1982. Role of electrophysiologic testing in managing patients who have ventricular tachycardia unrelated to coronary artery disease. Am J Cardiol 50: 165–171.
14. Rahilly GT, Prystowsky EN, Zipes DP, Naccarelli GV, Jackman WM, Heger JJ. 1982. Clinical and electrophysiologic findings in patients with repetitive monomorphic ventricular tachycardia and otherwise normal electrocardiogram. Am J Cardiol 50: 459–468.
15. Chapman JH, Schank JP, Crampton RS. 1975. Idiopathic ventricular tachycardia: an intracardiac

electrical, hemodynamic and angiographic assessment of six patients. Am J Med 59: 470–480.

16. Veltri EP, Platia EV, Giffith LVC, Reid PR. 1985. Programmed electrical stimulation and long term follow up in asymptomatic NSVT. Am J Cardiol 56: 309–314.

17. Fulton DR, Chung KJ, Tabakin BS, Keane JF. 1985. Ventricular tachycardia in children without heart disease. Am J Cardiol 55: 1328–1331.

18. Fauchier JP, Cosmay P, Desveaux B. 1984. Troubles du rhythme ventriculaire du sujet sain sans cardiopathie apparente. Info Cardio 8: 747–770.

19. Garson A Jr. 1987. Ventricular arrhythmias in the young. Clinical and experimental findings. In: Ventricular Tachycardias, from Mechanism to Therapy, E. Aliot and R. Lazzara Ed., Martinus Nijhoff Publishers, Dordrecht.

20. Coumel P, Leclercq JF, Attuel P, Rosengarten M, Milosevic D, Slama R, Bouvrain Y. 1980. Tachycardies ventriculaires en salves. Etudes electrophysiologique et thérapeutique. Arch Mal Coeur 73: 153–164.

21. Coumel P, Leclercq JF, Slama R. 1985. Repetitive monomorphic idiopathic ventricula tachycardia. In: Cardiac electrophysiology and arrhythmias, D.P. Zipes and J. Jalife Ed., Grune and Stratton, Orlando: 457–468.

22. Pietras RJ, Lam W, Bauernfiend R, Sheikh A, Palileo E, Strasberg B, Swiryn S, Rosen KM. 1983. Chronic recurrent right ventricular tachycardia in patients without ischemic heart disease: clinical, hemodynamic and angiographic findings. Am Heart J 105: 357–366.

23. Buxton AE, Waxman HL, Marchlinski FE, Simson MB, Cassidy DM, Josephson ME. 1983. Right ventricular tachycardia: clinical and electrophysiologic characteristics. Circulation 68: 917–927.

24. Buxton AE, Marchlinski FE, Doherty JV, Cassidy DM, Vassallo JA, Flores BT, Josephson ME. 1984. Repetitive monomorphic ventricular tachycardia: clinical and electrophysiologic character- istics in patients with and patients without organic heart disease. Am J Cardiol 54: 997–1002.

25. Zimmermann M, Maison Blanche P, Cauchemez B, Leclercq JF, Coumel P. 1986. Determinants of the spontaneous ectopic activity in repetitive monomorphic idiopathic ventricular tachycardia. J Am Coll Cardiol 7: 1219–1227.

26. Gallavardin L. 1922. Extrasystolie ventriculaire à paroxysmes tachycardiques prolongés. Arch Mal Coeur 15: 298–306.

27. Parkinson J, Papp C. 1947. Repetitive paroxysmal tachycardia. Br Heart J 9: 241–262.

28. Dimond EG, Hayes HL. 1960. Benign paroxysmal ventricular tachycardia: report of a case. Ann Intern Med 53: 1255–1260.

29. Denes P, Wu D, Dhingra RG. 1976. Electrophysiologic studies in patients with chronic recurrent ventricular tachycardia. Circulation 54: 229–236.

30. Palileo EV, Ashley WW, Swiryns S, Bauernfiend RA, Strasberg B, Petropoulos AT, Rosen KM. 1982. Exercise provocable right ventricular out flow tract tachycardia. Am Heart J 104: 185–193.

31. Belhassen B, Shapira I, Pelleg A, Copperman I, Kauli N, Laniado S. 1984. Idiopathic recurrent sustained ventricular tachycardia responsive to Verapamil: an ECG electrophysiologic entity. Am Heart J 108: 1034–1036.

32. German LDG, Packer DL, Bardy GH, Gallagher JJ. 1983. Ventricular tachycardia induced by atrial stimulation in patients without symptomatic cardiac disease. Am J Cardiol 52: 1202–1207.

33. Lin FC, Finley CD, Rahimtoola SH, Wu D. 1983. Idiopathic paroxysmal ventricular tachycardia with a QRS pattern of right bundle branch block and left axis deviation: a unique clinical entity with specific properties. Am J Cardiol 52: 95–100.

34. Klein GS, Millman J, Yee R. 1984. Recurrent ventricular tachycardia responsive to Verapamil. P.A.C.E. 7: 938–948.

35. Fauchier JP, Desveaux B, Cosnay P, Raynaud P, Philippe L, Itti R. 1985. Troubles du rhythme ventriculaire complexes du sujet jeune. Arch Mal Coeur 9: 1333–1343.

36. Josephson ME, Horowitz LN, Farshidi A, Spielman SR, Michelson EL, Greenspan AM. 1979. Recurrent sustained ventricular tachycardia. E. Pleomorphism. Circulation 59: 459–468.

37. Coumel P, Leclercq JF, Attuel P, Maison Blanche P. 1984. The QRS morphology in post myocardial infarction ventricular tachycardia. A study of 100 tracings compared with 70 cases of idiopathic ventricular tachycardia. Eur J Cardiol 5: 792–805.

38. Rosenbaum MB. 1969. Classification of ventricular extrasystoles according to form. J Electrocardiology 2: 289–298.

39. Vetter V, Josephson ME, Horowitz L. 1981. Idiopathic sustained ventricular tachycardia in children and adolescents. Am J Cardiol 47: 315–322.

40. Wu D, Kou HC, Hung JS. 1981. Exercise triggered paroxysmal ventricular tachycardia: a repetitive rhythmic activity possibly related to after depolarisation. Ann Int Med 95: 410–414.

41. Breithardt G, Becker R, Seipel L, Abenroth RR, Ostermeyer J. 1981. Non invasive detection of late potentials in man: a new marker for ventricular tachycardia. Eur Heart J 2: 1–11.

42. Simson MB. 1981. Identification of patients with ventricular tachycardia after myocardial infarction from signals in the terminal QRS complex. Circulation 64: 235–242.

43. Berbari EJ, Scherlag BJ, Hope RR, Lazzara R. 1978. Recording from the body surface of arrhythmogenic ventricular activity during the ST segment. Am J Cardiol 41: 697–702.

44. Buxton AE, Simson MB, Falcone R, Dresden C, Marchlinski FE, Waxman HL, Josephson ME. 1984. Signal averaged ECG in patients with nonsustained ventricular tachycardia: identification of patients with potential for sustained ventricular arrhythmias. J Am Coll Cardiol 3: 495 (abstract).

45. Brugada P, Wellens HJJ. 1984. Programmed electrical stimulation of the human heart. In: Tachycardias, Mechanisms, Diagnosis, Treatment, M.E. Josephson and H.J.J. Wellens Ed., Lea and Febiger, Philadelphia, p. 61–89.

46. Terrier de la Chaise A, Brembilla-Perrot B, Balaud A, Morizot P, Cherrier F, Pernot C. 1987. Correlation potentiels tardifs de surface et arythmies ventriculaires déclenchables (à propos de 115 cas). Arch Mal Coeur 80: 177–183.

47. Perrot B, Thiel B, Cherrier F, Faivre G. 1984. Résultats de l'application systématique des méthodes de stimulation ventriculaire. Arch Mal Coeur 3: 262–272.

48. Brembilla-Perrot B, Terrier de la Chaise A, Pichene M, Pernot C, Cherrier F. 1986. Valeur diagnostique du test à l'Isuprel dans les tachycardies d'effort. Arch Mal Coeur 3: 309–313.

49. Sugrue DD, Holmes DR, Gersh BJ, Edwards WD, Mc Laran CJ, Wood DL, Osborn MJ, Hammil SL. 1984. Cardiac histologic findings in patients with life threatening ventricular arrhythmias of unknown origin. J Am Coll Cardiol 4: 952–957.

50. Wellens JJ. 1978. Value and limitation of programmed electrical stimulation of the heart in the study and treatment of tachycardias. Circulation 57: 845–853.

51. Touboul P, Claveyrolas R, Huerta F, Porte J, Delahaye JP. 1975. Tachycardie ventriculaire induite par des battements supraventriculaires prématurés à complexe QRS normal. Arch Mal Coeur 68: 969–976.

52. Zipes DP, Foster PR, Troup PJ, Pederson D. 1978. Atrial induction of ventricular tachycardia reentry versus triggered automaticity. Am J Cardiol 44: 1–8.

53. Wellens HJJ, Bar FW, Farre J, Ross DL, Weiner I, Vanagt EJ. 1980. Initiation and termination of ventricular tachycardia by supraventricular stimuli. Am J Cardiol 46: 576–582.

54. Cranefield PF. 1977. Action potentials, after potentials and arrhythmias. Circ Res 41: 415–423.

55. Yeh BK,, Lazzara R. 1977. Genesis of triggered and spontaneous automaticity by norepinephrine and isoproterenol in ventricular myocardium. Fed Proc 36: 1660–1668.

56. Leclercq JF, Rosengarten MD, Attuel P, Coumel P, Slama R. 1981. L'extrasystolie ventriculaire idiopathique: une parasystolie ventriculaire droite non protégée du rhythme sinusal. Arch Mal Coeur 74: 1249–1261.

57. Fontaine G, Guiraudon G, Frank R, Vedel J, Grosgogeat Y, Cabrol C, Facquet J. 1977. Stimulation studies and epicardial mapping in ventricular tachycardia: study of mechanisms and selection for surgery. In: Reentrant arrhythmias, H.E Kulbertus Ed., M.T.P. Publishers: Lancaster: 334–350.

58. Marcus FI, Fontaine G, Guiraudon G, Frank R, Laurenceau JL, Malergue MC, Grosgogeat Y. 1982. Right ventricular dysplasia: a report of 24 cases. Circulation 65: 384–399.
59. Pietras RJ, Mautner R, Denes P, Wu D, Dhingra R, Towne W, Rosen KM. 1977. Chronic recurrent right and left ventricular tachycardia: comparison of clinical and angiographic findings. Am J Cardiol 40: 32–37.
60. Kennedy HL, Pescarmona JE, Bouchard RJ, Goldberg RJ, Caralis DG. 1982. Objective evidence of occult myocardial dysfunction in patients with frequent ventricular ectopy without clinically apparent heart disease. Am Heart J 104: 57–65.
61. Morgera T, Salvi A, Alberti E, Silvestri F, Camerini F. Morphological findings in apparently idiopathic ventricular tachycardia. An echocardiographic haemodynamic and histologic study. Eur Heart 6: 323–334.
62. Vignola PA, Aonuma K, Swaye PS, Rozanski JJ, Blanstein RL, Benson J, Gosselin AJ, Lister JW. 1984. Clinically silent myocarditis and ventricular tachycardia. Circulation 70 (II): 403 (abstract).
63. Strain JE, Grose RM, Factor SM, Fisher ID. 1983. Result of endomyocardial biopsy in patients with spontaneous ventricular tachycrdia but without apparent structural heart disease. Circulation 68: 1171–1181.
64. Van Hoogenhuyze D, Olsen E, Crook B, Van de Brand M. 1981. Myocardial biopsy in patients with ventricular tachycardia. Am J Cardiol 47: 499 (abstract).
65. Dungan WT, Garson A Jr, Gillette PC. 1981. Arrhythmogenic right ventricular dysplasia: a cause of ventricular tachycardia in children with apparently normal hearts. Am Heart J 102: 745–750.
66. James TN, Marilley RJ, Marriot HJL. 1975. De subitaneis mortibus. XI. Young girl with palpitations. Circulation 51: 743–748.
67. Kennedy HL, Whitlock JA, Sprague M, Kennedy LJ Buckingham TA, Golberg RJ. 1985. Long term follow-up of asymptomatic healthy subjects with frequent and complex ventricular ectopy. N Engl J Med 312: 193–197.

9. Right ventricular dysplasias

G. FONTAINE*, F. FONTALIRAN*, E. MARTIN DE LA SALLE**,
A. PAVIE***, C. CABROL, G. CHOMETTE and Y. GROSGOGEAT
* Service de Rythmologie et de Stimulation Cardiaque, du Professeur
Y. Grosgogeat, Hopital Jean Rostand, 39 rue Jean Le Galleu, 94200 Ivry, France
** Service d'Anatomo-Pathologie, du Professeur G. Chomette,
CHU Pitie-Salpetriere, 47 Boulevard de l'Hôpital, 75013 Paris, France
*** Service de Chirurgie Cardiovasculaire, Service du Pr. Cabrol,
CHU Pitie-Salpetriere, 93 Boulevard d l'Hôpital, 75013 Paris, France

Definition

The term 'arrhythmogenic right ventricular dysplasia' has been proposed in 1977 during an attempt to classify 3 cases of ventricular tachycardia resistant to medical treatment and surgically cured [1]. In these patients, the surgical treatment which consisted of a simple ventriculotomy performed in the area of origin of ventricular tachycardia [2] proved to be effective. The surgical procedure was guided by epicardial mapping. The pathological and histological studies of two adult cases of Uhl anomaly has been reported one year later in two patients suffering from chronic recurrent ventricular tachycardia [3]. In a review of the antiarrhythmic surgery in 1979, the pathology and histology of arrhythmogenic right ventricular dysplasia are mentioned and briefly described from the result of direct observation and histological study of peroperative samples.

All of them showed the appearance of a thick layer of fatty tissue and fibrosis in right ventricular regions in which the wall was particularly thin [4]. In the middle of this tisue some strands of surviving cardiomyocytes partially degenerated could be seen. The histological structure of this tissue was compatible with the electrophysiological phenomena of ventricular postexcitation observed by epicardial mapping, endocavitary electrophysiological studies, and from the surface tracing [1, 2, 5–8]. On a more general approach, the term 'right ventricular dysplasia' reviewed in 1982 incorporated other alterations mainly located at the level of the right ventricular myocardium including Uhl's anomaly, and not obligatorily associated to cardiac arrhythmias [9]. However, the differences between ventricular dysplasia and Uhl's anomaly are opposed both from a clinical and histological standpoint, although at this latter level some similarities were observed [10]. Analogies between histological findings and mechanism of the ventricular tachycardia in both arrhythmogenic right ventricular dysplasia and the border zone of myocardial infarction have been underlined in 1984. These two completely different clinical conditions are in agreement with the appearance and the dynamic behaviour of delayed potentials [11]. In a recent paper based on three complete heart histology, we have added lipomatosis cordis with the preceding entities [12]. In a more recent editorial, this concept has been further extended [13].

This work deals with observations obtained from seven total hearts with right ventricular dysplasia, suggest a new classification of these cases from a pathological and histological standpoint [13].

Origin of the entire hearts

In a series of 7 patients constituting the background of this work, one patient (N° 4) previously operated died after 6 years, of a noncardiac cause. Another entire heart has been more recently obtained in three patients (N° 1, 2, 3). This was related to the fact that the fulguration procedure, which is generally extremely well tolerated, has been extended to the treatment of critical cases beyond operability, in which the general condition was from the beginning extremely poor. This was particularly the case of two patients who died, one of a noncardiac cause (N° 2), i.e. severe pulmonary infection present before the fulguration procedure; the other (N° 3) had a final evolution of a severe form of the disease in which it was not possible to evaluate the effect of the fulguration procedure. However, at the beginning of our experience a third patient died of low cardiac output during a fulguration session when the haemodynamic coverage was not properly achieved (N° 1). This attempt was indicated for recurrences of rapid ventricular tachycardia seven years after an effective antiarrhythmic surgical treatment.

Two hearts were from patients who have had heart transplants and in whom a primary cardiomyopathy led to congestive cardiac failure combined with ventricular rhythm disorders. One developed progressive cardiac failure (N° 6). The N° 5 patient's brother died suddenly.

In one case of Uhl's anomaly (N° 7) the death in the hospital allowed a necropsic examination. This case which has been already partially reported [3] has been added to this series in order to rediscuss its relationship with dysplasia.

The aim of this retropective study is to compare the pathological and histological features obtained from these seven hearts which confirm the previously reported data of macroscopic and microscopic level but which also introduce new ones. We will try to delineate the limits of a new series of pathological entities in order to underline the wide spectrum of pathological situations which are entering the quite confusing boundaries, including the different forms of arrhythmogenic right ventricular dysplasia, adipomatosis cordis, idiopathic dilated cardiomyopathy and Uhl's anomaly.

Pathological study

The pathological study of these seven cases shows:
– Qualitative data which are present in all of them.
– Some particularities specific for some of them.

Macroscopic abnormalities

Right cavities dilatation
It is mainly located at the level of the right ventricle and could be appreciated between 20 to 40%. The fresh specimen had the same aspect seen during antiarrhythmic surgery, at the time of haemodynamic discharge, as the free wall of the right ventricle in its mid portion. This free wall is almost completely covered by abnormal fatty tissue hiding the normal brown-red aspect of the subepicardial normal myocardium. Only the area located at the anterior aspect of the right ventricle seems normal.

Thinness of the right ventricular myocardium
After a section, this wall is particularly impressive because of the thinness of the myocardium, ranging around one millimeter instead of the three millimeters which are generally observed in a normal free right ventricular wall. The trabeculations seem more marked, which could be probably the result of the decrease in thickness of the parietal wall. In some area, especially in the infundibulum, the myocardium is almost completely absent and is almost exclusively replaced by abnormal fatty tissue (N° 1). The layers of this abnormal adipose tissue have the same thickness through the wall. This adipose tissue contains small arteries which are clearly visible and more frequent and of larger diameter than what it would have been possible to find in normal adipose tissue observed in some area of the heart like the AV grooves.

Dense subendocardial fibrosis
This is the most striking new observation. Zones of dense whitish fibrosis with polycyclic boundary are found on the endocardium of the right ventricle in the paraseptal area of the apex, over some trabeculations; and also on the moderator band (N° 1, 3, 6). This fibrosis appears in a completely unpredictable way on myocardium which looks otherwise completely normal. Its topography is not related to the dysplastic zones. After cut, this fibrotic tissue looks to be set down on the endocardium which appears as an abrupt localised increase in its thickness.

Trabeculations
The trabeculations of the right ventricle look particularly visible and hypertrophied. Especially the moderator band prolonged by the conus muscle is clearly

individualized. The first ones could explain some patterns obtained during the angiography, like fissuring aspect of the infundibular area, the second could explain the lacunar picture sometimes observed on angiographies in the infundibular area (N° 1, 2, 3).

However, as indicated above, this could be related to the fact that the normal structures are definitely emphasized because of the thinness of the parietal wall (N° 6).

The right ventricular endocardium
In most of the cases it looks normal, with exception of some areas of fibrosis already mentioned. However in one case (N° 2), on the fresh specimen the central part of the endocardium showed a yellow-orange homogeneous colour. The histology showed that it was the result of fibrous (and not adipose) infiltration of all the endocardium without any plaque of fibrosis in this particular area.

The left ventricular wall
In two cases (N° 4, 5) the free wall of the left ventricle is covered by a thick layer of fatty tissue ranging from 20 to 50% of the wall. In one case (N° 4), this layer of fatty tissue is quite regular all over the left ventricle, in the other (N° 5) the adipose tissue seems to penetrate deeply toward the endocardium in some places.

Microscopic analysis

Histological data common to all the cases

They are located at the level of the right ventricle

The right ventricular wall
Most of the ventricular wall is constituted by a particular kind of tissue. At the first view, it is possible to see adipocytes of normal structure both in size and pattern. They constitute 30 to 90% of the wall thickness (Fig. 1-A and B, Fig. 2-A). However, from place to place, their limits are strengthened by zones of fibrosis which are thick and isolated. In the middle of this tissue, it is possible to see some strands of cardiomyocytes of varying size, sometimes interconnected,

---

Figure 1. (Case N° 3). A: Typical aspect of arrhythmogenic right ventricular dysplasia at the level of the right ventricle. The endocardium is on the right side, the epicardium on the left. Strands of cardiomyocytes are upcoming from the subendocardial layers toward the middle of the wall within fibroadipose tissue and turning around two vessels with a normal wall (G = 40×). B: Enlarged view of the connecion between the strands of cardiomyocytes and the subendocardial muscle (G = 120×). C: In the same patient, it is possible to observe on the left ventricle interstitial fibrosis which is surrounding strands of cardiomyocytes cut transversally (G = 320×).

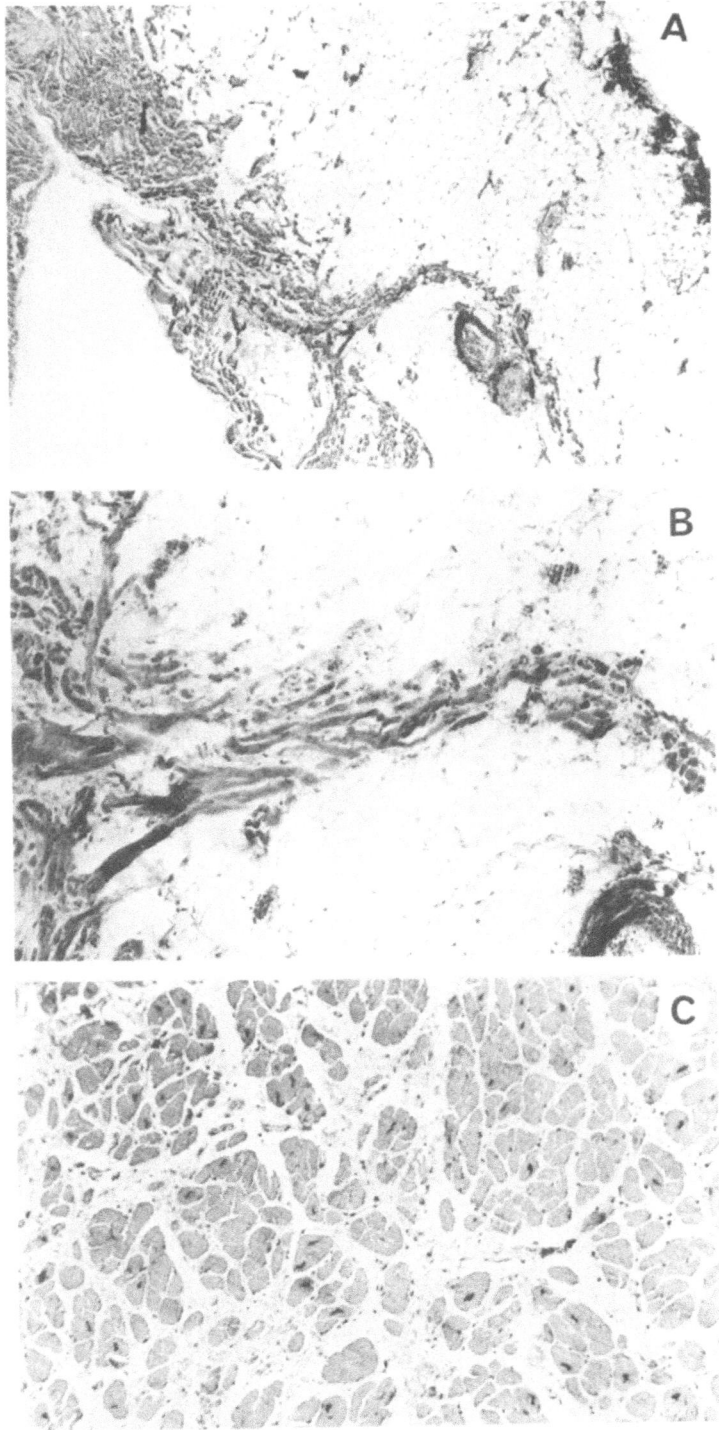

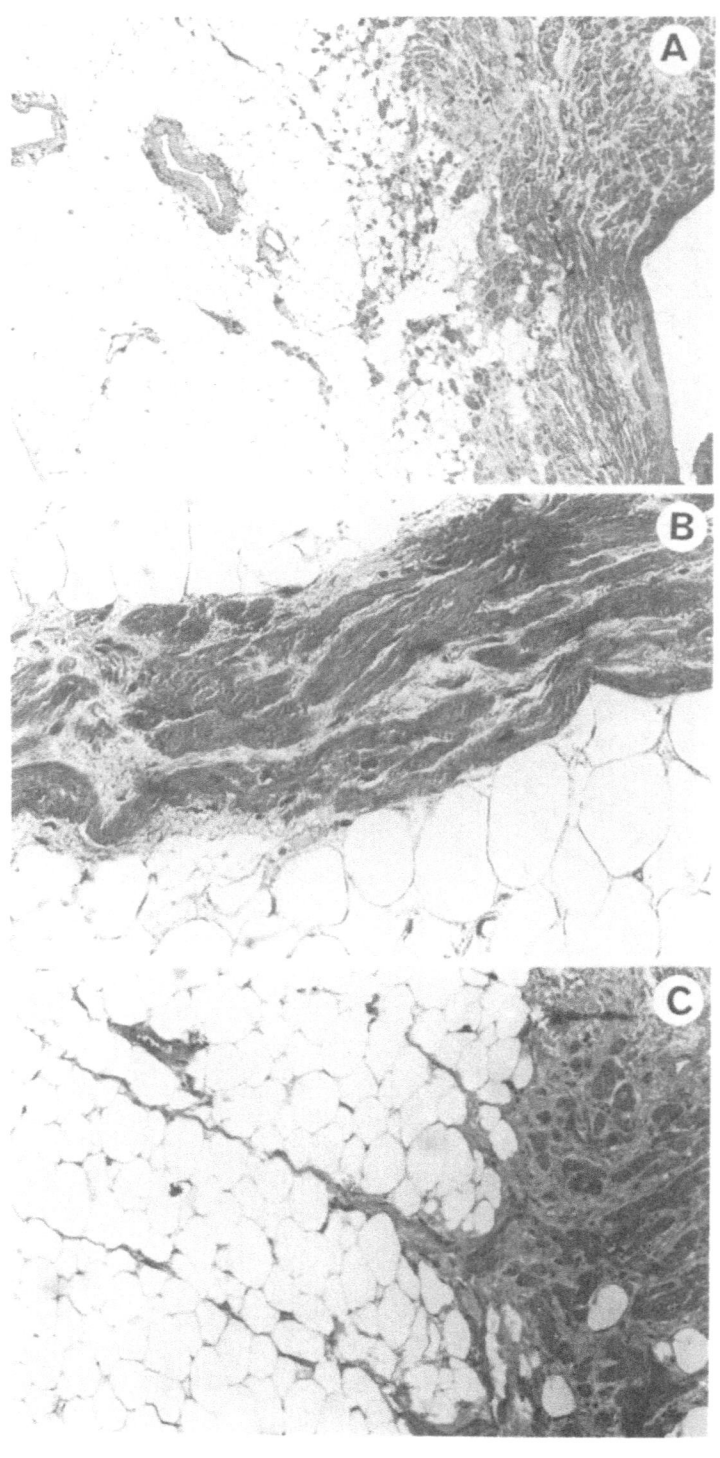

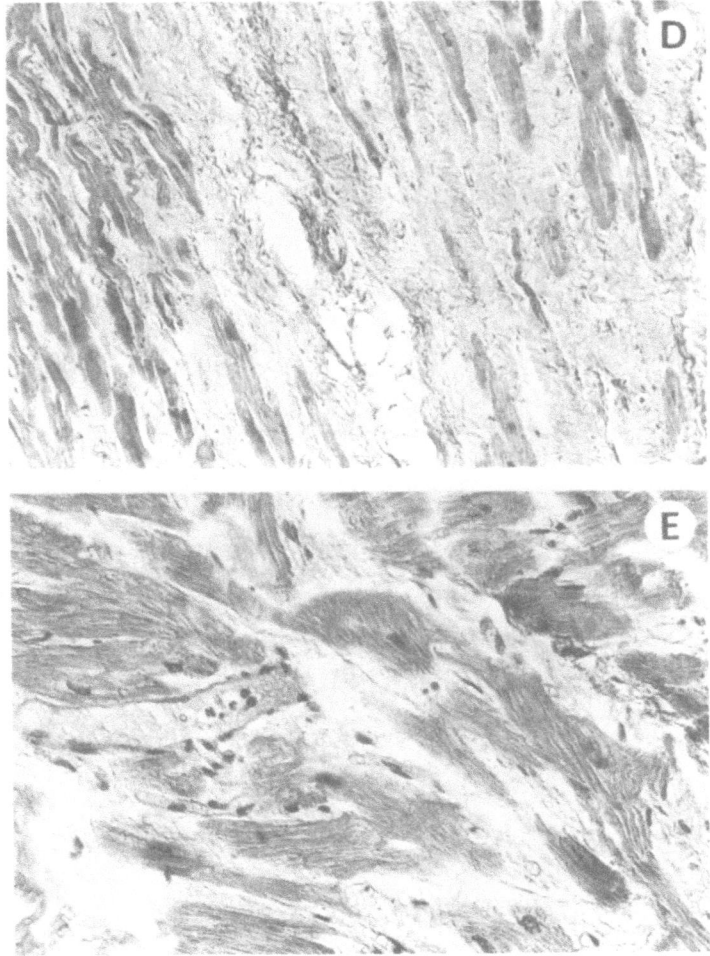

Figure 2. (Case N° 2). A: Typical aspect of arrhythmogenic right ventricular dysplasia within subendocardial layers and almost complete disappearance of cardiomyocytes in the mediomural and subepicardial layers. One of the two vessels has a media which is slightly thickened. Note the relative importance of fibrosis compared to the data presented in Fig. 1 (G = 40×). B: Layers of cardiomyocytes imbeded in a zone of fibrous tissue which is quite moderate when it is located adjacent to adipose cells (G = 320×). C: Strands of fibrous tissue running between adipocytes. In the middle of the fibrous tissue, it is possible to recognize some cardiomyocytes. Note also the sclerosis which is surrounding the strands of cardiomyocytes at the lower part of this figure (G = 130×). D: Same patient: left ventricle. Interstitial fibrosis which is quite important. Strands of cardiomyocytes exhibit signs of degenerescence with irregular aspect of cardiomyocytes in the inferior part of the figure (G = 130×). E: Acidophilic nuclei with nuclear dystrophy and some adipocytes. Same sample at a higher amplification (G = 320×).

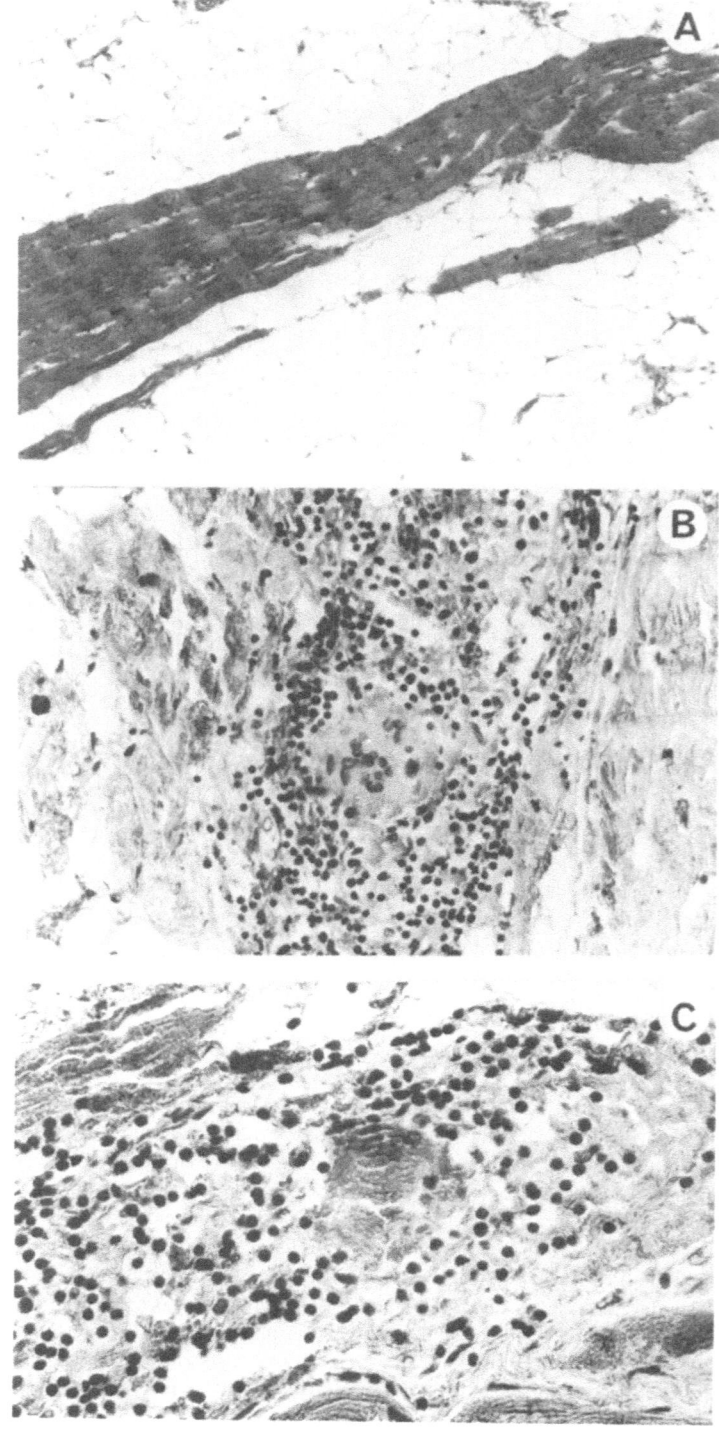

Figure 3. (Case N° 1). A: Strands of cardiomyocytes cut longitudinally in the middle of adipose tissue. On this figure, the main characteristics of right ventricular dysplasia and quasi-total absence of interstitial fibrosis. B: Same patient: thick fibrosis with existence of large number of lymphocytes in the middle of the picture. It is possible to see some giant cells with asteroïd nodules (G = 320×). C: Lymphoplasmocytary infiltration. Myocytes on the way of degenerescence (G = 320×).

other times in obvious connection with subendocardial myocytes (Fig. 1-A). These cardiomyocytes are constituted by one or several cellular layers, are or not surrounded by a small amount of fibrosis (Fig. 2-B and Fig. 3-A). In other places they are deeply imbeded in fibrous tissue (Fig. 2-D).

They could show or not nuclear or cytoplasmic distorsions. It is, finally, possible to observe in all cases, in the middle of the adipose tissue, obviously abnormal vessels with a thickened wall (Fig. 4, Fig. 5-B, Fig. 6-C). These vessels are frequently constituted by two or three layers of leiomyocytes of different directions. Sometimes, the thickness of the wall is such that the lumen is difficult to see. The leiomyocytes of the vascular wall generally show a longitudinal organization parallel to the main axis of the vessel. When the lumen is clearly visible, it is frequently excentrated (Fig. 5-B).

The endocardium

The plaques of thick fibrosis which are particularly striking during the macroscopic examination are constituted by the increase in the thickness of the subendocardial tissue by connective tissue. In some places, cardiomyocytes are imbedded in fibrosis and in that case they show abnormalities in the size of nuclei

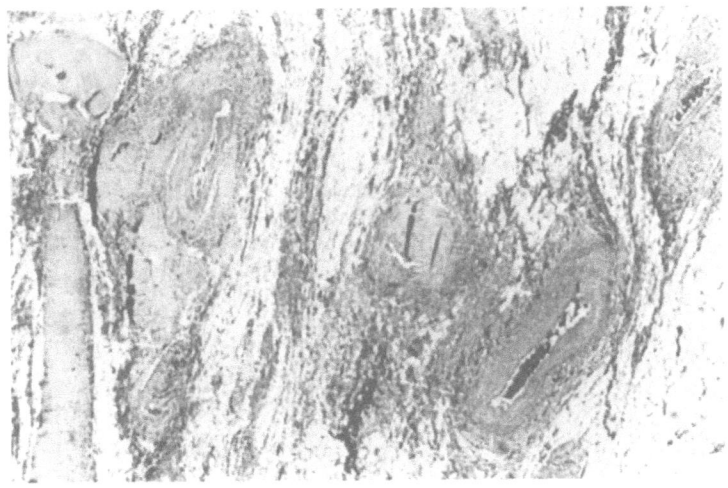

Figure 4. (Case N° 4). Case of adipomatosis cordis with major infiltration of fatty tissue within the left ventricle. Appearance of vessels with a very thick media. Many areas of interstitial fibrosis are oriented toward a particular direction (G = 40×).

122

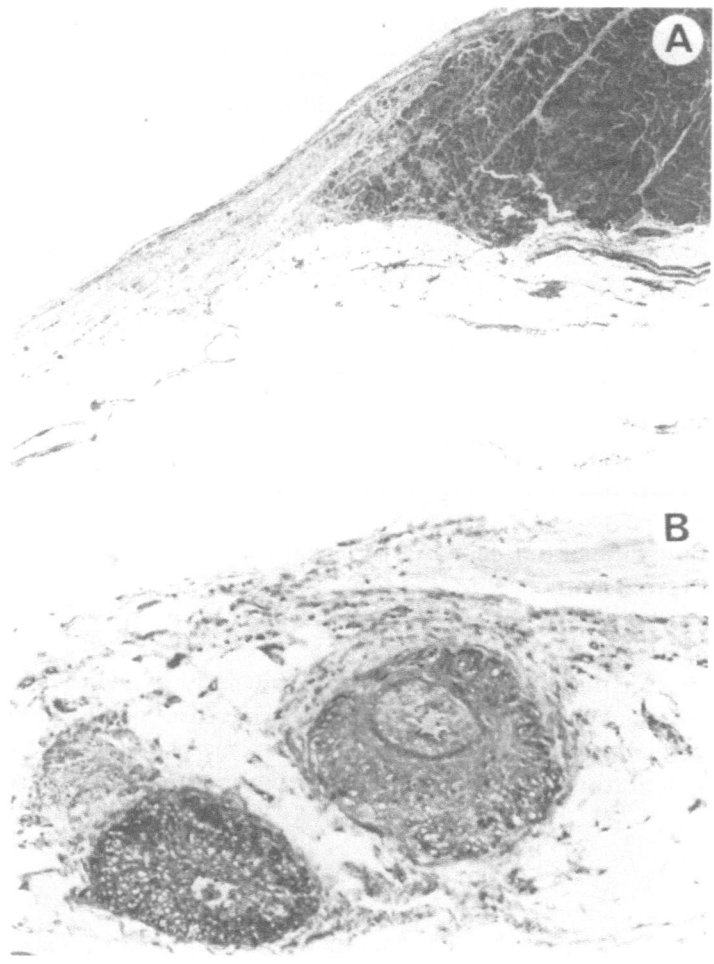

Figure 5. (Case N° 7). A: Typical aspect of Uhl's anomaly with a complete interruption of myocardium which is replaced by fibroadipose tissue with a complete absence of cardiomyocytes within this tissue. Note the major thinness of the wall (G = 40×). B: Same patient. Appearance in the abnormal zone of two vessels with a very thickened media. Note also the major thickness of the intima with the internal elastic boundary which is clearly visible (G = 120×).

→

Figure 6. (Case N° 6). A: Note the very irregular aspect of some cardiomyocytes during fibrous degenerescence. Within an area of major amount of connective tissue, the fibrosis is quite irregular and some lymphoplasmocytes can be seen (G = 320×). B: Strands of myocytes interspersed with areas of fibrous tissue and dystrophic nuclei (G = 520×). C: Large area of subendocardial fibrosis which is crossed by a very thick vessel in the adjacent subendocardium (G = 120×).

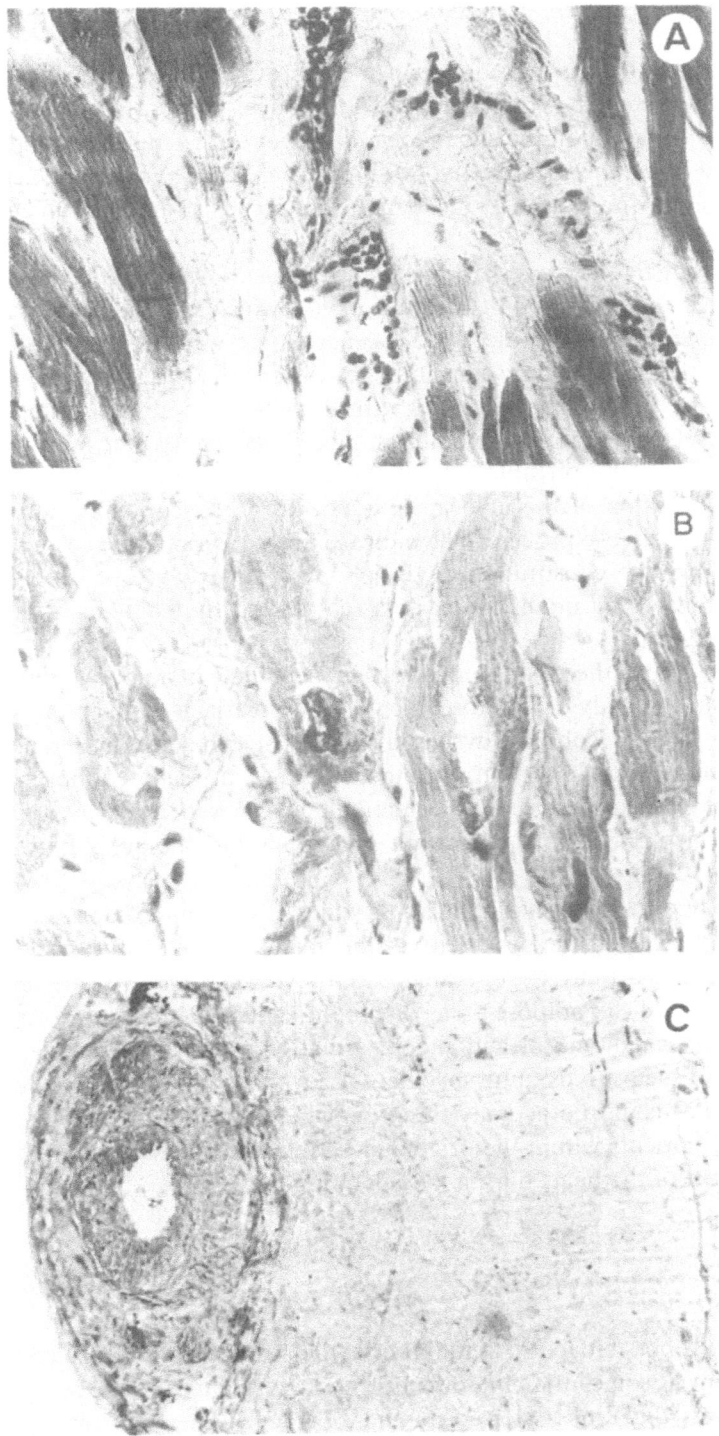

and cytoplasmic structure. In some places, no cardiomyocyte can be seen (Fig. 6-C).

In other areas, there is a predominance of fibrous tissue. The density of this connective tissue could be very variable. The myocytes located beneath the thick fibrous tissue are found in the subendocardial layer of the right ventricular free wall. In some cases, these cardiomyocytes are completely normal, but generally they are frequently infiltrated by the conjonctive tissue upcoming from endocardial layers (Fig. 1-C).

We think that these strands of cardiomyocytes surviving within the adipose tissue are only the remnants of cardiomyocytes which have developed a progressive degeneration with time. This degeneration is most of the time adipose and in some other cases mainly constituted by fibrous tissue [10]. This hypothesis is reinforced by the finding of vessels with a thickened wall [10]. These distal coronary vessels are surprising by their number and their aspect, within such a kind of fatty tissue. It is possible to think that these vessels were originally aimed at the vascularisation of the myocardium and have been modified during the evolution of the disease process. The increase in their number is only apparent. On the contrary the constitution of the parietal leiomyocytes is probably the result of a nonspecific modification as a reaction to the changes in the local circulatory behaviour.

The appearance of these cardiomyocytes in the middle of adipose tissue makes a very typical anomaly. Therefore the term dysplasia is appropriate, since, according to Stanley Robbins, dysplasia signifies stricto sensu a 'deranged development'. However, in the current medical usage, the same author indicates that it is also used to describe either epithelial or mesenchymal tissue, which shows atypical proliferation as a result of chronic inflammatory or irritating process [14].

Finally, the pericardium has a thickness which is variable from case to case.

Despite the fact that the specificity of this histological structure which combines strands of partially degenerated cardiomyocytes bordered by layers of fibrosis in the middle of adipose tissue due to the replacement of cardiomyocytes constituting the mediomural and subepicardial layers, it needs to be further elucidated and seems to us quite specific. Discovery of this structure within the dysplastic zones could be actually the only coherent feature which permits to classify these patients within the original description exclusively based on macroscopic aspect of the heart during the operation [1].

Specific features of each case

In case N° 1 it is possible to see at the level of the right cavity and also on the left ventricular cavity, some inflammatory infiltrates with giant cells, the cytoplasm of which contains sometimes asteroïd nodules (Fig. 3). Other infiltrates are constituted only by lymphoplasmocyte cells, infiltrating either the fat or the muscular and fibrous tissue (Fig. 3-C).

Case N° 2 seems to be quite particular due to definite large participation of the connective tissue in addition to the wide spectrum of its pattern (Fig. 2-A, C, D). In some cases, the fibrous tissue is thick and hyalin. In other cases, it shows a dense pattern, in other places, this connective tissue is very weak and discrete. In addition, on the left side, in some places, data suggesting primary cardiomyopathy are found and it is possible to note the presence of lymphoplasmocyte infiltrates (Fig. 2-E). The pattern of primary cardiomyopathy is however very localised and this case could be on the border line between dysplasia and idiopathic dilated cardiomyopathy.

Case N° 3: in addition to the typical pattern of arrhythmogenic right ventricular dysplasia, some layers of fatty tissue are penetrating deeply in the base of the septum.

In case N° 4 in which ethylic liver cirrhosis is present, it is observed a fatty infiltration of myocardium which also involves the left ventricle. At this level, myocytes are quite irregular, imbeded in a hyalin fibrous tissue. However, it is obviously possible to consider that this patient could have had an ethylic cardiomyopathy.

In case N° 6, it is possible to see the infiltration of fatty tissue within the left ventricle, accompanied by some extent of fibrosis.

In the case of Uhl's anomaly, N° 7, a very large amount of fibrous tissue is found in the subendocardial area (Fig. 5-A). The pericardium seems also thickened. Between these two layers, there is no strand of cardiomyocytes. However, it is possible to observe many vessels which are obviously abnormal. Some of them cut obliquely, could suggest the pattern of cardiomyocytes, which could be located within the relatively small amount of fatty tissue separating the two areas of the epicardium and the subendocardium.

Table 1. ARVD = Arrhythmogenic right ventricular dysplasia. VT = Ventricular Tachycardia. IDC = Idiopathic dilated cardiomyopathy.

	Diagnosis	Arrhythmia	Comments
1. DUV	ARVD	VT	Operated for VT 7 years previously
2. MIC	ARVD	VT	Involvement of the left ventricle
3. ALI	ARVD	VT	Involvement of both ventricles
4. GON	ARVD	VT	Operated for VT 7 years previously
5. LEF	IDC	O	Post tranplant (sudden death in family)
6. GUY	IDC	O	Recipient heart removed at cardiac transplantation
7. GRO	Uhl	VT	Adult form of Uhl's Anomaly + VT

Comments

The study of these seven complete hearts of right ventricular dysplasia finally shows some data which are more varied than those which have been only deduced from peroperative samples, which were limited to the area of origin of ventricular tachycardia.

It is therefore possible to individualise a series of histological patterns from which it is more appropriate to understand the cardiological description concerning the clinical description of these patients, their electrocardiographic appearance, their echocardiographic and angiocardiographic features, etc . . .

It is, however, necessary to keep in mind that these subgroups are probably artificial oversimplifications, and that there should exist an intermediate spectrum between the previously individualised types, leading to a wide spectrum of possibilities [15].

Arrhythmogenic right ventricular dysplasia

This syndrome is characterised by a normal left ventricle from a pathological and histological standpoint [9]. The free wall of the right ventricle is covered by an important layer of fatty tissue. The amount of myocardium looks quite small located in the subendocardial layers, and is striking by its small amount as compared with the importance of fatty tissue due to the degeneration of myocytes which are sometimes able to survive within the fat. We have seen that this degeneration of myocytes is mainly involving the subepicardial layers. Some strands of cardiomyocytes partially degenerated are still present within the fat. They show a particular structure, exchanging connections with the normal subendocardial layers. These fibers are almost always surrounded by a thin layer of fibrous tissue. However, some plaques of thick fibrous tissue with polycyclic limit could be observed from place to place on the endocardium. Within this fibrous tissue, it is frequently possible to observe some strands of surviving cardiomyocytes.

In right ventricular dysplasia, the topography of the lesions is typical: they are mainly located in the places which have been called the triangle of dysplasia, i.e. the infundibulum, the apex and the diaphragmatic zone located below the tricuspid valve [9]. The natural evolution of this disease is not clearly known. From the histological standpoint, the comparison between several cases and the histology suggesting several degrees of evolution in the same heart has suggested a pathogenetic mechanism [10].

The review of the literature allows us to find histological description of what we have called myofat. For instance, the case of one patient operated for ventricular arrhythmias [16] and a case intitled hypoplasia of the right ventricular myocardium [17] were reported. Others suggest the retrospective diagnosis of the disease, as in the report of Virmani et al who presented in 1982 the data concerning three patients who died suddenly during effort (two of them during sportive effort) and in whom no symptoms were reported before death [18]. In these cases, the thinness of the myocardium of the right ventricle showed features which were extremely suggestive, and were compared with previous reports concerning Uhl's anomaly. However, Virmani et al stressed that the amount of fatty infiltration observed in their cases has not been found in cases of Uhl's anomaly. In the patients in whom a typical pattern of arrhythmogenic right ventricular dysplasia showed an increase of the thickness of the myocardial wall, there is a definite amount of adipose tissue, while in Uhl's anomaly there is a definite decrease in the thickness of the right myocardial wall which explains the term 'parchment heart' [19].

Arrhythmogenic right ventricular dysplasia with left ventricular involvement

In our first cases [1] we were struck by the fact that in some patients it was possible to see abnormal potential on the epicardium of the left ventricle during epicardial mapping in sinus rhythm, despite the fact that this ventricle looked normal. The dysplastic process could therefore invade the subepicardial layers of the left ventricle, especially in the left paraseptal areas both on the anterior and posterior wall. In one of our cases (N° 3) strands of adipose tissue were clearly visible in the lower part of the interventricular septum. In another patient, it was possible to see the definite involvement of fibrous tissue within the left subendocardial layers.

However it is impressive to see the relatively large amount of fibrous tissue on the subendocardial left side of the heart, as compared to the predominant transformation in fatty tissue on the subepicardial and mediomural layers on the right ventricle. The same pathological process could therefore lead to differentiation mainly oriented toward the transformation in fibrous tissue on the left side, and toward adipose tissue on the right. The distinction between primary cardiomyopathy could, therefore, be quite difficult and could be suspected clinically only if there is a definite involvement of the left ventricular function [20–24].

On the other hand, it has not yet been possible for us to see a case in whom subendocardial sclerosis of the left ventricle could be found with the same isolated pattern at the level of the right ventricle. This situation could be at least theoretically suggested by some forms of primary ventricular cardiomyopathy or myocarditis with arrhythmogenic foci, located in the right ventricle [12, 25].

Adipomatosis cordis

With the exception of adipomatosis found in the obese people or old women, the 'essential adipomatosis' is characterised by fatty degeneration or fatty infiltration of myocardium which is located in a homogenous pattern on both ventricles [26]. The aspects observed in the right ventricle are quite comparable to those of arrhythmogenic right ventricular dysplasia [12].

At the level of the left ventricle, it is possible to observe a deep penetration of fat within layers of myocytes with a thick layer of fatty tissue at the epicardial level. However, in these cases, fibrosis is minor. The topography of this adipose tissue suggests that the fat is extending toward the mediomural and even subendocardial layers. In our experience, the most predominant clinical pattern was related to an isolated cardiac failure suggesting a familial cardiomyopathy in one case, combined in the other with runs of right ventricular tachycardia.

Ventricular tachycardia originating from the high part of the right septum

On a heart which looks clinically normal, the arrhythmia is characterised in most cases by ventricular extrasystoles which could be very symptomatic and badly tolerated. The morphology of these extrasystoles is typical, they activate the ventricles according to an axis oriented from upward to downward [27]. They are generally considered as benign. In some cases, these extrasystoles could increase in frequency, could lead to bigeminism, doublets, triplets. At a higher degree, it is possible to observe runs of paroxysmal attacks of ventricular tachycardia of short duration [28, 29]. In very rare cases, it is possible to observe episodes of nonsustained ventricular tachycardia which could with time lead to sustained episodes, over several hours, and even several days. The myocardium being basically healthy, these attacks do not seem to be life-threatening but sometimes they could be extremely incapacitating [30]. Like the extrasystoles previously described, with which they are almost always associated, these tachycardias are characterised by a typical pattern with a major R wave in Lead III and VF [29].

These tachycardias are generally impossible to initiate by programmed pacing, and it is also very rare to stop them with the same technique of stimulation. Few cases which have undergone epicardial mapping have shown the presence of delayed or fragmented potentials not only around the site of origin of the arrhythmia but also far away on the free wall of the right ventricle [31]. We are aware of three cases, in whom this arrhythmia was studied over a long period of time, which have been finally considered as arrhythmogenic right ventricular dysplasia cases. One of them has even been operated by another group (L.S. Dreifus, personal communication, 1985). However, up to now we have not been able to examine the complete heart of a patient in this kind of category.

Uhl's anomaly

We have had the opportunity to observe some adult forms of Uhl's anomaly. Two hearts have been studied [3]. In this case, the main feature is a major dilatation of the right ventricular cavity, and secondly an extreme thinness of its wall, which is, in most of the cases, completely replaced by a tissue which is mainly fibrous, sometimes referred as 'parchment heart'. In our operated case, it was possible to see the flow of blood within the cavity. This fibrous tissue is mixed with some layers of adipocytes. The muscular tissue of the myocardium has almost completely disappeared on the anterior and lateral aspect of the right ventricular free wall, and it is only in the area of insertion of the tricuspid papillary muscle or the diaphragmatic aspect of the right ventricle that it is possible to find some layers of myocardium which are close to normal.

This situation looks close to the old description of the heart, which pertained to the Osler collection and was briefly described in his textbook on medicine published in 1920 [32] and which was displayed in the Museum of Pathology of the McGuill University of Montreal. This heart, which we have not been able to trace, has been probably lost during the fire which destroyed the department of Mary Abbott in the mid Sixties. However, credit has to be given to Dr Harold Segall from Montreal who made a very pleasant description of this specimen, which remains unique in the literature because the thinness of the wall was extending to the four chambers including the septum. The author did not hide his surprise to see that this patient, who died suddenly during a moderate effort walking up a smooth slope, was able to survive with such a heart up to his mid-forties [33].

Cases of Uhl's anomaly of the adult complicated by ventricular arrhythmias are quite rare [34]. However in addition to this generalised form involving all of the right ventricle, localised forms have been described which were located at the level of the pulmonary infundibulum or restricted to the anterior aspect of the right ventricle. For all these cases, the main feature was an extreme thinness of the myocardial wall suggesting the parchment heart, the relatively small amount of adipose tissue and the absence of myocardium in the areas involved by the disease process [35–39].

In most of these cases of arrhythmogenic right ventricle, the common denominator consists in the existence of an arrhythmogenic substrate which is located at the level of the right ventricle, and which is not related to coronary artery disease and of which the prognosis is mainly dependent on ventricular arrhythmia. We have seen the histopathological features which could explain the possibility of desynchronisation of ventricular activation leading to tachycardia and degeneration to ventricular fibrillation [40]. The fact that cardiomyocytes are dissociated is one of the main characteristics indispensible for the establishment of intramyocardial circus movement which could be observed at any level within the heart. The role played by fibrosis is particularly well known in the border zone of myocardial infarction scars. The role played by the infiltration of myocardium by fatty tissue is more recent and not so completely elucidated. In a superb synthesis, which shows their immense knowledge in the field of pathology and histoloy of cardiac arrhythmias, Bharati and Lev have underlined the probable role played by this tissue in a patient who died suddenly [15].

We have, for our part, been informed of what is accepted as sudden death in five patients in whom the diagnosis of arrhythmogenic right ventricular dysplasia or related syndrome has been established, and in whom only two have been resuscitated. Other groups have established a relation between sudden death in some young patients and some sportsmen and this disease [16, 18, 41].

In addition, some familial cases have been reported. Siblings are generally involved in the same disease [42–47].

This description of the main aspects of the arrhythmogenic right ventricle may suggest that there are some entities which could be individualised [48, 49]. However, some of them may only represent different aspects within the same disease process, of which the pathophysiological mechanisms and kinetics are presently incompletely understood.

Limitation of the study

This retrospective study is mainly limitated by the non systematic protocol used to study the anatomic and histologic specimens, and the way the samples were taken. It seems to us extremely important to go further in this study on the upcoming base, following pathological and histologcal approaches:
- Extension of the lesions at the level of the two ventricles and the septum which could be systematically studied.
- Topography of the lesion with special attention to both epicardium and endocardium.
- Nature and proportion of the main components: cardiomyocytes, fibrosis, adipose tissue.

It is, in fact, the quantitative character of these lesions and their spread all over the myocardium which are important to give more pathological and histological data, which are of the utmost importance to better understand the disease process of this fascinating subset of cardiomyopathies.

References

1. Fontaine G, Guiraudon G, Frank R, Vedel J, Grosgogeat Y, Cabrol C, Facquet J. 1977. Stimulation Studies and Epicardial Mapping in Ventricular Tachycardia: Study of Mechanisms and Selection for Surgery. In – Reentrant Arrhythmias – H.E. Kulbertus Ed. MTP Pub. Lancaster: p. 334–350.

2. Frank R, Fontaine G, Vedel J, Mialet G, Sol C, Guiraudon G, Grosgogeat Y. 1978. Electrocardiologie de quatre cas de dysplasie ventriculaire droite arythmogene. Arch Mal Coeur 71: 963–972.

3. Vedel J, Frank R, Fontaine G, Drobinski G, Guiraudon G, Brocheriou C, Grosgogeat Y. 1978. Tachycardies ventriculaires recidivantes et ventricule droit papyrace de l'adulte. (A propos de deux observations anatomo-cliniques). Arch Mal Coeur 71: 973–981.

4. Fontaine G, Guiraudon G, Frank R. 1979. Mechanism of Ventricular Tachycardia with and without Associated Chronic Myocardial Ischaemia: Surgical Management Based on Epicardial Mapping. In – Innovations in Diagnosis and Management of Cardiac Arrhythmias – O.S. Narula Ed. William & Wilkins Pub. Baltimore: p. 516–545.

5. Fontaine G, Guiraudon G, Frank R. 1978. Intramyocardial Conduction Defects in Patients Prone to Ventricular Tachycardia. I – The Postexcitation Syndrome in Sinus Rhythm. In – Management of Ventricular Tachycardia. Role of Mexiletine – E. Sandoe, D.G. Julian, J.W. Bell Ed. Excerpta Medica Pub. Amsterdam: p. 39–55.

6. Fontaine G, Guiraudon G, Frank R. 1978. Intramyocardial Conduction Defects in Patients Prone to Ventricular Tachycardia. II – A Dynamic Study of the Post-Excitation Syndrome. In – Management of Ventricular Tachycardia. Role of Mexiletine – E. Sandoe, D.G. Julian, J.W. Bell Ed. Excerpta Medica Pub. Amsterdam: p. 56–66.

7. Fontaine G, Guiraudon G, Frank R. 1978. Intramyocardial Conduction Defects in Patients Prone to Ventricular Tachycardia. III – The Post-Excitation Syndrome during Ventricular Tachycardia. In – Management of Ventricular Tachycardia. Role of Mexiletine – E. Sandoe, D.G. Julian, J.W. Bell Ed. Excerpta Medica Pub. Amsterdam: p. 67–79.

8. Fontaine G, Guiraudon G, Frank R, Tereau Y, Fillette F, Chomette G, Grosgogeat Y. 1982. The Pathophysiology of Chronic Disturbances of Ventricular Rhythm. In – Cardiac Electrophysiology Today – A. Masoni, P. Alboni Ed. Academic Press Pub. London: p. 251–271.

9. Marcus FI, Fontaine G, Guiraudon G, Frank R, Laurenceau JL, Malergue MC, Grosgogeat Y. 1982. Right Ventricular Dysplasia: a Report of 24 Cases. Circulation 65: 384–399.

10. Fontaine G, Tereau Y, Frank R, Guiraudon G, Fillette F, Chomette G, Grogogeat Y. 1982. Dysplasie ventriculaire droite arythmogene et maladie de Uhl. Arch Mal Coeur 75: 361.

11. Fontaine G, Frank R, Tereau Y, Fillette F, Chomette G, Rossi L, Grosgogeat Y. 1984. Correlazioni anatomo-patologiche ed elettrofisiologiche nei pazienti affetti da tachicardie ventricolari croniche recidivanti. In – Le nuove frontiere delle aritmie – F. Furlanello ed. Piccin Pub. Padova: p. 253–269.

12. Chomette G, Koulibaly M, Linares-Cruz E, Fontaine G, Grosgogeat Y, Cabrol C. 1986. Dysplasie arythmogene. Parentees nosologiques avec le syndrome de Uhl et la lipomatose. A propos ce trois observations anatomo-cliniques. Arch Anat Cytol Path 34: 46–50.

13. Fontaine G, Fontaliran F, Chomette G. 1986. Il ventricolo destro aritmogeno. G Ital Cardiol 16: 1–3.

14. Robbins SL, Cotran RS, Kumar V. 1984. Pathologic Basis of Disease – W.B. Saunders Co Pub. Philadelphia: p. 34.

15. Bharati S, Lev M. 1983. Arrhythmogenic Ventricles. Pace 6: 1035.

16. Olsson SB, Edvardsson N, Emanuelsson H, Enestrom S. 1982. A Case of Arrhythmogenic Right Ventricular Dysplasia with Ventricular Fibrillation. Clin Chem 5: 591–596.

17. Bharati S, Feld A.W., Bauernfeind RA, Kattus AA, Lev M. 1983. Hypoplasia of the Right Ventricular Myocardium with Ventricular Tachycardia. Arch Pathol Lab Med 107: 249–253.

18. Virmani R, Robinowitz M, Clark MA, McAllister HA. 1982. Sudden Death and Partial Absence of the Right Ventricular Myocardium. Arch Pathol Lab Med 106: 163–167.

19. Uhl HS. 1952. A Previously Undescribed Congenital Malformation of the Heart: Almost Total Absence of the Myocardium of the Right Ventricle. Bull John Hopkins Hosp 91: 197–205.

20. Reiter MJ, Smith WM, Gallagher JJ. 1983. Clinical Spectrum of Ventricular Tachycardia with Left Bundle Branch Morphology. Am J Cardiol 51: 113–121.

132

21. Rowland E, McKenna WJ, Sugrue DD, Barclay R, Foale RA, Krikler DM. 1984. Ventricular Tachycardia of Left Bundle Branch Block Configuration in Patients with Isolated Right Ventricular Dilatation. Clinical and Electrophysiological Features. Br Heart J 51: 15–25.
22. Cherrier F, Floquet J, Cuilliere M, Neimann JL. 1979. Les dysplasies ventriculaires droites. A propos de 7 observations. Arch Mal Coeur 72: 766–773.
23. Manyari DE, Klein GJ, Gulamhusein SS, Kostuk WJ, Boughner DR, Guiraudon G, Wyse DG, Mitchell LB. 1983. Arrhythmogenic Right Ventricular Dysplasia: a Generalized Cardiomyopathy. Circulation 68: 251–257.
24. Fitchett DH, Sugrue DD, Mac Arthur CG, Oakley CM. 1984. Right Ventricular Dilated Cardiomyopathy. Br Heart J 51: 25–30.
25. Trigano JA, Nasta H, Michaud JL, Houel J, Jouven JC, Jouve A, Torresani J. 1983. Tachycardie ventriculaire rebelle par dysplasie ventriculaire droite. Un cas de guerison chirurgicale rapporte a 6 ans de l'intervention. Arch Mal Coeur 76: 852–857.
26. Letac B, Tayot J, Barthes P. 1977. Infiltration graisseuse du coeur et maladie de Uhl. (A propos d'une observation de lipomatose cardiaque). Arch Mal Coeur 70: 107–113.
27. Rosenbaum MB. 1969. Classification of Ventricular Extrasystoles According to Form. J Electrocardiol 2: 289.
28. Gallavardin L. 1922. Extrasystole ventriculaire a paroxysmes tachycardiques prolonges. Arch Mal Coeur 15: 298.
29. Parkinson J, Papp C. 1947. Repetitive Paroxysmal Tachycardia. Br Heart J 9: 241.
30. Kennedy HL, Whitlock JA, Buckingham TA, Kennedy LJ, Goldberg RJ. 1983. Five to Ten Year Follow-up of Apparently Healthy Subjects with Frequent and Complex Ventricular Ectopy. Circulation 68: SUP-III, 107.
31. Fontaine G, Guiraudon G, Frank R, Tereau Y, Pavie A, Cabrol C, Chomette G, Grosgogeat Y. 1984. Surgical Management of Ventricular Tachycardia Not Related to Myocardial Ischemia. In – Tachycardias: Mechanisms, Diagnosis and Treatment – M.E. Josephson, H.J.J. Wellens Ed. Lea & Febiger Pub.: P. 451–473.
32. Osler. 1905. The Principles and Practices of Medicine – D. Appleton and Co. Pub. 1: 820.
33. Segall HN. 1950. Parchment Heart (Osler). Am Heart J 40: 948–950.
34. Bharati S, Ciraulo DA, Bilitch M, Rosen KM, Lev M. 1978. Inexcitable Right Ventricle and Bilateral Bundle Branch Block in Uhl's Disease. Circulation 57: 636–644.
35. Rizzon P. Sindrome di Uhl. 1965. Cuore e Circulazione 49: 121–135.
36. Suguira M, Hayashi T, Ueno K. 1970. Partial Absence of the Right Ventricular Muscle in an Aged. Jpn Heart J 11: 582–585.
37. Reeve R, Mac Donald CD. 1964. Partial Absence of the Right Ventricular Musculature: Partial Parchment Heart. Am J Cardiol 14: 415–419.
38. Gould L, Gutman B, Carrasco J, Lyon AF. 1967. Partial Absence of the Right Ventricular Musculature, a Congenital Lesion. Am J Med Sci 42: 636–641.
39. Montella S, Soresi V, Calo S. 1969. Absence partielle congenitale du myocarde ventriculaire droit chez le nourrisson (un cadre anatomo-clinique particulier de l'anomalie de Uhl). Arch Mal Coeur 62: 1183–1195.
40. Ursell PC, Fenoglio JJ, jr. 1982. Structural Basis of Ventricular Tachycardia. In – Ventricular Tachycarda. Mechanisms and Management – M.E. Josephson Ed. Futura Publishing Co. New York: p. 151.
41. Furlanello F, Bettini R, Cozzi F, Del Favero A, Disertori M, Vergara GS, Durante GB, Guarnerio M, Inama G, Thiene G. 1984. Ventricular Arrhythmias and Sudden Death in Athletics. Ann NY AcadSci 427: 253–279.
42. Froment R, Perrin A, Loire R, Dalloz CL. 1968. Ventricule droit papyrace du jeune adulte par dystrophie congenitale. A propos de 2 cas anatomo-cliniques et de 3 cas cliniques. Arch Mal Coeur 61: 477–503.
43. Lassabe G, Sacrez A, Bareiss P, Wolff F, Toledano C, Germain R. 1981. Forme familiale de

dysplasie ventriculaire droite. Ann Cardiol Angeiol 30: 331–335.

44. Waynberger M, Courtadon M, Peltier JM, Ducloux G, Jallut H, Slama R. 1974. Tachycardie ventriculaire familiale. A propos de 7 cas. Nouv Presse Med 3: 1857–1860.

45. Diggelmann U, Baur H.R. 1984. Familial Uhl's Anomaly in the Adult. Am J Cardiol 53: 1402–1403.

46. Voigt J, Agdal N. 1982. Lipomatous Infiltration of the Heart. An Uncommon Cause of Sudden, Unexpected Death in a Young Man. Arch Pathol Lab Med 106: 497–498.

47. Ruder MA, Winston SA, Davis JC, Abbott JA, Eldar M, Scheinman MM. 1985. Arrhythmogenic Right Ventricular Dysplasia in a Family. Am J Cardiol 56: 799–800.

48. Thiene G. 1985. Ventricolo destro aritmogeno: displasia, malattia o sindrome? G Ital Cardiol 16: 13–15.

49. Morgera T, Salvi A, Alberti E, Silvestri F, Camerini F. 1985. Morphological Findings in Apparently Idiopathic Ventricular Tachycardia. An Echocardiographic Haemodynamic and Histologic Study. Eur Heart J 6:323–334.

10. Ventricular arrhythmias in the young: clinical and experimental findings

ARTHUR GARSON, JR.*

*The Lillie Frank Abercrombie Section of Cardiology, Department of Pediatrics,
Baylor College of Medicine, Houston, Texas*
* Dr. Garson is an Established Investigator of the American Heart Association, Dallas, Texas

Abstract

Adults and children have similarities as well as differences in their ventricular arrhythmias. The most similar are the definition of the arrhythmias; although the rate of ventricular tachycardia in an infant may be as high as 500/minute with a QRS duration of 40 msec. Also similar are the techniques of intracardiac electrophysiology study. However, there are major differences in the etiology, prognosis and treatment of ventricular arrhythmias in children. There are four major areas of difference. 1) Idiopathic incessant ventricular tachycardia occurs in nfants less than the age of three years. It does not respond to conventional investigational antiarrhythmic agents. The majority of patients have Purkinje cell tumors causing the tachycardia. These tumors cannot be detected by echocardiography or angiography. Electrophysiologically directed surgery is curative. 2) In children with ventricular tachycardia who are thought to have an otherwise normal heart, the heart is usually not 'normal'. When anatomic and hemodynamic cardiac catheterization is performed in these patients, in 70% either arrhythmogenic right ventricle or congestive cardiomyopathy is found. If the heart is truly normal, the prognosis is excellent. On the other hand, children with arrhythmogenic right ventricle or congestive cardiomyopathy, especially those who have exercise-related ventricular tachycardia, may die suddenly. 3) The idiopathic long QT syndrome occurs more commonly in children than adults. Sudden death may occur without preceding symptoms and treatment is recommended for even the asymptomatic child who has the diagnosis of prolonged QT syndome (in addition to the long QT interval, the diagnosis of the syndrome requires either a positive family history, bradycardia, deafness, or typical T wave morphology). 4) Patients who have had repair of congenital heart disease die suddenly due to ventricular arrhythmias. Treatment of these arrhythmias based on results of the Holter have resulted in a significant decrease in morality. The drugs that are successful in the treatment of arrhythmias in these patients (phenytoin, mexiletine) are different from the traditionally effective drugs in adults with ischemic heart disease. This observation has led to the hypothesis that the cellular mechanism of the initiating ventricular arrhythmias in patients after repair of congenital heart disease (triggered activity) may be different from the mechanism in those with ischemic heart disease (reentry). This hypothesis is extended to other patients with the common findings of ventriculr hypertrophy, cellular disarray and fibrosis such as aortic stenosis/aortic insufficiency, hypertrophic cardiomyopathy and systemic arterial hypertension. This hypothesis applies to all patients regardless of their age, perphaps pointing out a major similarity in arrhythmia mechanism. Therefore, the differences between children and adults may be less than is immediately apparent.

Introduction

The electrocardiographic and electrophysiologic definitions for ventricular arrhythmias in adults and children are identical. However, considering electrocardiographic morphology, ventricular tachycardia occurs at much more rapid rates with narrower QRS complexes in children. For example, Figure 1 demonstrates sustained, monomorphic ventricular tachycardia at a rate of 500/minute with a QRS duration of 40 milliseconds. Different from adults, in children ventricular tachycardia may have a more rapid rate than supraventricular tachycardia. Despite the more rapid rates, the performance and interpretation of intracardiac electrophysiology studies are also relatively similar.

However, the major differences between adults and children are demonstrated in consideration of the conditions associated with the ventricular arrhythmias, their prognosis and the treatment. Under the age of three years, by far the most common diagnosis is 'incessant idiopathic' ventricular tachycardia. In the childhood and young adult age group, the majority are thought to have a 'normal' heart, although many do not. Also in this age group, there are increasing numbers of patients with ventricular arrhythmias with congenital heart disease, most after intracardiac repair of their defects. There are also increasing numbers of patients with prolonged QT intervals recognized as the cause of ventricular tachycardia. It is in these four areas that the ventricular arrhythmias of children differ from adults who have mainly coronary artery disease. These form the basis for the remainder of the discussion.

'Incessant idiopathic' ventricular tachycardia

Our first case was the most instructive. At six months of age, she was noted by her pediatrician to have a 'rapid heart rate'. The rate had returned to normal by the time an electrocardiogram was obtained. She was entirely asymptomatic and remained asymptomatic until the age of 15 months when she was taken to the local

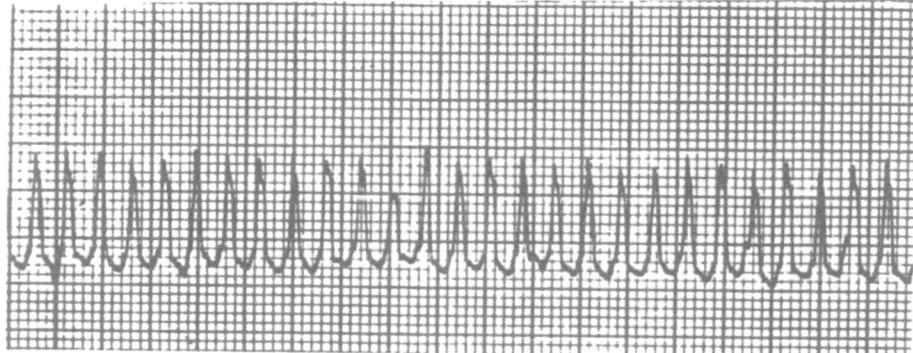

Figure 1. Rapid ventricular tachycardia in an infant. The rate is 500 per minute. AV dissociation is apparent on the right of the tracing. There are two fusion beats.

emergency room for lethargy, pallor and shortness of breath. Her heart rate was found to be 300/minute. The diagnosis was made of 'supraventricular tachycardia with aberration'. She was given intravenous digoxin for this arrhythmia and within minutes had ventricular fibrillation. She was defibrillated but remained in this tachycardia throughout most of the day and night for three weeks. The tachycardia was not responsive to conventional antiarrhythmic drugs. At the age of 18 months, she was transferred to Texas Children's Hospital and the diagnosis of ventricular tachycardia was made (Figure 2). On echocardiography and cineangiography she had reduced left ventricular function but no anatomic abnormality was seen. At the age of 19 months, she underwent electrophysiology study. The diagnosis of ventricular tachycardia was confirmed with the earliest site of endocardial activation at the left ventricular apex. The tachycardia could be terminated with premature ventricular extrastimuli, but it returned after several sinus beats. Because of continued tachycardia and low cardiac output, she was taken to the operating room with the idea of ablating that area of the heart. To our surprise, a small (5 mm × 12 mm) gray patch was found on the epicardial surface at the left ventricular apex. Removal of this lesion resulted in sinus rhythm. On pathologic examination, the gray area was entirely made up of large, pale staining cells with the general characteristics of Purkinje cells [1]. The patient is now six and a half years after the operation. She remains in sinus rhythm without medication.

Incessant idiopathic ventricular tachycardia is a disease of infancy. We have encountered 20 cases, all under the age of 26 months when first presenting with a tachyarrhythmia (the mean age was 10 months). There were significantly more females than males (13/7). Of the 20 patients, six had undergone an episode of cardiopulmonary arrest (four of whom had ventricular fibrillation when given digitalis for the incorrect diagnosis of supraventricular tachycardia with aberration), nine presented with congestive heart failure due to the incessant tachycar-

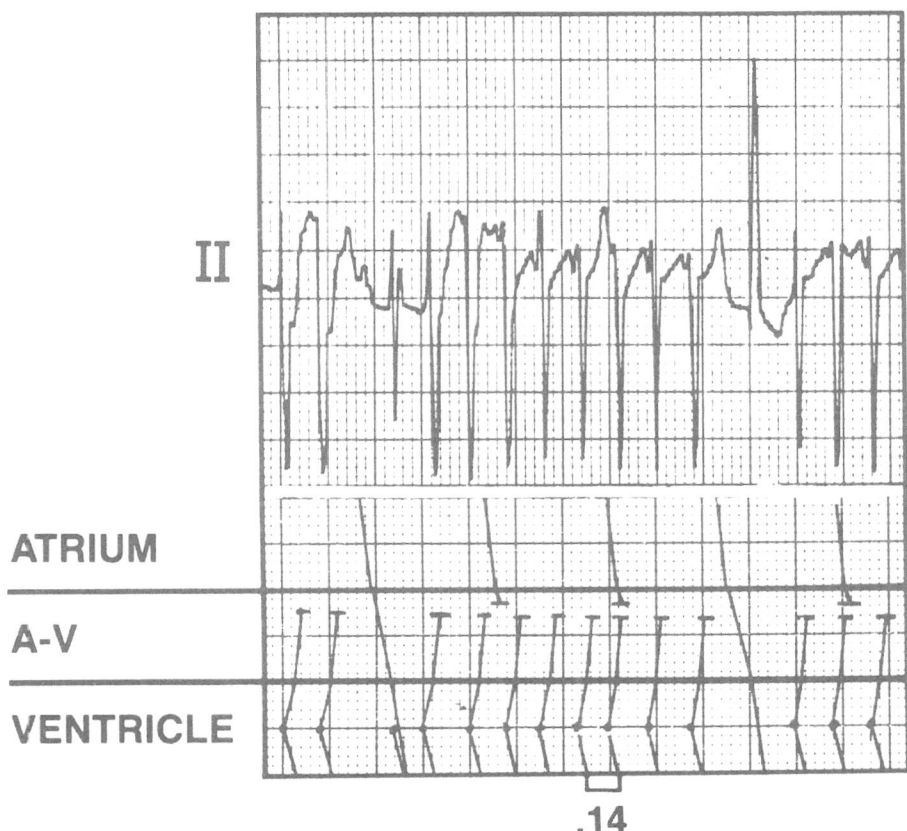

II

ATRIUM

A-V

VENTRICLE

.14

Figure 2. Ventricular tachycardia satisfying all adult criteria. A ladder diagram is shown below the tracing. There is AV dissociation. There is a sinus capture beat (8th beat) and a fusion beat (6th beat). Despite the QRS duration of 60 msec, this was documented to be ventricular tachycardia originating from the left ventricular apex.

dia and only five were asymptomatic but were found to have a rapid heart rate. The rate of the ventricular tachycardia ranged from 170 to 440/minute (mean 260/ minute). The most common QRS morphology was that of right bundle branch block with left axis deviation (9/20), but all the different varieties of bundle branch block were seen in individual patients. In 18/20, the tachycardia morphology was always the same; in two, there was more than one morphology of different sustained monomorphic ventricular tachycardias. At electrophysiology study, the morphology of the QRS complex generally corresponded to the site of earliest endocardial activation. The most common single location was the posterior left ventricular free wall (6/20), followed by the left ventricular septum. Overall, 13/20 were in the left ventricle, four were in the right ventricle and three spread throughout the endocardium of both the right and the left ventricles. All 20 patients had endocardial mapping, and 17 had introduction of premature stimuli and rapid pacing. In 13 of the 17, the tachycardia could be terminated briefly by premature stimuli.

All 20 had been tried on multiple conventional antiarrhythmic drugs (mean 3.2 per patient), and 12 had received amiodarone. All drugs had failed to appreciably affect either the rate of the tachycardia or the amount of the day the patient spent in tachycardia. Accordingly, all 20 were taken to the operating room. At surgery, epicardial and endocardial mapping was again repeated. At the site of earliest activation, 15/20 were found to have a tumor (13 Purkinje cell tumors, two rhabdomyoma). One patient had no visible findings but on biopsying the area of earliest activation, chronic myocarditis was found. Two patients were found to have only nonspecific fibrosis and two patients, early in the series, had no biopsy performed. All patients had excision of the site of earliest endocardial and/or epicardial activation as well as cryoablation of the surrounding tissue.

Immediately after surgery, all 20 patients were in sinus rhythm. Two patients died early in the postoperative period, one from a severe neurologic insult that occurred at the time of a cardiopulmonary arrest due to the ventricular tachycardia before surgery; the other had removal of extensive tumor in the endocardium of both the right and left ventricles and died postoperatively of low cardiac output. The other 18 patients are alive and in sinus rhythm in follow-up from two months to six years, (mean 1.2 years). Only two are on antiarrhythmic drugs. The reduced ventricular function that had been present preoperatively resolved in 14 of the 15 patients.

In conclusion, a rapid incessant tachycardia with a QRS morphology different from the sinus was likely to be due to ventricular tachycardia, not supraventricular tachycardia. In one published series, only two percent of children with supraventricular tachycardia had supraventricular tachycardia with aberration [3]. We have found that incessant ventricular tachycardia in infants less than three years of age was likely to be due to a tumor, despite a normal echocardiogram and angiocardiogram. The most common type of tumor was the 'Purkinje cell tumor'. This has previously been reported only in pathologic series involving sudden death in children [4, 5]. Since incessant ventricular tachycardia did not respond to medical therapy and was treated successfully with operation, we recommend that surgery be considered early in the course of these patients.

Ventricular tachycardia in children with a 'normal heart'

While it is known that premature ventricular contractions in children with an otherwise normal heart have an entirely benign outcome [6], the findings are different in ventricular tachycardia. Deal et al [7] recently reported 24 patients with ventricular tachycardia, six to 21 years old. All were thought to have a normal heart. Symptoms, most often syncope or presyncope, occurred in 67% of the patients; in nine, these symptoms were related to exercise. The most common morphology was left bundle branch block (18/24), and the rate ranged from 130–300/minute. During electrophysiology study, sustained monomorphic tachycardia could be induced in 11/18. Only 2/7 patients who received isoproterenol had but tachycardia appeared during the infusion. The site of earliest activation was in the right ventricle in 15/17.

While all the patients were initially thought to have a normal heart, on echocardiography, 26% were found to have an abnormality in either the right or left ventricle with either dilation, reduced ejection fraction or both. During cardiac catheterization, 70% of the patients were found to have an abnormality: half had arrhythmogenic right ventricular dysplasia and the other half had early left ventricular congestive cardiomyopathy. Therefore, the echocardiogram was not sensitive enough to detect the abnormalities in children. Dunnigan et al. [8] found that in all six of their children that presented with sustained monomorphic ventricular tachycardia, at cardiac catheterization, half had evidence of congestive cardiomyopathy and the other half had evidence of a restrictive cardiomyopathy. In four of the six patients, the cardiac muscle biopsy was felt to be abnormal with increased areas of fibrous tissue. However, there was no specific cardiac pathologic diagnosis made on the biopsy.

The prognosis for ventricular tachycardia in children with a normal heart depends entirely on whether the heart is found to be normal at cardiac catheterization. We [9] found in a series of 15 children with ventricular tachycardia who had a normal heart proven at cardiac catheterization, in an average follow-up of five years, there were no deaths and only two patients had symptoms – both with palpitations. On the other hand, Deal et al. [7] found that two of their 23 patients with ventricular tachycardia died suddenly. However, both had been symptomatic, both had exercise-induced ventricular tachycardia, both had ventricular tachycardia induced during electrophysiology study and neither had a normal heart at cardiac catheterization. In a review of the other 106 published cases of ventricular tachycardia in children thought to have a normal heart, only 31 had had cardiac catheterization. Of these 106 patients, there were three deaths, none had had prior cardiac catheterization; one had been known to have syncopal episodes, and one had arrhythmogenic right ventricular dysplasia at autopsy. There was no information about the third patient. In the 103 survivors, two concepts emerged: ventricular tachycardia in patients with a normal heart is resistant to treatment with traditional antiarrhythmic drugs. The arrhythmia was also persistent throughout follow-up, only disappearing in approximately 20% of the patients.

In conclusion, in a child, ventricular tachycardia is usually an indicator of an abnormal heart (usually either arrhythmogenic right ventricular dysplasia or congestive cardiomyopathy). Therefore, we recommend that all children with ventricular tachycardia have a hemodynamic and angiographic cardiac catheterization. In our series of nine patients with ventricular tachycardia and a truly normal heart who had electrophysiology study, we were unable to induce even a single non-bundle branch reentry beat in any patient [9]. Deal et al. [7] found similarly that the patients with a truly normal heart did not have inducible arrhythmias, while those with arrhythmogenic right ventricular dysplasia or congestive cardiomyopathy with clinical ventricular tachycardia did have ventricular tachycardia induced during electrophysiology study. Therefore, it is possible that induction of ventricular tachycardia during electrophysiology study may also be an indicator of an abnormal heart. Since both children that died suddenly reported by Deal et al. [7] had inducible sustained ventricular tachycardia, it is possible that this implies a poor prognosis in this patient group. Therefore, it may be that electrophysiology study should be recommended in these patients. Finally, if the heart is entirely normal at cardiac catheterization and angiography, if the patient is asymptomatic, if the tachycardia is not exercise related and cannot be induced during electrophysiology study, then the prognosis for the patient is excellent and treatment may not be necessary.

Idiopathic long QT syndrome

Since the idiopathic long QT syndrome is congenital, and since it causes sudden death, it is likely to be more prevalent in children than adults. Nonetheless, the problems and the diagnosis of the *syndrome* are as difficult in children as adults. For example, it is known that all patients with a prolonged QT interval may not be at risk of sudden death, and conversely there may be some patients with the syndrome, who are at risk of sudden death, who have a normal QT interval. Therefore, Schwartz [10] has proposed certain 'major' and 'minor' criteria for the diagnosis of the syndrome. The major criteria are: 1) A corrected QT interval (Bazett's formula [11]) greater than 0.44 seconds; 2) Family members with the long QT syndrome; 3) Syncope related to noise or anger. The minor criteria are: 1) Congenital deafness; 2) Bradycardia; 3) Large, notched T waves; 4) T wave alternans. For the diagnosis of the syndrome, Schwartz requires two major criteria, or one major and two minor criteria. In children, we would modify the requirement to allow the diagnosis of the syndrome in any patient with a prolonged corrected QT interval and one minor criterion.

We have recently reported 26 children with a corrected QT interval greater than 0.44 seconds. This did not necessarily represent patients with the true 'syndrome', however it described the spectrum of patients who have an abnormal electrocardiogram [12]. The age at the diagnosis of the prolonged QT interval ranged from one week to 27 years (with a mean of 12 years). The initial presentation was a cardiac arrest in two, syncope in 12 and palpitations in four. Eight patients were asymptomatic: three had the diagnosis made on an electrocardiogram obtained for bradycardia and five on an electrocardiogram obtained because another family member had a prolonged QT interval. On the electrocardiogram, 15 of the 26 patients had a corrected QT interval greater than 0.50. All of these patients ha either syncope (9/15) or a positive family history (9/15), or both (6/15). In comparison, 11 patients had a corrected QT interval les than 0.50. Syncope occurred in four, a positive family history in five or both syncope in the patient and a positive family history in two patients. In follow-up of our 26 children, there were four sudden deaths. All of these patients had a corrected QT interval greater than 0.50. Only one of the four was known to be taking a beta blocker at the time of treatment. Conversely, the majority of the patients have been taking either beta blockers, or phenytoin. After beginning this treatment, six of the seven patients with prior episodes of syncope had a cessation in syncopal episodes; the seventh required a pacemaker and left Stellate ganglionectomy for elimination of symptoms.

In conclusion, children with the prolonged QT interval syndrome can present with a cardiac arrest or sudden death without preceding symptoms. Therefore, we recommend that in children with a diagnosis of the prolonged QT *syndrome,* treatment be instituted whether or not the child is symptomatic. We would begin treatment with a beta blocking agent. While there are not numerous patients reported taking long-acting beta blockers, we have maintained five such patients on atenolol; there have been no symptoms and no sudden deaths in these patients. Additionally, the class Ib agents (phenytoin, mexiletine, tocainide) have all been reported to be effective in treating this syndrome [13, 14]. In the presence of continued symptoms while taking medication, the next step is implantation of a pacemaker, especially if the child has bradycardia. A great number of patients with a prolonged QT develop torsade-de-pointes following a bigeminal cycle. It is thought that the compensitory pause following the premature beat is part of the pathophysiology of the rapid tachyarrhythmia that follows. Therefore, if a pacemaker is implanted and the long pause is prevented following a premature beat, this may reduce or eliminate episodes of torsade-de-pointes [15]. The final possible treatment for such patients is left Stellate ganglionectomy [16]. There has been controversy over the success of this operation. Most patients continue to take beta blockers even after surgery. In children, the operation has not been performed sufficiently frequently to make a conclusion as to its success.

Ventricular arrhythmias after repair of congenital heart disease

In the 1960's, intracardiac repair of congenital cardiac defects began to occur routinely. There was a great deal of enthusiasm as children who had previously been cyanotic began to enjoy completely normal lifestyles. However, in the 1970's it became apparent that some of these children were dying suddenly late after the operation. The majority of the sudden deaths occurred in patients where the repair involved incision or suturing in the ventricle. The more complex the lesion, the higher incidence of late sudden death. For example, in lesions involving a right ventriculotomy, sudden death occurs in 1–2% of the postoperative ventricular septal defect, approximately 5% of postoperative tetralogy of Fallot and 18% of postoperative truncus arteriosis with single pulmonary artery [17–19]. On the left side of the heart approximately 3% of children die suddenly after aortic valvotomy or aortic valve replacement [20].

The largest body of information has been collected about postoperative tetralogy of Fallot. Ventricular arrhythmias are common after this operation. On routine electrocardiogram, 10% of the patients have premature ventricular contractions, and 30% have ventricular arrhythmias in association with a treadmill exercise test. On Holter, the incidence of ventricular arrhythmias is 50% with 9% of the patients having nonsustained ventricular tachycardia [18, 21, 22]. During electrophysiology study, using a protocol with paired premature ventricular extrastimuli, and burst pacing at two sites in the right ventricle, 26% of the patients had nonsustained ventricular tachycardia and 10% sustained ventricular tachycardia [23]. There is a general correlation between patients who have syncope, a high grade of ventricular arrhythmias on the Holter and inducible nonsustained ventricular tachycardia at electrophysiology study. However, in a specific patient, there may be discordance among all three tests. For example, asymptomatic patients with entirely no arrhythmia on the Holter may have inducible sustained ventricular tachycardia; conversely, a syncopal patient with only infrequent single uniform premature ventricular contractions on the Holter may have absolutely no arrhythmia induced during electrophysiology study.

Both spontaneous and inducible ventricular arrhythmias are related to abnormal hemodynamics. The prevalence of premature ventricular contractions on routine electrocardiogram is 8% in patients with a right ventricular systolic pressure less than 40 mm Hg but increases to 30% in patients with a right ventricular systolic pressure greater than 90 mm Hg [24]. In addition, patients with inducible nonsustained or sustained ventricular tachycardia in general have had either elevated right ventricular systolic or end-diastolic pressures. However, again, in a specific patient, ventricular arrhythmias may exist in the presence of an excellent hemodynamic repair. The other factors related to the presence of ventricular arrhythmias are age at operation and increased duration since surgery. These two factors are not independent since 20 years ago many more operations were done on older children than they are now. In fact, however, mathematical analysis reveals that the more significant factor is the increased duration since surgery. This implies that as children who have had repair of tetralogy enter adulthood, the incidence of ventricular arrhythmias will continue to rise [24].

Sudden death is related to preceding ventricular arrhythmia. In our series [18], 38% of those patients with premature ventricular contractions on routine electrocardiogram died suddenly between one and 10 years after the operation. The relationship of sudden death to abnormal hemodynamics is evident: 100% of our patients who died suddenly had both right ventricular systolic pressure over 60 mm Hg and right ventricular end-diastolic pressure greater than 8 mm Hg.

Approximately 15 years ago, it was suggested that late complete AV block was responsible for these sudden deaths and that the pattern of right bundle branch block – left hemiblock indicated a high risk [25]. In retrospect, all of the patients with sudden death in that study also had ventricular arrhythmias and more recent reports have demonstrated that the majority of patients who later died suddenly did not have preceding right bundle branch block – left anterior hemiblock, but had ventricular arrhythmias [26]. The final demonstration of the relationship between sudden death and ventricular arrhythmias is that treatment of the ventricular arrhythmias abolishes sudden death [24]. Since 1978, we have treated all patients after repair of tetralogy of Fallot who had greater than Lown Grade 2 ventricular arrhythmias on Holter. Our goal of treatment has been an absolute reduction of premature ventricular contractions to less than 10 uniform premature ventricular contractions per hour, regardless of the frequency or type of ventricular arrhythmia before treatment. Of our 484 patients who have had repair of tetralogy, we have treated 44. In 42 of the 44, a successful drug was found by our criteria and none of these paients died. Both of the patients without successful treatment died as well as seven of the 21 who were untreated [24].

The drugs we have found effective in treating ventricular arrhythmias in these patients have largely been the class Ib agents: phenytoin and mexiletine [27, 28]. In our treated patients, phenytoin was successful in 88%, mexiletine in 89% and quinidine in 14%. We have chosen to manage patients based on the Holter, firstly because this management has been shown to be effective, but secondly because the patient population is different than the usual adult patient. Very few of our patients present with symptomatic, sustained ventricular tachycardia and so there is not the urgency for treatment required in the adult population, many of whom have been resuscitated from a sudden cardiac arrest. In any of our patients who have symptomatic episodes, if there is a great deal of ambiant ectopy, they are treated based on the Holter reduction of ventricular arrhythmia. On the other hand, a symptomatic patient with very little ambiant ectopy will undergo repeated electrophysiology studies while taking different antiarrhythmic drugs orally. A problem with chronic drug – electrophysiology studies in these patients is that even symptomatic patients who have had repair of congenital cardiac defects and clinical ventricular tachycardia may not have inducible, sustained ventricular tachycardia. Also, especially in the young age group, the acceptability of chronic studies by parents and children is low. It is not acceptable to leave a chronic catheter in a small child who is likely to remove it rather forcefully. The final reason for the low utilization of chronic drug-electrophysiology studies is that there is a relatively poor correlation between control of the arrhythmia on the Holter and lack of inducibility in the electrophysiology laboratory. In our Holter studies, we demonstrated a high degree of control of ventricular arrhythmias using Ib agents. On the other hand, in drug-electrophysiology studies, among 20 patients reported [29, 30], in only 11 patients could any drug be found which eliminated the induction of sustained ventricular tachycardia: quinidine or procainamide were successful in 1/12, phenytoin in 5/12 (despite 9/12 without ventricular arrhythmia on the Holter while taking phenytoin), and propranolol 5/11. Since it is likely that phenytoin is an effective agent that suppresses ventricular arrhythmias on the Holter and also prevents sudden death, the observation that patients taking phenytoin are still inducible in the catheterization laboratory may place phenytoin in the similar category as amiodarone, where the clinical findings and the electrophysiology findings are not necessarily similar.

In conclusion, in patients after repair of tetralogy of Fallot and other similar lesions, ventricular arrhythmias and sudden death are related. The risk of sudden death is likely to be higher than the reported 5% since it is now known that the incidence of ventricular arrhythmias increases with each succeeding year after surgery. The actual data will be difficult to obtain since a large number of these patients are now being treated for their ventricular arrhythmias. One difference in these patients from their adult counterparts is that, at least in this particular problem, it appears that sudden death can be prevented by treatment with antiarrhythmic drugs.

Therefore, it is apparent that some patients with ventricular arrhythmias require drug treatment. It is not yet established which patients, in particular, require treatment. The criterion of treating those with Lown Grade 2 arrhythmias or greater, clearly results in over-treatment. More specific criteria are needed. At some institutions, only those with inducible, sustained ventricular tachycardia during electrophysiology study are treated [31]. Since the prognostic ability of a positive or a negative electrophysiology study has not yet been demonstrated, the treatment of patients based upon the electrophysiology study may be premature. Finally, it has been suggested that only symptomatic patients be treated [32]. This is also unlikely to solve the problem since many patients with palpitations have no arrhythmia and over half of the patients with sudden death after tetralogy of Fallot repair were completely asymptomatic before their deaths [33]. Hopefully, with further prospective study, the relative value of the Holter and the electrophysiology study will be ascertained and a rational plan for treatment of specific patients can be devised.

At present, suppression of ventricular arrhythmias on the Holter appears to be an adequate way of assessing treatment of these patients. Further follow-up will be necessary to determine if chronic electrophysiologic drug testing is preferable. Finally, the agents that are successful in suppression of ventricular arrhythmias in these patients are different from those traditionally used in adult patients with ischemic heart disease and ventricular arrhythmias. This observation forms the basis for the following hypothesis.

Nonischemic ventricular arrhythmias in children and adults: a unifying hypothesis

The observation that the class Ib agents (phenytoin and mexiletine) are effective in treating arrhythmias in patients after repair of congenital heart disease, and that the class Ia agents (quinidine and procainamide) are not effective, has led to a great deal of discussion. This is because the adult with ischemic heart disease and ventricular arrhythmias has generally the opposite findings with a good response to quinidine and a poor response to phenytoin. The explanation for these findings may have important implications. There are three possibilities: 1) The ages of the patients are different; 2) The drugs act differently; 3) The diseases produce different mechanisms of ventricular arrhythmias.

In attempting to explain the difference in drug response on the basis of the age of the patient, it is important to recognize that the majority of the patients being treated for ventricular arrhythmias after repair of congenital heart disease are not children. The majority of them are over 15 years of age and many are over 30 years of age. Therefore, it is difficult to ascribe the success of phenytoin to the fact that it is more effective in children. Furthermore, it has recently been shown that both phenytoin and quinidine have similar cellular electrophysiologic effects on neonatal and adult Purkinje fibers [34].

Certainly, the class Ia and class Ib agents are different in electrophysiologic effects. While both block the sodium channel, quinidine increases the action potential duration and phenytoin has either no effect or may decrease the action potential duration. However the most interesting difference between the drugs is with respect to delayed afterdepolarizations and triggered activity. Both phenytoin and mexiletine have been shown to decrease delayed afterdepolarizations while quinidine may actually cause an increase in delayed afterdepolarizations and lead to sustained triggered activity [35–37]. Therefore, if the ventricular arrhythmias in patients after repair of congenital heart disease were initiated by delayed afterdepolarizations, the observation that phenytoin is effective and quinidine is not effective in the treatment of the clinical arrhythmias could be consistent with the mechanism of delayed afterdepolarizations as the cause of the arrhythmias.

A final possibility for the explanation of the differential drug effect is that the underlying substrate of postoperative congenital heart disease is electrophysiologically different from myocardial infarction. The features of postoperative tetralogy of Fallot are hypertrophy, cellular disarray (in the region of the infundibulum), a large ventriculotomy incision and, in the majority, right ventricular dilation due to postoperative pulmonary insufficiency. This is potentially different from the patients with coronary disease who suffers a myocardial infarction and has ventricular tachycardia related to the infarct scar.

In order to examine the possible cellular mechanisms involved in arrhythmias after repair of tetralogy of Fallot, we have created a dog model. This involves creation of a 'pre-op' tetralogy for the first part of the animal's life by banding the pulmonary artery (causing increased right ventricular pressure) and performing a pulmonary artery to the left atrium anastomosis (causing cyanosis). After approximately four months, the animals are 'corrected' on cardiopulmonary bypass, undergo de-banding, closure of the anastomosis and right ventriculotomy. The animals are then observed for the next six months with repeated 24-hour electrocardiograms and electrophysiology studies.

In preliminary experiments done on animals with continued elevated right ventricular systolic pressure after repair, we have found ventricular arrhythmias. On 24-hour electrocardiogram in several animals the coupling interval of the premature beat was directly related to the preceding cycle length, suggesting a possible mechanism of triggered activity [38]. In one animal during electrophysiology study, the inducing cycle length was directly related to the rate of the induced ventricular tachycardia, another possible finding in triggered activity [39].

Therefore, our early animal studies are suggestive that delayed afterdepolarizations could be involved in the initiation of ventricular arrhythmias in patients after repair of tetralogy of Fallot. This finding is strengthened by the recent report of delayed afterdepolarizations in patients after repair of tetralogy of Fallot. Benito et al. [40], performed monophasic action potential recordings in 10 patients after intracardiac repair of tetralogy of Fallot. All had greater than Lown Grade 2 ventricular arrhythmias on Holter. In six of the 10, delayed afterdepolarizations were found and initiated spontaneous ventricular arrhythmias in the electrophysiology laboratory.

Therefore, in attempting to explain the observation that the class Ib drugs are effective in treatment of ventricular arrhythmias after repair of tetralogy of Fallot, we arrive at the hypothesis that the reason for the difference in drug response is that the cellular mechanism for the initiation for the ventricular arrhythmias may be different in patients after repair of tetralogy than in those with myocardial infarction.

However, this hypothesis does not only apply to patients after repair of tetralogy of Fallot. There are other diseases that have in common the features of ventricular arrhythmia, sudden death, hypertrophy and cellular disarray. Additional features include the presence of areas of fibrosis, either native or surgically induced, and possibly cardiac dilation. Diseases which fit these general criteria are aortic stenosis/aortic insufficiency (both pre and postoperative), hypertrophic cardiomyopathy (both unoperated and after septal myotomy/myectomy), and finally systemic hypertension. There is additional evidence supporting the hypothesis that delayed afterdepolarizations are involved in the initiation of arrhythmias in these patients as well. Firstly, in both pre and postoperative patients with aortic stenosis/aortic insufficiency, phenytoin and mexiletine are effective in treatment of ventricular arrhythmias [20, 27, 28]. In children with hypertrophic cardiomyopathy, both phenytoin and verapamil have been shown to be effective in the treatment of ventricular arrhythmias [41, 42]. Finally, the patient reported by Zipes et al., who was thought on the basis of intracardiac electrophysiology study to have ventricular tachycardia due to delayed afterdepolarizations and triggered activity, had systemic hypertension [43]. Moreover, in rats with experimentally induced systemic hypertension, delayed after-depolarizations have been found by cellular electrophysiologic studies to be the likely cause of their ventricular arrhythmias [44].

The unifying hypothesis is that patients with hypertrophy, cellular disarray, and areas of scarring have a different cellular mechanism for ventricular arrhythmias (involving delayed afterdepolarizations and triggered activity) than patients with ischemic heart disease and myocardial infarction (involving reentry), regardless of their age. This difference in mechanism, rather than the difference in age, explains the differential effect of certain drugs in children and adults with ventricular arrhythmias.

While this hypothesis accounts for the electrophysiologic observations, we must go further to explain how the disease process leads to the initiating ventricular arrhythmia that then ends in irreversible ventricular fibrillation and sudden death.

Returning to the situation after repair of tetralogy of Fallot, it has been found that ventricular tachycardia originates in areas adjacent to large areas of scar. This is not necessarily in the right ventricular outflow tract in the area of the ventriculotomy, but may also be in fibrotic areas surrounding the ventricular septal defect patch or the infundibular resection [45]. In one patient, the reentrant ventricular tachycardia was mapped and found to progress around the entire area of the ventriculotomy incision as a macro-reentrant circuit [46]. In our experimental animals, we found ventricular tachycardia related to the ventriculotomy, but the findings are more consistent with a micro-reentrant circuit at the edge of the ventriculotomy rather than macro-reentry involving the entire incision.

Regardless, in certain situations, there are ventricular arrhythmias that have their site of origin near large fibrous areas. If the fibrous areas are reduced, such as in patients with no right ventriculotomy, the ventricular arrhythmias have been found to be reduced [47]. In our experimental model, we have also found that a simple ventriculotomy is not likely to lead to ventricular arrhythmias [48]. However, with the addition of persistently elevated right ventricular systolic and/or diastolic pressure to the ventriculotomy, ventricular arrhythmias do occur in these animals [49]. On pathologic examination, the ventriculotomy incision in animals with normal right ventricular hemodynamics had microscopically straight and smooth borders with little irregularity. On the other hand, animals with a ventriculotomy that healed in the presence of elevated right ventricular systolic and end-diastolic pressure had a much irregular appearance with fibrous tissue extending at right angles like 'fingers' into the surrounding myocardium. It is possible that a more irregular scar is the genesis of the ventricular arrhythmias. It might be that, electrophysiologically, the cells in the region of these fibrous extensions could be altered and lead to triggered activity. This is currently under investigation in our animal model.

The initiating premature ventricular beat must become ventricular tachycardia. It is known that postoperative tetralogy patients with ventricular tachycardia have areas of slow conduction in the right ventricle. This has been demonstrated both during intracardiac electrophysiologic study where the electrograms in the region of the right ventricular outflow tract and the summit of the ventricular septum are wide and fragmented [50]. This has also been demonstrated by the presence of 'late potentials' recorded by signal averaged electrocardiography in postoperative tetralogy patients who have ventricular tachycardia. There are significantly more late potentials in postoperative tetralogy patients with ventricular tachycardia compared to those with single premature beats or those without any ventricular arrhythmias. If a single premature beat that was originated by a delayed afterdepolarization encountered such an area of slow conduction, it is certainly possible that this could then lead to a reentrant ventricular tachycardia. As well, it is possible the fibrosis in the outflow tract and summit of the ventricular septum, similar to a myocardial infarction, leads to denervation of distal (inferior) parts of the ventricles. This could further create inhomogenous areas leading to reentry.

Once the reentry circuit is begun, it is likely that a hypertrophied, enlarged right ventricle will continue to sustain the ventricular tachycardia. It has been shown that with a decrease in volume, caused by Valsalva maneuver, termination of ventricular tachycardia may occur [51]. It is likely that the opposite could occur with an enlarged, dilated right ventricle leading to continuation of the arrhythmia.

It is important next to account for the progression of sustained ventricular tachycardia to ventricular fibrillation. As discussed previously, it is unlikely for a patient with a completely normal heart who has ventricular tachycardia, to have ventricular fibrillation or sudden death. On the other hand, the patient after repair of tetralogy of Fallot, especially one with abnormal hemodynamics, is at a markedly increased risk of ventricular fibrillation and sudden death. There are three possible explanations for this finding. Firstly, there is a primary electrical reason. It has been demonstrated that in the presence of large areas of delayed conduction, patients with ventricular tachycardia are more likely to have ventricular fibrillation [52]. The second explanation is hemodynamic. In our experimental model, we have found that in dogs with pulmonary stenosis and elevated right ventricular pressure, in response to rapid ventricular pacing at 300 beats/minute (simulating ventricular tachycardia) the *left* ventricle became ischemic. It is known that ischemia is a potent stimulus to ventricular fibrillation [53]. In addition, it has been reported that animals with hypertrophy, such as that found in tetralogy of Fallot, are more likely to have ventricular fibrillation with ischemia than animals without hypertrophy. To bring this closer to a clinical correlation, Palik et al. [55], have reported that in patients with high right ventricular pressures after repair of defects similar to tetralogy of Fallot, there is both right and left ventricular dysfunction. It is possible that the cause of this dysfunction is intermittent ischemia. The third possible cause of degeneration of ventricular tachycardia to ventricular fibrillation is elevated serum catecholamines. In our experimental model, we have found that in the animals with a pulmonary artery band, during rapid ventricular pacing, the serum norepinephrine increases markedly. This does not occur in normal animals. The elevated norepinephrine could be of cardiac origin released in association with ischemia; alternatively, it could be of adrenal origin in response to reduced cardiac output. Nonetheless, the increase in norepinephrine in the presence of ventricular tachycardia could certainly predispose to ventricular fibrillation [56].

Finally, we must account for the observation that some postoperative tetralogy patients who are found to be in ventricular fibrillation are very difficult to defibrillate. It is known that in the presence of ventricular hypertrophy, the ventricular defibrillation threshold is increased and successful eventual defibrillation is less common than in the non-hypertrophied heart [57]. This is certainly the case in postoperative tetralogy of Fallot where right ventricular hypertrophy rarely, if ever, regresses [58].

In summary, if we begin with a patient who has a disease characterized by hypertrophy, cellular disarray, areas of scarring and abnormal hemodynamics, it is likely that cells in the irregular border zone surrounding a scar will have delayed afterdepolarizations and triggered activity. This can cause single premature ventricular beats, or sustained ventricular tachycardia. Areas of slow conduction and inhomogeneity could then allow the single premature beat to become a reentrant ventricular tachycardia. In the presence of a large right ventricle, the first few beats of ventricular tachycardia are likely to sustain. Sustained ventricular tachycardia may then undergo degeneration to ventricular fibrillation on an electrical basis because of fragmented conduction, or due to ischemia or increased serum norepinephrine. In the presence of hypertrophy, the fibrillating heart is difficult to defibrillate and sudden death may result.

This hypothesis applies to diseases in all aged patients, not just children. Perhaps an understanding of this process will lead to improved survival for children as well as adults with nonischemic ventricular arrhythmias. In some ways, perhaps children are more like 'little adults'.

References

1. Garson A, Gillette PC, Titus JL, Hawkins EP, Kearney D, Ott D, Cooley DA, McNamara DG. 1984. Surgical treatment of ventricular tachycardia in infants. N Engl J Med 310: 1443–45.
2. Gillette PC, Smith RT, Garson A, Mullins CE, Gutgesell HP, Goh TH, Cooley DA, McNamara DG. 1985. Chronic supraventricular tachycardia: A curable cause of congestive cardiomyopathy. J Am Med Assoc 253: 391–92.
3. Garson A, Gillette PC, McNamara DG. 1981. Supraventricular tachycardia in children: Clinical features, response to treatment and long-term follow-up in 217 patients. J Pediatr 98: 875–82.
4. James TN, Beeson CW, Sherman EB. 1975. De Subitaneis Mortibus: XIII Multifocal Purkinje cell tumors of the heart. Circulation 52: 333–44.

5. Ferrans VJ, McAllister HA, Haese WH. 1976. Infantile cardiomyopathy with histiocytoid change in cardiac muscle cells: Report of six patients. Circulation 53: 708–19.

6. Jacobsen J, Garson A, Gillette PC, McNamara DG. 1978. Premature ventricular contractions in normal children. J Pediatr 92: 36–8.

7. Deal BJ, Miller SM, Prechel D, Scagliotti D, Gallastegui L. 1985. Ventricular tachycardia in the young without overt heart disease. Circulation 72 (Suppl III): 340.

8. Dunnigan A, Pierpont ME, Smith SA, Breningstall G, Benditt DG, Benson DW, Jr. 1984. Cardiac and skeletal myopathy associated with cardiac dysrhythmias. Am J Cardiol 53(6): 731–7.

9. Garson A, Gillette PC, Porter CJ, McNamara DG. 1982. Ventricular tachycardia in children with a normal heart. Circulation 66 (Suppl II): 170.

10. Schwartz PJ. 1985. Idiopathic long QT syndrome: progress and questions. Am Heart J 109 (2): 399–411.

11. Bazett HC. 1918. Analysis of the time relations of electrocardiograms. Heart 7: 353–8.

12. Ross BA, Garson A, McNamara DG. 1984. Factors affecting outcome in children with long QT syndrome. Circulation 70 (Suppl II): 320.

13. Bricker T, Garson A, Gillette PC. 1984. A history of seizures in the family associated with sudden cardiac deaths. Am J Dis Chld 138: 866–8.

14. Takamizawa K, Takao A. 1985. Mexiletine for successful treatment of the long QT syndrome. Proc Second World Congress of Pediatric Cardiology 101.

15. Kay GN, Plumb VJ, Arcinigas JG, Henthorn RW, Waldo AL. 1983. Torsade-de-pointes: the long – short initiating sequence and other clinical features. J Am Coll Cardiol 2: 806–17.

16. Locati E, Schwartz PJ, Moss AJ, Crapton RS. 1985. Long-term survival after left cervico-thoracic sympathectomy in high risk long QT syndrome patients with refractory ventricular arrhythmias. J Am Coll Cardiol 7: 235.

17. Moller JH, Patton C, Varco RL, Lillehei CW. 1985. Postoperative ventricular septal defect: 24–30 years follow-up of 232 patients. Proc Second World Congress of Pediatric Cardiology: 20.

18. Garson A, Nihill MR, McNamara DG, Cooley DA. 1979. Status of the adult and adolescent following repair of tetralogy of Fallot. Circulation 59: 1232–40.

19. Fyfe DA, Driscoll DJ, Danielson GK, Mair DD. 1985. Truncus arteriosus with single pulmonary artery: influence of pulmonary vascular obstructive disease on early and late operative results. J Am Coll Cardiol 5: 1168–72.

20. Garson A, Smith RT, Moak JP, Ross BA, McNamara DG. 1985. Sudden death in children related to ventricular arrhythmias. J Am Coll Cardiol 5: 130B–4B.

21. Garson A, Gillette PC, Gutgesell HP, McNamara DG. 1980. Stress-induced ventricular arrhythmias after tetralogy of Fallot repair. Am J Cardiol 46: 1006–12.

22. Kavey RE, Blackman MS, Sondheimer HM. 1982. Incidence and severity of chronic ventricular dysrhythmias after repair of tetralogy of Fallot. Am Heart J 103 (3): 342–50.

23. Garson A, Porter CJ, Gillette PC, McNamara DG. 1983. Induction of ventricular tachycardia during electrophysiologic study after repair of tetralogy of Fallot. J Am Coll Cardiol 1: 1493–1502.

24. Garson A, Randall DC, McVey P, Smith RT, Moak JP, Gillette PC, McNamara DG. 1985. Prevention of sudden death after repair of tetralogy of Fallot: treatment of ventricular arrhythmias. J Am Coll Cardiol 6: 221–7.

25. Wolff GS, Rowland TW, Ellison RC. 1972. Surgically induced right bundle branch block with left anterior hemiblock. Circulation 45: 587–93.

26. Fuster V, McGoon DC, Kennedy MA. 1980. Long-term evaluation (12–22 years) of open heart surgery for tetralogy of Fallot. Am J Cardiol 46: 635–40.

27. Garson A, Kugler JD, Gillette PC, Simonelli A, McNamara DG. 1980. Control of late postoperative ventricular arrhythmias with phenytoin in young patients. Am J Cardiol 46: 290–4.

28. Moak JP, Gillette PC, Garson A. 1984. Mexiletine: an alternative to dilantin for pediatric ventricular arrhythmias. Circulation 70 (Suppl II): 207.

29. Kugler JD, Cheatham JP, Gumbiner CH, Hofschire PJ, Latson LA. 1985. Results of phenytoin

and propranolol drug electrophysiology studies for ventricular tachycardia in patients having repaired lesions with tetralogy of Fallot physiology. Circulation 72 (II): 341.

30. Deal BJ, Miller SM, Scagliotti D, Gallastegiu JM. 1985. Electrophysiologic drug testing in ventricular arrhythmias following tetralogy of Fallot repair. Circulation 72 (II): 197.

31. Byrum CJ, Sondheimer HM, Kavey REW, Blackman MS. 1985. Ventricular arrhythmia nontherapy guided by electrophysiologic tesing. Am Heart J 110: 707.

32. Deanfield JE, Franklin RCG, Dickie S, McKenna W, Gersony W, Hallidie-Smith K. 1985. Prognostic significance of ventricular arrhythmias after repair of tetralogy of Fallot: a prospective study. Proc Second World Congress of Pediatric Cardiology: 14.

33. Deanfield JE, McKenna WJ, Hallidie-Smith KA. 1980. Detection of late arrhythmia and conduction disturbance after correction of tetralogy of Fallot. Br Heart J 44 (3): 248–53.

34. Spinelli W, Rosen M. 1986. Developmental and use-dependent effects of phenytoin on neonatal and adult Purkinje fibers. J Am Coll Cardiol 7: 123.

35. Rosen MR, Gelband H, Merker C, Hoffman BF. 1973. Mechanisms of digitalis toxicity: effects of ouabain on phase four of canine Purkinje fibers transmembrane potential. Circulation 47: 681–6.

36. Amerini S, Carbonin P, Cerbai E, Giotti A, Mugelli A, Pahor M. 1985. Electrophysiological mechanisms for the antiarrhythmic action of mexiletine on digitalis, reperfusion and reoxygenation-induced arrhythmias. Br J Pharmacol 86 (4): 805–15.

37. Tseng G, Wit AL. 1985. Arrhythmogenic effects of quinidine on triggered activity in atrial muscle. Circulation 72 (Suppl III): 380.

38. Moak JP, Rosen MR. 1982. The effects of pacing on ouabain-induced sustained rhythmic activity. Circulation 66 (Suppl II): 79.

39. Johnson N, Danilo P, Wit A, Rosen MR. 1985. Response to pacing of triggered activity occurring in catecholamine-treated canine coronary sinus. Circulation 72 (Suppl III): 381.

40. Benito F, Aguado AG, Fernandez A, Moreno F. 1985. Delayed afterdepolarizations in patients post-repair of tetralogy of Fallot: could be considered a mechanism in the genesis of ventricular arrhythmias? Proc Second World Congress of Pediatric Cardiology: 111.

41. Spicer RL, Rocchini AP, Crowley DC, Rosenthal A. 1984. Chronic verapamil treatment in young adult patients with hypertrophic cardiomyopathy. Am J Cardio 53: 1614–19.

42. Gillette PC, Garson A. 1977. Electrophysiologic and pharmacologic characteristics of automatic ectopic supraventricular tachycardia. Circulation 56: 571–75.

43. Zipes DP, Foster PR, Troup PJ, Pedersen DH. 1979. Atrial induction of ventricular tachycardia: reentry versus triggered automaticity. Am J Cardiol 44 (1): 1–8.

44. Aronson RS. 1981. Afterpotentials and triggered activity in hypertrophied myocardium from rats with renal hypertension. Circ Res 48: 720–8.

45. Kugler JD, Pinsky WW, Cheatman JP, Hofschire PJ, Mooring PK, Fleming WH. 1983. Sustained ventricular tachycardia after repair of tetralogy of Fallot: new electrophysiologic findings. Am J Cardiol 51 (7): 1137–43.

46. Harken AH, Horowitz LN, Josephson ME. 1980. Surgical correction of recurrent sustained ventricular tachycardia following complete repair of tetralogy of Fallot. J Thorac Cardiovasc Surg 80 (5): 779–81.

47. Kawashima Y, Matsuda H, Hirose H, Nakano S, Shirakura R, Kobayashi J. 1985. Ninety consecutive corrective operations for tetralogy of Fallot with or without minimal right ventriculotomy. J Thorac Cardiovasc Surg 90 (6): 856–63.

48. Moak JP, Garson A. 1986. Late electrophysiologic effects of experimental right ventriculotomy. J Am Coll Cardiol 7: 49.

49. Garson A. 1984. Ventricular arrhythmias after congenital heart surgery: a canine model. Pediatr Res 18: 1112–20.

50. Deanfield J, McKenna W, Rowland E. 1985. Local abnormalities of right ventricular depolarization after repair of tetralogy of Fallot: a basis for ventricular arrhythmia. Am J Cardiol 55 (5): 522–5.

51. Waxman MB, Wald RW, Finley JP, Bonet JF, Downar E, Sharma AD. 1980. Valsalva termination of ventricular tachycardia. Circulation 62 (4): 843–51.
52. Cassidy DM, Vassallo JA, Miller JM, Josephson ME. 1985. Differences in endocardial electrophysiologic characteristics in coronary artery disease patients with ventricular tachycardias versus cardiac arrest. Circulation 72 (Suppl III): 160.
53. Benchimol A, Matsuo S, Wang TF. 1972. Phasic coronary arterial flow velocity during arrhythmias in man. Am J Cardiol 29: 604–15.
54. Tepper D, Sarda MA, Capasso JM, Somberg JC. 1986. Does hypertensive hypertrophy cause myocardial electrical instability? J Am Coll Cardiol 7: 111A.
55. Palik I, Graham TP, Burger J. 1986. Ventricular function in patients with obstructed right ventricular pulmonary artery conduits. J Am Coll Cardiol 7: 201A.
56. McRae JR, Wagner GC, Rogers MC. 1974. Paroxysmal familial ventricular fibrillation. J Pediatr 84: 515–20.
57. Fyke FE, Vlietstra RE, Danielson GK, Beynen FM. 1983. Verapamil for refractory ventricular fibrillation during cardiac operations in patients with cardiac hypertrophy. J Thorac Cardiovasc Surg 86 (1): 108–11.
58. Reduto LA, Berger HJ, Johnstone DE. 1978. Radionuclide assessment of exercise right and left ventricular performance following total correction of tetralogy of Fallot. Circulation 58: 145–50.

11. Late ventricular tachycardia after repair of tetralogy of Fallot

F. MARÇON and C. PERNOT

Because of recent advances in surgical techniques and postoperative care, the number of patients surviving correction of congenital heart defects is becoming significant and the long-term sequelae of these repairs are assuming greater importance. Long-term electrophysiologic consequences of repair of tetralogy of Fallot (TOF) include atrioventricular and intraventricular conduction defects, sinus node dysfunction and ventricular arrhythmias. An increasing amount of evidence suggests that malignant ventricular arrhythmias are a cause of late sudden death in patients after repair of TOF and apparented malformations with obstruction of the right ventricular outflow tract (ventricular septal defect associated with pulmonary valve stenosis, double outlet right ventricle, truncus arteriosus). Recent attention, therefore, has been focused on the detection, prevention and treatment of ventricular arrhythmias in these patients.

Incidence

In regard to its incidence in adults, ventricular tachycardia is a rare event in children and adolescents in whom premature ventricular contractions (PVC's) are more frequently observed than clinical ventricular tachycardia. Ventricular tachycardia following surgical repair of TOF is at the present time one of the most common causes of ventricular tachycardia observed by pediatric cardiologists (33 per cent in our experience) and will probably, in future, be encountered more and more by adult cardiologists because of increasing incidence with increasing follow-up.

Reported incidences of ventricular dysrhythmia after surgical repair of TOF vary from 5 to 50% according to the method of detection (standard ECG, exercise stress testing, Holter monitoring) [1–10]. Among 72 patients with operated TOF, Kavey [7] detected ventricular arrhythmia by 24 h ambulatory monitoring and/or exercise testing in 30 patients (42%) of whom nine only (14%) had PVC's on the standard ECG. Likewise, Garson [11] reported ventricular arrhythmia induced by treadmill exercise in 31 (30%) of 104 patients who underwent treadmill exercise testing at a mean age of 13,8 years, an average of 7 years after repair of TOF. Only 15 patients had ventricular arrhythmia at rest. 24 h ambulatory monitoring and exercise testing are more sensitive methods for detecting ventricular arrhythmias than routine electrocardiography and therefore are recomended for all patients after repair of TOF.

Prognosis

In contrast with the clinically well tolerated and benign 'primitive' ventricular dysrhythmias observed in children with a normal heart, ventricular dysrhythmias following surgical repair of TOF have generally a poor prognosis and may be associated with sudden death.

Sudden death is now a recognized late event after repair of TOF. Garson [12], in a review of patients with sudden death observed in the section of pediatric cardiology at the Texas Children's Hospital and related to prior arrhythmias, has shown that post-operative congenital heart disease is, with unoperated congenital heart disease (35%), the most frequent condition associated with late sudden death, before palliated congenital heart disease (17%), unoperated acquired heart disease (7%) and long-QT syndrome (5%). Post-operative TOF only account for 11% of the total of late sudden deaths. In all large series of repaired TOF, sudden death is noted with a reported incidence varying from 0.8 to 5.5 per cent [2, 4, 5, 7, 13]. Attention was initially focused on the possibility of late complete atrioventricular block from progressive damage to the proximal conduction system. This concept arose when the electrocardiographic pattern of right bundle branch block and left axis deviation was found in a proportion of patients after intracardiac repair of TOF [14]. A poor prognosis was reported for patients with these conduction defects [15] and for those who had experienced transient perioperative complete atrioventricular block [16, 17], but has not been confirmed by others [5, 18–20]. Deanfield's [21] pathologic study of conduction system in three patients who died suddenly after repair of TOF showed that in every case the atrioventricular node, atrioventricular bundle and left bundle branch were undamaged and that complete atrioventricular block was probably not the cause of the death. The role of late complete atrioventricular block in late sudden death after corrective surgery of TOF has certainly been overemphasized and still arises occasionally. Moreover, progress in surgical techniques to preserve conduction system and the development of pacemaker implantations seem to have had no influence on the incidence of late sudden death after surgical repair of TOF.

On the other hand, recent reports strongly suggest that patients with manifest ventricular arrhythmias are at higher risk of sudden death: a high incidence of ventricular arrhythmias has been demonstrated in postoperative patients with

TOF and has been associated with sudden death in retrospective and prospective series [4–7, 9, 10, 22–24]. The mortality rate for patients with ventricular dysrhythmias, detected on exercise testing and/or ambulatory monitoring, is higher than for patients without. In the Kavey's series [7], the overall mortality for the entire study group was 5.5% though the mortality rate for patients with proven potentially malignant ventricular dysrhythmias was 33%, comparable to similar groups reported by others [2, 4, 23]. Among the 488 patients of Garson et al. [9], followed up for more than 1 month after repair of TOF (mean follow-up time 6.1 years), nine died suddenly: each one of the nine had PVC's on routine electrocardiogram, whereas PVC's occurred in only 12% (p<0.0001) of patients who did not die suddenly. Moreover, Garson et al. [9] have demonstrated that sudden death after repair of TOF could be markedly reduced using an agressive treatment program aimed at abolition of PVC's from the routine and 24 hours electrocardiogram.

Etiologic factors

The specific etiology of ventricular dysrhythmias occurring in patients with TOF after surgery is unknown but it is clear that no single abnormality causes ventricular arrhythmias in these patients.

Hemodynamic factors

Poor hemodynamic result after corrective surgery is held to be an important factor predisposing to ventricular arrhythmias by the majority of authors [1, 4, 11, 22, 23]. Patients with PVC's on routine electrocardiogram, exercise testing and 24 hours ambulatory monitoring have a significantly higher systolic right ventricular pressure ($\geqslant 60$ mm Hg) [1, 4, 7, 25]. In general, the higher the right ventricular systolic pressure, the greater the number of patients with PVC's, the greatest prevalence occurring with a right ventricular systolic pressure greater than 60 mm Hg [4, 9]. The right ventricular end-diastolic pressure has been also related, but less significantly, to PVC's [9]. In a previous study [23], we have compared hemodynamic results in 6 patients with documented ventricular tachycardias after intracardiac repair of TOF (4 patients), or similar malformation (2 patients), with the results of 44 patients without dysrhythmia. Results are listed in Table 1. The two groups did not differ by age at the time of surgical repair, by the surgical technique and the duration of follow-up. Incidence of intraventricular or atrioventricular conduction defects was similar in both groups. A residual systolic pressure gradient between pulmonary artery and right ventricle superior to 30 mm Hg and a recurrent ventricular septal defect (QP : QS $\geqslant 1.5 : 1$) were significantly more frequent in patients with ventricular tachycardia. The combination of ventricular tachycardia and poor hemodynamic result was associated in this study with a mortality rate of 33%. These results are comparable to major comparable studies [7, 9] but are not in concordance with others [5, 10, 26]. Therefore, if no relation between PVC's and increased right ventricular systolic pressure was observed by Deanfield et al. [5], ventricular arrhythmias were related by these authors to decreased right ventricular ejection fraction by nuclear angiography [24]. Likewise, in a first report, Kavey et al. [7] were unable to correlate ventricular dysrhythmias with a poor hemodynamic result, but a further study of this group [27] demonstrated that patients with ventricular arrhythmias after corrective surgery of TOF had a significantly more marked right ventricular enlargement and a significantly lower left ventricular ejection fraction measured by radionuclide angioscintigraphy, the right ventricular ejection fraction being lower, but not significantly ($p < 0.10$). Thus, alteration of right or left ventricular functions, or both, could be also factors of importance to predispose to ventricular arrhythmias. Radionuclide imaging at rest but preferentially at exercise [28, 29, 30] has been suggested as an accurate assessment of the surgical results and prognosis but further studies are needed to standardize protocols [28].

Postoperative pulmonary valve insufficiency is common after surgical repair of

Table 1. Comparative data between patients with and without ventricular tachycardia after complete surgical repair of tetralogy of Fallot.

	VT	no VT	
Number of patients	6	44	
Age of surgery	6 ± 2 yrs	7.8	NS
Duration of follow-up	8 ± 2.5 yrs	8.7	NS
Surgical repair			
Infundibular patch	4 (70%)	33	NS
Ventriculotomy	5 (83%)	40	NS
Functional class			
NYHA	I (5/6)	I (42/44)	NS
Mitral valve prolapse	1 (17%)	6 (14%)	NS
Standard ECG			
RBBB	6 (100%)	42 (95%)	NS
RBBB + LAD	3 (50%)	17 (39%)	NS
First-degree block	1 (17%)	5 (11%)	NS
Catheterization data			
PA-RV gradient >30 mm Hg	3 (50%)	4 (9%)	p<0.05
Recurrent VSD (QP/QS >1.5 : 1)	3 (50%)	3 (7%)	p<0.02
Recurrent VSD + PA-RV gradient	3 (50%)	0	p<0.001
Pulmonary valve insufficiency	3 (50%)	16 (36%)	NS

Abbreviations: VT = ventricular tachycardia; NYHA = New-York Heart Association; PA-RV gradient = pulmonary artery-right ventricle gradient; VSD = ventricular septal defect; RBBB = right bundle branch block; LAD = left axis deviation.

TOF both in patients with and without ventricular dysrhythmias and has been not related to ventricular arrhythmias [4, 23]. Therefore, because there were no other causes established in patients with an extremely dilated, poorly contracting right ventricle, it is possible that pulmonary insufficiency contributed to the problem, and that with longer follow-up pulmonary insufficiency might lead to ventricular arrhythmias [29].

Timing of surgery and follow-up

The presence of PVC's is strongly related to the duration of follow-up. Patients with such complexes have a significantly longer follow-up than those without in large series [9–11]. With increasing age at follow-up there is a steadily increasing incidence of PVC's and such complexes have been observed in up to one third of patients of 30 years and older [9]. There is also an increased incidence of later development of PVC's with increasing patient age at repair [7, 9, 10]. Which of both factors is the most significant for later ventricular dysrhythmias is unsettled question at the present time. Referring to Garson et al. [9], the duration of follow-up is probably the most significant factor, but the recent series of 22 patients of Martin [32], operated on before 2 years of age without late ventricular dysrhythmia for a follow-up of 10 years or more, seems to be in contrast with this concept. Finally, patients who experienced ventricular dysrhythmias are significantly older at the time of study in all series, however longer is the duration of follow-up, postoperatively or preoperatively. These findings suggest that the onset of ventricular dysrhythmias is age-related and long term follow-up for rhythm evaluation is necessary whether patients have been operated upon after 2 years of age or not.

Other factors

Reintervention, particularly for recurrent ventricular septal defect, is a well-etablished influencing factor for development of ventricular dysrhythmias [7]. Occasionally, other factors, like mitral valve prolapse [10], may have contributed to ventricular dysrhythmias. In a personal case, recurrent ventricular tachycardia was caused by a voluminous post-infarct left ventricular aneurism, secondary to surgical injury of anomalous left-anterior descending coronary artery originating from the right coronary artery.

Mechanisms of ventricular tachycardia

Ventricular tachycardia using the ventriculotomy scar as macro-reentrant circuit was convincingly demonstrated by Horowitz et al. [33], who reported the cessation of ventricular tachycardia when a transverse incision was made across the prior ventriculotomy scar at reoperation. This mechanism is probably less common than originally thought. Several reports [10, 26, 29] in which the earliest site of ventricular activation was mapped at numerous areas in the right ventricle (rather than just the outflow tract) support the idea that almost any area can be arrhythmogenetic. Myocardial fibrosis has been observed in patients who died suddenly after intracardiac repair [21, 34]. In the pathologic study of Deanfield et al. [21], fibrosis was present, in varying degrees, in the different right ventricular sites of the three examined hearts. In each case the right ventriculotomy site was extensively replaced by fibrous tissue. It is easy to imagine how ventricular arrhythmia might originate in the presence of fibrosis of the right ventricular myocardium, with localised slowing of conduction favouring the development of reentry circuits. Thus, the myocardial fibrosis could be part of the natural history of the uncorrected heart with tetralogy of Fallot, or related to the operation and postoperative hemodynamic status.

Because the arrhythmias can be induced during electrophysiologic study [26, 31, 33, 35, 37], it can be inferred that they are due to either a reentry or a triggered mechanism, or both [37]. Why certain patients with similar measured parameters have ventricular tachycardia and other ones do not, and why certain postoperative patients tolerate ventricular tachycardia with few symptoms and other die suddenly, are the subjects of continuing investigations [38]. As virtually all patients who have been reported to die suddenly had an elevated right ventricular systolic pressure [1, 4, 25], it may be that those without right ventricular outflow tract obstruction tolerate ventricular tachycardia, while those with residual obstruction who develop ventricular tachycardia rapidly undergo hemodynamic and electrophysiologic deterioration, that may be manifest as sudden death. This concept might probably be extended to the patients with impaired ventricular function.

Prevention and treatment

Since it appears that the majority of late sudden deaths after corrective surgery of TOF are related to ventricular arrhythmias, the question of prevention of late ventricular arrhythmias is of first importance in these patients.

Prevention of ventricular arrhythmias can be considered first at the time of surgery or secondly after intervention. On the basis of presumed pathophysiologic mechanisms producing ventricular arrhythmias in these patients, primary prevention of ventricular arrhythmias may include: lower age at intervention (under two years), amelioration of myocardial protection during operation, production of as small an area of ventrculotomy and outflow resection as possible to give a small scar, reduction of the right ventricle systolic pressure and prevention of pulmonary valve insufficiency. But improvement of hemodynamic results comes up against certain technical difficulties which cannot be relieved. So achievement of low right ventricle systolic pressure is often inconsistent with a small outflow tract resection or trivial pulmonary valve regurgitation. In some cases it is not possible to reduce the right ventricular obstruction any further because of small distal pulmonary arteries. In like manner, reintervention for residual obstruction in order to reduce right ventricular systolic pressure creates a new scar which can be consistently considered as a risk factor for arrhythmias. However, the achievement of a good hemodynamic result is clearly not the entire answer to the problem of the prevention of ventricular arrhythmias, since some patients with a low pressure have ventricular arrhythmias and some of those with a high pressure do not.

Postoperatively, prevention of ventricular arrhythmias and sudden death is based upon the detection and treatment of patients at higher risk. Routine postoperative hemodynamic catheterization for all patients with tetralogy of Fallot or apparented malformations (double outlet right ventricle, pulmonary stenosis or atresia associated with ventricular septal defect, truncus arteriosus . . .) is recommended within 1 to 2 years of operation, since assessment based on clinical variables is unreliable in estimating the success of operation. In our institution, complete electrophysiologic study (sinus node function, A-V conduction, right ventricular pacing) is performed during the same period. If possible, evaluation by radionuclide angiography of ventricular function (right or left ventricular ejection fractions, right and left ventricular volume ratio) should be made at the time of catheterization, at rest and on exercise. The patients with a good or excellent hemodynamic result (right ventricular systolic pressure <50 mm Hg, no recurrent ventricular septal defect, mild pulmonary valve insufficiency, normal right and left ventricular ejection fractions, right and left ventricular volume ratio <2) do not require a frequent evaluation. If the hemodynamic result is poor and/or a residual, surgically accessible defect is found, reoperation should be considered. Some residual lesions such as proximal pulmonary artery branch stenosis or supravalvular pulmonary stenosis may be treated by percutaneous angioplasty [39]. If surgery is not attempted, the patient should be monitored frequently for dysrhythmias, especially PVC's. All postoperative patients should have, at the time of cardiac catheterization, a resting ECG, exercising test and ambulatory 24 hours electrocardiographic monitoring. If ventricular arrhythmia is not detected, scanning with resting ECG, exercising test and ambulatory 24 hours monitoring is repeated annually. If ventricular arrhythmia is detected by one of these means, treatment should be considered. Garson et al. [9] recommend that the following should be treated with antiarrhythmic drugs: (a) any patient with syncope, and/or more than 10 uniform PVC's per hour, or any multiform PVC's, couplets or ventricular tachycardia; (b) any patient with an elevated right ventricular systolic pressure or reduced right ventricular contractility who also has more than infrequent uniform premature

160

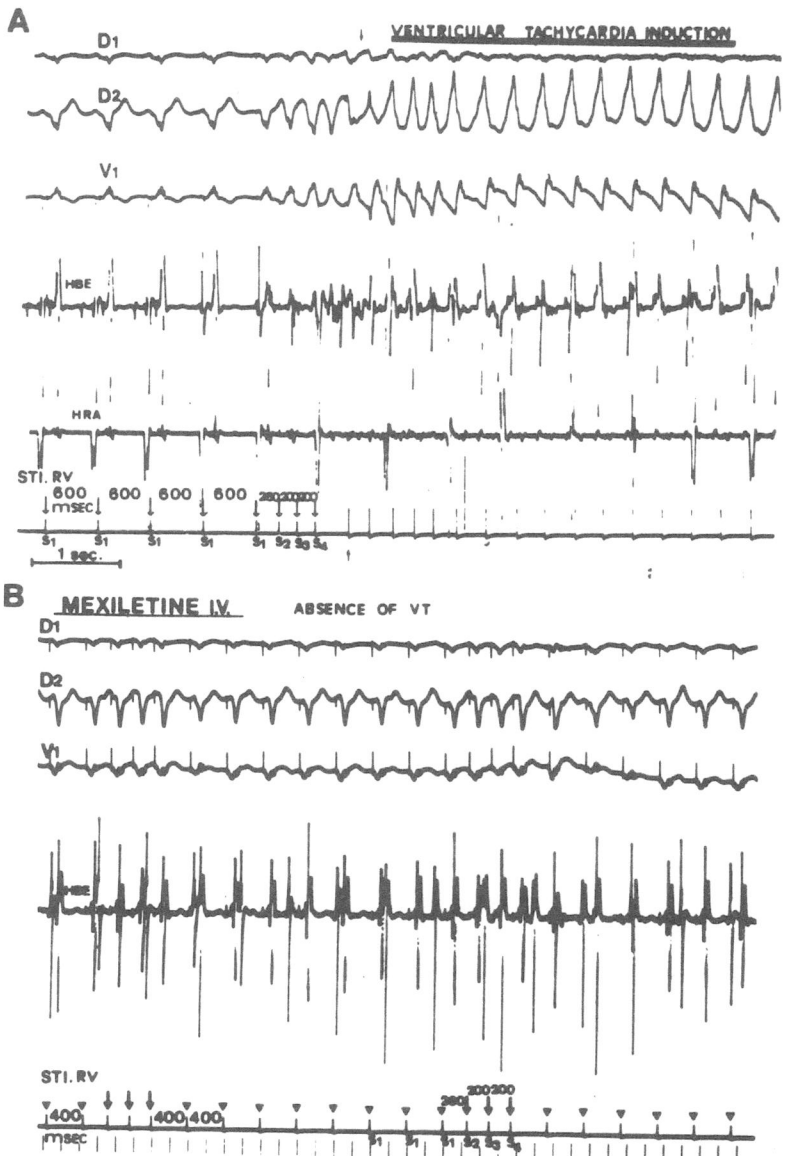

Figure 1. Recording during electrophysiologic study in a 16-year-old girl with spontaneous recurrent sustained ventricular tachycardia after repair of TOF. A. Induction of sustained ventricular tachycardia by 3 programmed extrastimuli (S2, S3, S4) introduced at right ventricular apex during right ventricular pacing (S1-S1 = 600 ms). B. After the intravenous adminitration of 375 mg of mexiletine over 45 minutes, ventricular tachycardia cannot be initiated by control protocol of right ventricular stimulation. No other coupling intervals or stimulation protocol produced ventricular tachycardia after mexiletine. Chronic oral treatment with mexiletine was institued: no recurrent ventricular tachycardia occured during a follow-up of 4 years. Abbreviations: D1, D2, V1 = surface ECG leads; HBE = His bundle electrogram; HRA = high right atrium; sti. RV = right ventricular stimulation; VT = ventricular tachycardia.

ventricular complexes on 24 hours electrocardiogram; (c) any patient with couplets or ventricular tachycardia on the 24 hours electrocardiogram without regard to a history of symptoms or hemodynamic findings. For these authors, current drug of choice is phenytoin which has been shown to be effective in treating such arrhythmias [40]. Compared with adult studies on ventricular arrhythmias and sudden deaths, the ventricular arrhythmias in these patients are rather easily controlled [9]. In addition, the spectrum of drugs that are effective is quite different from that in adults. Thus phenytoin and mexiletine are very effective, and propranolol relatively effective, in these postoperative patients with tetralogy, whereas quinidine is relatively unsuccessful. Amiodarone should be given to patients with arrhythmias unresponsive to conventional treatment [41]. Although the symptomatic effects of this drug in children are comparatively mild, the long-term effects of the drug are unknown and, therefore, amiodarone is recommended only for refractory arrhythmias.

The usefulness of electrophysiologic study is still uncertain. At the present time, electrophysiologic study is indicated in patients with syncope and in selected patients with ventricular tachycardia when pharmacologic and pacing regimens failed to prevent recurence of tachycardia, to determine the mechanism and the site of origin of the tachycardia before its surgical resection [42]. Electrophysiologic study also is helpful to select an effective antiarrhythmic drug in patients with spontaneous recurrent ventricular tachycardia (Fig. 1) [26, 43–45]. If successful in preventing induction of ventricular tachycardia, the drug is then given orally. In the asymptomatic patients, the value of such a study remains to be determined, but the induction of sustained ventricular tachycardia should be considered as a risk factor for spontaneous ventricular tachycardia and sudden death, and treatment should be recommended.

References

1. James FJ, Kaplan S, Chou TC. 1975. Unexpected cardiac arrest in patients after surgical correction of tetralogy of Fallot. Circulation 52: 691–695.
2. Quattelbaum TG, Varghese PJ, Neill CA, Donahoo JS. 1976. Sudden death among postoperative patients with tetralogy of Fallot. A follow-up study of 243 patients for an average of twelve years. Circulation 54: 289–293.
3. Gillette PC, Yeoman MA, Mullins CE, McNamara DG. 1977. Sudden death after repair of tetralogy of Fallot. Electrocardiographic and electrophysiologic abnormalities. Circulation 56: 566–571.
4. Garson A, Nihill MR, McNamara DG, Cooley DA. 1979. Status of the adult and adolescent after repair of tetralogy of Fallot. Circulation 59: 1232–1240.
5. Deanfield JE, Mc Kenna WJ, Hallidie-Smith KA. 1980. Detection of late arrhythmia and conduction disturbance after correction of tetralogy of Fallot. Br Heart J 44: 248–253.
6. Wessel HU, Bastanier CK, Parel NH, Berry TE, Cole RB, Muster AJ. 1980. Pronostic significance of arrhythmia in tetralogy of Fallot after intracardiac repair. Am J Cardiol 46: 843–848.
7. Kavey REW, Blackman MS, Sondheimer HM. 1982. Incidence and severity of chronic ventricular dysrhythmias after repair of tetralogy of Fallot. Am Heart J 103: 342–350.

8. Tamer D, Wolff GS, Ferrer P, Pickoff AS, Casta A, Metha AV, Garcia O, Gelband H. 1983. Hemodynamics and intracardiac conduction after operative repair of tetralogy of Fallot. Am J Cardiol 1: 552–556.
9. Garson A, Randall DC, Gillette PC, Smith RT, Moak JP, Mc Vey P, McNamara DG. 1985. Prevention of sudden death after repair of tetralogy of Fallot: treatment of ventricular arrhythmias. J Am Coll Cardiol 6: 221–227.
10. Matina D, Mouly A, Massol J, Gatau-Pelanchon J, Blin D, Langlet F, Levy S, Monties JR, Gerard R. 1985. Troubles du rhythme ventriculaire après réparation de tétralogie de Fallot. A propos de 59 cas. Arch Mal Coeur 78: 103–110.
11. Garson A, Gillette PC, Gutgesell HP, McNamara DG. 1980. Stress-induced ventricular arrhythmia after repair of tetralogy of Fallot. Am J Cardiol 46: 1006–1012.
12. Garson A, McNamara DG. 1985. Sudden death in a pediatric cardiology population, 1958 to 1983: relation to prior arrhythmias. J Am Coll Cardiol 5: 134B–137B.
13. Katz NM, Blackstone EH, Kirklin JW, Pacifico AD, Bargeron LM. 1982. Late survival and symptoms after repair of tetralogy of Fallot. Circulation 65: 403–410.
14. Kulbertus HE, Coyne JJ, Hallidie-Smith KA. 1969. Conduction disturbances before and after surgical closure f ventricular septal defect. Am Heart J 77: 123–131.
15. Wolff GS, Rowland TW, Ellison RC. 1972. Surgically induced right bundle branch block with left anterior hemiblock. Circulation 45: 587–593.
16. Moss AJ, Klyman G, Emmanouilides GC. 1972. Late onset complete heart block. Am J Cardiol 30: 884.
17. Krongrad E. 1978. Prognosis for patients with congenital heart disease and postoperative intraventricular conduction defects. Circulation 57: 867–869.
18. Cairns JA, Dobell ARC, Gibbons JE, Tessler I. 1975. Prognosis of right bundle branch block and left anterior hemiblock after intracardiac repair of tetralogy of Fallot. Am Heart J 90: 549–554.
19. Downing JW, Kaplan S, Bove KE. 1972. Postchirurgical left anterior hemiblock and right bundle branch block. Br Heart J 34: 263–270.
20. Steeg CN, Krongrad E, Davachi F, Bowman FO, Malm JR, Gersony WM. 1975. Postoperative left anterior hemiblock and right bundle branch block following repair of tetralogy of Fallot: clinical and etiologic consideration. Circulation 51: 1026–1029.
21. Deanfield JE, Ho SY, Anderson RH, McKenna WJ, Allwork SP, Hallidie-Smith KA. 1983. Late sudden death after repair of tetralogy of Fallot: a clinicopathologic study. Circulation 67: 626–631.
22. Kobayashi J, Hirose H, Ivakano S, Matsuda H, Shirakura R, Kawashima Y. 1984. Ambulatory electrocardiographic study of the frequency and cause of ventricular arrhythmia after correction of tetralogy of Fallot. Am J Cardiol 54: 1310–1313.
23. Cloez JL, Khalife K, Weber JL, Aliot E, Marçon F, Pernot C. 1984. Tachycardies ventriculaires tardives après correction chirurgicale d'une cardiopathie congénitale. Incidence, sévérité et facteurs prédictifs. Arch Mal Coeur 77: 534–542.
24. Deanfield JEV, Franklin R, McKenna WJ, Dickie S, Gersony W, Hallidie-Smith KA. 1985. Prognostic significance of ventricular arrhythmia after repair of tetralogy of Fallot. A prospective study. (Abstract). Br Heart J 53: 676.
25. Fuster V, McGoon DC, Kennedy MA, Ritter DG, Kirklin JW. 1980. Long-term evaluation (12 to 22 years) of open heart surgery for tetralogy of Fallot. Am J Cardiol 46:635–642.
26. Kugler JD, Pinsky WW, Cheatham JP, Hofchire PJ, Mooring PK, Fleming WH. 1983. Sustained ventricular tachycardia after repair of tetralogy of Fallot: new electrophysiologic findings. Am J Cardiol 51: 1137–1143.
27. Kavey REW, Thomas FD, Byrum GJ, Blackman MS, Sondheimer HM, Bove EL. 1984. Ventricular arrhythmias and biventricular dysfunction after repair of tetralogy of Fallot. J Am Coll Cardiol 4: 126–131.
28. Reduto AL, Berger HJ, Johnstone DE, Hellenbrand W, Wackers FJT, Whittemore R, Cohen LS,, Gottschalk A, Zaret B. 1980. Radionuclide assessment of right and left ventricular exercise

reserve after total correction of tetralogy of Fallot. Am J Cardiol 45: 1013–1018.

29. Parrish MD, Graham TP, Born ML, Jones J. 1982. Radionuclide evaluation of right and left ventricular function in children: validation of methodology. Am J Cardiol 49: 1241–1247.

30. Brunotte F, Marçon F, Cloez JL, Laurens MH, Itty C, Robert J, Pernot C. 1985. Apprt des radio-isotopes à l'étude de la fonction ventriculaire droite et gauche dans la tétralogie de Fallot opérée. Arch Mal Coeur 78: 771–776.

31. Garson A, Porter CJ, Gillette PC, McNamara DG. 1983. Induction of ventricular tachycardia during electrophysiologic study after repair of tetralogy of Fallot. J Am Coll Cardiol 1: 1493–1502.

32. Martin R, Khagani A, Radley-Smith R, Yacoub M. 1985. Patient status 10 or more years after primary total correction of tetralogy of Fallot under the age of 2 years (Abstract.). Br Heart J 53: 666.

33. Horowitz LN, Vetter VL, Harken AH, Josephson ME. 1980. Electrophysiologic characteristics of sustained ventricular tachycardia occurring after repair of tetralogy of Fallot. Am J Cardiol 46: 446–452.

34. Marin-Garcia J, Moller JH. 1977. Sudden death after operative repair of tetralogy of Fallot. Br Heart J 39: 1380–1385.

35. Mehta AV, Sanchez GR, Donner RM, O'Riordan AC, Black IFS. 1983. New electrophysiologic findings after repair of tetralogy of Fallot (Abstract.). J Am Coll Cardiol 1 (suppl. 2): 614.

36. Vetter VL, Horowitz LN. 1982. Electrophysiologic results of repair of tetralogy of Fallot. Am J Cardiol 49: 999–1003.

37. Gillette PC, Garson A. 1981. Intracardiac electrophysiologic studies: use in determining the site and mechanisms of dysrhythmias. In: Gillette PC, Garson A (eds) Pediatric Cardiac Dysrhythmias. New York: Grune and Stratton, 77–120.

38. Garson A. 1984. Ventricular dysrhythmias after congenital heart surgery: a canine model. Pediatr Res 18: 1112–1120.

39. Lock JE, Castaneda-Zuniga WR, Fuhrman BP, Bass JL. 1983. Balloon dilatation angioplasty of hypoplastic and stenotic pulmonary arteries. Circulation 67: 962–967.

40. Garson A, Kugler JD, Gillette PC, Simonelli A, McNamara DG. 1980. Control of late postoperative ventricular arrhythmias with phenytoin in young patients. AmJ Cardiol 46: 290–294.

41. Garson A, Gillette PC, McVey P, Hesslein PS, Porter CJ, Angell LK, Kaldis LC, Hittnner HM. 1984. Amiodarone treatment of critical arrhythmias inn children and young adults. J Am Coll Cardiol 4: 749755.

42. Harken AH, Horowitz LN, Josephson ME. 1980. Surgical correction of recurrent sustained ventricular tachycardia following complete repair of tetralogy of Fallot. J Thorac Cardiovasc Surg 80: 779–781.

43. Horowitz LN, Josephson ME, Farshidi A, Spielman SR, Michelson EL, Greenspan AM. 1978. Recurrent sustained ventricular tachycardia. 3. Role of the electrophysiologic study in selection of antiarrhythmic regimens. Circulation 58: 986–997.

44. Josephson ME, Horowitz LN. 1979. Electrophysiologic approach to therapy of recurrent sustained ventricular tachycardia. Am J Cardiol 43: 631–642.

45. Kugler JD, Bansal AM, Cheatham JP, Pinsky WW, Moorine PK, Hofschire PJ. 1985. Drug-electrophysiology studies in infants, children and adolescents. Am Heart J 110: 144–154.

12. Drug-induced torsades de pointes: clinical and experimental observations bearing on mechanism

WARREN M. JACKMAN, KAREN J. FRIDAY, BELA SZABO,
EUGENE PATTERSON, ETIENNE M. ALIOT, and RALPH LAZZARA
From the Department of Medicine, University of Oklahoma Health Sciences Center and the Veterans Administration Medical Center, Oklahoma City, Oklahoma, USA

Torsades de pointes associated with the administration of quinidine or other class 1A antiarrhythmic agents, phenothiazines, or tricyclic antidepressants is a very distinctive and unusual ventricular tachyarrhythmia. It occurs in the setting of pronounced QTU interval prolongation and has a characteristic pause-related pattern of initiation [1–6]. The incidence of this arrhythmia does not seem to increase with increasing severity of ventricular disease, and may occur in patients with seemingly normal hearts [6–8]. Similarly, the incidence does not seem to increase with increasing drug dose. Torsades de pointes typically occurs at usual or low doses and serum drug levels [3–5, 9–14], and may occur after months of uncomplicated drug therapy without the appearance of other known inciting factors, such as hypokalemia and hypomagnesemia [5, 6, 15]. Susceptible patients have a high risk of recurrence of this arrhythmia upon exposure to any of the other drugs which broaden the T wave and enhance the U wave [5, 14, 16–21], whereas the majority of patients will not develop torsades de pointes regardless of the number of agents tried.

The mechanism of drug-induced torsades de pointes is still uncertain. The prevailing hypothesis attributes the broad TU complex to a marked variability in the degree to which the drug prolongs repolarization in ventricular myocardium (Fig. 1) [3, 22–32]. This heterogeneity of repolarization times creates a 'dispersion of refactoriness' [33, 34] which forms the substrate for reentry. A premature ventricular impulse, originating during the relative refractory period, propagates slowly through the incompletely recovered myocardium and around regions with the longest refractory periods, forming a functional reentrant circuit (Fig. 2). The twisting QRS morphology for which the syndrome is named [35] is not a consistent finding [1, 6] and may result from a gradual migration of this functional reentrant circuit or from the presence of two (or more) discrete reentrant circuits with similar rates competing for dominance [35–38]. In the latter condition, the gradual change in the QRS morphology would be attributed to fusion complexes with a progressive change in the contribution of the two (or more) foci.

A new hypothesis proposes that the late component of the TU complex, which

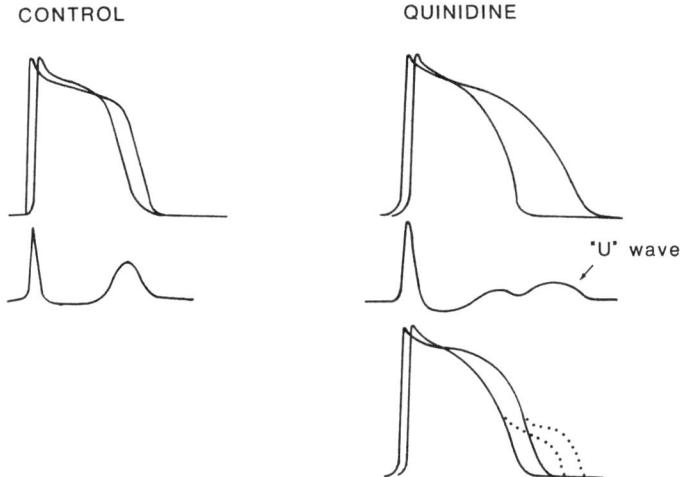

Figure 1. Two hypotheses for the genesis of the broad TU wave produced by quinidine and similar agents in drug-induced torsades de pointes. *Left:* Upper tracings simulate transmembrane potentials in the ventricular myocardium and lower tracing simulates a lateral precordial electrocardiogram. The normal T wave is related to asynchronous repolarization of the ventricular myocardium, represented by a difference in the time of phase 3 of the two action potentials. *Right:* The late component of the TU complex (U wave) may result from the very late repolarization of some region(s) of the myocardium, represented by the widest action potential in the top tracings. Alternatively, the broad TU wave may represent both prolonged repolarization and early afterdepolarizations, connoted by the dotted lines in the lower tracings.

we will refer to as the U wave, represents a summation of early afterdepolarizations occurring throughout the myocardium (Fig. 1) [1, 6, 40–43]. Ventricular extrasystoles and ventricular tachycardia are attributed to triggered firing. The complex morphological patterns observed during the tachycardia are thought to result from variability in the number and locations of the sites of triggered firing as well as variability in firing rates. The afterdepolarization hypothesis is based on a canine model of torsades de pointes using cesium chloride [39, 40, 42, 43] which, like quinidine, depresses the repolarizing potassium currents [44, 45].When CsCl is administered intravenously to anesthetized dogs the sinus rate slows, prominent U waves develop, and bursts of rapid, polymorphic ventricular tachycardia emerge and appear to be associated with the largest U waves (Fig. 3). *In vitro,* cesium produces early afterdepolarizations and triggered firing both of which are enhanced at slow rates (Fig. 4) [39, 41]. Bradycardia-dependent early afterdepolarizations and triggered firing have now also been shown for quinidine when combined with low potassium [46].

It is difficult, if not impossible, to firmly establish the mechanism of a clinical tachycardia. However, any proposed mechanism should be capable of accounting for all of the specific features of that tachycardia. Many of the features of drug-induced torsades de pointes mentioned above are consistent with either the

A.   B.

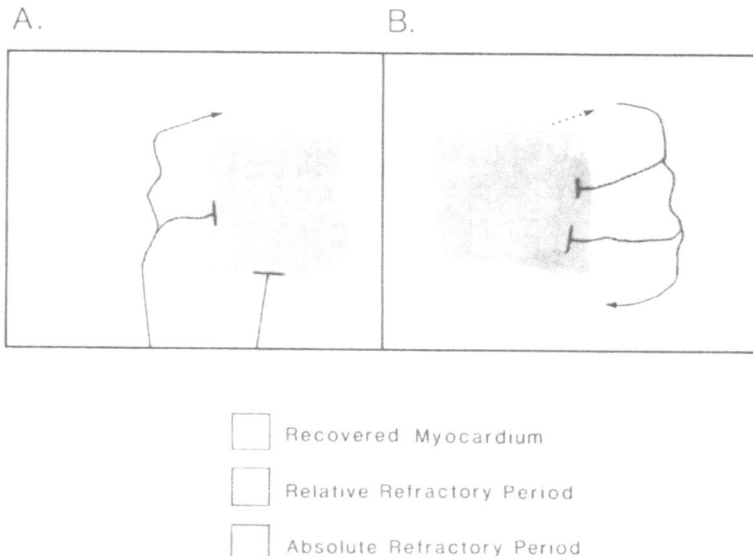

☐ Recovered Myocardium

☐ Relative Refractory Period

☐ Absolute Refractory Period

Figure 2. Schematic representation of the initiation of reentry by a premature ventricular impulse encountering heterogeneously recovered myocardium. *Panel A:* The straight lines at the bottom represent a premature ventricular impulse propagating through fully recovered myocrdium. The shaded area on the right represents myocardium which is still within the absolute refractory period. The stippled area on the left represents myocardium within the relative refractory period. The early impulse fails to excite the myocardium in the shaded zone. Perpendicular lines indicate conduction block. The impulse slowly traverses the stippled zone and begins to travel in a clockwise pattern as shown in *panel B.* The area which was penetrated by the original wavefront now becomes the completely refractory zone around which the reentrant impulse propagates.

reentry or triggered firing hypothesis. The most specific features of this unique arrhythmia are in the pattern of tachycardia initiation. The following description refers to torsades de pointes associated with the administration of quinidine and similar agents. The same pattern, termed pause-dependent torsades de pointes [1, 6], can also be manifested with hypokalemia, hypomagnesemia, and bradyar-rhythmias [13, 23, 27, 47–58]. This is in contrast to catecholamine-provoked torsades de pointes, often occurring in the absence of a pause, which will not be discussed. The Jervell and Lange-Neilsen syndrome [59] and Romano-Ward syndrome [60, 60a] are prototypic, but there are many variants of the 'adrenergic-dependent long QT syndromes' [6, 61].

The initiation of drug-induced torsades de pointes is consistently linked to a pause or sudden deceleration in the ventricular rhythm [1, 3–5]. The pause produces a large, bizarre U wave (Fig. 5A). The first ventricular complex emerges relatively late, during the U wave (Fig. 5C). An etiologic relationship between the pause-enhanced U wave and the tachycardia is suggested by the observation that increasing U wave amplitude is often associated with longer and

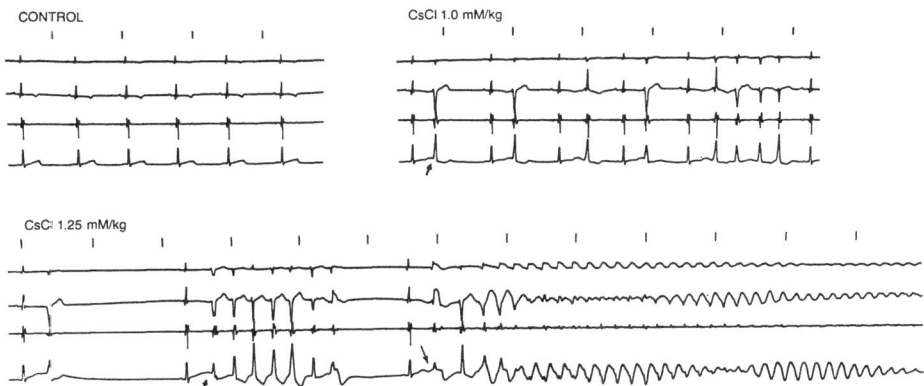

Figure 3. Induction of abnormal TU waves and torsades de pointes by cesium. Cesium chloride was administered intravenously to a dog while electrocardiographic leads I, II, III, and V2 (top to bottom) were recorded. The control recordings are shown at the top left and the effects of cesium chloride (1 mM/kg) shown at the top right. The *arrow* denotes an abnormal U wave interrupted by a ventricular extrasystole. In the lower panel, with a higher cesium dose (1.25 mM/kg), the TU abnormality is exaggerated after a long pause (*lower arrow*) and is followed by a short burst of polymorphic ventricular tachycardia. This short burst is followed by another pause which leads to a more prominent U wave (*upper arrow*) and sustained ventricular tachycardia with twisting morphology, closely mimicking the pause-dependent long QT syndromes in man. *From* Brachmann J, Scherlag BJ, Rosenshtraukh LV, and Lazzara R. 1983. Bradycardia-dependent triggered activity: relevance to drug-induced multiform ventricular tachycardia. Circulation 68: 846–856, with permission.

faster episodes of tachycardia (Figs 6 and 7) [1, 8]. The U wave amplitude is directly related to both the pause duration (Fig. 8) and the pre-pause ventricular rate (Fig. 9) [6]. These two factors combine to produce a positive feedback loop which perpetuates the arrhythmia in a bigeminal pattern. A pause in the ventricular rhythm of any etiology, such as that produced by the premature atrial complex in figure 10, results in an enhanced post-pause U wave and the emergence of a ventricular extrasystole. Each ventricular extrasystole, in turn, produces a short or 'fast' cycle followed by a compensatory pause. This results in another enhanced post-pause U wave and another ventricular extrasystole, etc. Eliminating sudden decelerations in the ventricular rhythm (Fig. 5, panel A and Fig. 7, panel A) and increasing the rate, such as by ventricular pacing (Figs 7–9), markedly decrease U wave amplitude and suppress the arrhythmia, further associating the arrhythmia and U wave. The U wave often oscillates in amplitude for several complexes following a pause or sudden deceleration [6]. While the oscillation in U wave amplitude may be apparent on the electrocardiogram (Fig. 9), it is usually easier to appreciate on intracardiac electrograms recorded with a low pass filter (Fig. 11).

The pivotal point separating the reentry and triggered firing hypotheses is whether the exaggerated U wave represents delayed repolarization of some

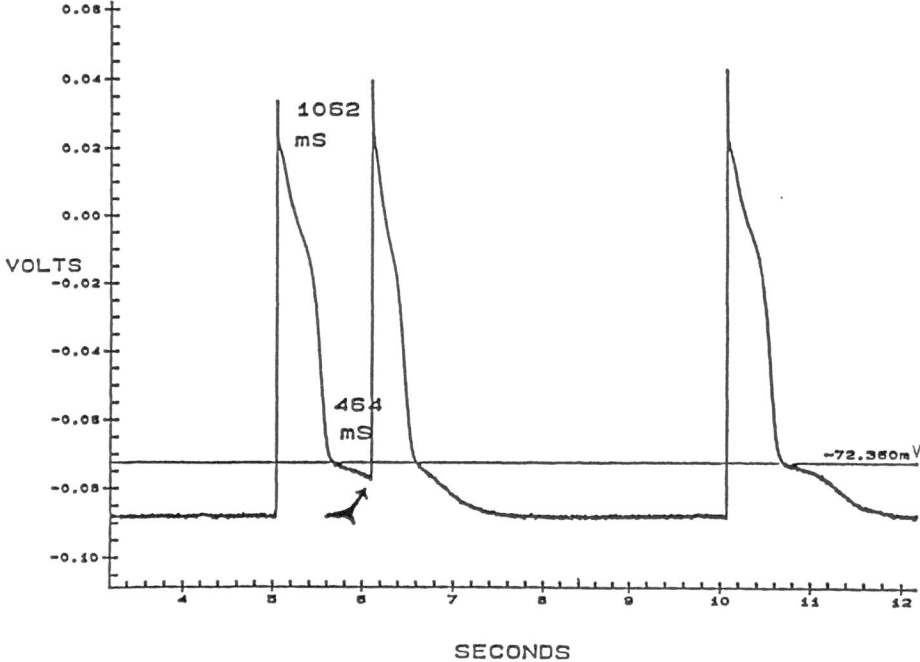

Figure 4. Cesium-induced early afterdepolarizations (EADs) and triggered firing. Microelectrode recording in canine Purkinje fiber superfused with Tyrode's solution containing 7 mM cesium chloride. First and third action potentials are electrically stimulated. When the stimulus cycle length was increased to 5 sec, EADs appeared but most did not fire. The first action potential shown in this figure was followed by an EAD which gave rise to a secondary, triggered action potential *(arrow)*. The diastolic interval between the stimulated and triggered action potentials was 464 msec, allowing recovery of the membrane currents.

→

Figure 5. Typical features of drug-induced torsades de pointes in a patient receiving disopyramide (150 mg every 6 hours) for atrial fibrillation. *A.* Striking post-pause U wave accentuation *(arrow)*. The U wave amplitude decreases progressively over the next two cycles. The QT interval (0.47 sec) is not significantly prolonged, considering the slow ventricular rate. *B.* Ventricular bigeminy associated with large 'post-pause' U waves *(arrow)*. *C.* Post-pause ventricular extrasystoles and torsades de pointes. Same monitor lead as panels A and B but gain is reduced. Note the first beat of the tachycardia is widely coupled (0.65 sec), emerging from the *largest* U wave. The T wave of that post-pause complex is barely perceptible, leaving the impression that the U wave is the T wave. *From* Jackman WM, Friday KJ, Anderson JL, Aliot EM, Clark M, Lazzara R. The long QT syndromes: A critical review, new clinical observations and a unifying hypothesis. Prog Cardiovasc Dis, in press.

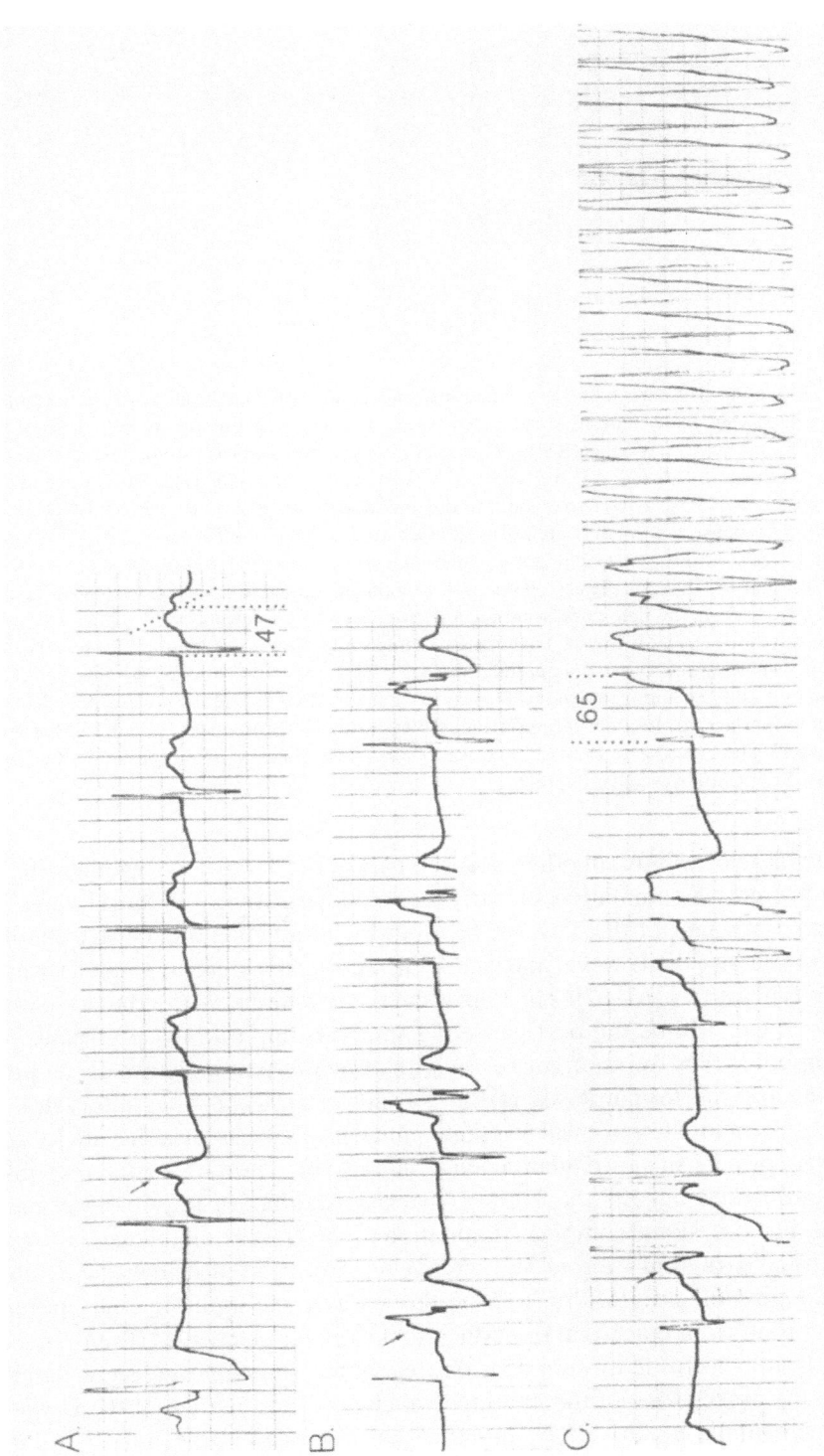

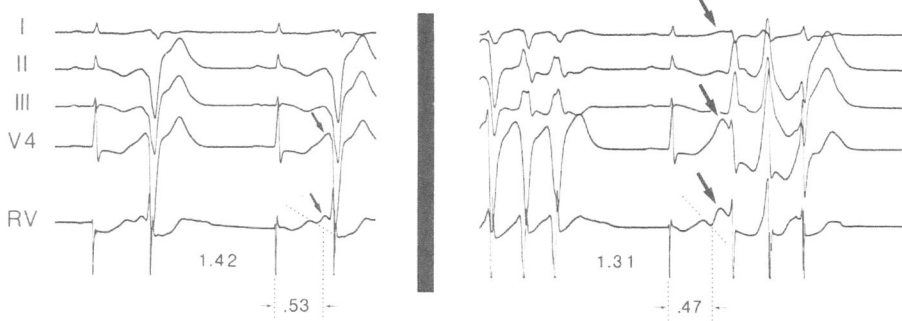

Figure 6. Relationship between U wave amplitude and number of sequential ventricular ectopic complexes in procainamide-induced torsades de pointes. Tracings from the top are ECG leads I, II, III, and V_4 and a right ventricular (RV) endocardial electrogram recorded from a bipolar catheter electrode (interelectrode spacing, 5 mm) using a filter bandwidth of 0.05–5000 Hz. The U wave of the endocardial electrogram (*arrow*) corresponds to the timing of the U wave on the surface ECG leads. The smaller post-pause U wave in the left panel is associated with one ventricular extrasystole, while the larger U wave in the right panel is associated with three sequential ventricular extrasystoles. Although the pause in the right panel (1.31 sec) is shorter than the pause in the left panel (1.42 sec), the faster pre-pause rate in the right panel is associated with a larger post-pause U wave. The faster pre-pause rate and shorter pause in the right panel is associated with a *shorter* post-pause QT interval (0.47 vs. 0.53 sec), showing the U wave amplitude may vary independently from the QT interval. The separation of T and U components of the TU wave is more pronounced on the endocardial electrogram than the surface electrogram. *From* Jackman WM, Friday KJ, Anderson JL, Aliot EM, Clark M, Lazzara R. The long QT yndromes: A critical review, new clinical observations and a unifying hypothesis. Prog Cardiovasc Dis, in press.

region(s) of myocardium, in other words, a part of the T wave, or whether the U wave represents a summation of early afterdepolarizations. If the U wave is simply a component of the T wave, factors which influence the T wave should similarly influence the U wave, and vice versa. A principal determinant of T wave duration is heart rate [62–67]. The longer the pause and the *slower* the pre-pause rate, the longer will be the post-pause QT interval. Importantly, post-pause U wave amplitude (and duration) increases with *faster* pre-pause rates. A faster pre-pause rate and shorter pause will result in a shorter post-pause QT interval, but often the post-pause U wave will be greater and will also be associated with longer and faster episodes of ventricular tachycardia (Fig. 6). This differential response to pre-pause rate suggests the T and U waves are different physiological phenomena. The occasional complete elimination of the U wave on regularization of the ventricular rhythm *without* an increase in rate, as seen in figure 7A, also suggests a physiological difference from the T wave. Monophasic injury potentials, recorded from epicardial or endocardial catheter electrodes (Franz silver-silver chloride electrode [68]) in dogs treated with cesium chloride show deflections on the downstroke of the potential which occur at the time of the U wave and appear similar to early afterdepolarizations recorded intracellularly in Pur-

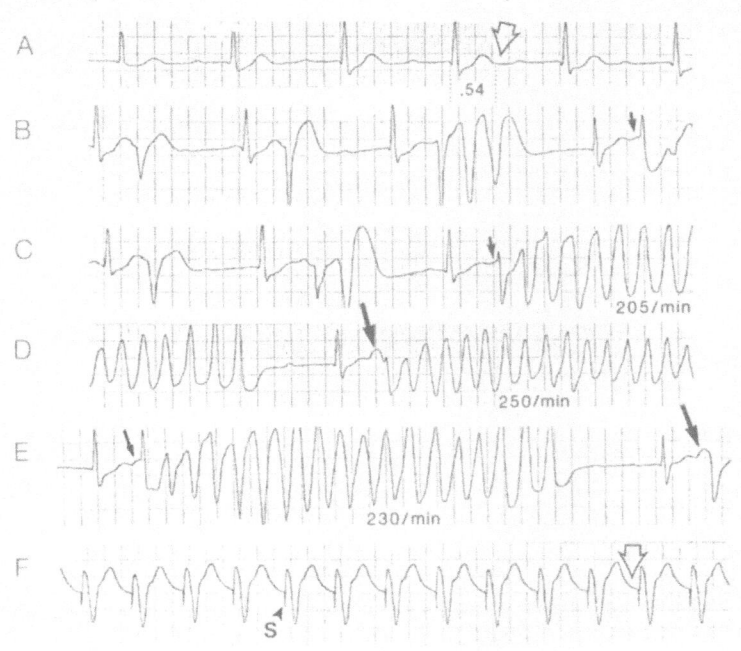

Figure 7. Relationship between U wave amplitude and ventricular tachycardia rate in imipramine-induced torsades de pointes. Panels A-E were recorded from the same monitor lead during a 45 minute period without intervention (not in chronological order). *Filled arrows* mark several post-pause U waves. Panels C, D and E show the initiation of three episodes of torsades de pointes with the mear. rate of the tachycardia listed below. The U wave amplitue associated with the initiation of the tachycardia is smallest in panel C, intermediate in panel E, and largest in panel D. Similarly, the mean tachycardia rate is slowest in panel C (205/min), intermediate in panel E (230/min), and fastest in pane: D (250/min). Panel A was recorded between the times of panel D and panel E and shows complete AV block and a junctional (or ventricular) escape rhythm at 47/min. Note that when the rhythm is regular, even though very slow, the U wave is minimal or absent (*unfilled arrow*) and the QT interval is not markedly prolonged for rate at 0.54 seconds. However, when the regularity of the rhythm is disturbed, such as by a ventricular extrasystole, short cycles followed by long cycles ('pauses') result in prominent U waves and ventricular extrasystoles or tachycardia (*filled arrows,* panels B-E). *Panel F,* recorded during temporary right ventricular pacing (100/min), shows a marked decrease in U wave amplitude (*unfilled arrow*). This was associated with complete resolution of the ventricular arrhythmia. *From* Jackman WM, Clark M, Friday KJ, Aliot EM, Anderson J, Lazzara R. 1984. Ventricular tachyarrhythmias in the long QT syndromes. Med Clin North Am 68: 1079–1109, with permission.

kinje fibers and myocardium exposed to cesium chloride (Figs 12–16) [43]. Similar deflections have been recorded in patients with pause-dependent torsades de pointes (Fig. 17) [69–71]. If the U wave represented late repolarization of discrete regions of myocardium, the monophasic injury potential would be expected to vary widely in duration in different regions of the heart, without the presence of the discrete late component.

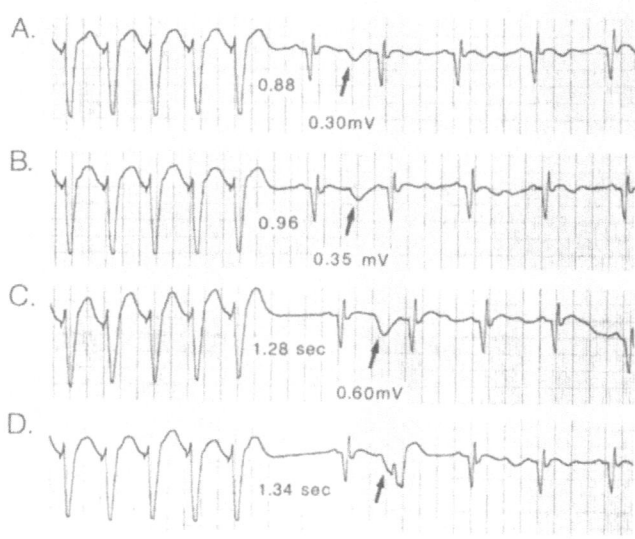

Figure 8. Relationship between pause length and U wave amplitude in a patient with quinidine-induced torsades de pointes. All four tracings were recorded from a mid-precordial lead at the end of a 45 second period of right ventricular pacing at a constant rate of 120/min. Panels A-D are arranged in order of increasing post-pacing escape ('pause') interval. As the pause increases from 0.88 sec in panel A to 1.28 sec in panel C, the U wave amplitude increases from 0.30 mV to 0.60 mV. The U wave following a longer pause of 1.34 sec is interrupted by a ventricular extrasystole, preventing measurement of its amplitude (panel D). These tracings show that, for the same pre-pause rate, increasing pause duration results in increasing post-pause U wave amplitude. Note the absence of U waves and only mild QT prolongation during right ventricular pacing. *From* Jackman WM, Friday KJ, Anderson JL, Aliot EM, Clark M, Lazzara R. The long QT syndromes: A critical review, new clinical observations and a unifying hypothesis. Prog Cardiovasc Dis, in press.

Several other points support the triggered firing hypothesis. One is centered on the genesis of the first beat of the tachycardia. In the reentry hypothesis, the pause results in an increase in the dispersion of refractoriness. A premature ventricular impulse, arising between the recovery times of the early and late repolarizing regions, is required to initiate reentry. However, this hypothesis does not account for the generation of this premature impulse or for the ventricular bigeminy which characteristically precedes the onset of overt torsades de pointes (Fig. 5B) [1, 6, 8]. In either situation, the normal ventricular impulse completing the pause occurs long after the end of the T and U waves and should encounter the myocardium in its most 'recovered' state, thereby failing to produce this first ectopic impulse by reentry. An exception would be if large regions of myocardium exhibited pause-dependent block. If significant myocardial phase 4 depolarization were the basis for the pause-dependent block, it might also be expected to produce widening of QRS complexes completing a pause and fre-

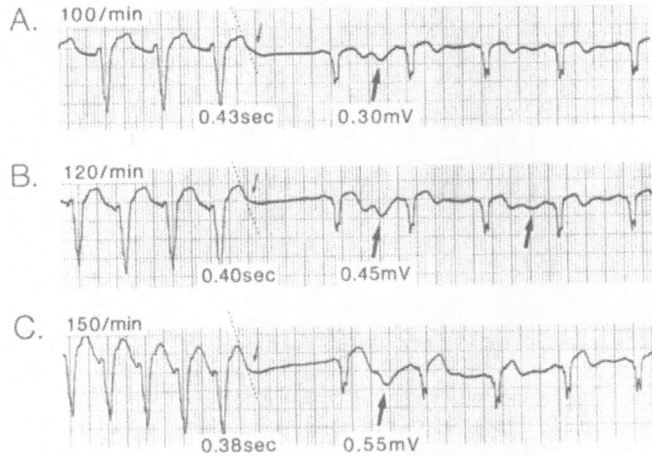

Figure 9. Relationship between pre-pause ventricular rate and post-pause U wave amplitude in same patient as figure 9. All tracings were recorded at the end of a 45 sec period of right ventricular pacing and all three tracings have approximately the same escape or 'pause' interval. As the right ventricular pacing rate increases from 100/min to 150/min in panels A to C, the QT interval of the paced complex decreases from 0.43 sec to 0.38 sec with decrease in the U wave amplitude (*small arrows*), while the post-pause U wave amplitude increases progressively from 0.30 mV to 0.55 mV (*large arrows*). Note the oscillation in U wave amplitude in the four complexes following the pause in panel B. *From* Jackman WM, Friday KJ, Anderson JL, Aliot EM, Clark M, Lazzara R. The long QT syndromes: A critical review, new clinical observations and a unifying hypothesis. Prog Cardiovasc Dis, in press.

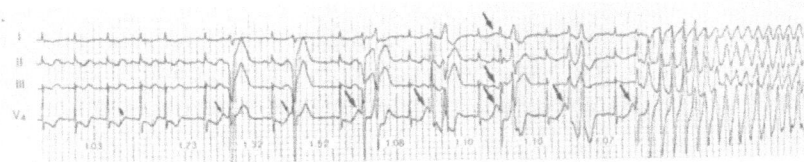

Figure 10. Accelerating feedback loop culminating in rapid ventricular tachycardia in a patient with procainamide-induced torsades de pointes. Patient same as in figure 6. Tracings from the top are ECG leads I, II, III, and V$_4$. At the left the rhythm is regular, and although slow (sinus cycle length = 1.03 sec) the U wave remains relatively small (*small arrow*). After four sinus complexes, a premature atrial complex occurs which results in a short cycle followed by a brief pause (1.23 sec). The post-pause U wave is larger (*second arrow*) and is associated with the appearance of the first ventricular extrasystole. Arrhythmia is then perpetuated in a bigeminal pattern with progressively increasing post-pause U wave amplitude (*arrows*) until sustained, rapid ventricular tachycardia occurs. As long as the ventricular rhythm was regular, as in the left of the tracing, there was no ventricular ectopy. However, any perturbation in ventricular cycle length, such as by the premature atrial complex, initiated ventricular extrasystoles which perpetuated bigeminally with rapid progression to sustained tachycardia or ventricular fibrillation. Temporary ventricular pacing at 100/min (not shown) completely suppressed all ventricular extrasystoles. *From* Jackman WM, Friday KJ, Anderson JL, Aliot EM, Clark M, Lazzara R. The long QT syndromes: A critical review, new clinical observations and a unifying hypothesis. Prog Cardiovasc Dis, in press.

174

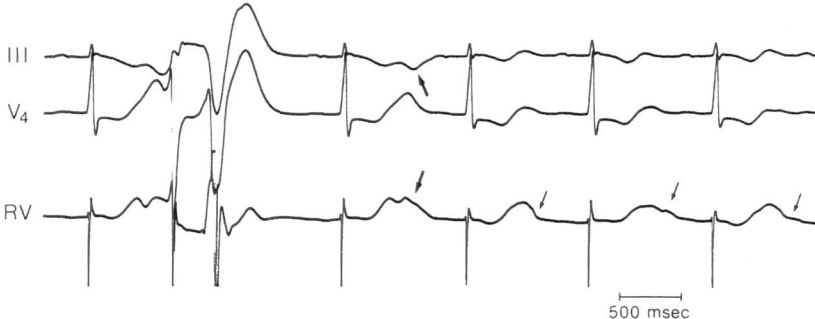

Figure 11. Oscillation of U wave amplitude following an abrupt deceleration of ventricular rate in procainamide-induced torsade de pointes. Same patient and format as figure 6 and 10. Enhanced U wave amplitude following the post-extrasystolic pause is apparent in the ECG leads as well as the right ventricular endocardial electrogram (*bold arrows*). Subsequent oscillation in U wave amplitude is evident on the endocardial electrogram (*fine arrows*), but not apparent on the surface ECG tracings. *From* Jackman WM, Friday KJ Anderson JL, Aliot EM, Clark M, Lazzara R. The long QT syndromes: A critical review, new clinical observations and a unifying hypothesis. Prog Cardiovasc Dis, in press.

quent ventricular 'escape' complexes. Neither QRS complex widening nor late diastolic ventricular extrasystoles are a consistent feature of this syndrome. The triggered firing hypothesis, on the other hand, easily explains the new appearance of pause-related ventricular extrasystoles, as the early afterdepolarizations in the cesium model are greatly enhanced by pauses [39, 41, 72].

Another factor supporting the triggered firing hypothesis is the marked exacerbation of this syndrome by hypokalemia [3–5], and the frequent suppression of the tachycardia by the acute administration of magnesium sulfate [73, 74]. Hypokalemia facilitates cesium and quinidine-induced triggered firing *in vitro* [41, 46, 72, 75].

A variant of the triggered firing hypothesis holds that susceptible patients differ from the remaining population by virtue of a defect in the repolarizing potassium currents, possibly due to altered genetic coding for potassium channels. Under normal circumstances the defective channels are capable of maintaining sufficient current to repolarize the cells and prevent triggered firing. The addition of quinidine or similar agents further depresses the repolarizing currents. The final insult is produced by the pause. Long cycles permit the sodium-potassium AT-Pase pump to reduce the potassium concentration just outside the cell membrane which further reduces the repolarizing potassium currents [76]. This allows the repolarizing currents to be overwhelmed by the usually lower amplitude inward currents which are present during the repolarization phase, producing early afterdepolarizations and triggered firing which are manifested clinically as U waves and ventricular tachycardia. Elimination of pauses by pacing eliminates the early afterdepolarizations and is reflected clinically by the loss of the U

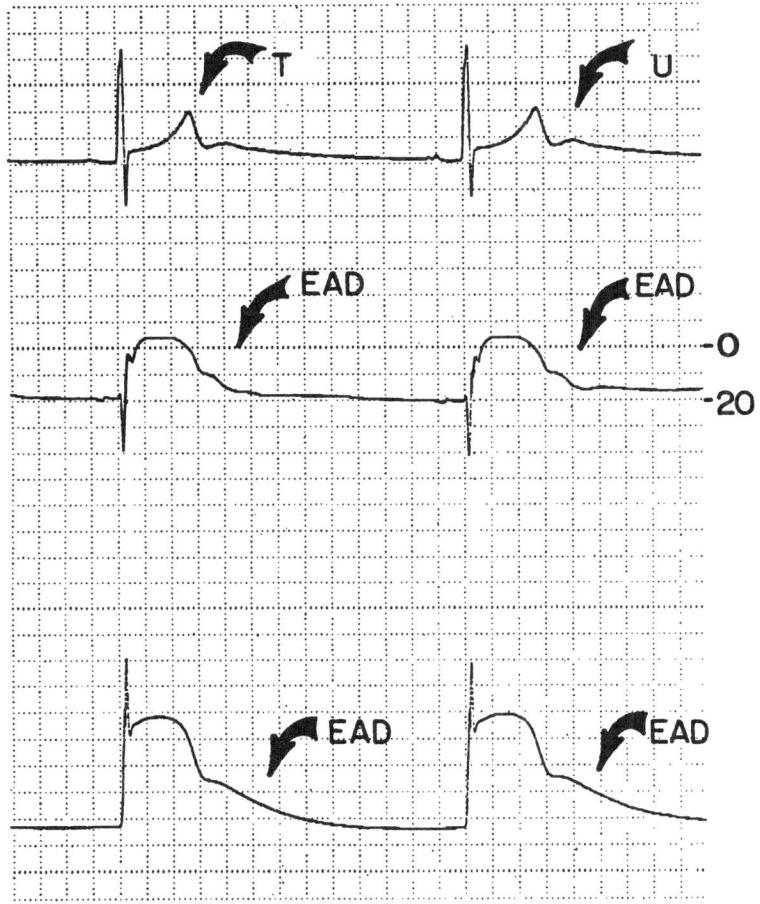

Figure 12. Monophasic injury potentials following cesium administration suggesting the U wave results from early afterdepolarizations. Tracings (top to bottom) are ECG lead V_2 and left ventricular epicardial and endocardial monophasic injury potentials recorded from a dog shortly after intravenous administration of cesium chloride, 1 mM/kg. Cesium produced slowing of the sinus rate and the appearance of U waves on the electrocardiogram. The monophasic injury potentials show a late deflection, during the U wave, which appears similar to the early afterdepolarizations (*EAD*) recorded *in vitro*.

wave. This variant of the triggered firing hypothesis may help to explain the observation that patients who develop torsades de pointes on receiving a class 1A antiarrhythmic agent are at high risk for torsades de pointes on exposure to another of the class 1A agents [5, 6, 14, 16–21].

Clinical observations provide only circumstantial evidence about the mechanism of a tachycardia. We believe that the features associated with the initiation of drug-induced torsades de pointes are more consistent with early afterdepolar-

176

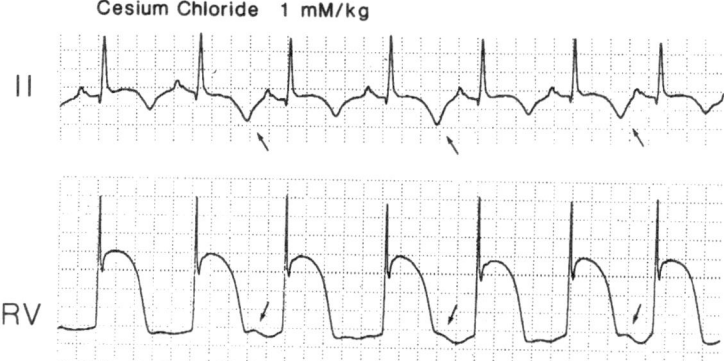

Cesium Chloride 1 mM/kg

II

RV

Figure 13. Monophasic injury potential during cesium-induced oscillation of the terminal phase of the TU wave (U wave). Cesium chloride, 1 mM/kg, was administered intravenously to an anesthetized dog. Tracings are ECG lead II and monophasic injury potential recorded from a catheter electrode in the right ventricle (RV). During alternate beats with the larger U wave (*arrows* in lead II), the monophasic injury potential has a discrete late component resembling an early afterdepolarizaton (*arrows*).

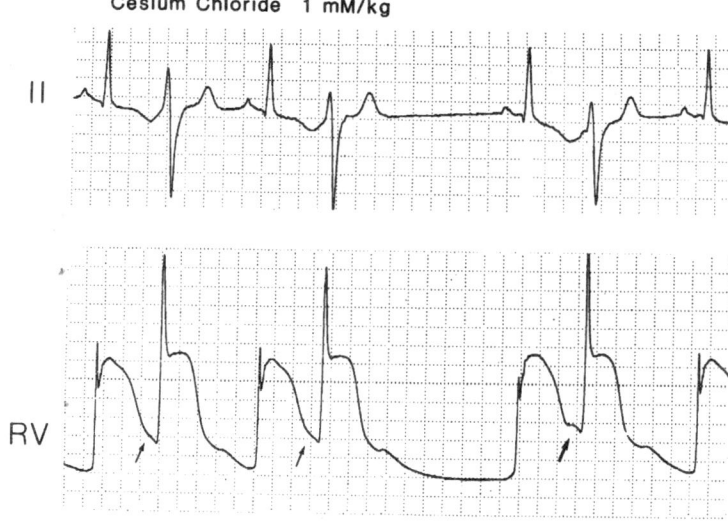

Cesium Chloride 1 mM/kg

II

RV

Figure 14. Monophasic injury potential during cesium-induced ventricular extrasystoles. The experiment and format are the same as shown in figure 13. The late component of the monophasic injury potential arises sooner and has larger amplitude (*arrows*) than in figure 13. The late component is further enhanced by the longer pause (*bold arrow*).

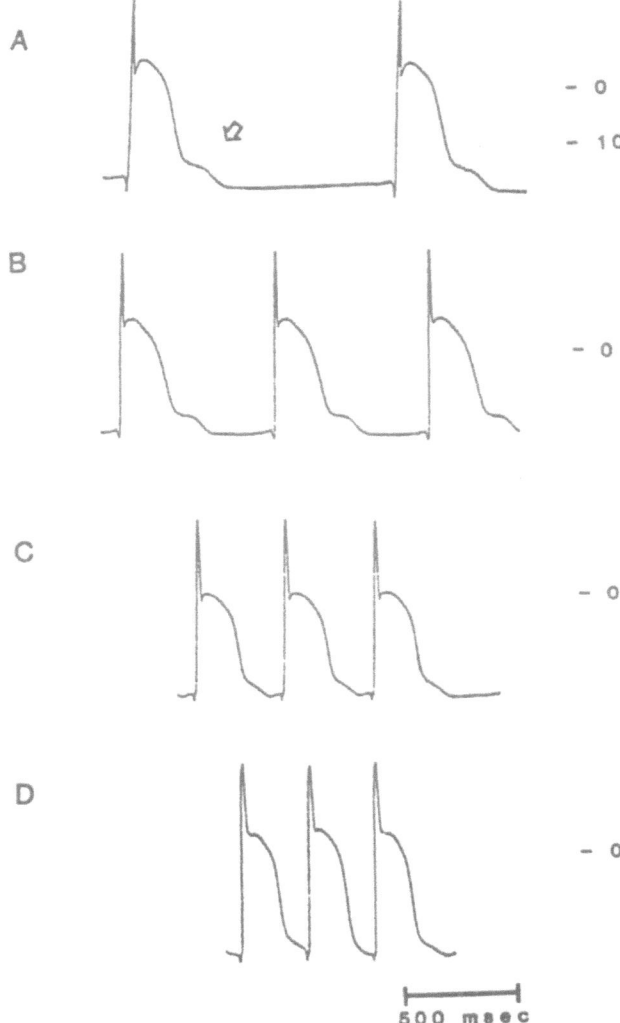

Figure 15. Effect of rate on cesium-induced afterdepolarizations *in vivo*. Tracings are monophasic injury potentials recorded from a left ventricular epicardial electrode in an open chest dog receiving cesium chloride, 1 mM/kg. Panels A-D were recorded during atrial pacing at cycle length 1200 msec, 700 msec, 400 msec, and 300 msec, respectively, showing progressive attenuation of the afterdepolarizations (*arrow*) at shorter cycle lengths. Note the similarity to the effect of pacing rate on U wave amplitude shown in figure 9. *From* Levine JH, Spear JF, Guarnieri T, Weisfeldt ML, de Langen CDJ, Becker LC, Moore EN. 1985. Cesium chloride-induced long QT syndrome: Demonstration of afterdepolarizations and triggered activity in vivo. Circulation 72: 1092–1103, with permission.

178

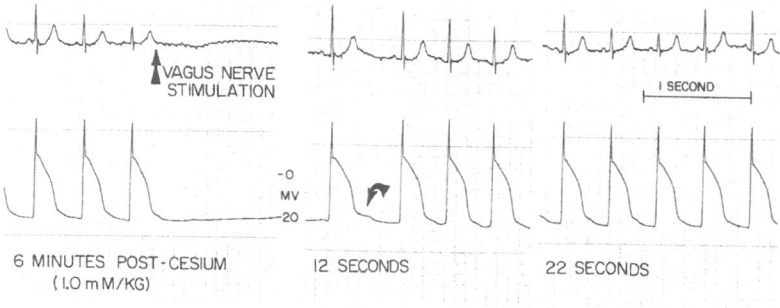

VAGUS NERVE
STIMULATION

I SECOND

-0
MV
-20

6 MINUTES POST-CESIUM
(1.0 m M/KG)

12 SECONDS

22 SECONDS

Figure 16. Effect of pause on cesium-induced early afterdepolarizations *in vivo.* Tracings are ECG lead V_2 and left ventricular endocardial monophasic injury potenial, recorded from a dog six minutes following administration of cesium chloride, 1 mM/kg. Left panel: A small U wave is apparent in lead V_2 with a correspondingly small deflection at the end of the monophasic injury potential. Vagal nerve stimulation produced a 12 second pause. The post-pause complex, shown in the middle panel, exhibits both an enhanced U wave in lead V_2 and an enhanced early afterdepolariation in the monophasic injury potential recording. Regularization of the rhythm following the pause is associated with a progressive decrease in the U wave amplitude and in the early afterdepolarization.

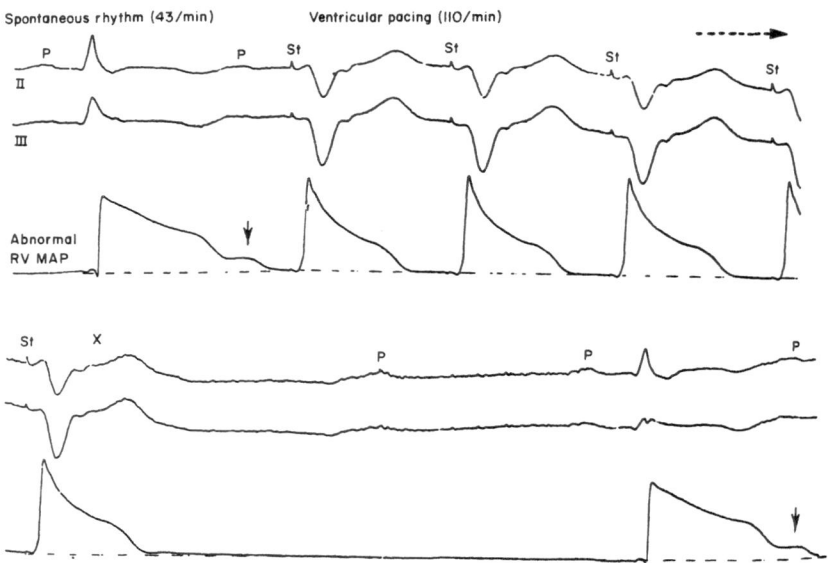

Spontaneous rhythm (43/min)   Ventricular pacing (110/min)

Figure 17. Monophasic injury potential in a patient with AV block induced torsades de pointes. Tracings are ECG leads II and III and monophasic injury potential recorded from a right ventricular endocardial suction electrode. A discrete late component is present in *post-pause* complexes (*arrows*), consistent with early afterdepolarizations. Note the similarity to the cesium-induced phenomenon in figure 16. *From* Bonatti V, Rolli A, Botti G. 1983. Recordings of monophasic action potentials of the right ventricle in long QT syndromes complicated by severe ventricular arrhythmias. Eur Heart J 4: 168–179, with permission.

izations and triggered firing then with reentry resulting from excessive dispersion of refractoriness. However, both mechanisms may be operative. Triggered firing may produce the initial tachycardia complexes which encounter heterogeneously recovered myocardium, initiating reentry which sustains the arrhythmia.

References

1. Jackman WM, Clark M, Friday KJ, Aliot E, Anderson J, Lazzara R. 1984. Ventricular tachyarrhythmias in the long QT syndromes. Med Clin North Amer 68: 1079–1109.
2. Denes P, Gabster A, Huang SK. 1981. Clinical, electrocardiographic and follow-up observations in patients having ventricular fibrillation during Holter monitoring. Role of quinidine therapy. Am J Cardiol 48: 9–15.
3. Kay GN, Plumb VJ, Arciniegas JG, Henthorn RW, Waldo AL. 1983. Torsade de Pointes: The long-short initiating sequence and other clinical features: Observations in 32 patients. J Am Coll Cardiol 2: 806–817.
4. Roden DM, Woosley RL, Primm RK. 1986. Incidence and clinical features of the qinidine-associated long QT syndrome: Implications for patient care. Am Heart J 111: 1088–1093.
5. Nguyen PT, Scheinman MM, Seger J. 1986. Polymorphous ventricular tachycardia: Clinical characterization, therapy and the QT interval. Circulation 74: 340–349.
6. Jackman WM, Friday KJ, Anderson JL, Aliot EM, Clark M, Lazzara R. The long QT syndromes: A critical review, new clinical observations and a unifying hypothesis. Prog Cardiovasc Dis, in press.
7. Moore MT, Book MH. 1970. Sudden death in phenothiazine therapy. A clinicopathologic study of 12 cases. Psychiatr Q 44: 384–402.
8. Ejvinsson G, Orinius E. 1980. Prodromal ventricular premature beats preceded by a diastolic wave. Acta Med Scand 208: 445–450.
9. Parkinson J, Campbell M. 1929. Quinidine treatment of auricular fibrillation. Quart J Med 22: 281–294.
10. Selzer A, Wray HW. 1964. Quinidine syncope: Paroxysmal ventricular fibrillation occurring during treatment of chronic atrial arrhythmias. Circulation 30: 17–26.
11. Moss AJ, Schwartz PJ. 1980. Delayed repolarization (QT or QTU prolongation) and malignant ventricular arrhythmias. Mod Concepts Cardiovasc Dis 51: 85–90.
2. Clark M, Lazzara R, Jackman WM. 1982. Torsades de Pointes: Serum drug levels and ECG warning signs. (abstr) Circulation 66 (Suppl II): II–71.
13. Fontaine G, Frank R, Grosgogeat Y. 1982. Torsades de Pointes: Defnition and management. Mod Concepts Cardiovasc Dis 51: 103–108.
14. Bauman JL, Baurenfeind RA, Hoff JV, Rosen KM. 1984. Quinidine syncope: Torsades de pointes due to quinidine: observations in 31 patients. Am Heart J 107: 425–30.
15. Reynolds EW, VanderArk CR. 1976. Quinidine syncope and the delayed repolarization syndrome. Mod Concepts Cardiovasc Dis 45: 117–122.
16. Maloney JD, Nissen RG, McColgan BS. 1980. Open clinical studies at a referral center: Chronic maintenance tocainide therapy in patients with recurrent sustained ventricular tachycardia refractory to conventional antiarrhythmic agents. Am Heart J 100: 1023–1030.
17. Wald RW, Waxman MB, Colman JM. 1981. Torsade de Pointes ventricular tachycardia: A complication of disopyramide shared with quinidine. J Electrocardiology 14: 301–308.
18. Keren A, Tzivoni D, Gottlieb S, Benhorin J, Stern S. 1982. Atypical ventricular tachycardia (Torsades de Pointes) induced by amiodarone: Arrhythmia previously induced by quinidine and disopyramide. Chest 81: 384–386.
19. Soffer J, Dreifus LS, Michelson EL. 1982. Polymorphous ventricular tachycardia associated with

normal and long QT intervals. Am J Cardiol 49: 2021–2029.

20. Shah A, Schwartz H. 1984. Mexiletine for treatment of Torsades de Pointes. Am Heart J 107: 589–591.

21. Clark M, Friday KJ, Anderson J, Jackman WM, Aliot E, Lazzara R. 1985. Drug induced torsades de pointes: High concordance rate among type IA antiarrhythmic drugs and amiodarone. (abstr) J Am Coll Cardiol 5: 450.

22. McRae JR, Wagner GS, Rogers MC, Canent RV. 1974. Paroxysmal familial ventricular fibrillation. J Pediatr 84: 515–518.

23. Krikler DM, Curry PVL. 1976. Torsade de Pointes, an atypical ventricular tachycardia. Br Heart J 38: 117–120.

24. Fowler NO, McCal D, Chou T, Holmes JC, Hanenson IB. 1976. Electrocardiographic changes and cardiac arrhythmias in patients receiving psychotropic drugs. Am J Cardiol 37: 223–230.

25. Jensen G, Sigurd B, Sandoe E. 1975. Adams-Stokes seizures due to ventricular tachydysrhythmias in patients with heart block: Prevalence and problems of management. Chest 67: 43–48.

26. Sclarovsky S, Strasberg B, Lewin R, Agmon J. 1979. Polymorphous ventricular tachycardia: Clinical features and treatment. Am J Cardiol 44: 339–344.

27. Steinbrecher UP, Fitchett DH. 1980. Torsade de Pointes: A cause of syncope with atrioventricular block. Arch Intern Med 140: 1223–1226.

28. DiSegni E, Klein HO, David D, Libhaber C, Kaplinki E. 1980. Overdrive pacing in quinidine syncope and other long QT interval syndromes. Arch Intern Med 140: 1036–1040.

29. Strasberg B, Sclarovsky S, Erdberg A, Duffy CE, Lam W, Swiryn S, Agmon J, Rosen KM. 1981. Procainamide-induced polymorphous ventricular tachycardia. Am J Cardiol 47: 1309–1314.

30. Kahn MM, Logan KR, McComb JM, Adgey AJJ. 1981. Management of recurrent ventricular tachyarrhythmias associated with QT prolongation. Am J Cardiol 47: 1301–1308.

31. Sclarovsky S, Lewin RF, Kracoff O, Strasberg B, Arditti A, Agmon J. 1983. Amiodarone-induced polmorphous ventricular tachycardia. Am Heart J 105: 6–12.

32. Tzivoni D, Keren A, Stern S. 1983. Torsades de Pointes versus polymorphic ventricular tachycardia. Am J Cardiol 52: 639–640.

33. Han J, Moe GK. 1963. Nonuniform recovery of excitability in ventricular muscle. Circ Res 14: 44-60.

34. Han J, Millet D, Chizzonitti B, Mo GK. 1966. Temporal dispersion of recovery of excitability in atrium and ventricle as a function of heart rate. Am Heart J 71: 481–487.

35. Dessertenne F. 1966. La tachycardie ventriculaire a deux foyers opposes variables. Arch Mal Coeur 59: 263–272.

36. Dessertenne F, Fabiato A, Coumel P. 1966. Les variations progressives de l'amplitude de l'electrocardiogramme. Actual Cardiol Angeol Internat 15: 241–258.

37. D'Alnoncourt CN, Zierhut W, Luderitz B. 1982. 'Torsade de pointes' tachycardia: Re-entry or focal activity? Br Heart J 48: 213–216.

38. Bardy GH, Ungerleider RM, Smith WM, Ideker RE. 1983. A mechanism of Torsades de Pointes in a canine model. Circulation 67: 52–59.

39. Brachmann J, Scherlag BJ, Rosenshtraukh LV, Lazzara R. 1983. Bradycardia-dependent triggered activity: relevance to drug-induced multiform ventricular tachycardia. Circulation 68: 846–856.

40. Jackman WM, Friday KJ, Scherlag BJ, Harrison LA, Berbari EJ, Clark M, Reynolds DW, Olson EG, Schechter E, Lazzara R. 1983. Torsades de Pointes: Clinical and experimental observations bearing on mechanism. (abstr) Clin Res 31: 193A.

41. Damiano BP, Rosen MR. 1984. Effects of pacing on triggered activity induced by afterdepolarizations. Circulation 69: 1013–1025.

42. Aliot E, Szabo B, Sweidan R, Lazzara R. 1985. Prevention of Torsades de Pointes with calcium channel blockade in an animal model. (abstr) J Am Coll Cardiol 5: 492.

43. Levine JW, Spear JF, Guarnieri T, Wiesfeldt ML, deLangen CDJ, Becker LC, Moore EN. 1985. Cesium chloride-induced long QT syndrome: Demonstration of afterdepolarizations and triggered activity in vivo. Circulation 72: 1092–1103.

44. Isenberg G. 1976. Cardiac Purkinje fibers: Cesium as a tool to block inward rectifying currents. Pfluegers Arch 365: 99–106.

45. Colatsky TJ. 1982. Mechanisms of action of lidocaine and quinidine on action potential duraton in rabbit cardiac Purkinje fibers. An effect on steady state sodium currents? Circ Res 50: 17–27.

46. Roden DM, Hoffman BF. 1985. Action potential prolongation and induction of abnormal automaticity by low quinidine concentrations in canine Purkinje fibers. Relationship to potassium and cycle length. Circ Res 56: 857–867.

47. Tamura K, Tamura T, Yoshida S, Inui M, Fukuhara N. 1967. Transient recurrent ventricular fibrillation due to hypopotassemia with special note on the U wave. Jap Heart J 8: 652–660

48. Loeb HS, Pietras RJ, Gunnar RM, Tobin JR. 1968. Paroxysmal ventricular fibrillation in two patients with hypomagnesemia: Treatment by transvenous pacing. Circulation 37: 210–215.

49. Raynaude R, Brochier M, Neel JL, Frauchier JP, Raynaud P. 1969. Tachycardie ventriculaire a foyer variable et dyskaliemie. Arch Mal Coeur 62: 1578–1598.

50. Curry P, Fithett D, Stubbs W, Krikler D. 1976. Ventricular arrhythmias and hypokalemia. Lancet 2: 231–233.

51. Levine SR, Crowley TJ, Hai HA. 1982. Hypomagnesemia and ventricular tachycardia: A complication of ulcerative colitis and parenteral hyperalimentation in a nondigitalized noncardiac patient. Chest 81: 244–247.

52. Topol EJ, Lerman BB. 1983. Hypomagnesemic Torsades de Pointes. Am J Cardiol 52: 1367–1368.

53. Schwartz SP, Orloff J, Fox C. 1949. Transient ventricular fibrillation. I. The prefibrillary period during established auriculoventricular dissociation with a note on the phonocardiograms obtained at such times. Am Heart J 37: 21–35.

54. Schwartz SP. 136. Studies on transient ventricular fibrillation. III. The prefibrillatory mechanism during established auriculo-ventricular dissociation. Am J Med Sci 192: 153–163.

55. Schwartz SP, de Sola, Pool N. 1950. Transient ventricular fibrillation. III. The effects of bodily rest, atropine sulfate, and exercise on patients with transient ventricular fibrillation during established auriculoventricular dissociation. Am Heart J 39: 361–386.

56. Dessertenne F. 1966. Considerations sur l'electrocardiogramme de la fibrillation ventriculaire. Arch Mal Coeur 59: 1421–1437.

57. Motte G, Coumel P, Abitol G, Dessertenne F, Slama R. 1970. Le syndrome QT long et syncopes par 'torsades de pointe'. Arch Mal Coeur 63: 831–853.

58. Slama R, Coumel R, Motte G, Gourdon R, Wayenberger M, Touche S. 1973. Tachycardies ventriculaires. Frontieres morphologiques entre les dysrythmies ventriculaires. Arch Mal Coeur 66: 1401–1411.

59. Jervell A, Lange-Nielsen F. 1957. Congenital deaf-mutism; functional heart disease with prolongation of the QT interval and sudden death. Am Heart J 54: 59–68.

60. Ward OC. 1964. A new familial cardiac syndrome in children. J Irish Med Assoc 54: 103–106.

61. Schwartz PJ. 1980. The long QT syndrome. In Sudden Death. Kulbertus HE, Wellens HJJ eds, Martinus Nijhoff Publishers, the Hague: 358–378.

62. Friderica LS. 1920. Duration of systole in electrocardiogram. Acta Med Scand 53: 469.

63. Lombard WP, Cope OM. 1919–20. Effect of pulse rate on the length of systoles and diastoles of the normal human heart in the standing position. Am J Physiol 49: 139–140.

64. Fenn GK. 1922. Studies in the variation of Q-R-S-T interval. Arch Intern Med 29: 441–448.

65. Adams W. 1936. Nomal duration of electrocardiographic ventricular complex. J Clin Invest 15: 335–342.

66. Blair HA, Wedd AM, Young AC. 1941. The relation of the QT interval to the refractory period, the diastolic interval, the duraion of contraction, and the rate of beating in the heart mucle. Am J Physiol 132: 157–175.

67. Bazett HC. 1920. An analysis of the time relations of electrocardiograms. Heart 7: 353–370.
68. Franz MR. 1983. Long-term recording of monophasic action potentials from human endocardium. Am J Cariol 51: 1629–1634.
69. Bonatti V, Finardi A, Botti G. 1979. Enregistrement des potentiels d'action monophasiques du ventricule droit dans un cos de QT long et alternance solee de l'onde U. Arch Mal Coeur 72: 1180–86.
70. Bonatti V, Rolli A, Botti G. 1983. Recording of monophasic action potentials of the right ventricle in long QT syndromes complicated by severe ventricular arrhythmias. Eur Heart J 4: 168–179.
71. Bonatti V, Rolli A, Botti G. 1985. Monophasic action potential studies in human subjects with prolonged ventricular repolarization and long QT syndromes. Eur Heart J 6 (Suppl D): 131–143.
72. Szabo B, Sweidan R, Scherlag BJ, Lazzara R. 1986. Cesium-induced late-coupled, triggered action potentials in Purkinje fibers. (abstr) JACC 7: 52A.
73. Tzivoni D, Keren A, Cohen AM, Loebel H, Zahavi I, Chenzbraun A, Stern S. 1984. Magnesium therapy for Torsades de Pointes. Am J Cardiol 53: 528–530.
74. Stern S, Keren A, Tzivoni D. 1984. Torsades de Pointes: Definitions, causative factors, and therapy: Experience with sixteen patients. Ann NY Acac Sci 427: 234–240.
75. Szabo B, Sweidan R, Scherlag BJ, Lazzara R. 1986. The mechanism of hyperpolarization induced triggered activity in guinea pig ventricular preparations. Abstract from X World Congress of Cardiology.
76. Kunze D. 1977. Rate-dependent changes in extracellular potassium in the rabbit atrium. Circ Res 41: 122–127.

13. Mechanisms of sudden death during Holter monitoring: A study of 74 cases

J.F. LECLERCQ, P. MAISONBLANCHE, B. CAUCHEMEZ, P. COUMEL
Department of Cardiology, Lariboisière Hospital, Paris, France

Summary

74 Holter recordings of sudden unexpected death (SD) were collected and analyzed by a computerized system, ATREC II.

Asystole caused SD in 17 aged, severely diseased patients (pts) (23%), by ischemic electromechanical dissociation rather than conduction disturbances.

Torsades de pointes (TdP) caused SD in 12 younger pts (16%). TdP were iatrogenic (class I-A drugs, hypokaliemia) and always preceded by long RR cycles and progressive 3-hour bradycardia (78.3 ± 2.6 to 60.2 ± 2.9 b/mn, p<0.001).

Ventricular fibrillation (VF) caused SD in 45 pts (61%). Almost all had coronary heart disease, but only 5 had ST segment changes before SD. In 34, VF followed a ventricular tachycardia (VT) lasting 30 sec if polymorphic and 3 min if monomorphic. In 11, primary VF was initiated by an R-on-T phenomenon or a pacemaker dysfunction. One-hour sinus tachycardia (82 ± 2.9 to 89.8 ± 3.7 b/min, p<0.001), or atrial arrhythmia (14 pts) were obvious predisposing factors. Long RR cycle in 20 cases, and shortening of coupling interval (446 ± 17 to 377 ± 13 ms, p<0.001) were immediate determinants of VT or VF. In 3 pts, antiarrhythmic drugs probably precipitated VF.

In conclusion, iatrogenicity and sympathetic drive are important determinants of SD. Betablockers combined with a tailored antiarrhythmic therapy and/or pacing suppression of compensatory pauses are probably useful. Automatic defibrillator is also appropriate, delivering usually DC shock during VT, before occurrence of VF.

Introduction

Sudden death (SD) in cardiac patients remains a major challenge for cardiologists in 1986. The mechanisms, the prediction and the prevention of SD are not yet perfectly defined. For several years, Holter monitoring has provided several examples of reorded sudden death (SD). In the literature, the published cases remain limited to a maimum of 10 to 20 per series, and few extensive studies of the determinants of the fatal event are available [7, 11, 14, 15, 16, 17]. However, knowing the mechanisms and the main determinants of SD appears useful to conceive an accurate prediction and/or prevention.

A cooperative study of the French working group on arrhythmias collected a number of SD recordings, and their analysis was performed uniformly in our institution [23]. The mechanism, as well as the main determinants of SD were particularly looked for: environmental rhythm, intervening factors in the hours preceding SD, initiating factor, terminal event.

Material and methods

We collected 89 tapes including SD, from 24 centers. In order to limit, as much as possible, our study to true unexpected SD, we excluded patients with recent myocardial infarction (before 21st day) or NYHA class-IV heart failure. Death was considered as sudden if occurring within 30 mn after the first symptom, and patients successfully resuscitaed by external DC shocks were included. 74 cases fulfilled these criteria and were retained for the study.

All tapes were analysed manually, including full disclosure on an optic-fiber system. 71/74 were 2-lead tapes. Computerized analysis was performed using the ATREC-II system [2].

The 74 patients were divided in 3 groups, according to the nature of the terminal event: (1) cardiac standstill; (2) torsades de pointes (TDP); and (3) ventricular fibrillation (VF).

Results

Table 1 shows the major findings in group I (cardiac standstill), which includes 17 patients (23%), 11 males and 6 females, aged (73.5 ± 2.4 yrs) (mean & SEM), with 5 out- and 12 in-hospital deaths. All patients except one had a known cardiac disease: in 13 an ischemic heart disease, in 2 an aortic stenosis, in 1 an atrial septal defect. Table 1 shows the major results of the tape analysis in this group. In 13/17 cases, the cardiac standstill was neither due to a paroxysmal SA nor an AV block, but to a progressive slowing of the atrial rate accompanied by a QRS widening, and terminated by an electromechanical dissociation. In the 4 other cases, SD was due to a conduction disorder: an AV block in 3 and a SA block in 1. A causal factor was found in 3 of these 4 cases: in one case the AV block was preceded by important ST segment changes, and in the 2 others SD occurred early after initiation of antiarrhythmic therapy (with flecainide and verapamil, respectively) and were, at least in part, of iatrogenic origin. Moreover, the role of a myocardial ischemia appears most important, as judged by the ST segment modifications in the minutes preceding SD: 11 of the electromechanical dissociations, and 1 of the AV blocks were clearly preceeded by ST segment changes. In fact, only one patient (the SA block) died from an isolated conduction disorder, without ischemia or iatrogenic factor, without apparent underlying heart disease.

Group II (TDP) includes 12 patients (16%), 7 females, 5 males (Table 2). They were younger than group I patients (66 ± 3 years, p = .06). Two died out of the hospital, and 10 SD occurred in the hospital (7 were successfully resuscitated). As seen in Table 2, only 4/12 had an underlying heart disease. The etiological factors were: – Class I-A antiarrhythmic drugs in 7/12 – Potassium depletion (diuretics) in 6/12 – Amiodarone therapy in 3/12. The two main determinants found in the Holter tape before the initial TDP were: a progressive bradycardia (78.3 ± 2.6 to 60.2 ± 2.9 b/mn during the 3 preceding hours, n = 12, p<.001) and a long-short cycle sequence related to a post-extrasystolic pause (12/12). The extrasystole responsible for pause may be atrial as well as ventricular, as shown by figure 1: the pause induced a huge deformation of the ventricular repolarization, then a ventricular premature beat occurred before the end of the repolarization, and TDP started. The importance of the bradycardia is also demonstrated by the predominance of TDP in the evening and night (7/12).

Table 1. Group I: Cardiac standstill.

	Sex	Age	Etiology	ST changes	Iatrogenic F	Mechanism	Remarks
1	M	69	CAD	–	Fléca-ïnide	AVB	2nd day of tt
2	M	84	CAD	+	–	EMD	Sinus brady
3	M	62	CAD		Véra-pamil	AVB	3rd day of tt
4	M	50	CAD	+	–	EMD	Sinus tachy.
5	F	73	CAD	–	–	EMD	–
6	F	84	CAD	+	–	AVB	–
7	M	80	CAD	+	–	EMD	PM for chronic AVB
8	F	58	Ao.ST	+	–	EMD	Sinus. brady.
9	M	75	CAD	+	–	EMD	Sinus. brady.
10	M	75	CAD	+	–	EMD	Sinus tachy.
11	F	79	Ao.ST	–	–	EMD	Atrial tachy.
12	F	82	CAD	+	–	EMD	Sinus tachy.
13	F	83	–	–	–	SAB	PAT
14	M	64	CAD	+	–	EMD	Sinus tachy.
15	M	75	CAD	+	–	EMD	Sinus tachy.
16	M	74	CAD	+	–	EMD	Sinus tachy.
17	M	82	CAD	+	–	EMD	Sinus brady.

186

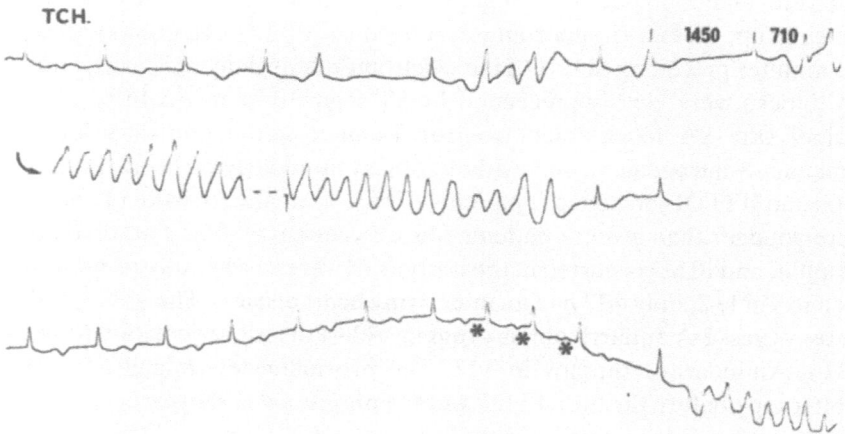

Figure 1. Torsades de pointes. Two episodes are initiated after a compensatory pause occurring respectively after ventricular (top) and atrial premature beats (stars, bottom). Note the monstruous deformation of the ventricular repolarization on the first beat after pause, leading to TdP.

Group III (VF) includes 45 patients (61%), 36 males and 9 females (Table 3). The mean age in this group was 65 ± 2.2 years (p = .02 vs group I, NS vs group II). 17 SD occurred out of the hospital and 28 in the hospital (only 8 could be resuscitated). All patients except 4 were known as coronary patients with healed myocardial infarction; 1 had aortic stenosis, and 1 a congenital long QT syndrome.

Table 2. Group II: Torsades de pointes.

	Sex	Age	Etiology	Iatrogenic factors	Heart rate		Long RR cycle
					h-3	h0	
1	M	54	–	Bepridil-Hypok.	70	40	+
2	F	69	–	Amiodarone-Hypok.	92	70	+
3	M	58	–	?	85	70	+
4	M	79	–	Quinidine	80	50	+
5	F	78	–	Quinidine-Hypok.	75	60	+
6	F	60	–	Quinidine	80	55	+
7	M	75	–	?	70 (PM)	70 (PM)	+
8	F	53	valvular	Amiodarone-hypok.	75	60	+
9	F	58	valvular	Quinidine	65	65	+
10	F	77	–	Quinidine	70	60	+
11	F	19	valvular	hypok.	85	50	+
12	M	65	C.A.D.	Disopyramide	92	72	+

Table 3. Group III.

	Preceding events									Initiating factors				Terminal event				Remarks
	ST changes	Atrial arrhythmia	Heart rate		Premature ventricular contractions					Long cycle	C.I.	New PVC	Salvo	VT/VF	Initial rate	Final rate	VT duration	
			h-1	3 min	N/mn	Poly-morph-ism	Short-est	C.I.	Runs									
1	-	Parox. AF	77	66	5	-	400	-	-	-	360	+	+	Mono. VT	240	240	40"	
2	+	-	75	<100	-	-	-	-	-	+	480	-	-	Poly. VT	200	240	30"	
3	-	Perm. AF	105	<116	1	+	500	-	-	+	360	-	-	Mono. VT	250	210	1'30"	QRS
4	-	-	56	63	2	-	460	+	-	-	460	-	-	Mono. VT	150	85	3'	Fléca.
5	-	-	102	<127	2	-	500	1	-	-	320	-	-	Mono. VT	140	180	7'	Fléca.
6	-	-	70	90	2	+	500	+	-	-	400	-	-	Poly. VT	250	200	6'	QRS
7	-	-	58	60	4	+	700	-	-	+	400	-	-	VF				
8	-	-	55	61	1	+	340	+	-	+	360	-	+ (5)	Mono. VT	320	380	1'	
9	+	-	60	57	-	-	-	-	-	+	300	-	-	VF				
10	+	-	120	<160	-	-	-	+	-	+	300	-	-	Poly. VT	240	300	15"	
11	-	-		60	1	-	360	-	-	+	320	-	+ (12)	Mono. VT	300	330	40"	
12	-	-		64	3	+	350	+	-	+	350	-	-	VF				
13	-	Perm. AF	104	<109	1	+	400	+	-	+	400	-	-	Mono. VT	200	200	40"	QRS
14	-	-	95	<102	1	-	360	+	-	-	320	-	-	Poly. VT	230	300	20"	
15	-	-	118	86	1	+	300	-	-	+	320	-	+ (8)	Mono. VT	280	280	3'	
16	-	APC's	70	70	2	-	380	-	-	+	280	-	-	Mono. VT	240	280	1'30"	
17	-	Perm. AF	80	71	3	+	380	+	-	+	360	-	+ (14)	Mono. VT	220	300	9'	
18	-	-	77	79	1	-	380	-	-	+	340	+	-	Mono. VT	300	300	6"	
19	+	-	62	74	10	-	440	-	-	+	420	+	-	Mono. VT	200	220	2'	
20	-	-	98	<100	1	+	380	+	-	-	320	+	-	Poly. VT	300	300	8"	
21	-	-	65	85	3	+	500	+	-	-	500	-	-	Mono. VT	120	100	4'	Fléca.
22	-	-	<103	103	-	-	-	-	-	-	360	-	-	Mono. VT	220	250	2'	

Table 3. (Continued).

	Preceding events										Initiating factors				Terminal event				Remarks
	ST changes	Atrial arrhythmia	Heart rate		Premature ventricular contractions					Long cycle	C.I.	New PVC	Salvo	VT/VF	Initial rate	Final rate	VT duration	
			h-1	3 min	N/mm	Polymorphism	Shortest	C.I.	Runs									
23	–	–	67	67	3	+	500	–	–	+	340	+	–	VF				P.M.
24	–	Perm. AF		80	2	+	600	–	–	–	600	+	+ (long)	Mono. VT	100	100	4'	QRS
25	–	–	86	95	1	–	360	–	–	+	280	–	+	Mono. VT	250	250	1'30"	
26	+	–	77	85	–	–	–	–	–	+	280	–	–	VF				
27	–	Perm. AF	100	<120	3	–	360	+	–	–	380	–	–	Mono. VT	200	240	4'	
28	–	Parox. AF	80	<100	5	+	700	+	–	–	360	–	–	Poly. VT	180	180	10"	
29	–	Parox AF	80	80	1	–	560	–	–	+	450	+	–	Poly. VT	170	140	30"	QRS
30	–	–	140	<158	–	–	–	–	–	–	300	–	+ (4)	Mono. VT	220	220	15'	
31	–	Perm. AF	80	90	3	+	400	+	–	–	320	–	–	Poly. VT	250	300	8"	
32	–	–	66	70	1	–	500	–	–	–	380	PM	–	VF				P.M.
33	–	APC's	73	88	–	–	–	–	–	–	600	+	–	Mono. VT	150	150	30"	
34	–	–	70	70	–	–	–	–	–	–	360	–	–	VF				
35	–	–	70	75	1	–	500	–	–	+	300	+	–	VF				
36	–	–	95	<115	–	–	–	–	–	–	440	–	–	Mono. VT	150	200	1'30"	
37	–	Parox. AF	92	<100	2	+	380	+	–	–	300	+	–	Poly. VT	250	270	20"	
38	–	APC's	94	92	–	–	–	–	–	+	360	–	–	Poly. VT	300	300	30"	
39	–	–	70	70	1	–	600	+	–	–	450	–	–	Mono. VT	190	210	2'	P.M.
40	–	–	70	70	1	+	500	–	–	–	550	–	–	Mono. VT	150	150	1'45"	P.M.
41	–	–	81	86	2	–	400	–	–	+	300	+	–	VF				
42	–	–	71	70	1	+	360	+	–	+	480	–	–	Poly. VT	250	330	9"	
43	–	Perm. FA	80	87	1	+	400	+	–	+	400	+	–	VF				P.M.
44	–	–	74	74	2	–	450	–	–	–	290	–	–	VF	–	–	–	
45	–	–	80	<130	3	+	400	–	–	–	400	–	–	Poly. VT	240	280	3'	

22/45 patients (49%) were treated by antiarrhythmic drugs for previous ventricular arrhythmias. 5 had had pacemaker implantation for AV block or marked bradycardia.

The terminal event: VF

SD due to VF usually follows an organized ventricular tachycardia (VT): only 11 patients died from immediate VF. In these cases, the coupling interval of the premature ventricular complexe (PVC) initiating VF is short: 340 ± 16 ms, realizing usually an R-on-T phenomenon. However, the majority of VF (34/45) follows a sustained VT, polymorphic in 12 cases, and monomorphic in 22.

The transformation of VT into VF: In case of VF following a sustained VT, the VT duration before its transformation into VF is 60 ± 30 sec for the polymorphic VT and 181 ± 44 sec for the monomorphic VT ($p = .06$). In 19 patients who had previous runs of VT, only one had a primary VF. In the other 18, the longest run of VT recorded before SD was shorter than the VT duration leading to VF: 46 ± 22 vs 453 ± 133 beats, $p<.01$. The transformation of VT into VF was preceded by an acceleration of the VT rate (219 ± 10 to 236 ± 12 b/mn, $n = 34$, $p<.001$). Figure 2 shows an example of the crucial importance of these two factors: a longer and faster VT leads to VF. In the presented case, the VT becomes sustained when its rate is higher than 300/mn. The transformation into VF occurred when VT rate reaches 370/mn. In addition, a third factor, i.e. a progressive widening of the QRS during the VT is present in 8 cases. 3 of them occurred early after introduction of flecainide, a new class-IC drug inducing an important delay in intraventricular conduction, and playing probably a favourizing role in the transformation into VF.

The precipitating factors of VT/VF: the initiating premature beat

Three characteristics of the initiation of VT of VF could be analysed and compared to preceding events: the coupling interval of the initiating PVC (RV1), the RR cycle preceding it, and the morphology of PVC.

The mean RV1 initiating VT or VF is 378 ± 12 ms for the whole group. It changes according to the type of the arrhythmia: 340 ± 16 ms for the 11 primary VF, 374 ± 19 ms for the 12 polymorphous VT, and 398 ± 20 ms for te 22 monomorphic VT ($p = .07$ between VF and monomorphic VT). A comparison between the RV1 of the initiating PVC to the shortest coupling interval of ventricular premature beat seen in the preceding hours shows a dramatic shortening: 377 ± 13 vs 446 ± 17 ms, $n = 35$, $p<.001$. In 8 of 22 patients with sustained monomorphic VT, the VT was not directly started by the initiating PVC, but by an initial salvo of different morphology. In two instances, VT or VF were induced

190

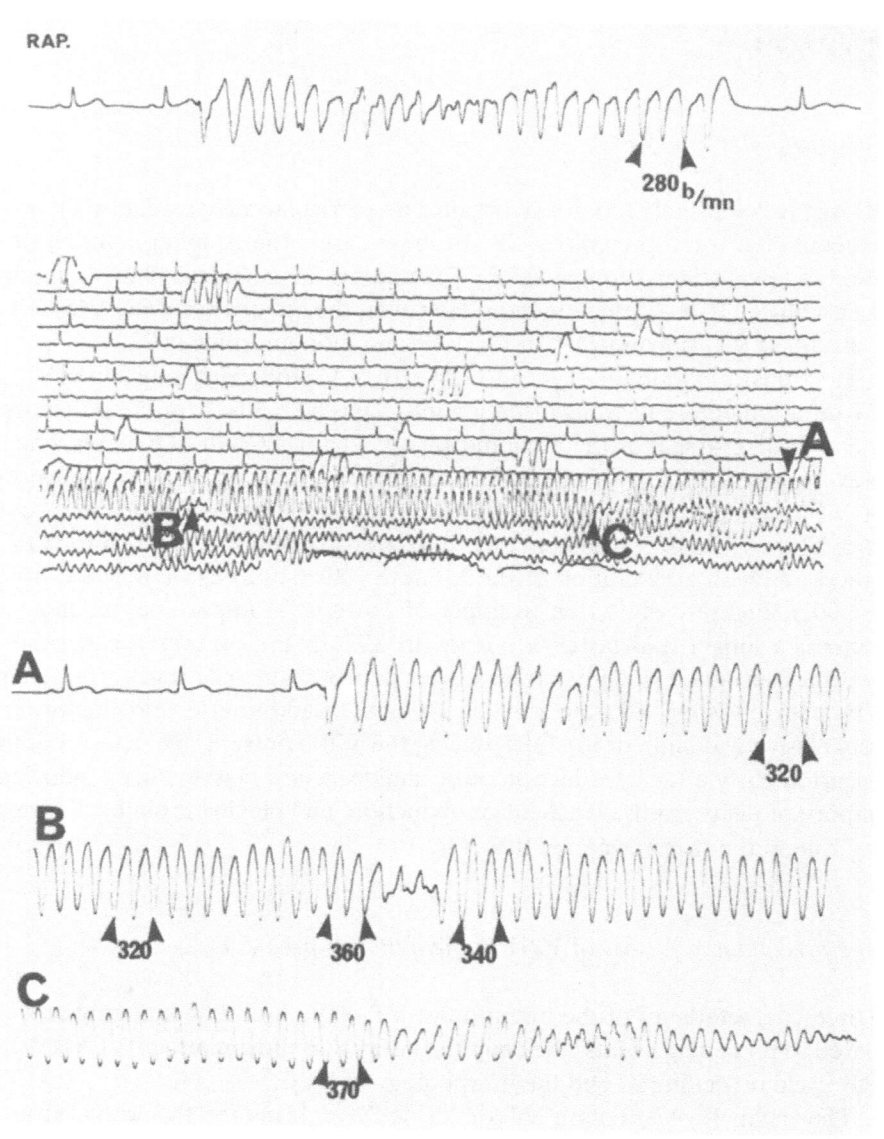

Figure 2. Sudden death by ventricular fibrillation following sustained monomorphic ventricular tachycardia in a coronary patient with frequent ventricular arrhythmias. The longest run of self-terminating VT (top) contained 25 QRS, and its maximal rate was 280 b/min. In A, a faster VT starts: its initial rate (320/min) increases till 360 (B), provoking a temporary disorganization, and again to 370 (C), leading to VF.

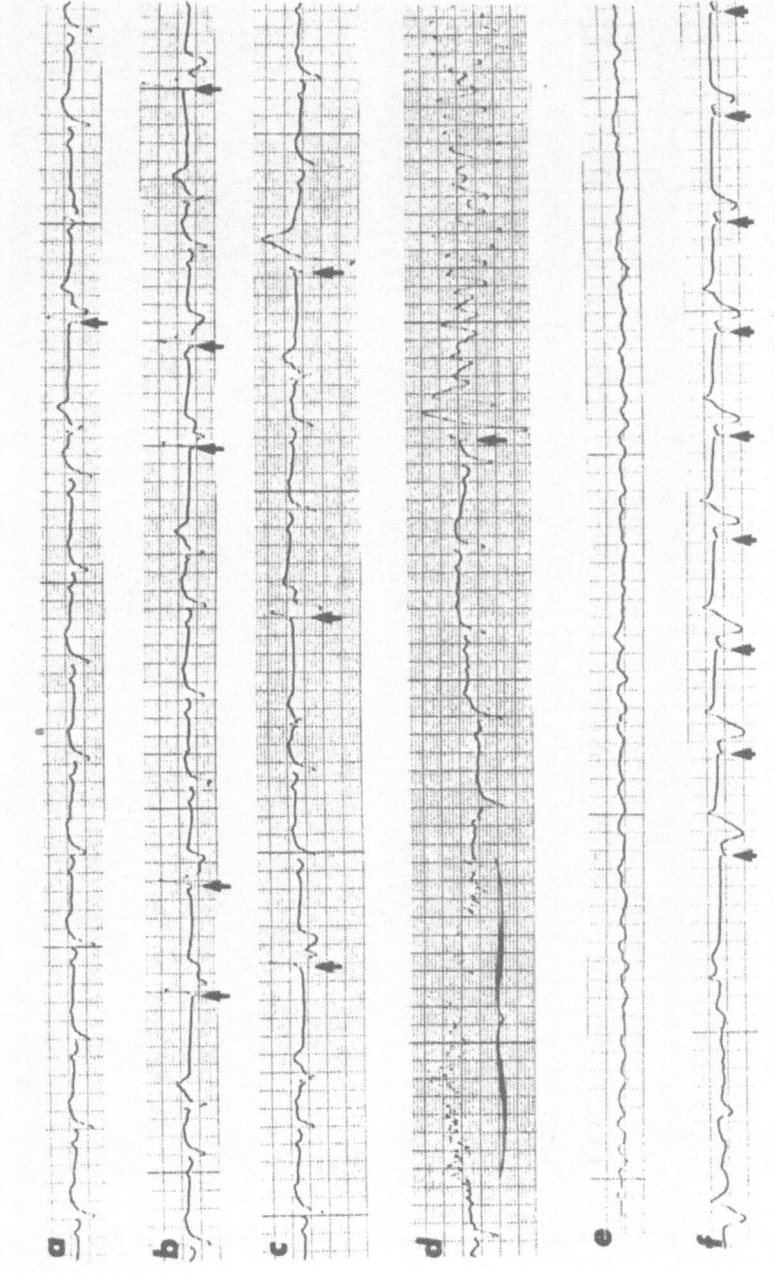

Figure 3. SD by VF triggered by a pacemaker sensing dysfunction. This bipolar PM senses usually accurately the spontaneous rhythm (arrows indicating spikes). In d, a few seconds after a strong parasite an inappropriate spike occurs within the repolarization starting a polymorphous VT, then VF. This one stops several minutes later, but PM gives only very enlarged QRS, without hemodynamic efficacy.

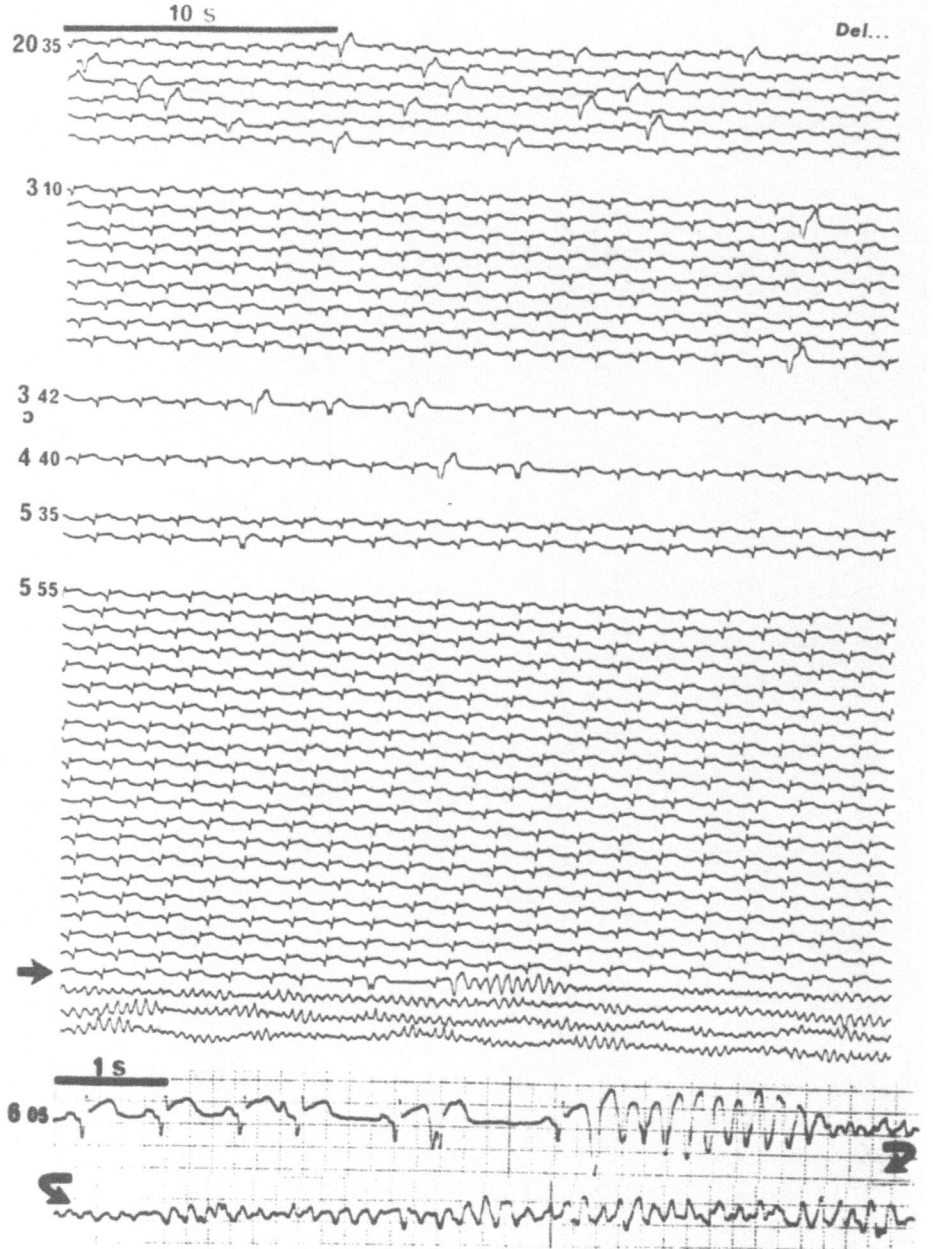

Figure 4. SD by VF initiated by a ventricular premature beat with short coupling interval (bottom). An atrial premature beat induced a compensatory pause, then a ventricular extrasystole which induced a longer pause, leading to a shortening of the coupling interval and to an R-on-T phenomenon. The unique sequence of 2 successive pauses before SD was seen at 3.42 a.m., but without significant shortening of the premature beat.

by a pacemaker dysfunction: in 1 case, the PM was able to detect spontaneous QRS in sinus rhythm, but not some types of ventricular premature beats and sustained VT was induced by a very short coupled extrastimulation after a spontaneous PVC. In the 2nd case (Figure 3), the sensing defect was unexpected, may be due to an interference, as suggested by the strong parasite a few seconds before the event.

A long RR cycle, usually due to a compensatory pause, i.e. exceeding by more than 25% the mean RR interval of the 5 preceding cycles, was present in 19 cases on one of the 2 cycles immediately preceding the initiating ventricular beat. In another case, this long RR cycle occurred during the sustained VT immediately before its acceleration into VF. This long RR cycle was then present in 20/45 cases (44%). Figure 4 shows an example of the determinant role of a succession of long RR cycles, allowing a decrease in the coupling interval of ventricular beats, and then an R-on-T phenomenon and a VF.

The morphology of the initiating PVC could be scrutinized in patients having a sufficient number of PVC's before SD. In 12 cases, the initiating PVC was never seen before SD, and appears 'new' in these patients. One case was directly triggered by a PM. Ten patients had no PVC's before SD. In 18 cases, the initiating PVC was present before SD, with usually a longer coupling interval, and in 4 cases, we cannot conclude for technical reasons. Figure 5 shows that the morphology of the PVC initiating VT leading to VF is clearly different from that of the usual PVC's in this patient. This 'new' type of PVC appears only 7 minutes before the VT, probably favoured by a sinus rate slowing.

The favoring factors in the hours before SD

In the hours preceding SD, two other determinants could be analyzed: the basic heart rate, and the ventricular premature beats.

We observed a significant increase in heart rate (sinus rate or ventricular rate for patients in chronic atrial fibrillation) during the last hour preceding SD: from 82 ± 2.9 to 89.8 ± 3.7 b/mn (n = 42, p<.001). In some cases, the cardiac acceleration is particularly obvious, as in the case of figure 6, in which a sinus tachycardia begins 10 mn before the initiation of VT, but in the majority of cases, the heart rate change is less pronounced, even if it is statistically significant.

Atrial arrhythmias were often encountered during the last hour before SD due to VF: 7 patients were in chronic atrial fibrillation, 5 had a paroxysmal sustained atrial arrhythmia starting less than 1 hour before SD, and in 3 the sustained VT was started by atrial premature beats. Thus in 14/45 patients (31%), atrial arrhythmia may play a role in the genesis of VF.

These two factors are often combined, as in the case of figure 7 in which the occurrence of VT is preceded by an increase of the ventricular response of the chronic atrial fibrillation.

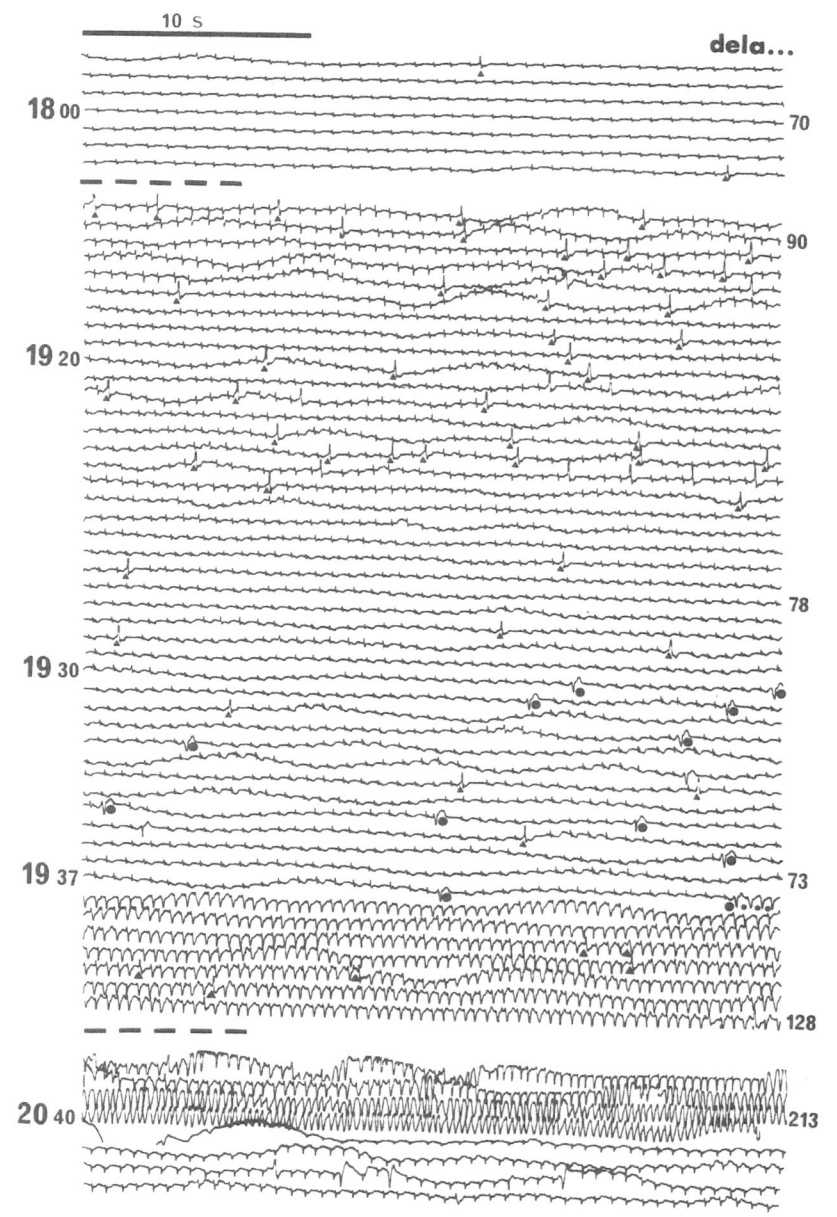

Figure 5. SD by VF after sustained monomorphic VT. This patient had only unifocal PVC's (tri-angles). After a sinus acceleration to 90/mn, inducing an increase of the usual PVC's, an abrupt slowing occurred, and a new type of PVC's (points) appeared at 19h30. Seven minutes later, this PVC started the VT. Note the similitude of morphology between this new PVC and the VT, and the persistence of the usual PVC's during the sustained monomorphic VT.

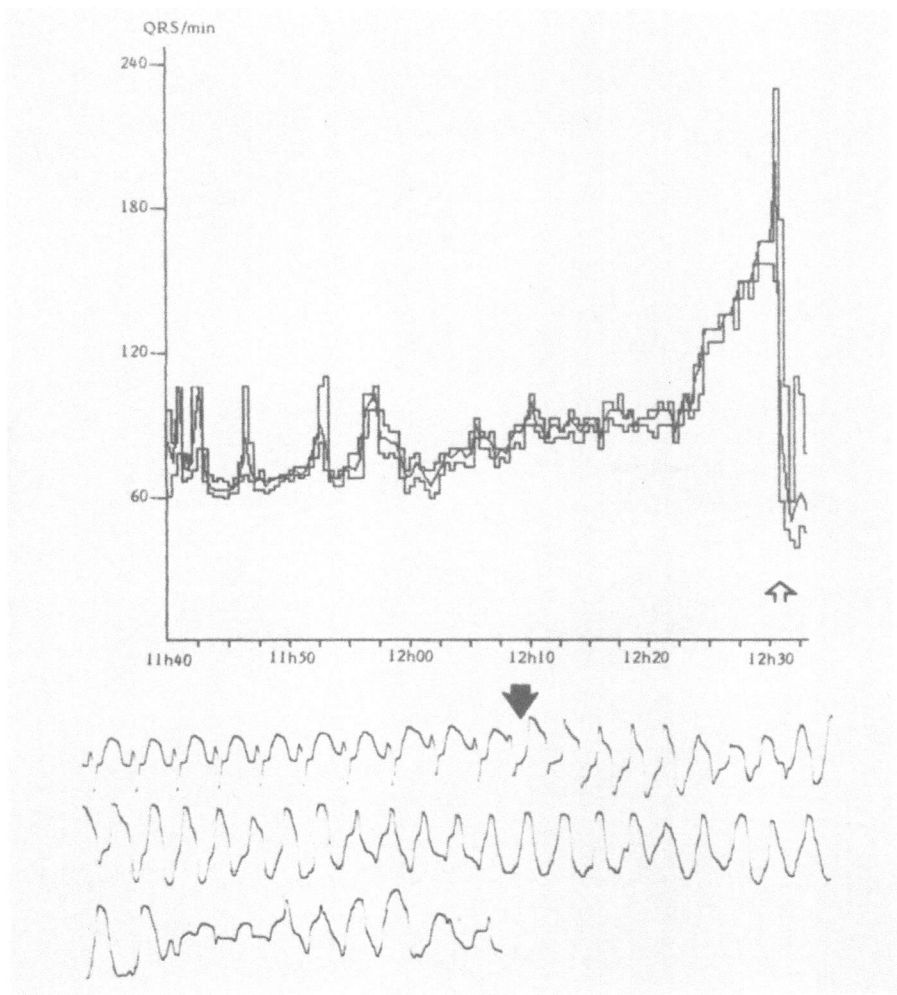

Figure 6. VF succeding to VT and announced by a progressive sinus tachycardia during the 10 preceding minutes: an exercise increases the sinus rate from 80 to 150/mn.

In contrast to the heart rate modifications, an increase in extrasystoles frequency was surprisingly rare: out of 45 patients, 10 had no ventricular premature beats in the 3 hours before SD, and only 11 of the other 35 had an increase of more than 50% in the last hour compared to the preceding two. Figure 8 is an example of one of these cases, with an obvious increase of both number and complexity, i.e. initial bigeminy, then runs of monorphic VT. One of these run induces the sustained VT, with a different morphology, and finally VF.

196

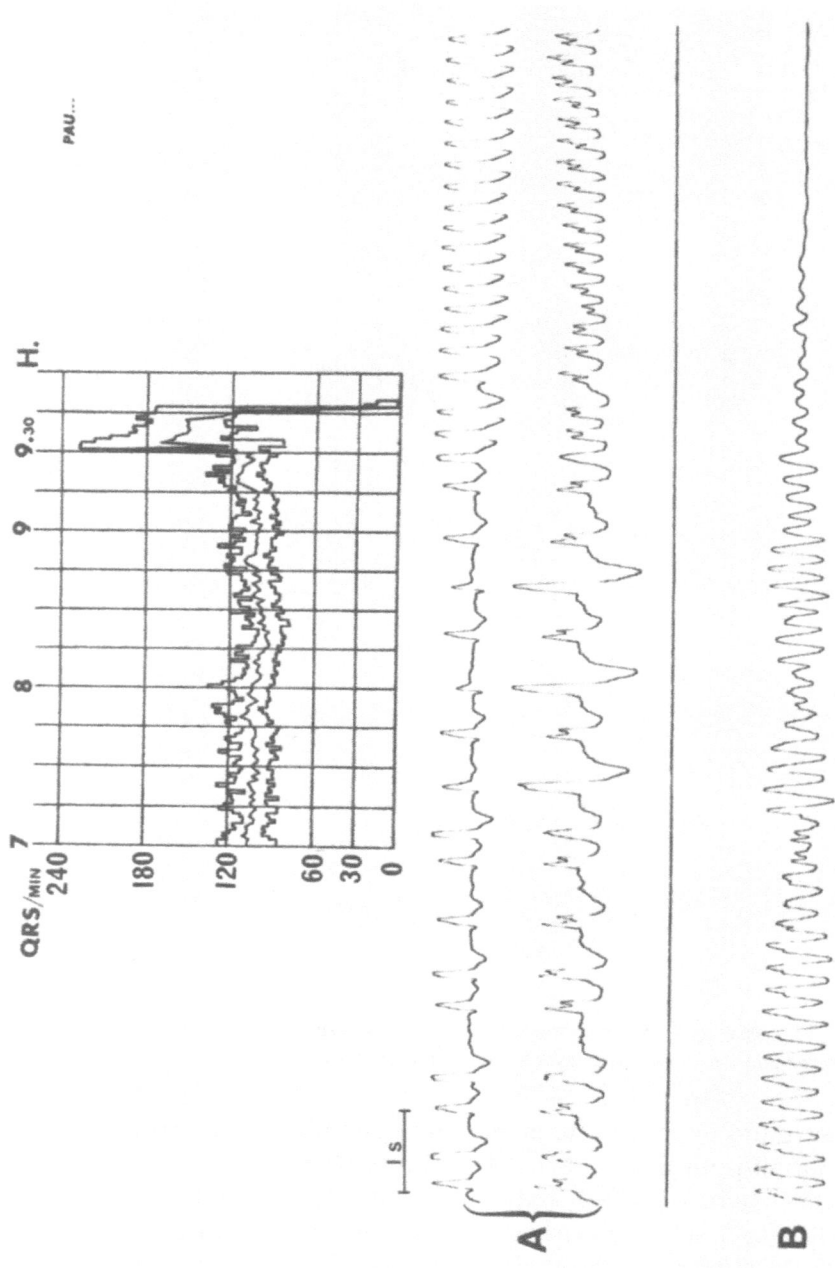

Figure 7. SD by VF after a sustained monomorphic VT in a patient with chronic atrial fibrillation. The ventricular response increases a few minutes before the VT, as seen in the heart rate curve (top).

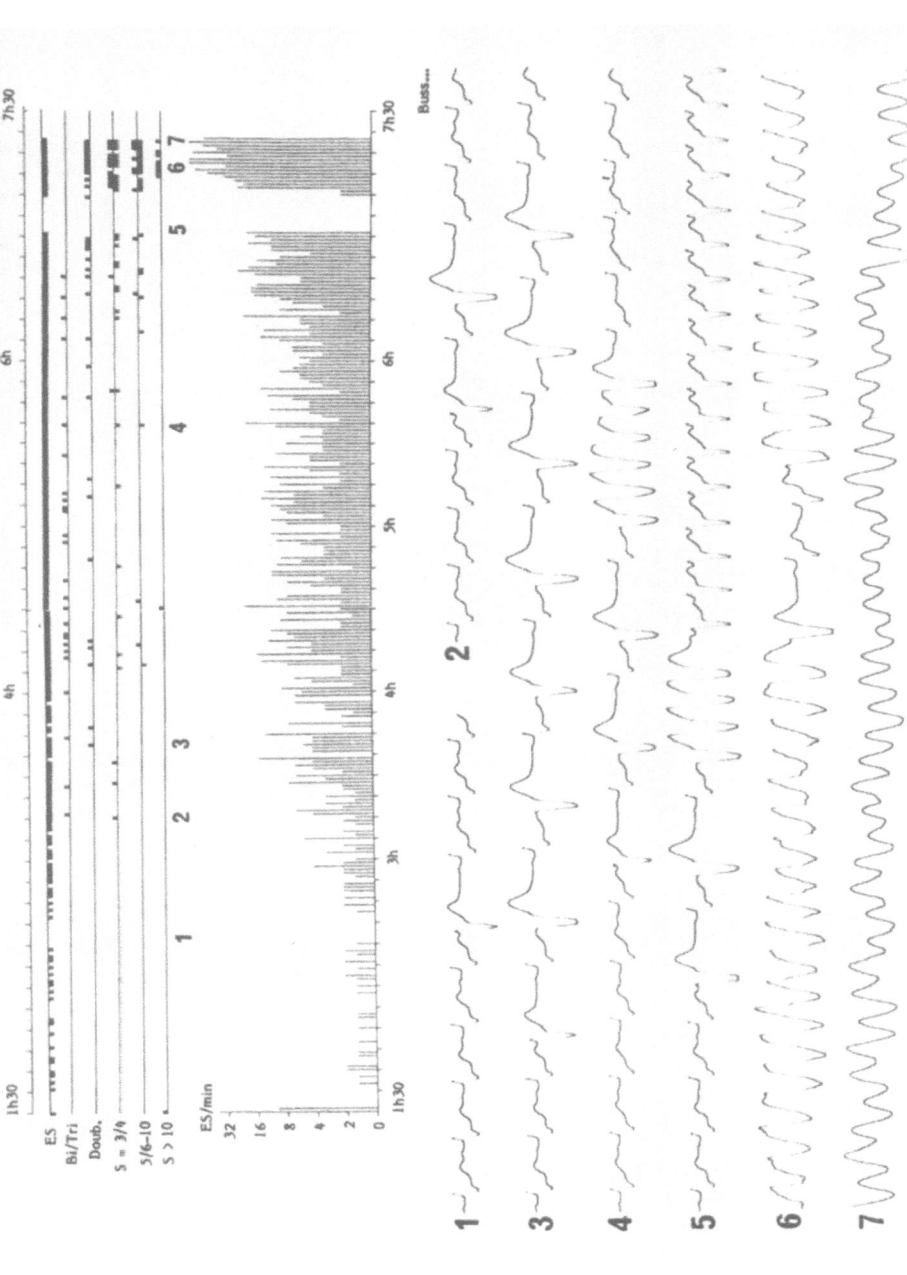

Figure 8. SD by VF succeding to VT and announced by an increase in the number and complexity of ventricular premature beats during the preceding 4 hours. The 3 last lines of the top diagram indicate the salvos of respectively 3 or 4, 5 to 10, and more than 10 QRS. Between 3 and 4 h, only short salvos are present. Longer runs appeared after 4 h and the sustained VT started at 6.30 am.

198

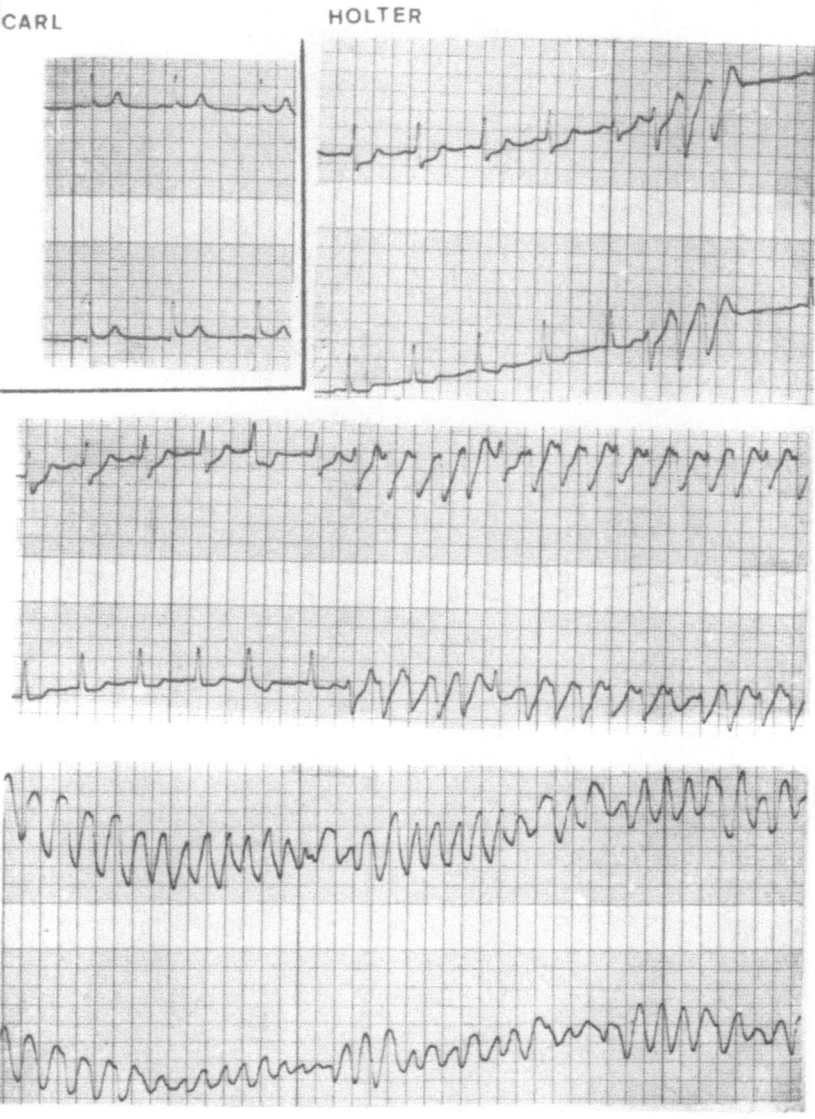

Figure 9. SD by VF succeeding to VT and preceded by an obvious myocardial ischemia with clearly visible ST segment depression. Note that the VT is also preceded by a long RR cycle by post-extrasystolic compensatory pause.

Contrasting with the heart rate increase in these coronary patients, ST segment changes were very unusual, seen only in 5 cases in the minutes preceding SD. Figure 9 shows an example of this kind of event: the VT is preceded by an obvious ST segment depression. But another precipitating factor is necessary to start the sustained VT, i.e. a long RR cycle in this case.

Thus, ST segment changes and increase of extrasystoles appears infrequent, and the major predisposing factor visible in the hour preceding SD is an increase of cardiac rate.

Discussion

The major findings of this analysis of 74 cases of recorded SD were the existence of 3 different terminal events: (1) cardiac standstill in 17 pts, frequently preceded by the evidence of ischemia; (2) TdP of iatrogenic origin in 12 pts; (3) ventricular tachyarrhythmias in 45 cases; a common determinant of which was a cardiac acceleration in the preceding hour, terminated by various combinations of accelerated VT, long-short RR cycles, and R-on-T phenomena.

Thus, the major mechanism of SD, particularly in coronary patients, is formed by ventricular tachyarrhythmias. This notion is also found in some preceding series [7, 11, 14, 17]. The role of cardiac standstill in the genesis of SD appears practically restricted to electromechanical dissociation and directly related to an ischemic process, in severely diseased patients. In contrast, VT or VF directly related to ischaemia is rare. Of course, one can argue that it was not detected by Holter monitoring, but why should it be different in groups I and III? Thus, at least in coronary patients, SD is usually due to an electrophysiological phenomenon, a sustained VT which leads to VF. This mechanism has been underlined in some series [11, 15] and is well correlated with the high incidence of SD in coronary patients with paroxysmal VT's [20]. The interindividual differences in the duration of VT leading to VF may represent a difference in the time necessary to reach the maximal rate compatible with organized VT. In a recent study of Stevenson & coll. [18] comparing coronary patients with aborted SD and those with sustained VT not leading to SD, the major difference found was a higher incidence of polymorphic VT, and a higher rate of the VT in case of monomorphic VT. Thus, the VT rate appears one of the major determinants of electrical instability leading to VF in coronary patients. The other recognized predisposing factor is the left ventricular dysfunction [10, 13]. The relationship between these 2 factors may be that the more the left ventricle is impaired, the more the patient is predisposed to fast VT.

The role of torsades de pointes in the genesis of SD should be clearly individualized. The 2 major determinants, bradycardia and long-short RR sequence, contribute to prolong and to make inhomogeneous the ventricular refractory period [1, 6, 8]. In the literature devoted to SD, the distinction between usual VF and Torsades de pointes is not always clear [4, 9]. This distinction appears of crucial importance as the determinants of either form of lethal arrhythmia, hence the therapeutic implications are different.

The prevention of SD remains a major challenge for cardiologists. If a therapy could be chosen logically, and not empirically as for the present time, it would be more beneficial, and less limited by side-effects. The lessons of studies on recorded sudden death are multiple:

– Iatrogenic factors (antiarrhythmic drugs, sensing pacemaker dysfunction) are not restricted to torsades de pointes: some asystoles or VF are favored by drugs which depress myocardial contractility and/or intraventricular conduction, and any pacemaker dysfunction is potentially dangerous. On the other hand, pacing may prevent long RR cycles, and antiarrhythmic drugs may prolong coupling intervals, two factors which constitute immediate determinants of VT/VF [8, 19]. In addition, pacing prevents torsades de pointes, and antiarrhythmic drugs may be useful for the control of paroxysmal atrial arrhythmias, which are not only markers but indeed determinants of VT/VF: a single atrial premature beat followed by a pause may precipitate the ventricular extrasystole which starts the VT or VF. A tailored therapy, adapted to individual cases is theoretically suitable, yet difficult to manage practically: any therapeutic weagon introduces its own possible iatrogenic consequences, and we cannot evaluate the real risk-benefit ratio.

– SD by VF could be accurately prevented by an implanted cardioverter-defibrillator. The time of response of this device (<30 sec) seems perfectly convenient in the vast majority of cases, permitting delivrance of the shock before a true VF. It agrees with the results published evidencing an increase in the rate survival [12].

– Myocardial ischemia is an important factor of cardiac tandstill, not of VT/VF. Its role appears quantitatively limited, and applies to aged and severely diseased patients. From the present experience, antianginal drugs or surgery thus seem to represent a small part in the prevention of SD.

– Finally, considering the determinant role of the increased sympathetic drive (reflected by the significant heart rate acceleration preceding VT/VF), the role of beta-blocking agents appears fundamental, only limited by hemodynamic considerations. In the literature, some other studies noted an increasing heart rate before SD [16]. However, considering the limited amount of increase (mean: 7 b/mn/hour), it is often necessary to use careful and computerized analysis to evidence it. It is important to realize that the apparent limited increase in the heart rate should not be taken as an argument against the important role of the sympathetic drive: a greater sensitivity of the arrhythmogenic mechanism to this factor necessarily implies a less marked (hence less evident) sinus acceleration before the event in predisposed patients. The results of prospective trials of beta-blockers after myocardial infarction, concluding to their preventive effect against SD [21, 22] is then consistently explained. This point contrasts with a poor antiarrhythmic effect of these drugs in terms of reduction of PVC's [5]. Further studies are probably necessary to determine which patients electively need beta-blocking drugs, since left ventricular function impairement simultaneously represents an indication (higher risk of SD) and a limitation of this therapy.

Acknowledgments

The authors wish to thank the following physicians who contributed to this multicentric study.
List of contributing centers:
Department of Cardiology, Lariboisière Hospital, Paris. (Pr Slama).
Cardiovascular Hospital Haut Lévèque, Bordeaux. (Pr Clementy).
Department of Cardiology, Brabois Hospital, Nancy. (Dr Brembilla-Perrot).
Péan Hospital, Paris. (Dr Ducardonnet).
Department of Cardiology, Trousseau Hospital, Tours. (Pr Fauchier).
Clinic of Béthune. (Dr Bens).
Department of Cardiology, General Hospital, Aix en Provence. (Dr Medvedowsky).
Department of Cardiology, General Hospital, Corbeil. (Dr Lardoux).
Hospital St Joseph, Lyon. (Dr Lopes).
Department of Cardiology, Universitary Hospital, Amiens. (Pr Quiret).
Department of Cardiology, General Hospital, Nimes (Dr Bosc).
Department of Cardiology, General Hospital, Angoulême. (Dr Flammang).
Department of Cardiology, Universitary Hospital, Nantes. (Pr Godin).
Department of Cardiology, General Hospital, Merlebach. (Dr Dambrine).

References

1. Browne KF, Prystowsky E, Heger JJ, Chilson DA, Zipes DP. 1983. Prolongation of the QT interval in man during sleep. Am J Cardiol 52: 55–59.
2. Coumel P, Leclercq JF, Maisonblanche P. 1984. Analysis of Holter tapes after myocardial infarction: are we looking to the right things? In 'The first year after myocardial infarction.' HE Kulbertus (ed), Futura publ., Mount Kisco N.Y., pp. 177–201.
3. Coumel P, Leclercq JF, Zimmerman M. The clinical use of Betablockers in the prevention of sudden death. Europ Heart J (in press).
4. Denes P, Gabster A, Huang SK. 1981. Clinical, electrocardiographic and follow-up observations in patients having ventricular fibrillation during Holter monitoring. Role of quinidine therapy. Am J Cardiol 48: 9–16.
5. Friedman LM, Byington RP, Capone RJ, Furberg CD, Goldstein S, Lchstein E. 1986. Effect of Propranolol in patients with myocardial infarction and ventricular arrhythmia. JACC 7: 1–8.
6. Kay GN, Plumb VJ, Arciniegas JG, Henthorn RW, Waldo AL. 1983. Torsades de pointes: the long-short initiating sequence and other clinical features: observations in 32 patients. JACC 2: 806–817.

7. Kempf FC, Josephson ME: Cardiac arrest recorded on ambulatory electrocardiograms. Am J Cardiol 53: 1577–1582.

8. Lehmann MH, Denker S, Mahmud S, Akhtar M. 1984. Postextrasystolic alterations in refractoriness of the His-Purkinje system an ventricular myocardium in man. Circulation 69: 1096–1102.

9. Lewis BH, Antman EM, Graboys TB. 1983. Detailed analysis of 24 hour ambulatory electrocardiographic recordings during ventricular fibrillation or torsades de pointes. JACC 2: 426–436.

10. Marchlinski FE, Buxton AE, Waxman HL, Josephson ME. 1983. Identifying patients at risk of sudden death after myocardial infarction: value of the response to programmed stimulation, degree of ventricular ectopic activity and severity of left ventricular dysfunction. Am J Cardiol 52: 1190–1196.

11. Milner PG, Platia EV, Reid PR, Griffith LSC. 1985. Ambulatory electrocardiographic recordings at the time of fatal cardiac arrest. Am J Cardiol 56: 588–592.

12. Mirowski M, Reid PR, Mower MM, Watkins L, Griffith LSC, Platia EV, Guarnieri T, Veltri R. 1985. Clinical experience with the automatic implantable cardioverter-defibrillator. PACE 8: A-58 (abstract).

13. Mukharji J, Rude RE, Poole K, Gustafson N, Thomas LJ et al. 1984. Risk factors for sudden death after acute myocardial infarction: two-year follow-up. Am J Cardiol 54: 31–36.

14. Nikolic G, Bishop RL, Singh JB. 1982. Sudden death recorded during Holter monitoring. Circulation 66: 218–225.

15. Panidis IP, Morganroth J. 1983. Sudden death in hospitalized patients: cardiac rhythm disturbances detected by ambulator electrocardiographic monitoring. JACC 2: 798–805.

16. Pratt CM, Francis MJ, Luck JC, Wyndham CR, Miller RR, Quinones MA. 1983. Analysis of ambulatory electrocardiograms in 15 patients during spontaneous ventricular fibrillation with special reference to preceding arrhythmic events. JACC 2: 789–797.

17. Roelandt J, Klootwijk P, Lubsen J, Janse MJ. 1984. Sudden death during longterm ambulatory monitoring. Europ Heart J 5: 7–20.

18. Stevenson WG, Brugada P, Waldecker B, Zehender M, Wellens HJJ. 1985. Clinical, angiographic, and electrophysiologic findings in patients with aborted sudden death as compared with patients with sustained ventricular tachycardia after myocardial infarction. Circulation 71: 1146–1152.

19. Swerdlow B, Axelrod P, Kolman B, Perry D, Merk R. 1983. Ambulatory ventricular tachycardia: characteristics of the initiating beat. Amer Heart J 106: 1326–1331.

20. Swerdlow CD, Winkle RA, Mason JW. 1983. Determinants of survival in patients with ventricular tachyarrhythmias. N Engl J Med 308: 1436–1442.

21. The Norvegian Multicenter Study Group. 1981. Timolol-induced reduction in mortality and reinfarction in patients surviving acute myocardial infarction. N Engl J Med 304: 801–807.

22. Beta-locker Heart Attack Trial Research Group. 1982. A randomized trial of propranolol in patients with acute myocardial infarction. I. Mortality results. JAMA 247: 1707–171.

23. Leclercq JF, Coumel P, Maisonblanche P, Cauchemez B, Zimmerman M, Chouty F, Slama R. 1986. Mise en évidence des mécanismes déterminants de la mort subite. Enquête coopéra tive portant sur 69 cas enregistrés par la méthode de Holter. Arch Mal Coeur 79: 1024–33.

14. Exercise stress testing in the management of ventricular tachycardias

R.W.F. CAMPBELL, Professor of Cardiology
P.B. ALABI, Research Associate
Academic Department of Cardiology, Freeman Hospital, Newcastle upon Tyne

Effects of exercise

Exercise, whether undertaken as a pleasurable pursuit or as a clinical investigation, produces important changes in cardiovascular dynamics. Exercise stress testing has become the most important non-invasive tool for the diagnosis and prognostication of coronary artery disease. However, exercise may be arrhythmogenic. With the onset of exercise there is withdrawal of vagal tone, an increase in sympathetic tone and an increase in levels of circulating catecholamines. These effects increase the rate of phase 4 diastolic depolarisation in the sinus node and accelerate AV nodal conduction. Cardiac frequency is increased and the temporal relationship of atrial and ventricular depolarisation is optimised for that frequency. However, the electrophysiological effects of exercise are more widespread than these influences on the sinus and AV node. Increased sympathetic tone and catecholamine release promote abnormal automatic behaviour, enhance triggered automaticity and may modify myocardial and His Purkinje circuits to favour reentrant activity. Latent re-entrant arrhythmias may also be precipitated through a change in 'trigger' events as when etopic beat frequency is increased. Although exercise produces haemodynamic change, these probably have little or no direct bearing on arrhythmogenesis. More important is the production by exercise of regional myocardial ischaemia which in turn can create an arrhythmogenic substrate.

Exercise and ventricular ectopic beats

In apparently normal subjects, ventricular ectopic beats are rarely detected by a conventional 12 lead electrocardiogram but are found in 50 to 80% of investigated population groups using dynamic electrocardiography [1, 2, 3]. During exercise stress testing approximately 30–40% of such individuals will show one or more ventricular ectopic beat [4]. The frequency of exercise induced ventricular ectopic beats is much higher in individuals with cardiac disease [5], being found in 70% or more of patients depending upon the exercise protocol and the nature of the underlying cardiovascular disease. Ischaemic heart disease is the condition most commonly associated with ventricular ectopic beats. The response of ectopic beat patterns to exercise differs markedly between patients with myocardial ischaemia and normal subjects. Ectopic beats detected at rest in normal subjects tend to disappear with exercise – a feature that has been suggested as typical of 'benign' ventricular ectopic beats [6]. By contrast, ventricular ectopic beats associated with ischaemic heart disease increase with exercise. Their role as prognosticators of future cardiac events is controversial but current evidence suggests that the lower the heart rate at which ventricular ectopic beats appear, the more ominous the prognosis [7]. Ventricular ectopic beats produced by exercise in normal subjects usually occur at high heart rates close to the end of a symptom limited test and with no ECG evidence of myocardial ischaemia.

The exercise modulation of ventricular ectopic beats may contain information related to underlying cardiovascular disease and to prognosis but there is no strong evidence to link ventricular ectopic beats with a propensity to ventricular tachycardia. Neither is there evidence that suppression of exercise ventricular ectopic beats by antiarrhythmic therapy is of prognostic benefit nor does this intervention appear relevant for individuals with ventricular tachycardia who, pari passu, have exercise related ventricular ectopic beats.

Exercise and ventricular tachycardia

Sustained ventricular tachycardia probably never occurs in normal individuals although dynamic electrocardiographic recordings occasionally document a few consecutive ventricular ectopic beats which technically satisfy a definition of ventricular tachycardia (3 or more ventricular ectopic complexes at a rate equal to or greater than 120 beats per minute) [1]. Ventricular tachycardia is usually associated with cardiovascular disease of which coronary artery disease is the most important type. Short self-terminating episodes of ventricular tachycardia beats commonly complicate the acute phase of myocardial infarction but it is in the late phase that clinically important sustained episodes of ventricular tachycardia are most likely to occur. There is increasing evidence that ventricular tachyarrhythmias are an important component of other cardiac conditions, including cardiomyopathies [8] and aortic stensosis [9]. Not all ventricular tachycardias are amenable to investigation by exercise stress testing.

Post myocardial infarction

Post myocardial infarction sustained ventricular tachycardia frequently is associated with a left ventricular aneurysm, is classically inducible by programmed electrical stimulation [10], but is unreliably precipitated by exercise stress testing.

Myocardial ischaemia

Ventricular tachycardia may be provoked by exercise in patients with coronary artery disease. It is important to differentiate whether this occurs as a direct consequence of the electrophysiological effects of exercise or occurs through a mechanism of induction of myocardial ischaemia. The relevance of this distinction is that if myocardial ischaemia is involved, management should be directed to this entity (coronary artery bypass grafting, angioplasty etc.) rather than to antiarrhythmic drugs. Sustained monomorphic ventricular tachycardia rarely complicates exercise-induced myocardial ischaemia, ventricular fibrillation or polymorphic ventricular tachycardia being more usual arrhythmogenic results.

Long QT syndromes

Patients with the rare but clinically important congenital long QT syndromes (Romano Ward and Jervell-Lange-Neilson) have a high incidence of sudden death with strong circumstantial evidence suggesting a ventricular tachyarrhythmia as the mechanism [11]. The history of a typical attack is for the patient, under conditions of stress or exercise, to collapse pulseless. Fortunately, in a high proportion of events the patient recovers, probably by self termination of a tachyarrhythmia. This implies that ventricular tachycardia or flutter rather than ventricular fibrillation is the mechanism. Exercise stress testing or noxious stimuli (classically auditory) may provoke these potentially life threatening arrhythmias which usually are not inducible by programmed electrical stimulation. Beta adrenoreceptor blockade and/or stellate ganglionectomy appear the only interventions of therapeutic benefit.

Mitral valve prolapse

Arguably one of the commonest cardiovascular diseases to afflict the human race, mitral valve prolapse is associated with cardiac arrhythmias including ventricular tachycardia and ventricular fibrillation [12]. These are extremely rare complications, which in affected subjects appear to be exercise related. As with the long QT syndrome, the tachyarrhythmias rarely are inducible by programmed electrical stimulation. Beta blocking drugs are reported to be of particular antiarrhythmic value.

Arrhythmogenic right ventricular dysplasia

Right ventricular dysplasia is attracting increasing attention, particularly with reports of a novel surgical management to control complicating ventricular tachyarrhythmias [13]. The arrhythmias often can be provoked by exercise but may also be inducible by programmed stimulation.

Catechol-related ventricular tachycardia in children

This rare condition of children may present as syncope on exercise and has been associated with a high incidence of sudden death [14]. It is postulated that the condition is due to an abnormal sensitivity of AV nodal and ventricular escape pacemakers and, in keeping with its exercise precipitation, there is evidence that beta adrenoreceptor blocking drugs are useful in clinical management. Programmed electrical stimulation is rarely helpful.

The foregoing indicate that exercise provoked ventricular tachycardia behaves differently from other types of ventricular tachycardia. Exercise related ventricular tachycardia can also be provoked by isoprenaline administration but is rarely precipitated by electrophysiological stimulation techniques. Exercise related ventricular tachycardia is associated with a variety of relatively unusual pathological conditions. Beta adrenoreceptor blocking drugs or, exceptionally, stellate ganglionectomy, are therapies of proven benefit.

Problems with exercise testing in the management of ventricular arrhythmias

Provocation of a ventricular tachyarrhythmia by programmed stimulation is usually highly reproducible. This underlies the value of electrophysiological studies in evaluating antiarrhythmic therapies in individual patients. Reproducibility of exercise related ventricular tachycardias by stress testing is poor. The reasons for this are unclear. Exercise is a very complex physiological event and the many changing factors may not follow the same time course in each test. The problem is particularly evident in ischaemia dependent arrhythmias perhaps because the development ischaemia and its electrophysiological consequences are unlikely to occur in exactly the same way during sequential tests. Repetitive exercise tests produce a training effect with a minor increase in exercise capacity and a sometimes impressive reduction in the frequency of ventricular arrhythmias [15]. Whether these effects truly reflect 'training' or are a manifestation of 'less stress' by familarity with the test procedure, is unclear. The low reproducibility of most exercise induced ventricular arrhythmias hinders the use of stress testing to investigate the therapeutic potential of antiarrhythmic drugs.

Exercise testing is not reliable as a screening test. Despite the spontaneous occurrence of exercise related ventricular arrhythmias in patients, formal exercise protocols often fail to reproduce natural events. This is a serious limitation of exercise stress testing as a screening tool for such patients as those with long QT syndromes etc.

Therapeutic uses of exercise testing in arrhythmia management

Despite problems of reliability and reproducibility, exercise testing may be the only method of characterising ventricular tachyarrhythmias occurring in some patients. Any ventricular tachycardia provoked by exercise should prompt consideration as to whether generation of ischaemia played a contributory role, in which case myocardial revascularisation should be considered as a part of the overall management. Identification of an exercise-provoked ventricular arrhythmia has the therapeutic implication that Vaughan Williams Class I antiarrhythmic drugs are often relatively ineffective, that inducibility by programmed electrical stimulation is unlikely and that beta blockers may be a useful management.

Exercise stress testing should be undertaken in all patients for whom long term antiarrhythmic therapy is prescribed as prophylaxis of a ventricular tachyarrhythmia. Although the test may be of little value for the initial selection of therapy, it is reassuring and clinically relevant to check that the chosen therapy is effective under physiological conditions other than rest or those at the time of an electrophysiological study.

Arrhythmogenic exercise protocol

Current exercise protocols have been devised for diagnosis and prognostication of coronary artery disease. They incorporate gradual increments in workload and allow periods of stabilisation. Isometric exercise is kept to a minimum. Were an arrhythmogenic protocol to be devised it likely would be substantially different, possibly including rapid development of workloads and encouraging an isometric contribution. As exercise related ventricular tachyarrhythmias attract more attention, there is a growing need to devise exercise protocols which increase the reliability and reproducibility of the test for provoking arrhythmias and for determining adequacy of administered therapy.

Acknowledgements

I should like to acknowledge the invaluable assistance of Miss Sue Murray in the preparation of this manuscript.

References

1. Brodsky M, Wu D, Denes P, Kanakis C, Rosen KM. 1977. Arrhythmias documented by 24 hour continuous electrocardiographic monitoring in 50 male medical students without apparent heart disease. Am J Cardiol 39: 390–395.
2. Sobotka PA, Mayer JH, Bauernfeind RA, Kanakis C, Rosen KM. 1981. Arrhythmias documented by 24 hour continuous ambulatory electrocardiographic monitoring in young women without apparent heart disease. Am Heart J 101: 753–759.
3. Fleg JL, Kennedy HL. 1982. Cardiac arrhythmias in a healthy elderly population. Detection by 24 hour ambulatory electrocardiography. Chest 81: 302–307.
4. McHenry PL, Fisch C, Jordan JW, Corya BR. 1972. Cardiac arrhythmias observed during maximal treadmill exercise testing in clinically normal men. Am J Cardiol 29: 331–336.
5. Poblete PF, Kennedy HL, Caralis DG. 1978. Detection of ventricular ectopy in patients with coronary heart disease and normal subjects by exercise testing and ambulatory electrocardiography. Chest 74: 402–407.
6. Jelinek MV, Lown B. 1974. Exercise stress testing for exposure of cardiac arrhythmia. Prog Cardiovasc Dis 166: 497–522.
7. Ivanova LA, Mazur NA, Smirnova TM, Sumerokov AB, Nazarenko VA, Svet EA. 1980. Electrocardiographic exercise testing and ambulatory monitoring to identify patients with ischaemic heart disease at high risk of sudden death. Am J Cardiol 45: 1132–1138.
8. McKenna WJ, Krikler DM, Goodwin JF. 1984. Arrhythmias in dilated and hypertrophic cardiomyopathy. Med Clin North Am 68: 983–1000.
9. Olshausen K, Schwarz F, Apfelbach J, Rohrig N, Kramer B, Kubler W. 1983. Determinants of the incidence and severity of ventricular arrhythmias in aortic valve disease. Am J Cardiol 51: 1103–1109.
10. Wellens HJJ, Brugada P, Stevenson WG. 1985. Programmed electrical stimulation of the heart in patients with life threatening ventricular arrhythmias. What is the significance of induced arrhythmias and what is the correct stimulation protocol? Circulation 72: 1–7.
11. Schwartz PJ, Periti M, Malliani A. 1975. The long Q-T syndrome. Am Heart J 89: 378–390.
12. Campbell RWF, Godman MG, Fiddler GI, Marquis RM, Julian DG. 1976. Ventricular arrhythmias in syndrome of balloon deformity of mitral valve. Definition of possible high risk group. Br Heart J 38: 1053–1057.
13. Marcus FI, Fontaine GH, Guiraudon G, Frank R, Laurencean JL, Malergue C, Grosgugeat Y. 1982. Right ventricular dysplasia: a report of 24 adult cases. Circulation 65: 384–398.
14. Coumel P, Fidelle J, Lucet V, Attuel P, Bouvrain Y. 1978. Catecholamine – induced severe ventricular arrhythmias with Adams-Stokes syndrome in children: report of four cases. Br Heart J 40: (Suppl) 28–37.
15. Sheps DS, Ernst JC, Briese FR, Lopez LV, Conde CA, Castellanos A, Myerburg RJ. 1977. Decreased frequency of exercise-induced ventricular ectopic activity in the second of two consecutive treadmill tests. Circulation 55: 892–895.

15. Malignant arrythmias during exercise testing: a French cooperative study

J.P. BROUSTET, H. DOUARD and B. MORA
Department of Exercise Testing, Hôpital Cardiologique du Haut Leveque – 33604 Pessac

There is no doubt that ventricular tachycardia (VT) and ventricular fibrillation (VF) do occur during exercise testing.

The use of DC countershock and of permanent monitoring of ECG has reduced the risk of death.

Initially, the aim of exercise ECG was to identify the patterns of exercise induced ischemia only in those patients in whom the diagnosis remained uncertain. Indeed the strong correlations established between the data from exercise testing and the prognosis, in terms of extent of coronary heart disease, extent of lesions and prediction of life expectancy, has changed exercise testing into a prognostic and decision-making tool. Therefore, the exercise tests have been performed by more and more severely diseased coronary patients. On the other hand, the generalization of early physical training after myocardial infarction is equivalent to many repeated exercise tests, sometimes at a high level, in more and more patients during the recovery phase of myocardial infarction of coronary revascularisation.

The aims of this investigation were:

1 – the determination of the rate and incidence of malignant arrythmias occurring during ET or during the early recovery phases of ET from 1975 to 1985;

2 – an attempt to delineate the profile of high risk patients for ET.

A detailed questionnaire was sent to the centers who wished to be included in the study, after a preliminary screening. Centers very specialized in arrhythmias were not retained.

Criteria for inclusion were:

a) – ventricular tachycardia (VT) or 'torsades de pointes' sustained for more than 30 seconds (with or without circulatory arrest);

b) – ventricular fibrillation (VF);

c) – cardiac arrest.

Results

A total of 458,000 ET were registered including 281,000 ET for diagnosis, assessment of therapeutic, decision for investigation, and 177,000 controlled training sessions (cardiac patients exclusively).

Among the first group the proportions of normal and diseased patients cannot be precisely determined: all the subgoups belonged to hospital departments of exercise testing and there was no center for sports or vocational medicine.

A ratio of one cardiac patient to one normal is probable. On the other hand, all the patients involved in training sessions were cardiac. Most of them had coronary hert disease and some had valvular surgery.

Among 458,000 exercise tests, 60 cases were retained according to the following classification:

– Diagnosis or evaluation tests: 49 with 4 deaths
– Training sessions: 11 with 2 deaths

The incidence of malignant arrythmias was 13/100,000 or 1/7,692 exercise tests and the death rate of 1.3/100,000 or 1/76,920 exercise tests.

The nature and evolution of malignant arrythmias are depicted in the following table:

Table 1.

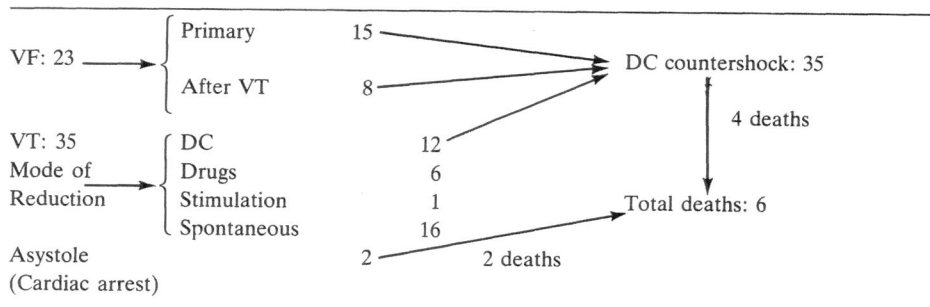

(Abbreviations: VF: ventricular fibrillation; VT: ventricular tachycardia).

Table 2. Patient characteristics.

Coronary heart disease (CHD)	42
Previous MI 39	
No MI 13	
Mitral valve prolapse (MVP)	6
Valvular stenosis aortic (AVS)	3
Right ventricle dysplasia (RVD)	4
Non obstructive hypertrophic myocardiopathy (NOHM)	1
Dilated myocardiopathy (MD)	4

There were 6 women and 54 men (mean age: 51 ± 11 (range 29–74 years) 19 were out-patients and 39 in-patients (2 unknown). 10 patients had a history of syncope, 33 patients received different anti-arrythmic drugs at the time of exercise test.

The occurrence of FV or TV was heralded in 29 of 56 cases by bouts of ventricular premature beating (VPB) in 10 cases, doublets in 1 case, bi or trigeminism in 4 cases, increase of isolated VPB in 14 cases. Among the coronary patients 11 had S-T elevation facing area of scar during exercise test, 17 had S-T segment depression $\geqslant 1$ mm. Chest pain preceded arrhythmia in 7 cases.

Evolution of survivors (n = 54)

31/60 carried out a new exercise test after anti-arrhythmic or surgical therapy or anti-ischemic drugs: one of them had a VT interrupted by manual percussion of sternum, one had VT interrupted by intravenous bolus of Amiodarone; a third one has a VT at the end of every maximal exercise test that he has carried out yearly over the last eight years!

The other 28 patients had no recurrence of severe arrhythmias.

The vital prognosis is the following: no information in 14 patients; 4 deaths occurred: two sudden deaths, one at rest, and one while the patient was on cycling uphill five years after TV and six years after resection of myocardial aneurysm; the duration of follow-up in 42 known survivors is 3.25 ± 2.9 years.

Information on six fatal cases

There were 4 men, 2 women; 2 were in-patients, 2 were out-patients. Two patients died during controlled training session: they were exercising on bicycles, as routinely practiced in France. Extrasystoles had preceded the fatality in 4 of 6 cases.

Five patients had myocardial infarction in phase II (2 cases) or in phase III (3 cases). The last patient had a mild aortic stenosis.

At autopsy, one of the coronary patients had myocardial hypertrophy and a venous by-pass grafted before the stenosis of the underlying coronary artery! Five of the six patients were taking drugs: Amiodarone (2) Dysopyramide (1) Procainmide (1), Propranolol (1). From the information provided by investigators, it was not possible to define a precise profile of the patients at high risk in exercise tests. Nevertheless age, poor left ventricular function, history of malignant arrhythmia, progressive widening of QRS during exercise, decrease of blood pressure and early elevation of S-T segment were mentioned.

The procedure of this cooperative study is certainly open to criticism: it is a retrospective study; the real prevalence of the disease is unknown; and the indications of ET surely differ between the different centers (for instance, ability to perform ET in AVS or arrhythmias investigation).

Nevertheless all the departments that we got in touch with did agree to this study, there was no refusal and we think that all severe injuries – including deaths – are really included.

It seems from these results that the incidence of severe arrhythmias, and especially death, are less common than some years ago. In 1971, Rochmis [6], in a large multicenter survey of complications of ET, found a mortality of 1/42,000 tests (study of 712,285 ET). In our study, the rate of mortality was about 1/77,000. The tests included run from 1975 to 1985, and we are not able to determine if the rate of events has decreased during the last 5 years. Probably if contra-indications of ET are better known and respected, this is counterbalanced by an enlargement of indications, that increases the risk of the procedure.

In interpretating estimates of incidence, it is important to recognize the characteristics of the population being tested. For Cobb, the relative risk of developing cardiac arrest with ET can be roughly estimated as 160 times greater than what might be expected to occur spontaneously, and only 6 times greater in cardiac rehabilitation programs [2]. Therefore, although all subjects included in rehabilitation programmes are cardiac, they are strongly selected before (80 per cent are coronary patients with a history of myocardial infarction).

Therefore the risk of severe incident appears minor, and ET must be considered – with respect for strict contra-indications – as a safe non-invasive test.

As for severe arrhythmias, comparison with other studies is more difficult because of variable data for inclusion; we restrained VF and VT not less than 30 seconds; the rate of 1/7,700 does not differ from the 1/2,000 to 1/13,000 previously reported [1, 3, 4, 5, 7, 8].

It seems, unfortunately, difficult as yet to diminish the incidence of morbidity and mortality of ET for this purpose, if heralded symptoms – such as decrease of blood pressure, precession of multifocal ventricular extrasystoles, early elevation of ST segment – are recognized and lead to the immediate cessation of the test, it appears that most accidents remain unforeseeable, even if always occurring in severe pathology.

Summary and conclusion

Among 458,000 exercise tests, including 177,000 during controlled cardiac rehabilitation, 60 malignant arrhythmias occurred (1/7600) of which 6 resulted in deat (1/77,000). Severe arrhythmias occurred in exercise phase in 4 cases and in the early recovery period in others.

Exercise testing may be considered as safe (low incidence of severe arrhythmias) but the prognosis of such event is worst (10% of deaths). The predictive value of heralding markers for malignant arrhythmias is very poor (flow specificity) while their strong sensitivity allows a good predictive value for absence of arrhythmia. This last statement explains and makes possible uncontrolled physical training in those patients who had an uneventful maximal exercise test.

Acknowledgements

The authors want to express their thanks to all the participants in the study who completed the detailed questionaires.

This study was carried out thanks to the cooperation of the following colleagues listed here by city in alphabetical order.

Agen: Daubèze; *Amiens:* Quiret, Jaubourg, Lesbre; *Avignon:* Joffre; *Bastia:* Mimi, Roux; *Beaumont:* Laffosse, Lloret; *Besancon:* Vial, Bassand; *Biarritz:* Béotti, Hourcade; *Bordeaux:* Broustet, Douard, Mora; *Boulogne:* Bardet; *Brest:* Penther; *Clermont-Ferrand:* Cassagnes; *Creil:* Librez, Joly; *Dommartin les toul.:* Goepfert, Maureria, Aliot; *Grenoble:* Mallion; *Hyeres:* Garaix, Roux; *Ivry:* Frank, Fontaine, Petitot; *Libourne:* Cottin; *Lille:* Lablanche, Bertrand; *Limoges:* Bensaïd; *Lyon* (Croix Rousse, Pradel, Saint Joseph: André-Fouet, Thizy, Pont, Tartulier, Saint Pierre, Gallavardin, Cahen, Quard); *Marseille:* Lévy, Gérard, Metge, Ebagosti, Torrésani†; *Nancy:* Brembilla-Perrot, Balaud, Pernot, Cherrier, Khalife, Gilgenkrantz; *Nantes:* Nicolas, Potiron-Josse; Nice: Roquebrune, Morand; *Orthez:* Sabaut; Paris (Bichat, Broussais, Cochin, Pitié, Tenon): Robert, Gourgon, Sellier, Dupérier, Degeorges, Réverdy, Grosgogeat, Witchitz; *Pau:* Mothes; *Perigueux:* Colin; *Quimper:* Guillou; *Reims:* Bajolet; *Rennes:* Lelong, Daubert, Gouffault; Rouen: Letac; *Toulouse:* Chollet, Bernadet; *Tours:* Brochier.

References

1. Brue RA, Kluge W. 1971. Defibrillatory treatment of exertional cardiac arrest in coronary disease. J Am Med Assoc 216: 653.
2. Cobb LA, Weaver WD. 1986. Exercise: a risk for sudden death in patients with coronary heart disease. JACC, 7 (n° 1): 215–9.
3. Detry JM, Abouantoun S, Wyns W. 1981. Incidence and prognostic implications of severe ventricular arrhythmias during maximal exercise testing. Cardiology 68 (Suppl 2): 35–43.
4. Hossack KF, Hartwig R. 1982. Cardiac arrest associated with supervised cardiac rehabilitation J Cardiac Rehabil 2: 402–8.
5. Irving JB, Bruce RA. 1977. Exertional hypotension and post exertional ventricular fibrillation. Am J Cardiol 39: 849–851.
6. Rohmis P, Blackburn H. 1971. Exercise tests. A survey of procedures, safety and litigation experience in approximately 170,000 tests. JAMA 217: 1061–1066.
7. Scherer D, Kaltenbach M. 1980. Frequency of life-threatening complications associated with exercise testing. Abstract book, 8th European Congress of Cardiology, PARIS, pp. 187.
8. Stuart R, Ellestad M. 1980. National survey of exercise stress testing facilities. Chest 77: 94–100.

16. The value of the 12 lead ECG in diagnosing ventricular tachycardia and in localizing its site of origin

HEIN J.J. WELLENS and PEDRO BRUGADA

Department of Cardiology, Academic Hospital of Maastricht, University of Limburg, Maastricht, the Netherlands

By correlating information from programmed electrical stimulation of the heart and intracardiac recordings with the 12 lead electrocardiogram we have improved our ability to predict the site of origin of a tachycardia showing a widened QRS complex [1–3]. That information is not only of value for diagnostic and prognostic reasons, but also because new methods of therapy like surgery and fulguration require a more exact localisation of the site of origin of the widened QRS complex.

Two topics will be discussed in this chapter. First, how to differentiate a ventricular from a supraventricular origin in the patient showing a tachycardia with a widened QRS complex. Second, after a ventricular origin has been established, how useful is the 12 lead ECG in localising the site of impulse formation in the ventricle.

The differentiation on the 12 lead ECG between a ventricular or a supraventricular origin of a tachycardia showing a widened QRS complex

We have learned that in the patient with a widened QRS complex the 12 lead ECG should be analysed in a very systematic way. By doing this it is frequently possible to select the correct diagnosis out of the different possibilities that may lead to a tachycardia with a widened QRS complex (Table 1). As shown in table 2 four steps should be taken consecutively.

Step 1: Is atrioventricular (AV) dissociation present during tachycardia?

Recognition of AV dissociation is usually not difficult (figure 1). But unfortunately AV dissociation is only present in approximately 50% of patients with ventricular tachycardia [2]. We conclude therefore that AV dissociation during a wide QRS complex tachycardia points to a ventricular origin of the arrhythmia, but presence of a relation beteen atrial and ventricular events does not rule out the possibility of a ventricular tachycardia.

Table 1. Possible causes of a regular tachycardia with a wide QRS complex

1) Supraventricular tachycardia with functional bundle branch block. This includes atrial tachycardia, atrial flutter with 2 to 1 atrioventricular conduction, A-V nodal tachycardia and a circus movement tachycardia with anterograde conduction over the AV node and ventriculo-atrial conduction over an accessory atrioventricular pathway.

2) Supraventricular tachycardia with pre-existent bundle branch block. Same types of tachycardia as mentioned under 1).

3) Supraventricular tachycardia with atrioventricular conduction over an accessory atrioventricular pathway. This includes atrial tachycardia, atrial flutter with 2 to 1 atrioventricular conduction, and a circus movement tachycardia with anterograde conduction over an accessory A-V pathway and retrograde conduction over the His bundle AV-node or a second accessory atrioventricular pathway.

4) Supraventricular tachycardia with anterograde conduction over a Mahaim fiber.

5) Ventricular tachycardia.

Table 2. Steps in the diagnosis of a wide QRS tachycardia.

1) AV dissociation?	Present	VT	
2) QRS width?	> 0.14 sec	VT	
		R/O	a) SVT with preexist. BBB
			b) SVT with anterogr. conduction over AP
3) Left axis deviation (left of −30°)?	Present favours	VT	
		R/O	a) SVT with preexist. BBB
			b) SVT with anterogr. conduction over Kent (septal or right sided) or Mahaim bundle
4) QRS configuration? RBBB shaped	V_1: mono- or biphasic QRS suggests VT V_6: R/S<1 suggests VT		
LBBB shaped	V_1–V_2: r_{tachy}<r_{sr} suggests SVT r_{tachy}>r_{sr} suggests VT notching downslope S wave suggests VT beginning QRS to nadir by 70 msec suggests VT		

Abbreviations: tachy = tachycardia; AV = atrioventricular; AP = accessory pathway; WPW = Wolff-Parkinson-White; CMT = circus movement tachyardia; AF = atrial fibrillation; SVT = supraventricular tachycardia; VT = ventricular tachycardia; sr = sinus rhythm; BBB = bundle branch block.

216

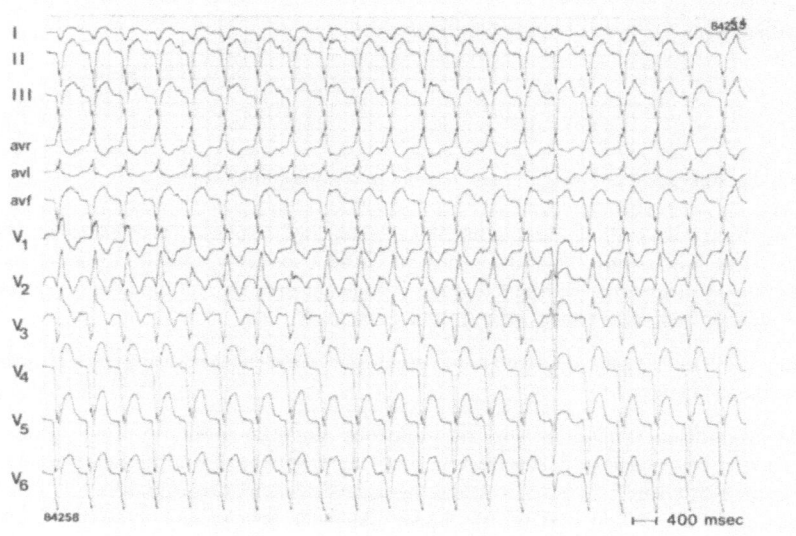

Figure 1. Ventricular tachycardia showing atrioventricular dissociation with occasional captures and fusion beats. Unfortunately, atrioventricular conduction of sinus beats during ventricular tachycadia is rare. A relatively slow rate ventricular tachycardia favours the occurrence of this phenomenon.

Step 2: What is the width of the QRS complex?

When we compared the width of the QRS complex in 100 cases of ventricular tachycardia and 100 cases of supraventricular tachycardia with aberrant intraventricular conduction, we found that all cases of supraventricular tachycardia with aberrant conduction had a QRS width of ≤0.14 sec, while 59% of cases with ventricular tachycardia has a QRS width of more than 0.14 sec [2]. These findings indicate that a QRS width of more than 0.14 sec is highly suggestive of a ventricular origin of the tachycardia. It is of interest, as recently reported by Coumel et al [4], that in coronary heart disease the average QRS complex is wider during ventricular tachycardia than the QRS complex of the patient with idiopathic ventricular tachycardia (171 ± 32 msec vs 135 ± 11 msec; $p < 0.001$). As pointed out [2] there are two situations in which a supraventricular tachycardia can have a QRS width of more than 0.14 sec. The first one is the patient having a supraventricular tachycardia in the presence of pre-existent bundle branch block, the second situation is a supraventricular tachycardia with atrioventricular conduction over an accessory atrioventricular pathway.

Step 3: Is marked deviation of the frontal axis present?

The majority of patients with ventricular tachycardia have a markedly abnormal QRS axis in the frontal plane. Independent of the QRS configuration (left or right bundle branch block like) the axis usually points superiorly. As emphasised by Coumel et al. [4] this is a typical finding in patients with ventricular tachycardia in the setting of a previous myocardial infarction. Patients with idiopathic ventricular tachycardia usually have (73%) a normal QRS axis in the frontal plane [4]. In discussing the importance of axis in the frontal plane in the differential diagnosis of the wide QRS tachycardia it is important to realise that a markedly abnormal axis can occur in patients with pre-existent bundle branch block during supraventricular tachycardia and in patients having during tachycardia atrioventricular conduction over an accessory pathway. In the latter situation marked left axis deviation can be found during anterograde conduction over a right sided or postero septal Kent bundle and marked right axis deviation in case of a left lateral Kent bundle.

Step 4: How is the configuration of the QRS complex?

The right bundle branch block shaped QRS complex
Many years ago Marriott described the differences in QRS configuration in lead V_1 between a supraventricular complex with right aberrant intraventricular conduction and an ectopic ventricular complex with a right bundle branch block like shape [5].

As Marriott pointed out a monophasic or biphasic QRS complex suggests an ectopic ventricular origin, while a triphasic QRS complex supports right aberrant intraventricular conduction.

Our own experience supports Marriott's observations [1]. We also found that lead V_6 is a very useful lead in making the distinction between a supraventricular complex with right aberrant atrioventricular conduction and a ventricular origin. Typically in the supraventricular complex with aberrant intraventricular conduction the QRS in V_6 starts with a Q-wave followed by an R-wave which is higher than the broad S-wave (figure 2). In contrast the ventricular ectopic complex shows in lead V_6 an R/S complex of less than 1 or a QS complex (figure 3).

The left bundle branch block shaped QRS complex
Unless a qR complex is present, which points to a ventricular origin, lead V_6 cannot be considered a useful lead to distinguish between a left aberrantly conducted supraventricular complex and an ectopic ventricular complex with a left bundle branch block shape.

Lead V_1 can be useful however. As shown in figure 4 during ventricular

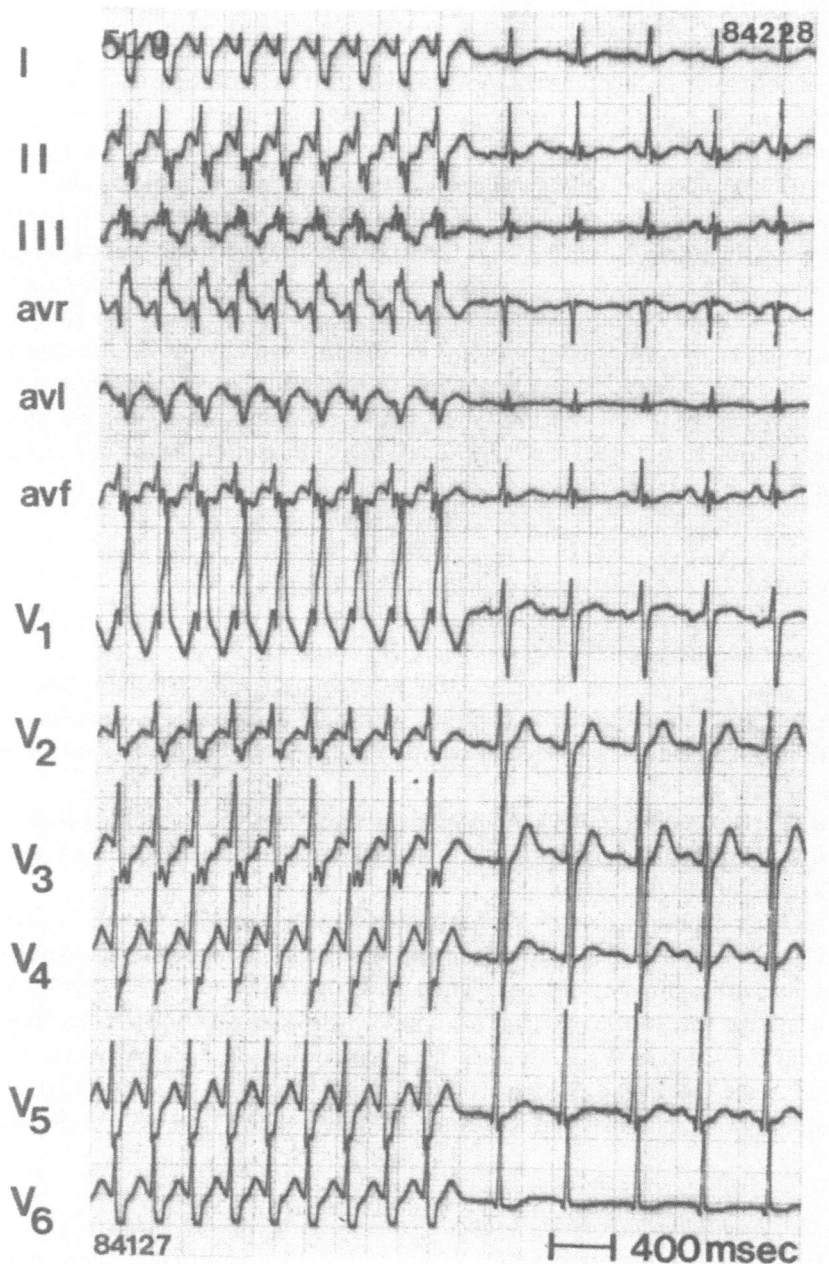

Figure 2. Example of functional right bundle branch block during a circus movement tachycardia with anterograde conduction over the AV node and retrograde conduction over an accessory atrioventricular pathway. The QRS complex in lead V_6 has the typical features described in the text.

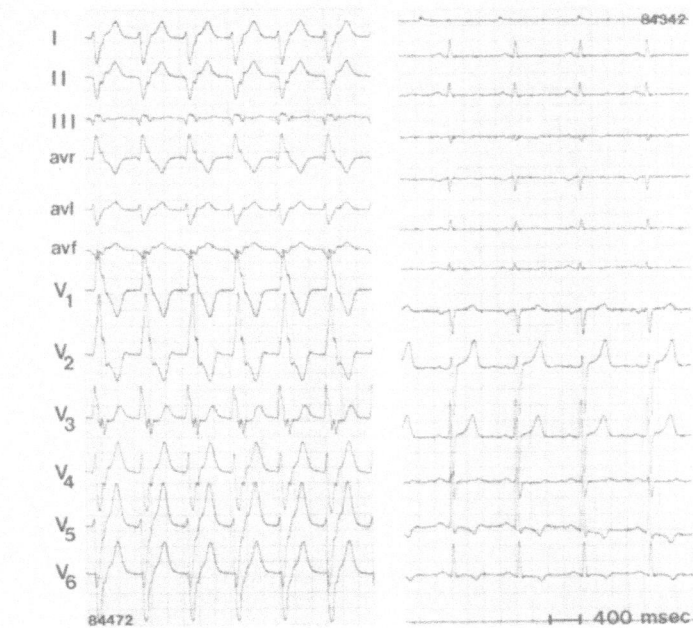

Figure 3. Ventricular tachycardia with a right bundle branch block shaped QRS complex. Note the r S complex in lead V₆.

tachycardia the QRS complex in V_1 (and frequently also in V_2) may show initial positivity broader and higher than the initial positivity during sinus rhythm. The reverse is usually the case in supraventricular tachycardia with left aberrant conduction. Apart from the initial portion of the QRS complex also a close look at the descending limb of the S-wave in lead V_1 and V_2 may be rewarding. In ventricular tachycardia the S-wave usually descends more slowly or shows notching in contrast to the more rapid descent of the S-wave in supraventricular tachycardia with left bundle branch block. Also a distance between the beginning of the QRS to the nadir of the S wave of more than 70 msec suggests a ventricular tachycardia.

The predictive value of the 12 lead ECG in differentiating between a ventricular and a supraventricular origin

When the above mentioned approach is used one is able to predict correctly the site of origin of tachycardia in 90% of patients with a regular tachycardia and a wide QRS complex [2]. In our experience mistakes are made in patients with pre-existent bundle branch block or atrioventricular conduction over an accessory

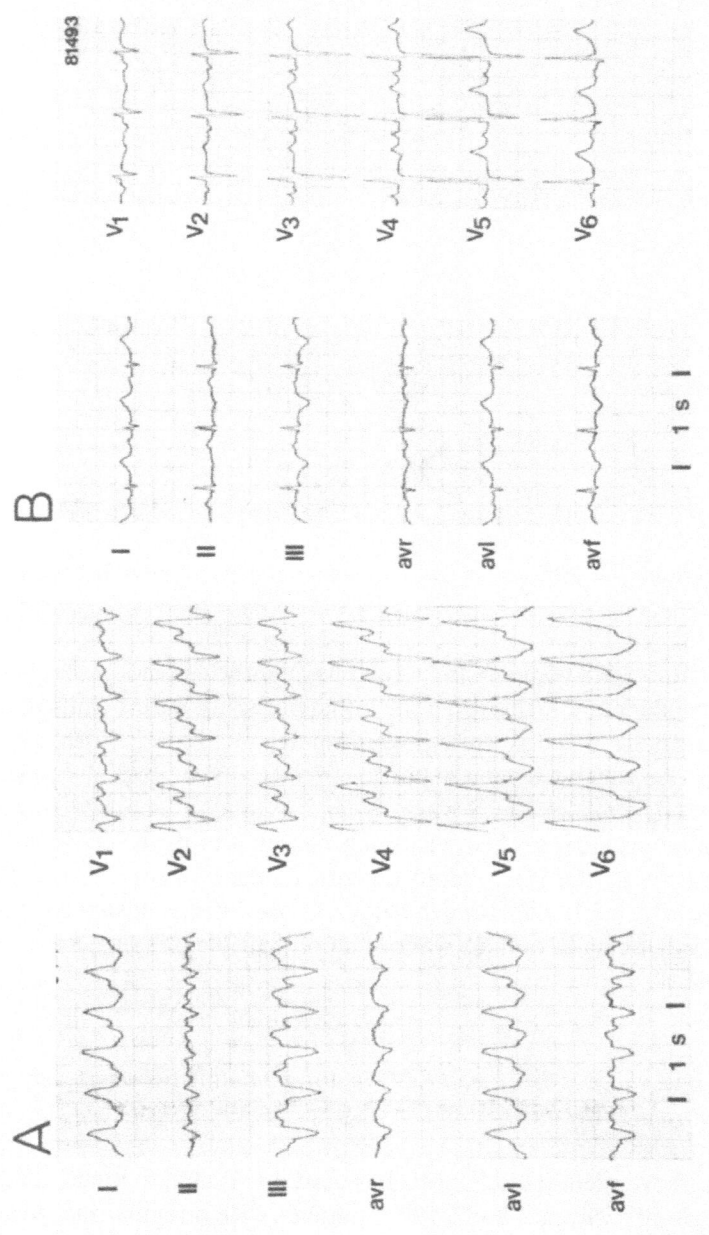

Figure 4. Ventricular tachycardia with left bundle branch block like configuration. The r wave in lead V_1 and V_2 is wider than the r wave during sinus rhythm.

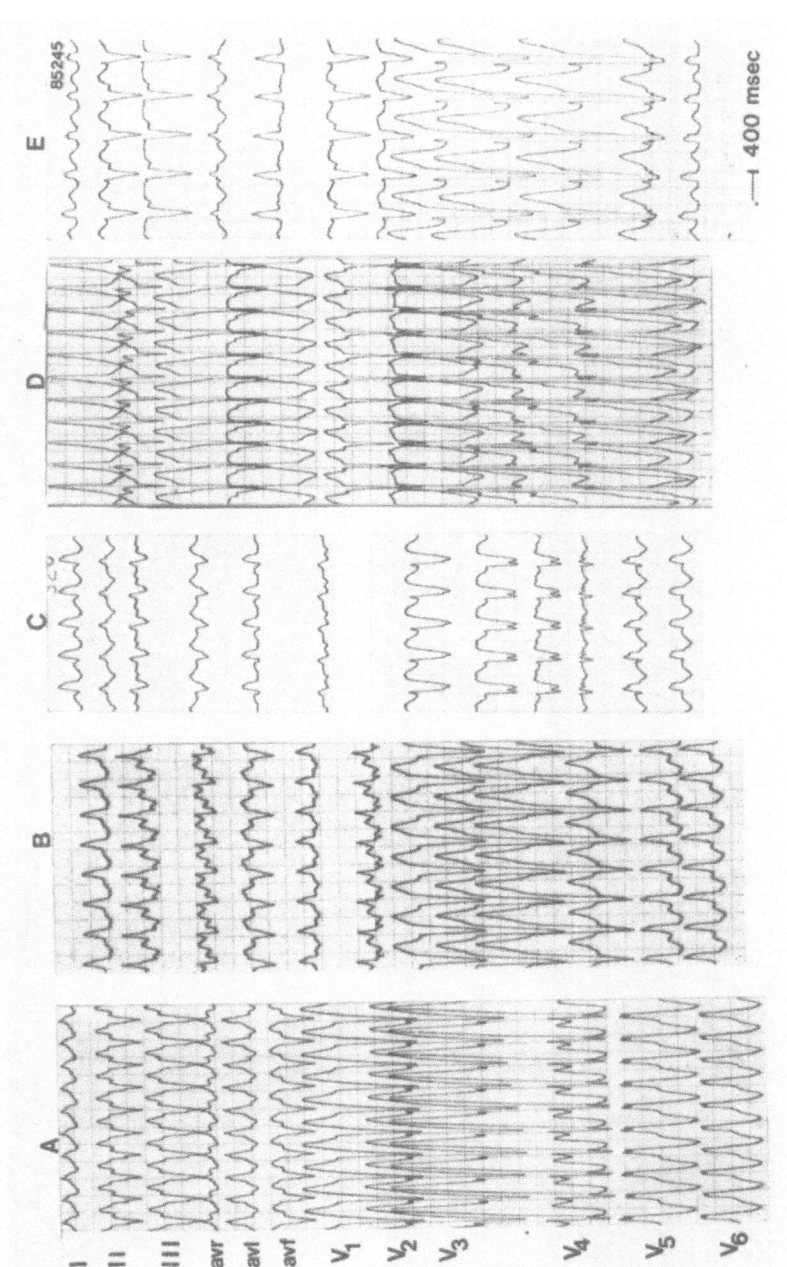

Figure 5. Five different patients all showing a regular wide QRS tachycardia with a left bundle branch block shaped QRS and a 1 to 1 relation between atrial and ventricular activity. See subsequent figures for explanation.

222

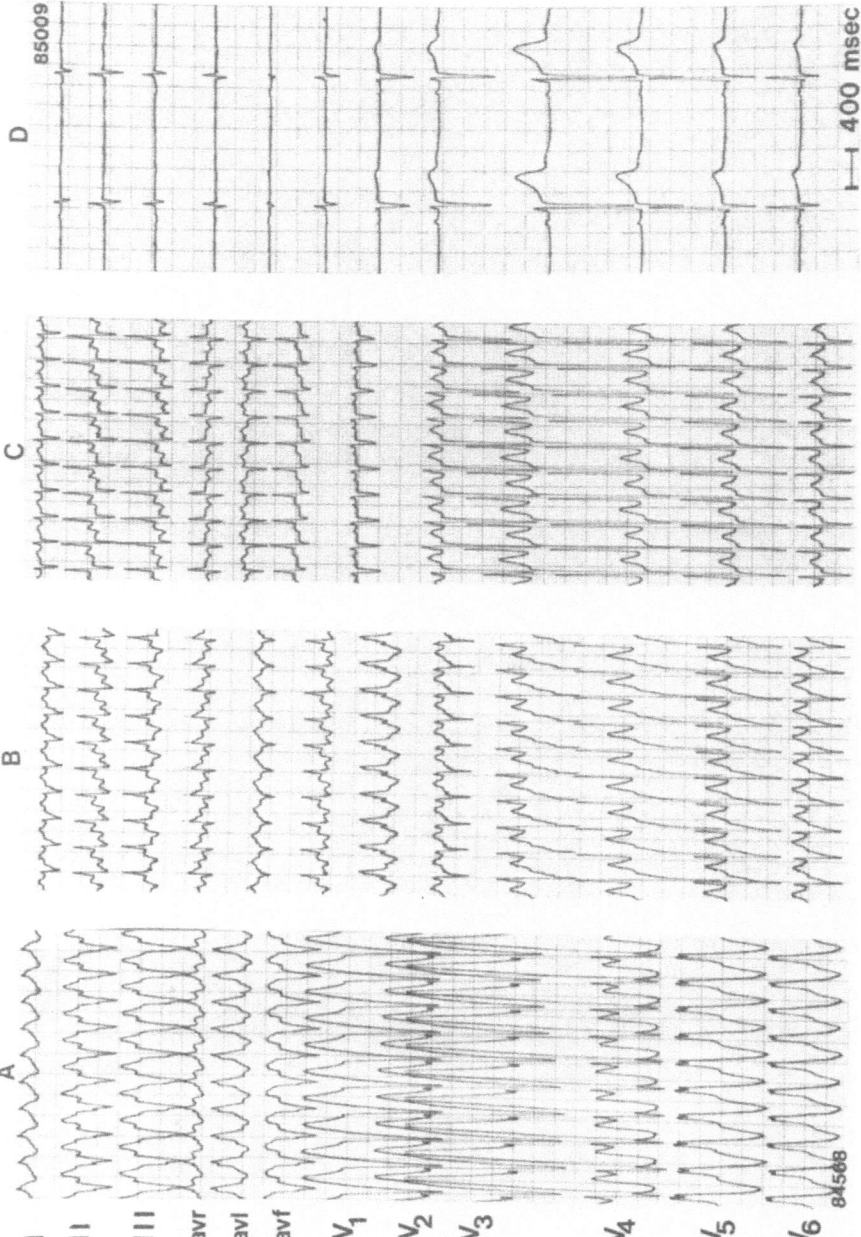

Figure 6. Patient of panel A of figure 5. The tachycardia shown in (A is an example of a circus movement tachycardia with anterograde conduction over the AV node, functional left bundle branch block and retrograde conduction over a septally located fastly conducting accessory pathway. Panel B shows the same type of tachycardia, but with functional right bundle branch block. In panel C non-aberrant conduction is present. Panel D gives the ECG during sinus rhythm.

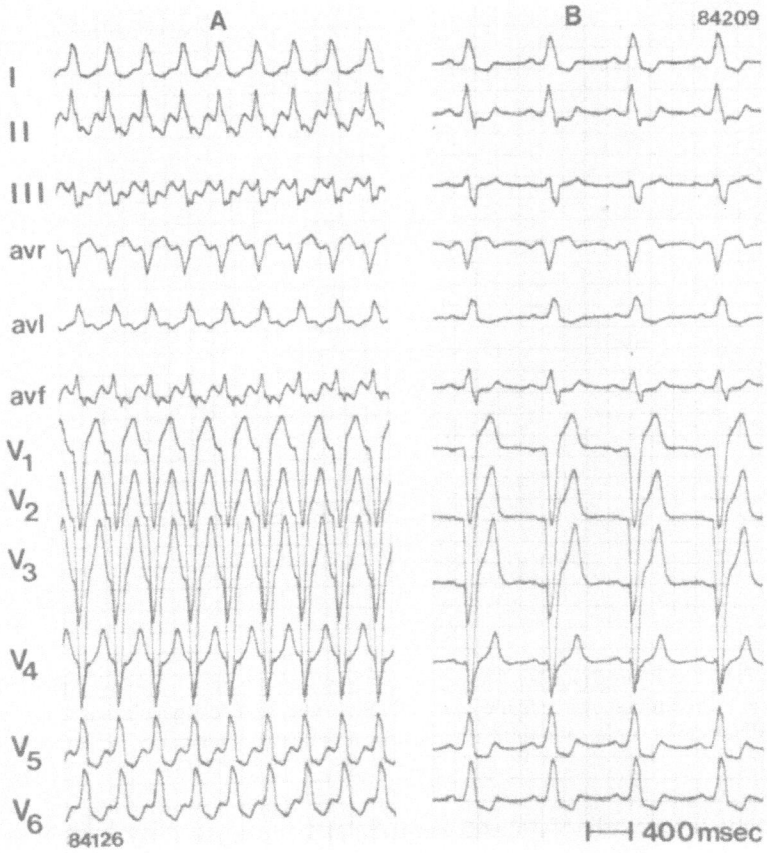

Figure 7. Patient of figure 5 panel B. The patient has a circus movement tachycardia with A-V conduction over the AV node, pre-existent left bundle branch block and retrograde conduction over a slowly conducting septally located accessory pathway (panel A). Panel B shows the ECG during sinus rhythm.

pathway [2]. The most difficult patient, however, is the patient presenting with a regular tachycardia with a left bundle branch block shaped QRS complex and a 1 to 1 relation between ventricular and atrial activity. This is shown in figure 5. As demonstrated in figure 6, panel A of figure 5 is from a patient with a circus movement tachycardia with anterograde conduction over the AV node, left bundle branch block and retrograde conduction over a rapidly conducting septally located accessory pathway. Panel B of figure 5 is from a patient with pre-existing left bundle branch block and a circus movement tachycardia using retrogradely a slowly conducting septally located accessory pathway (see figure 7). Panel C of figure 5 shows a ventricular tachycardia from a patient with an old anteroseptal infarction (figure 8). Panel D of figure 5 is an example of a circus

224

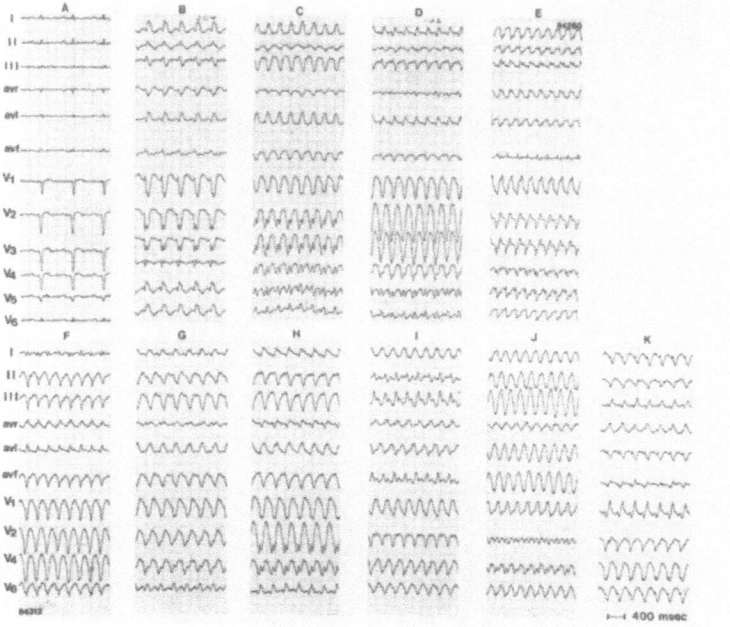

Figure 8. Patient of figure 5 panel C. The patient had an old anteroseptal infarction. Panel B shows the ventricular tachycardia shown in figure 8 panel C. Nine other types of a regular sustained ventricular tachycardia could be initiated in this patient during programmed stimulation of the heart.

movement tachycardia with atrioventricular conduction over a right sided accessory pathway (figure 9). Panel E of figure 5 represents a patient with atrioventricular conduction over a Mahaim fiber (figure 10). These examples demonstrate that the 12 lead electrocardiogram during a wide QRS tachycardia does not always allow to make the correct diagnosis. The figures 6 to 10 illustrate, however, that the combination of the ECG during tachycardia and the ECG during sinus rhythm usually brings sufficient information. We believe that in 1986 only rarely intracardiac electrophysiologic studies are required to differentiate between a supraventricular origin and a ventricular origin of a tachycardia showing a widened QRS complex.

The relation between te site of origin and the QRS configuration in ventricular tachycardia

In 1981 Josephson et al. [3] reported on the relation between QRS configuration and site of origin as determined during endocardial mapping in a large series of patients with ventricular tachycardia on the basis of coronary heart disease. They

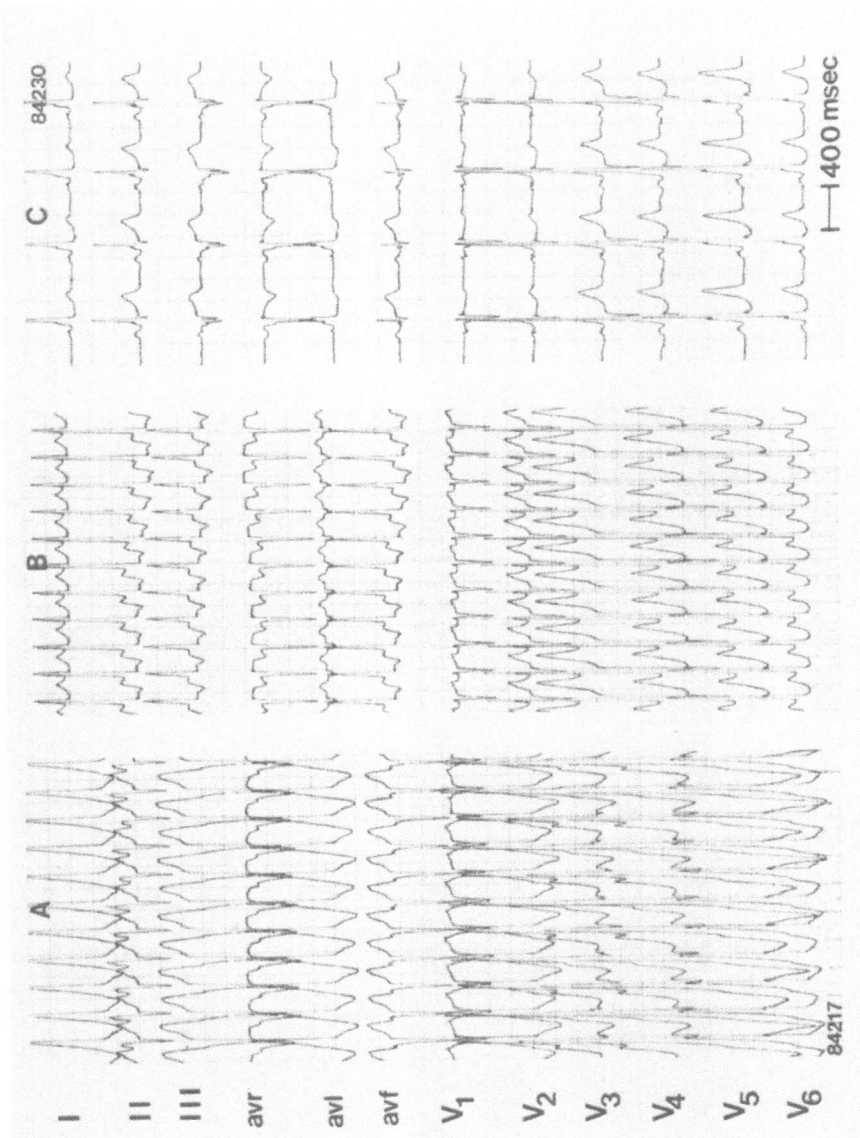

Figure 9. Patient of figure 5 panel D. The tachycardia was based on a circus movement tachycardia with atrioventricular conduction over an accessory pathway and retrograde conduction over the His bundle – AV node (panel A). Panel B shows the orthodromic circus movement tachycardia also seen in this patient. Panel C is the ECG during sinus rhythm.

226

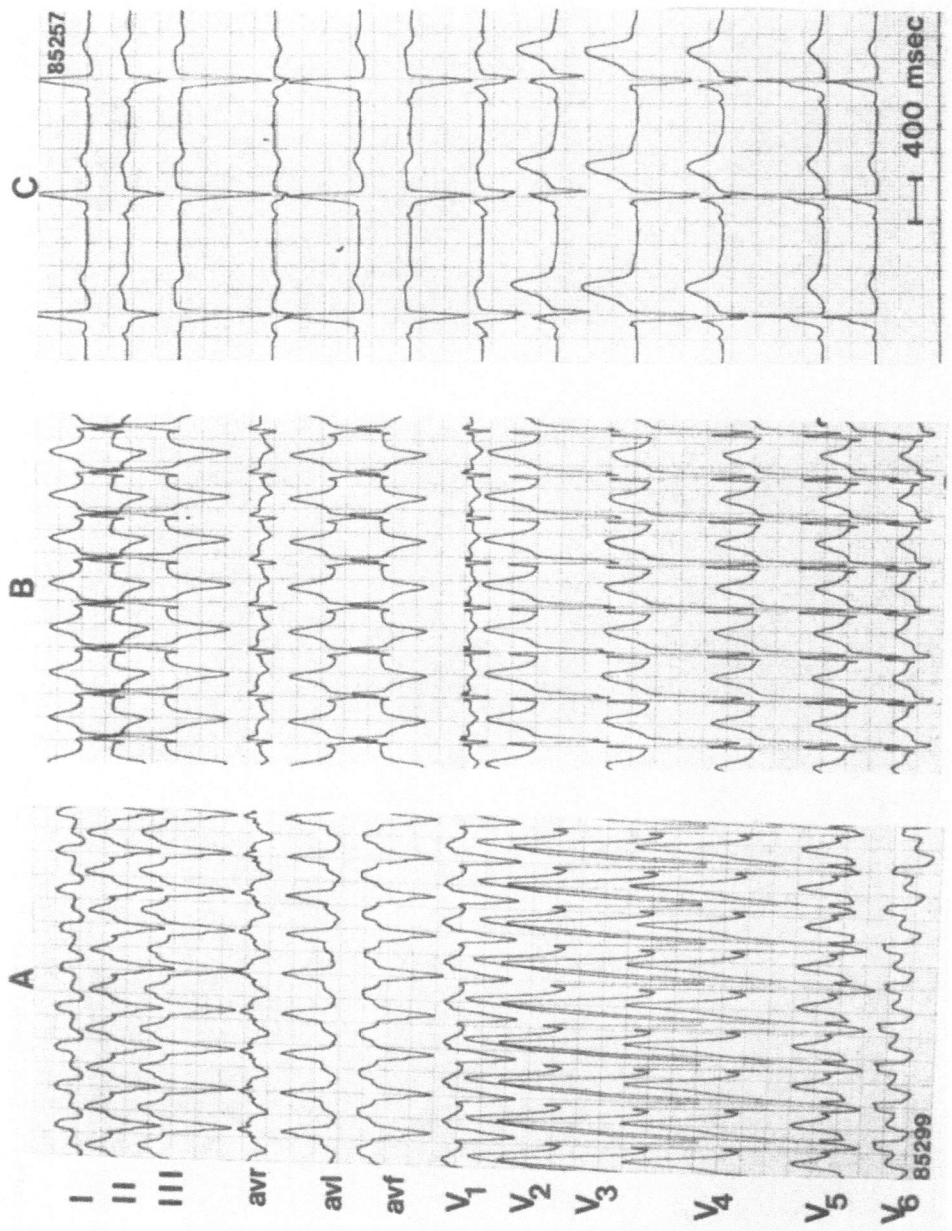

Figure 10. Patient of figure 5 in panel E. In this patient with a septal accessory atrioventricular pathway (panel C) the tachycardia pathway (panel A) used anterogradely a Mahaim fiber and retrogradely the septally located Kent bundle. The patient also had an orthodromic circus movement tachycardia with anterograde conduction over the AV node and retrograde conduction over the septally located Kent bundle (panel B).

found that in general the axis in the frontal plane relates to superior-inferior location, but does not distinguish an apical from a basal origin.

Ventricular tachycardia showing a left bundle branch block like configuration

Josephson et al. [3] pointed out that in coronary heart disease VT with a left bundle branch block (LBBB) shape originates from the septal or paraseptal sites in the left ventricle. They conclude that:
1) A concordant QS pattern in the precordial leads point to an origin of VT in the anteroseptal region (fig. 11)
2) Q waves in I and V_6 in the presence of a superior axis indicate an origin along the inferior aspect of the anterior septum (fig. 8, panel H)
3) R waves in I, V_2 to V_6 are specific for a posterior septal or paraseptal origin

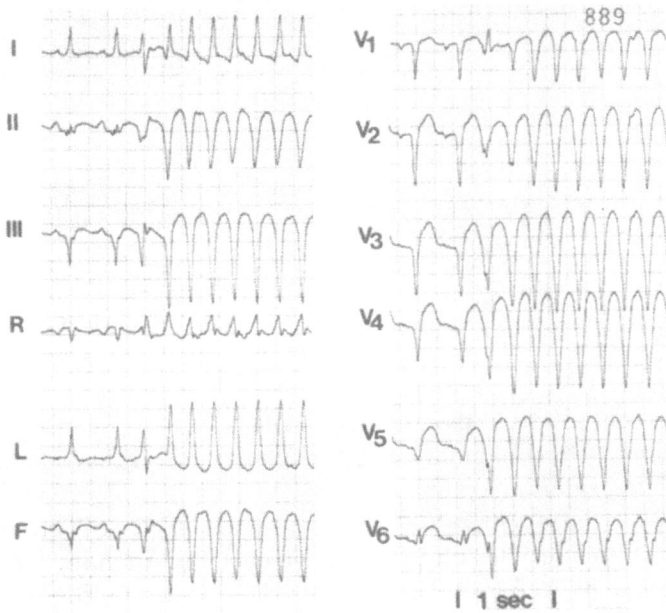

Figure 11. A ventricular tachycardia in a patient with an old inferior and old anteroseptal infarction showing a concordant QS pattern in the precordial leads. Endocardial mapping pointed to an origin of VT in the anteroseptal region.

228

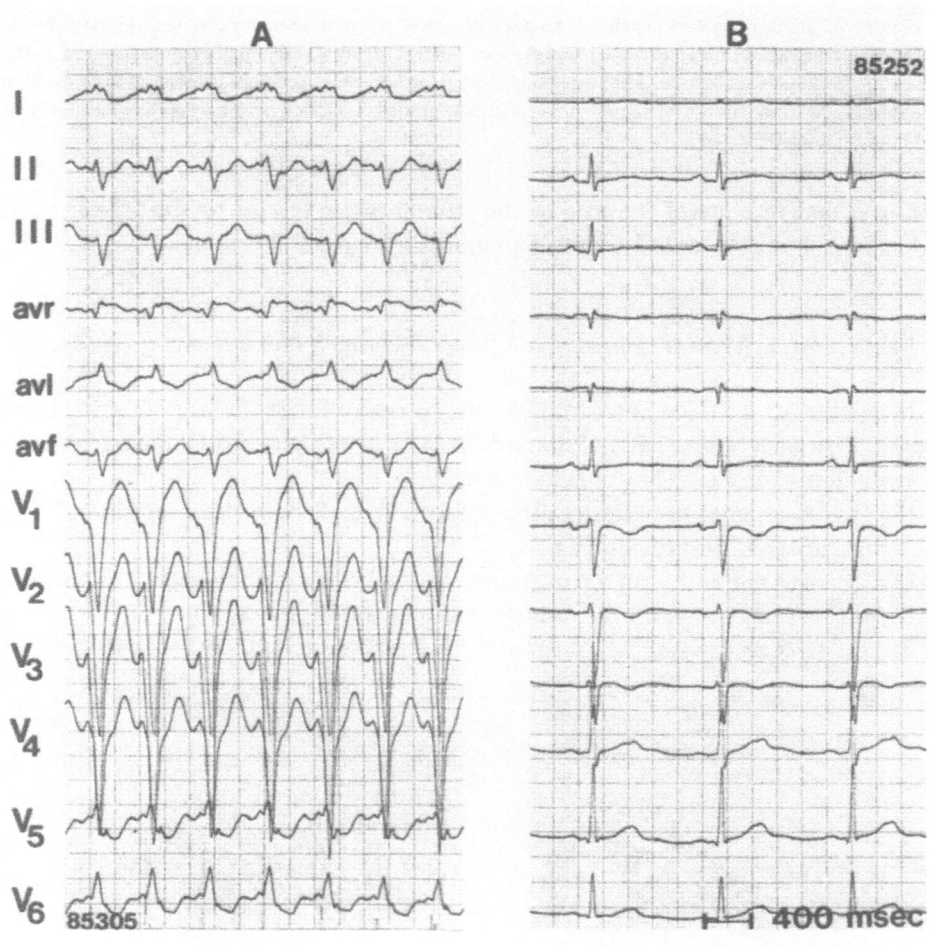

Figure 12. A ventricular tachycardia in a patient with right ventricular dysplasia. The site of origin was in the apex of the right ventricle.

    regardless of the axis in the frontal plane (fig. 4)
4) A VT with LBBB configuration and an inferior axis arises from the superior aspect of the anterior septum.

Although not found by Josephson and colleagues [3] it is likely that also in coronary heart disease VT with LBBB shape may arise from the infarcted right ventricle as recently reported by Karaqueuzian [6] in the dog heart. In non coronary heart disease LBBB shaped VT originates in the right ventricle. Fig. 12 is an example of a VT arising in the apex of the right ventricle in a patient with right ventricular dysplasia. Typically VT arising in the outflow tract of the right ventricle has a LBBB shape with an inferior axis.

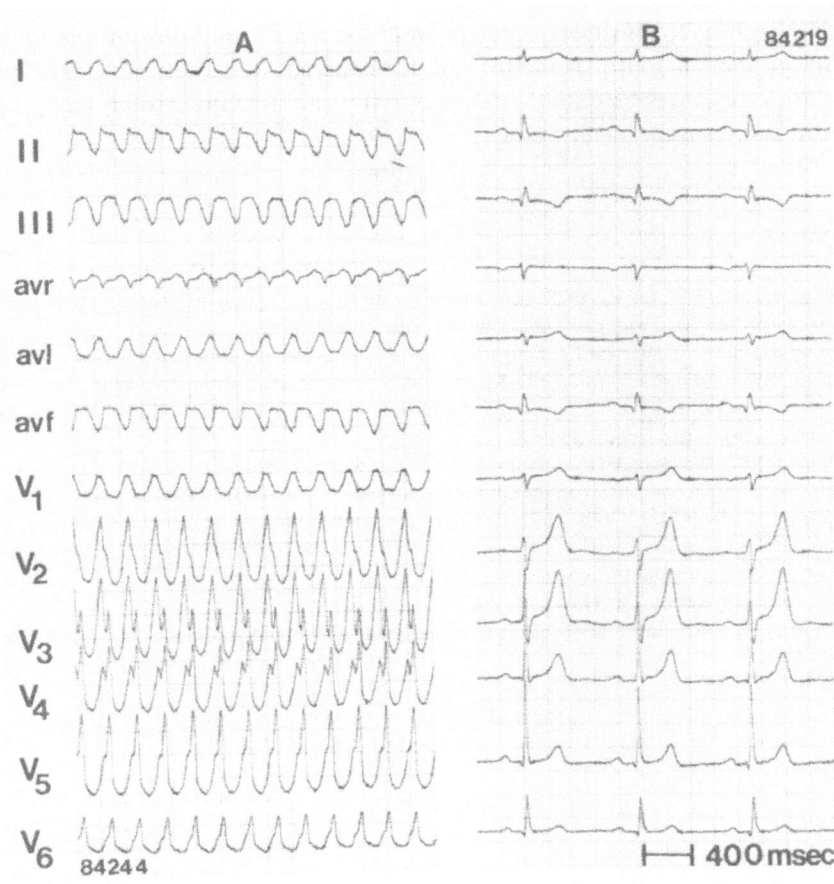

Figure 13. Ventricular tachycardia in a patient with an old inferior myocardial infarction. The site of ventricular impulse formation was in the inferioposterior paraseptal area of the left ventricle.

Ventricular tachycardia with a right bundle branch block shape

Josephson [3] indicated that:
1) A QR or QS in lead I, with Q waves in the precordial leads suggests an anteroapical origin (fig. 1)
2) A concordant R pattern in the precordial leads indicates a left posterior origin (fig. 13)
3) Reliable differentiation between an apical and anterolateral origin in patients showing an R wave in V_1 and an rS or qS in lead V_6 is not possible.

The above indicates that the 12 lead ECG can be of help in *suggesting* the site of origin of a ventricular tachycardia. It should be stressed (as done by Dr. Josephson) that endocardial or intramural conduction delay from scars, hypertrophy or primary electrical disturbances may prevent the use of the QRS morphology to reliably predict that site. If identification of the site of origin of a ventricular tachycardia becomes essential for appropriate therapy endocardial mapping is required for accurate localisation.

References

1. Wellens HJJ, Bär FW, Lie KI. 1978. The value of the electrocardiogram in the differential diagnosis of a tachycardia with a widened QRS complex. Am J Med 64: 27.
2. Wellens HJJ, Bär FW, Vanagt EJ, Brugada P, Farré J. 1981. The differentiation between ventricular tachycardia and supraventricular tachycardia with aberrant conduction. The value of the 12 lead electrocardiogram. In: What's new in electrocardiography? Wellens HJJ, Kulbertus HE (Eds), Martinus Nijhoff, The Hague: 184–199.
3. Josephson ME, Waxman HL, Marchlinski FE, Horowitz LN, Spielman SR. 1981. Relation between site of origin and QRS configuration in ventricular rhythms. In: What's new in electrocardiography? Wellens HJJ, Kulbertus HE (Eds). Martinus Nijhoff, The Hague: 200–228.
4. Coumel P, Leclercq JF, Attuel P, Maisonblanche P. 1984. The QRS morphology in post-myocardial infarction ventricular tachycardia. A study of 100 tracings compared with 70 cases of idiopathic ventricular tachycardia. Eur Heart J 5: 792.
5. Marriott HJL. 1970. Differential diagnosis of supraventricular and ventricular tachycardia. Geriatrics 25: 91.
6. Karaqueuzian HS, Sugi K, Ohta M, Fischbein MC, Mandel WJ, Peter T. 1986. Inducible sustained ventricular tachycardia and ventricular fibrillation in conscious dogs with isolated right ventricular infarction: Relation to infarct structure. JACC 7: 850–858.

17. Regional phase mapping of radionuclide gated biventriculograms in patients with sustained ventricular tachycardia

D. LE GULUDEC*, C. SEBAG*, M. BOURGUIGNON**,
H. VALETTE**, P. MERLET**, A. SIRINELLI*, J.M. DAVY*,
A. SYROTA**, G. MOTTE*
* Service de cardiologie, Hôpital Antoine Béclère, 157, rue de la Porte de Trivaux
– 92140 Clamart, France
** Service Frédéric Joliot, Département de biologie du C.E.A.,
91400 Orsay, France

Knowledge of origin site of sustained ventricular tachycardia (VT), and its spatial relationship with regional myocardial abnormalities, are often useful to predict pathophysiology of VT, and to guide surgical or electrical therapy. It usually requires a cardiac catheterization for angiography and/or endocardial mapping. Functional images of gated equilibrium radioventriculography (GERV) can provide non invasive data on ventricular activation. The phase pattern of the first harmonic of Fourier analysis may represent the sequence of ventricular contraction, which follows the sequence of intra-ventricular conduction. It has been used to study abnormalities of ventricular electromechanical activation as they are observed in bundle branch block [1–2] pacemaker rhythms [3–8], Wolff-Parkinson-White syndrome [9–14] and VT [15–18]. We studied the ability of Fourier analysis to locate the onset of ventricular activation during VT,and to determine the etiology of VT in 6 patients.

Methods

Patients

Criteria for inclusion were the following: history of ECG documented paroxysmal monomorphic sustained VT; induction and termination of the same VT during programmed stimulation (PS); hemodynamically stable, well tolerated VT.

Six patients entered the study, four males and two females, age ranging from 25 to 72 years (mean 52,5). All patients underwent echocardiography, cardiac catheterization for ventricular angiography, and coronarography, to characterise their heart disease. The diagnosis was arrhythmogenic right ventricular (RV) dysplasia (ARVD n = 2) dilated cardiomyopathy(n = 1),ischemic heart disease with inferoapical aneurysm (n = 1), cardiac hydatic cyst (n = 1); in one patient no cardiac abnormality could be found. All patients were on anti-arrhythmic therapy which did not prevent clinical VT induction, but decreased the heart rate and made the VT hemodynamically more suitable for GERV.

Electrophysiologic studies (EPS)

EPS were performed before GERV acquisition.Multiple electrode catheters were placed, through the femoral vein, at right atrium, atioventricular junction in His bundle position, right ventricular apex and pulmonary infundibulum. Sustained VT was induced by 1,2 or 3 premature ventricular stimuli during sinus rhythm or ventricular pacing. VT was stopped by ventricular extrastimuli or by overdrive.

Gated blood acquisition and processing

GERV was successively performed during sinus rhythm (SR), RV pacing, and sustained VT. Data were collected after intravenous injection of 20 mC of in vitro 99 m technetium labelled red blood cells with an Anger camera (Siemens ZLC 75) with high sensitivity colimator, in line with a dedicated computer (Sopha S4000). Each acquisition lasted 5 min, gated on the R waves, 16 images per cardiac cycle were stored on a disk memory in a 64 × 64 matrix resolution. After equilibrium of the tracer in the vascular space, images were acquired in the 30° to 40° left anterior oblique projection which allowed the best separation of right and left ventricles ('best septal incidence'). The gated series of images were corrected for undersampling, resulting in slight variation in heart rate. Each study was first displayed in cine mode to assess technical adequacy. Data were then smoothed with a three dimensional space and time filter, reducing random variation of radionuclide decay. Ventricular regions of interest were drawn automatically,checked for accuracy and manually corrected if necessary on aortic and pulmonary valve plane using black and white display and amplitude and phase image of Fourier analysis [19]. Ejection fraction (EF) was calculated using three regions of interest (end-diastolic, end-systolic and background regions). Regional wall motion was evaluated from amplitude image and regional EF.

Fourier analysis

Using Fourier theorem, each pixel's time-activity curve was fitted with a single cosine function, at the fundamental frequency, which period is equal to RR interval. Each cosine function can be fully characterised by two parameters:

amplitude, which is the maximum variation of each pixel's cosine, and phase, which represent the shift in time of a given pixel's cosine. Phase data are expressed in degrees from 0° to 360° through out the RR interval, with 180° defined to be that of a cosine function whose maximum occurs at the peak of QRS. Results of Fourier analysis are displayed in 3 images: amplitude image (by colour coding the value of amplitude in each pixel), phase image (by colour coding the value of phase in each pixel), and the phase distribution histogram whose axis represents phase angle (3° per channel) and y axis the number of pixels in each channel. Pixel whose amplitude value is less than 5% of maximum were excluded from phase analysis. A flexible colour scale can be translated along the phase histogram, and dilated to make earliest phase pixels more evident. Phase data were also displayed cinematically. Normal phase image in SR shows an homogeneous ventricular pattern with a narrow peak histogram, and earliest phases in proximal septum.

Correlation

Phase pattern of each acquisition (SR, RV pacing, and VT), were examined by 3 independent observers. VT origin on phase mapping was determined as the earliest phase area and correlated with ECG pattern of VT (QRS morphology and axis). Moreover the relationship between VT origin in GERV and wall motion abnormalities in SR-GERV were analysed. In all cases interpretation of earliest phase area was easy and the same for the 3 observers.

Results

The patients data are resumed in Table 1.

Patient no 1 was a forty-three year old woman with arrhythmogenic RV dysplasia and normal LV and coronary arteries, as demonstrated by cardiac angiography. During SR, ECG was normal, without any right bundle branch block (RBBB). She suffered from recurrent monomorphic VT characterized by left bundle branch block (LBBB) pattern with left axis deviation ($-60°$) at a rate of 205 beats/min (Fig. 1). She was on anti-arrhythmic therapy (amiodarone 2000 mg/week). During SR, scintigraphic data visualized hypokinesia of the free wall of a dilated RV and Fourier analysis demonstrated a large area of decreased amplitude and delayed phase on RV free wall, while the remainder of the two ventricles were synchronous with normal wall motion. During pacing at RV apex, areas of earliest phase were located at the RV apex and right ventricular septum. During VT, pixels of earliest phase were located on right ventricular anterior wall, at the border of the dyskinetic area at rest (Fig. 2). From there, phase progressed toward the remainder of RV and LV, the latest area being the

234

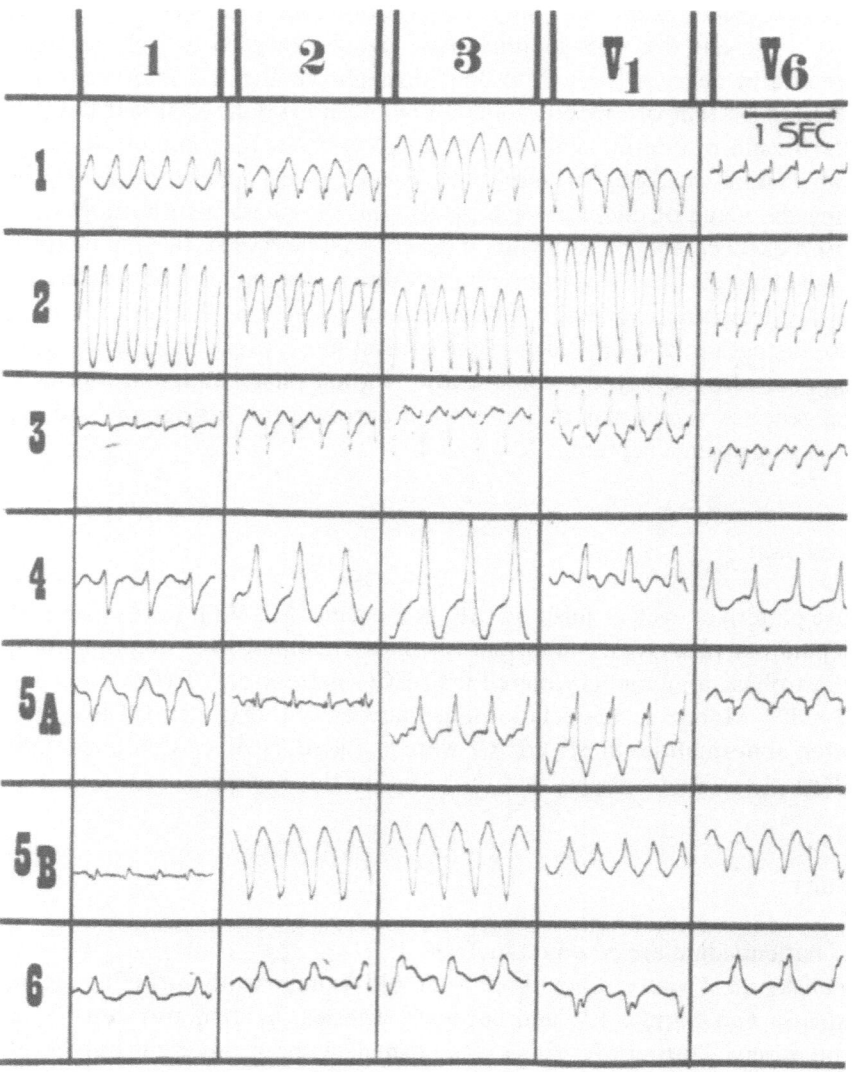

Figure 1. Electrocardiograms during ventricular tachycardia. Shown are ECG leads I, II, III, V1, and V6 during seven VT morphologies in six patients. Two different tachycardia were imaged in patient no. 5.

Figure 2. Patient no. 1 data (ARVD). A: GERV performed in 40° left anterior oblique projection. Sum image (upper left), amplitude image of the first harmonic of Fourier analysis (lower left), phase image and histogram (lower and upper right). Color scale is visualized on histogram (in order of increasing phase: blue, green, yellow, orange, red, purple). B: Phase images (left) and histograms (right) during right ventricular stimulation (upper) and VT (lower). C: Phase image and histogram during VT with ventricular mask and dilated color scale, for better visualization of pixels of earliest phases.

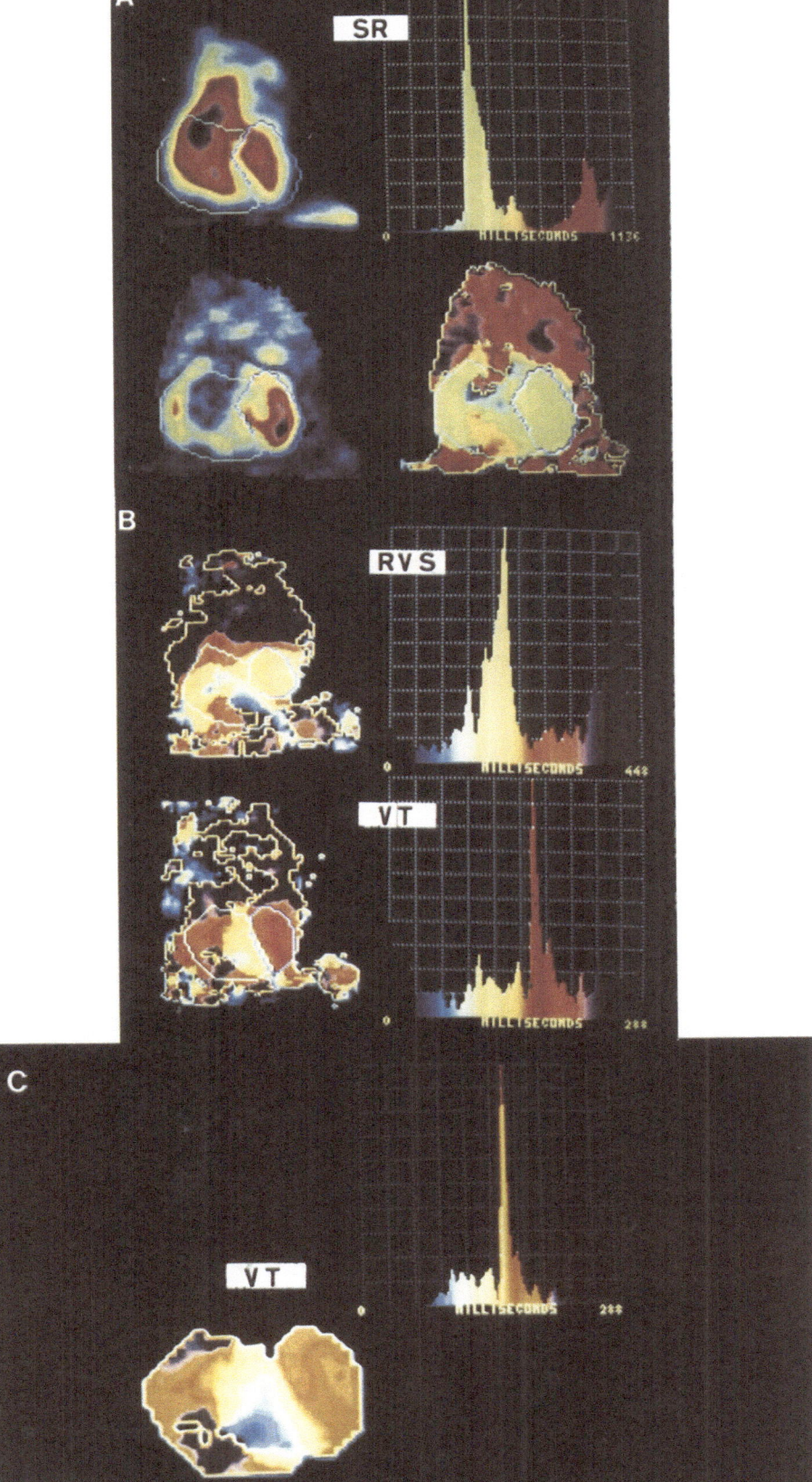

236

SINUS RHYTHM

VENTRICULAR
TACHYCARDIA

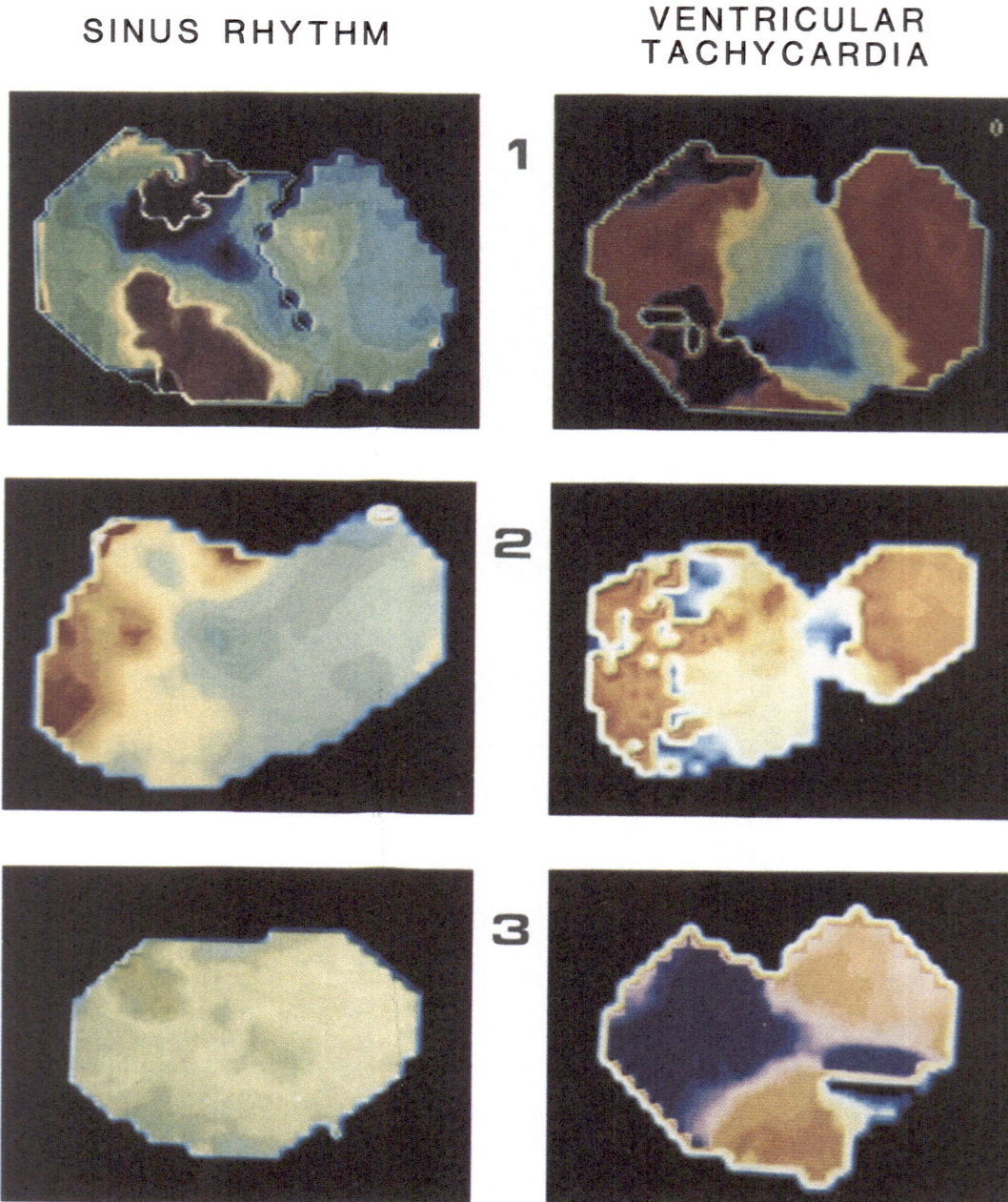

Figure 3. Phase images of the two ventricles during sinus rhythm (left) and ventricular tachycardia (right) in six patients. Two different tachycardia were imaged in patient no. 5. Color scale is the same as described in Fig. 2.

SINUS RHYTHM

VENTRICULAR
TACHYCARDIA

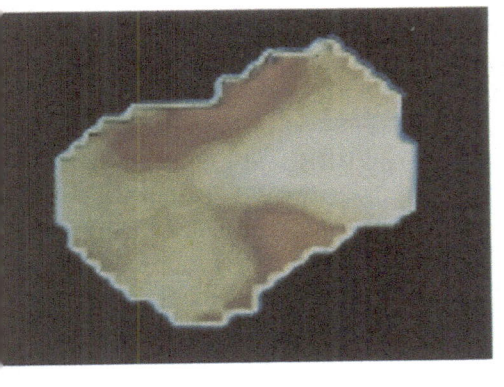
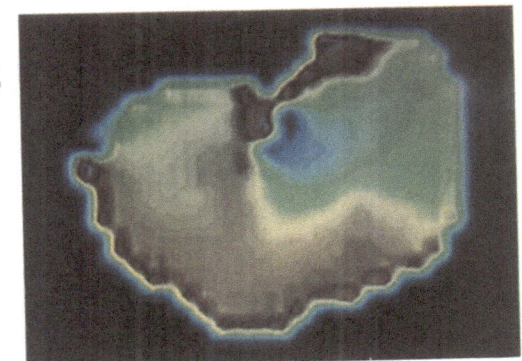

4

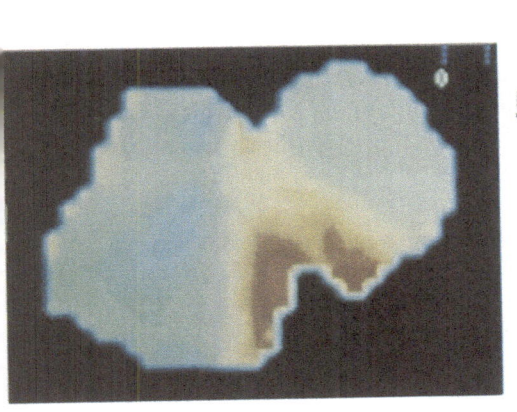

A

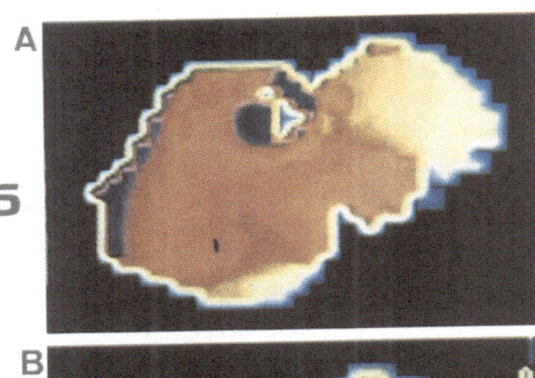

5

B

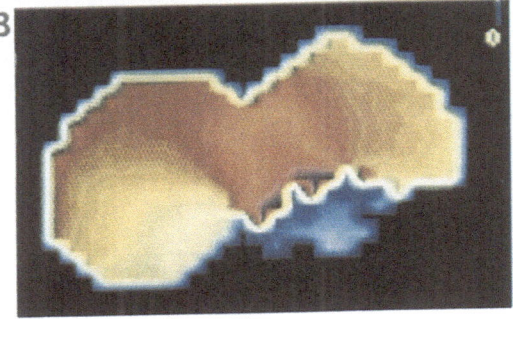

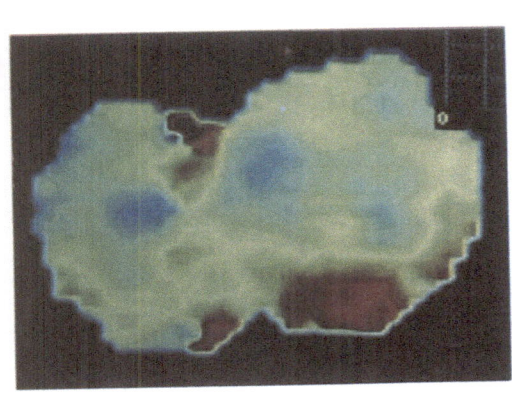

6

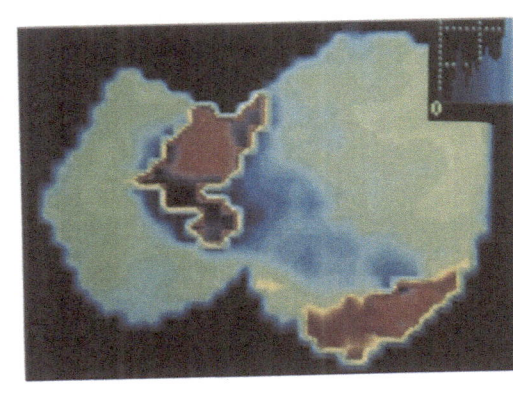

abnormal free wall of RV. However, most of the LV had latter phase than most of the RV, corresponding to the electrocardiographic LBBB pattern.

Patient no 2 was a 25 year-old man with an history of recurrent VT and ARVD proven by cardiac angiography. This case was previously reported [23] because GERV first suggested the diagnosis of ARVD, while echocardiography was normal. During SR, ECG was normal without any BBB and GERV showed hypokinesia of the free wall of a dilated RV. Fourier analysis demonstrated decreased amplitude and phase delay of this area. During ventricular pacing at the RV apex, earliest phases were located at the RV apex, but with persistant delay in dyskinetic area. During VT, ECG showed LBBB pattern with left axis deviation ($-45°$) and rate at 260/min (Fig. 1) and endocardial mapping showed that this VT originated under the infundibular area. Points of earliest phase were located at the infundibulum, at the limit between the normal and abnormal areas as defined during SR (Fig. 3).

Patient no 3 was a 44 year-old man whose complete investigation (including echocardiography, exercice testing, thallium 201 myocardial scintigraphy, right and left cardiac catheterisation and coronary angiography) revealed a normal heart. He presented with recurrent VT, occurring each time he omitted to take his anti-arrhythmic therapy (propafenone 600 mg/day). ECG, as well as GERV, were normal in SR. During ventricular pacing, phase pattern was concordant

Table 1. Patients' data. G.E.R.V.: gated equilibrium radio ventriculography; L.B.B.B.: left bundle branch block pattern during ventricular tachycardia; R.B.B.: right branch block pattern during ventricular tachycardia; L.V.: left ventricle; R.V.: right ventricle.

Diagnosis	G.E.R.V. (sinus rythm)		Ventricular Tachycardia		
			ECG		Phase
			Morphology	Rate	
1 R.V. dysplasia	Amplitude ↘ Phase delay	R.V. free wall	LBBB Axis-60°	205/mn	Upper limit of dyskinetic area
2 R.V. dysplasia	Amplitude ↘ Phase delay	R.V. free wall	LBBB Axis-45°	260/mn	Inferior limit of dyskinetic area
3 Normal heart	Normal		RBBB Axis-70°	190/mn	L.V. apex
4 Idiopathic dilated Cardiomyopathy	Heterogeneous amplitude R.V. phase delay: (R.B.B.B.)		RBBB Axis+100°	110/mn	L.V. septum
5 Hydatic cyst	Amplitude ↘↘ Phase opposition	L.V. and R.V. apex	A) RBBB Axis+140°	145/mn	L.V. lateral free wall
			B) RBBB Axis-80°	185/mn	L.V. apex
6 L.V. aneurysm	Amplitude ↘↘ Phase opposition	L.V. apex	LBBB Axis+40	100/mn	Upper limit of dyskinetic area

with ventricular activation sequency. VT was characterised by RBBB and left axis deviation ($-70°$) and heart rate of 190/min (Fig. 1). Points of earliest phase were located at the left ventricular apex with RV phase delay concordant with electrical RBBB (Fig. 3).

Patient no 4 was a 60 year-old woman with idiopathic congestive cardiomyopathy. Cardiac catheterization showed diffusely reduced wall motion and normal coronary arteries. During SR, QRS was wide with a RBBB and a left axis, while VT was characterized by RBBB pattern and rightward axis ($+100°$) (Fig. 1). She took antiarrhythmic therapy (amiodarone 2000 mg/week) which failed to prevent induction of VT but slowed its rate at 110/mn. Isotopic ejection fraction of LV was 32% in sinus rhythm and 24% during VT. Phase pattern during SR showed RV delay due to RBBB and heterogenous LV phase due to regional wall motion abnormalities. During ventricular pacing, RV presented the earliest phases while LV abnormalities worsened. During VT, areas of earliest phase were located at the upper part of left septum (Fig. 3).

Patient 5 was a 71 year-old man with recurrent VT. Echocardiography, cardiac angiography and scanner showed a large liquid tumour at the cardiac apex related to an hydatid cyst. After surgery, histological examination confirmed this diagnosis. During SR, QRS morphology was normal. GERV showed a lack of radioactivity near the apex of both ventricle. Fourier analysis showed decreased amplitude and phase delay, which persisted during ventricular pacing. During clinical VT, a RBBB pattern was observed, with right axis ($+140°$). Two different VT were induced by PS: one of them was the same as the clinical VT (A); the other one (B) had RBBB pattern and left axis deviation ($-80°$) (Fig. 1). Both were concordant with phase mapping, which located the origin of VT-A in the lateral wall of left ventricle near the apex, and the origin of VT-B at the apex of the left ventricle (Fig. 3). Both originated at the border of the cyst. After surgical ablation of the cyst, there were no recurrence of either spontaneous or induced VT, and GERV was normal.

Patient no 6 was a 72 year-old man with three vessels coronary artery disease and infero posterior aneurysm visualised by cardiac catheterisation. ECG showed sequelae of inferior myocardial infarction and functional RBBB when the heart rate was over 100/min. Spontaneous and induced VT had LBBB pattern and axis at $+40°$, at a slow rate of 100/min (Fig. 1), related to amiodarone therapy (2000 mg/week). During SR, GERV showed dilated ventricles with poor kinetic, decreased LV ejection fraction (20%) and amplitudes; the phase pattern showed a large area of opposite phase in the infero apical left ventricle, corresponding to the aneurysm. During VT, EF decreased to 14%. Areas of earliest phase were located at the anteroseptal border of the aneurysm; the LV phases preceded the RV phases; this delay of RV phases was inconsistent with electrical LBBB pattern (Fig. 3).

Discussion

Accuracy of the phase mapping

Fourier phase imaging seems to be sensitive in characterising abnormal pattern of ventricular activation in our serie.

In patients with heart disease (5/6) phase data showed a close spatial relationship between the origin of VT and regional wall motion abnormalities. This fact is consistent with previous electrophysiologic and scintigraphic reports [2, 25] concerning VT related to LV aneurysm, originating from the border zone of dyskinesia. Fewer reports are available concerning VT related to ARVD [20–23]; our findings suggest – for the first time with GERV – that spatial relationship could be similar for right ventricular dyskinesia.

In 5/6 patients, VT-phase mapping was consistant with VT-QRS pattern, and with endocardial mapping of right ventricle in the only patient it was done. Left ventricle endocardial mapping is not currently done in our patients, unless surgical therapy is planned. In one patient with an apical aneurysm (no 6) phase mapping seems to be more consistent with the probable origin of the VT than electrocardiographic findings: earliest phases are located in LV at the border of the aneurysm while ECG shows a LBBB pattern. Josephson et al. [24–25] have determined with endocardial mapping that LBBB pattern is very frequently related with a LV origin in patients with coronary artery disease and regional wall motion abnormalities [24]. The phase mapping in our patient is closely consistent with this fact. In patient no 3, two different electrical patterns of VT seems to be in agreement with two different emergences of electrical activation on phase mapping, both located at two opposite borders of the heart cyst. Swiryn et al. [15] related the case of one patient with two different VT but the same origin on phase mapping, with differing progression to the remainder of the ventricles. When pleiomorphic tachyardia exist, phase mapping seems to be able to distinguish between different foci or only one focus with differents ways of activation. This is an important finding when surgical or catheter ablation therapy is planned [26].

Table 2. Correlations between Fourier phase pattern and ventricular pacing location determined by X-rays in patients with permanent pacemakers or during mapping.

Author	Patients	Pacing	Correlation
Frais 1981	5	5	X-rays: 4
Friedman 1981	8	8	Epicardial mapping: 8
Turner 1982	14	15	Endocardial mapping: 13
Botvinick 1982	8	8	X-rays: 8
Bashore 1983	13	36	Endocardial mapping: 36
Links 1985	12	25	Endocardial mapping: 20

The ability of Fourier phase mapping to identify the origin of conduction abnormalities has been studied by several authors during bundle branch block [1–2], Wolff-Parkinson-White syndrome [9–14] and ventricular pacing [3–8]. Table 2 shows the good assessment (80 to 100%) of the ventricular activation origin by phase mapping during pacing, in the literature: correlations were done by X-ray location of electrodes for patients with permanent pacemaker [3–6], or during endo or epicardial mapping [4, 7, 8].

Only a few studies of phase mapping during VT have been reported [15–18, 23]. Table 3 shows good accuracy of phase mapping in locating origin of VT. Correlation with ECG findings and location of wall motion abnormalities was done for the first time by Swiryn and coworkers [15]. Pre or per surgical enocardial or epicardial mapping was latter used by several authors [16–18]. Correlations were fairly good in all reports.

Technical considerations

GERV with first harmonic Fourier analysis is actually a valid routine procedure in nuclear cardiology [27]. However, acquisition during VT has specific problems of feasibility. The procedure requiring a cardiac caheter to induce VT, is not completely non invasive. Most electrophysiology laboratories do not have a portable gamma-camera and VT must be induced in a nuclear medicine division, which is an unusual and less secure place than a cardiology laboratory. GERV acquisition requires 5 min of monomorphic, electrically and hemodynamically stable VT, which is not the case for all patients. The number of patients in whom procedure can be performed is increase by the use of anti arrhythmic drugs, which slow the VT rate. However a good selection of patients must be done.

Precise accuracy suffers from several technical limits. Phase image is a two dimensional projection of three dimensional events, and only one view is done. Superimposition of the cardiac structures limits the precision for determining areas of earliest phases, specially when they are located on the inferior wall.

Table 3. Correlations between Fourier phase pattern and ECG or mapping findings during VT. (W.M.A. = wall motion abnormalities).

Author	Patients	Correlation
Swiryn 1982	6	ECG: 4/6 W.M.A.: 6/6 Endocardial mapping: 1/1
Turner 1982	3	Endocardial mapping: 3
Dae 1982	2	Endocardial and Epicardial mapping: 2
Mac Carthy 1983	6	Endocardial mapping: 6

Other views might be useful but increase time of acquisition during VT. Tomographic acquisition of GERV is not suitable for the same reason.

Random noise can sometimes alter the quality of Fourier analysis; in patients with very low ejection fraction and large ventricular dysfunction, amplitude of cycle changes in activity is in the same order as random noise. However, the acquisition time of 5 min and the use of spatial and temporal filters make it a rare problem.

Some authors [8–15] noted, at high heart rate, difficulties in determining the beginning and end of activation sequence, which they termed 'wraparound'. We have not observed such problems in our short series. However, the computer is triggered by the peak of QRS; although it is identical for each acquired cycle and for all pixels, it does not correspond exactly to the onset of ventricular depolarization. Consequently areas of very early depolarization can be missed. The shorter the cycle length, the larger is the phase lost corresponding to the increment between onset of depolarization and R wave trigger. It would certainly be useful to use list mode acquisition in order to redefine afterwards the trigger used to gate the study, with a time shift from the usual R wave trigger.

Using only the first harmonic of Fourier transformation is another source of imprecision. Previous studies have shown that most of the temporal information of a time activity curve is contained in the fundamental frequency. Recently, some authors have tested the use of multiharmonic analysis to modelise each pixel's time activity curve [28–32]. Such multiharmonic analysis may optimise parametric images of GERV specially in patients with poor LV function and during sustained VT.

The temporal resolution depends on the number of images per cardiac cycle, and the representation of phase data. 16 images/RR is commonly considered as a good compromise between temporal resolution, statistical quality of images, and acquisition time. Color scale used (256 colors levels) and histogram (over 360 degrees, 1 channel in 1/360 of RR) seems satifactory.

Table 4. Left ventricular ejection fraction value during sinus rhythm (SR) and sustained ventricular tachycardia (VT).

	SR		VT	
	LV EF	Rate/mn	LV EF	Rate/mn
No 1	56%	53	50%	205
No 2	70%	75	61%	260
No 3	61%	83	59%	190
No 4	32%	72	24%	110
No 5	60%	82	40%	150
No 6	20%	56	14%	101

Another artefact results from lateral motion of great vessels or of the heart, changing the activity curve without changing the real volume. Such artefacts can be easily identified near the valves, and on amplitude images, and should not alter the analysis. The influence of regional wall motion abnormalities on phase pattern should be considered. Phase pattern characterises the change in radioactivity during cardiac cycle and so reflects mechanical events. In normal heart the sequence of mechanical events is closely related to the electrical depolarization; phase delay may represent either abnormal kinetic or abnormal depolarization. However, Botvinick et al [33] have previously shown that phase data may keep its ability to reflect abnormal activation even when abnormal contraction exist. Our experience reported here is that phase disturbance in SR does not mask the origin of VT but may modify the extension of activation to the remainder of ventricles, as estimated by phase analysis.

Conclusion

Phase mapping of GERV seems accurate in the management of patients with clinically well tolerated VT. It helps to determine the etiology of VT. Then it is able to dtermine the origin site of ventricular tachycardia in both LV and RV. It can establish the spatial relationship between wall motion abnormalities in SR, and the emergence of VT. It can serve as a guide for endo or epicardial mapping, resulting in shortening of these tests. It can help to distinguish unifocal from multifocal tachycardias. This findings can be used successfully to aid surgical or electrical therapy.

References

1. Frais MA, Botvinick EH, Shosa DW. 1982. Phase image characterizaton of ventricular contraction in left and right bundle branch block. Am J Cardiol 50: 95.
2. Swiryn S, Pavel D, Byrom E, Witham D, Meyer-Pavel C, Windham C, Handler B, Rosen K. 1981. Sequential regional phase mapping of cardionuclide gated bioventriculograms in patients with left bundle branch block. Am Heart J 102: 1000.
3. Frais MA, Botvinick EH, O'Connell JW, Shosa DW, Scheinmann NM, Hattner RS. 1981. The phase image: an accurate means of detecting and localizing abnormal foci of ventricular activation. J Nucl Med 22: 18.
4. Byrom E, Swiryn S, Pavel D, Meyer-Pavel C, Handler B, Rosen K. 1981. Correlation of phase image patterns with various cardiac activation patterns induced by pacing (abstract). J Nucl Med 22: 18.
5. Turner DA, Von Behren PL, Ruggie NT, Hauser RG, Denes P, Messer JV, Fordham EW, Groch MW. 1982. Non invasive identification of initial site of ventricular contraction by least square phase analysis of radionuclide cine angiograms (abstract). Circulation 65: 1511.
6. Botvinick EH, Frais MA, Shosa DW, O'Connell NW, Pacheco-Alvarez A, Scheinman C, Hattner R. 1982. An accurate means of detecting and characterizing abnormal patterns of ventricular activation by phase image analysis. Am J Cardiol 50: 289.

7. Bashore TM, Stine RA, Shaffer P, Bush CA, Leier CV, Schaal SF. 1982. The non invasive localisation of ventricular ectopy using radionuclide phase imaging (abstract). Circulation 66: II-125.

8. Links JM, Raichlen JS, Wagner HN, Reid PR. 1985. Assessment of the site of ventricular activation by Fourier analysis of gated blood-pool studies. J Nucl Med 26: 27.

9. Chan W, Kalff V, Mac Donald D, Rabinovitch M, Jenkins J, Thrall J, Pitt B. 1983. Topography of preemptying ventricular segments in patients with Wolff-Parkinson-White syndrome using scintigraphic phase mapping and oesophaeal pacing. Circulation 67: 1139.

10. Rakovec P, Kranjec I, Fettich J, Fidler V, Pungercar D, Janezic A, Porentz M, Varl B. 1983. Localization of accessory pathways in Wolff-Parkinson-White syndrome by phase imaging. Cardiology 70: 138.

11. Nakajima K, Bunko H, Tada A, Tonami N, Taki J, Nanbu I, Hisada K, Misaki T, Iwa T. 1984. Tomographic phase analysis to detect the site of accessory conduction pathway in Wolff-Parkinson-White syndrom (abstract). J Nucl Med 25: 86.

12. Nakajima K, Bunko H, Tada A, Taki A, Tonami N, Hisada K, Misaki T, Iwa T. 1984. Phase analysis in patients with Wolff-Parkinson-White syndrom with surgically proved accessory conduction pathways. J Nucl Med 25: 7.

13. Aliot E, Laurens MH, Thouvenot P, Brunotte F, Prestat MP, Zannad F, Gilgenkrantz JM, Robert J. 1985. L'image de phase des ventriculographies isotopiques: contribution à l'étude du syndrome de Wolff-Parkinson-White. Arch Mal Coeur 8: 1166.

14. Dormehl I, Bitter F, Henze E, Adam WE, Wersmuller P. 1985. An evaluation of the diagnostic efficacity of phase analysis of data from radionuclide ventriculograms in patients with Wolff-Parkinson-White syndrom. Eur J Nucl Med 11: 150.

15. Swiryn S, Pavel D, Byrom E, Bauernfeind R, Strasberg B, Palileo E, Lam W, Wyndham C, Rosen K. 1982. Sequential regional phase mapping of radionuclide gated biventriculograms in patients with sustained ventricular tachycardia: close correlation with electrophysiologic characteristics. Am Heart J 103: 319.

16. Podrid PJ, Ziekonka J, Lown B, Holman BL, Carr S, Young J, Biflock L. 1980. The use of radioventriculography for localizing the site of origin of ventricular tachycardia (abstract). Circulation (suppl. 3) 62: 1148.

17. Mc Carthy DM, Makler PT, Waxman HL, Buxton AE, Marchlinski FE, Horowitz LN, Spielman SR, Alavi A, Josephson ME. 1983. Fourier phase image during ventricular tachycardia: relationship to endocardial site of origin (abstract). JACC 1: 712.

18. Dae MN, Botvinick EH, Scheinmann MH, Morady FJ, Davis JA, Schechtmann N, Frais M, Faulkner D, O'Connell W. 1984. Correlation of scintigraphic phase maps with intra-operative epicardial/endocardial maps in patients with activation disturbances (abstract). J Nucl Med 21: 80.

19. Goris ML, Mc Killop JH, Briandet PA. 1981. A fully automated determination of the left ventricular region of interest in nuclear angiocardiography. Cardiovasc Intervent Radiol 4: 117.

20. Fontaine G, Guiraudon G, Franck R, Coutle R, Dragodanne C. 1976. Epicardial mapping and surgical treatment in six cases of resistant ventricular tachycardia not related to coronary artery disease. In: the conduction system of the heart. Wellens HJJ, Lie KL, Janse MJ (eds). Philadelphia, Lea Fibiger, 545.

21. Marcus FI, Fontaine GH, Guiraudon G, Franck R, Laurenceau JL, Malergue C, Grosgogeat Y. 1982. Right ventricular dysplasias. A report of 24 cases. Circulation 65: 384.

22. Rossi P, Massumi A, Gillette P, Hall RJ. 1982. Arrhythmogenic right ventricular dysplasia: clinical features diagnostic techniques and current management. Am Heart J 103: 415.

23. Bourguignon MH, Sebag C, Le Guludec D, Davy JM, Slama M, Motte G, Syrota A. 1986. Arrhythmogenic right ventricular dysplasia demonstrated by phase mapping of gated equilibrium radio ventriculography. Am Heart J 111: 997.

24. Josephson ME, Horowitz LW, Waxman HL, Cain ME, Spielman SR, Greenspan AM, Marchlinski FE, Ezri MD. 1981. Sustained ventricular tachycardia: role of the 12-lead electrocardiogram in localizing site of origin. Circulation 64: 257.

25. Josephson ME, Horowitz LN, Fanshidi A, Spear JF, Kastor JA, Moore EN. 1978. Recurrent sustained ventricular tachycardia. II. Endocardial mapping. Circulation 57: 440.
26. Horowitz LN, Josephson ME, Harken AM. 1980. Ventricular resection guided by epicardial and endocardial mapping for treatment of recurrent ventricular tachycardia. N Engl J Med 302: 589.
27. Links JM, Douglass KH, Wagner HN. 1980. Patterns of ventricular emptying by Fourier analysis of gated blood pool studies. J Nucl Med 21: 978.
28. Cramer JA, Ehrhardt JC, Collins SM. 1981. Second harmonic analysis in the asessment of ventricular contraction patterns from radionuclide images. In: Frontiers of Engineering in Health care. Cohen BA (ed). Houston. IEEE Ingineering in Medicine and Biology Society 97.
29. Wendt RE, Murphy PH, Clark JW, Burdine JA. 1982. Interpretation of multigated Fourier functional images. J Nucl Med 23: 715.
30. Bacharach SL, Green MV, Vitale D. 1983. Optimum number of harmonics for fitting cardiac volume curves (abstract). J Nucl Med 24: 17.
31. Mukai T, Tamaki N, Yonekura Y. 1983. Optimum order harmonics of Fourier analysis in multigated blood pool studies (abstract). J Nucl Med 24: 17.
32. Machac J, Horowitz SF, Broder D, Goldsmith SJ. 1984. Accuracy and precision of regional multiharmonic Fourier analysis of gated blood-pool images. J Nucl Med 25: 1294.
33. Botvinick EH, Dunn R, O'Connell W, Shosa D, Tucker C, Herfkens R. 1980. The phase image-its relationship to patterns of contraction and conduction. Circulation (suppl. III) 65: 551.

18. Methods and results of noninvasive detection of ventricular late potentials

EDWARD J. BERBARI, LEONARD DECARLO, KAREN J. FRIDAY, and WARREN M. JACKMAN
University of Oklahoma Health Sciences Center and Veterans Administration Medical Center, Oklahoma City, Oklahoma, USA

Introduction

In 1973, Boineau and Cox [1] showed that electrograms from ischemic regions of the canine heart were delayed and fractionated. Waldo and Kaiser [2] described bridging of the diastolic interval with low level electrical activity. Then Scherlag et al. [3], Hope et al. [4], Williams et al. [5] and El-Sherif et al. [6, 7], all working in the same laboratory, evolved an animal model for monitoring and relating this delayed or continuous electrical activity to the generation of ventricular arrhythmias. A wide variety of observations verified the relationship between late potentials and ventricular arrhythmias. These included patterns such as 2 : 1 block in the ischemic/infarct zone as well as progressive beat-by-beat prolongation of late potentials evolving to continuous electrical activity anteceding ectopic ventricular discharges and ventricular tachycardia. Other studies [8–10] also described prolongation and conduction block of late potentials as a function of heart rate and drugs. Multi-electrode epicardial mapping by El-Sherif et al. [11] and Wit et al. [12] has further verified these late activated areas as the substrate of reentry. An editorial comment by Josephson and Wit [13] clearly emphasizes the role of continuous electrical activity in defining reentry as a mechanism of ventricular tachycardia. Initial studies in man on late potentials were reported by Josephson et al. [14] and Fontaine et al. [15] which were recorded from the endocardial and epicardial surface, respectively, of patients with ventricular tachycardia.

The first recording of late potentials from the body surface was made from dogs in 1978 [16]. This study demonstrated the feasibility of recording late potentials from the body surface and showed that these potentials corresponded to potentials recorded directly from epicardial electrodes in dogs with myocardial infarctions. Prolongation of late potentials was measured on the epicardial and body surface as a function of the heart rate. The original study also linked the late potentials with the presence of arrhythmias. These two results led to studies in which the goals were to identify some of the functional characteristics of surface recorded late potentials not only as a function of heart rate but in combination with lidocaine or epinephrine infusion [17–20].

A report by Simson et al. [21] described several enhancements to the technique such as the use of a bidirectional digital filter to reduce phase shift of the filters and the use of the vector magnitude recording derived from the X, Y, and Z leads. (This methodology is the most popular in the clinical laboratories). The attempt was made to correlate the duration of the surface late potentials with the epicardial late potentials in dogs following myocardial infarction. There was a good correlation (r = .93), but the linear regression line did not pass through the origin nor did it have a slope of 1.0 implying that the surface recording did not record the full extent of late potentials. A similar preliminary finding was presented by Blake et al. [22].

The earliest studies in man were done to verify the presence of late potentials in patients following a myocardial infarction or those with ventricular tachycardia. Rozanski, et al. [23] recorded late potentials in patients with ventricular aneurysms and ventricular tachycardia. Following anuerysmectomy and the resultant abolition of ventricular tachycardia, the late potentials could no longer be detected. A similar study by Marcus et al. [24] did not find the abolition of late potentials to be a primary indication of surgical success in treating ventricular tachycardia but in all cases in which late potentials were abolished so was the ventricular tachycardia. Simson et al. [25] studied patients shortly after myocardial infarction and found a correlation between late potentials and the subsequent development of ventricular tachycardia. Breithardt et al. [26] found a similar correlation, but in another study also concluded that late potentials per se were not predictive of sudden death [27]. Denes et al. [28] have shown that late potentials were a reliable, reproducible marker for distinguishing patients with ventricular tachycardia from normal subjects. Cain et al. [29] have shown that the frequency content and not just duration/amplitude measurements of late potentials accurately separates those with and without inducible ventricular tachycardia. More recently in an abstract report Cain et al. [30] have also shown that spectral changes in the late potential frequency content following antiarrhythmic drug therapy is also predictive of the drug's efficacy. Simson et al. [31] also studied the effects of antiarrhythmic drugs on late potentials. The late potentials were not abolished by the antiarrhythmic drug even when the drug proved effective in preventing sustained ventricular tachycardia. Since they had already shown a relationship between late potentials and inducible ventricular tachycardia they may have been predisposed to look for the abolition of late potentials as an indicator of drug efficacy rather than configuration changes in late potential waveform. A multivariable study by Kanovsky et al. [32] compared late potentials, Holter monitoring and cardiac catheterization. They concluded that late potentials alone provide independent information for identifying patients with ventricular tachycardia after myocardial infarction. It was in concert with these other tests that 85% of patients were correctly identified (sensitivity 81%, specificity 90%).

Methods

There are very few aspects of recording late potentials which are system specific. Most modern mini or micro computer systems can be programmed to perform a variety of analysis methods. The system described below is one of several that has been developed in our laboratory. We will begin with a brief description of the hardware and describe some aspects of the system software.

An orthogonal X, Y, Z bipolar lead set is used. The X electrodes are positioned along the mid auxiliary line at the level of the 4th intercostal space. The Y lead is positioned along the mid clavicular line. The upper electrode is placed in the region of sub-clavicular space the lower electrode is placed in the lower abdominal region. The anterior Z electrode is positioned at the intersection of the 4th intercostal space and the mid-clavicular line and the posterior Z lead is positioned at the reflection of the anterior electrode on the back. The positive electrode sites are leftward, inferior and anterior. The ECG preamplifiers are of a low noise design with a high CMRR (>120 dB) and are battery operated. The data shown in this report were bandpass filtered (6 dB/oct) between 100 and 300 Hz with analog filters. More recent systems rely on digital filters. The gain of the amplifiers was maximized to allow the signal to cover the dynamic range of the 12 bit A/D converter of ± 5 volts. A sampling rate of 2000 Hz per channel was used. A total of 5 signals were digitized: A low gain, unfiltered lead, the high gain bandpass filtered X, Y and Z leads, and the output of a hardwired QRS detector. Figure 1 is a block diagram of this front end. Note that the signal into channel 1 depended on the lead selected for input to the QRS detector. The QRS detector produced a 2 msec pulse during the QRS and was not designed to reject abnormal or varying QRS complexes. The software used a correlation algorithm to select specific QRS complexes and to properly align them prior to inclusion in the average. A template surrounding the QRS detect point was chosen from the first beat and used for aligning and beat selection of all subsequent beats. Figure 2 shows a diagram of this scheme. The time of interest (TOI) is the ST segment region in which late potentials are most commonly recorded.

The computer used in this study was a MASSCOMP MC-560. This is a multimicroprocessor system with dedicated microprocessors for I/O handling, computing, and graphics display. With this type of architecture a real time Unix operating system becomes possible.

The software is divided into two functions: 1) data acquisition and signal averaging and 2) data analysis. In the data acquisition phase, the system will average a specified number of beats. The 4 ECG tracings along with the variables specific to the average, e.g., number of beats, gain, sampling frequency, etc., are saved for the analysis program. The MASSCOMP graphics system displays up to 830 points in the X axis. The software uses 800 points, which at a sampling rate of 2000 Hz results in a 400 msec window of the ECG.

One aspect of late potentials which we wanted to study was the effect of heart

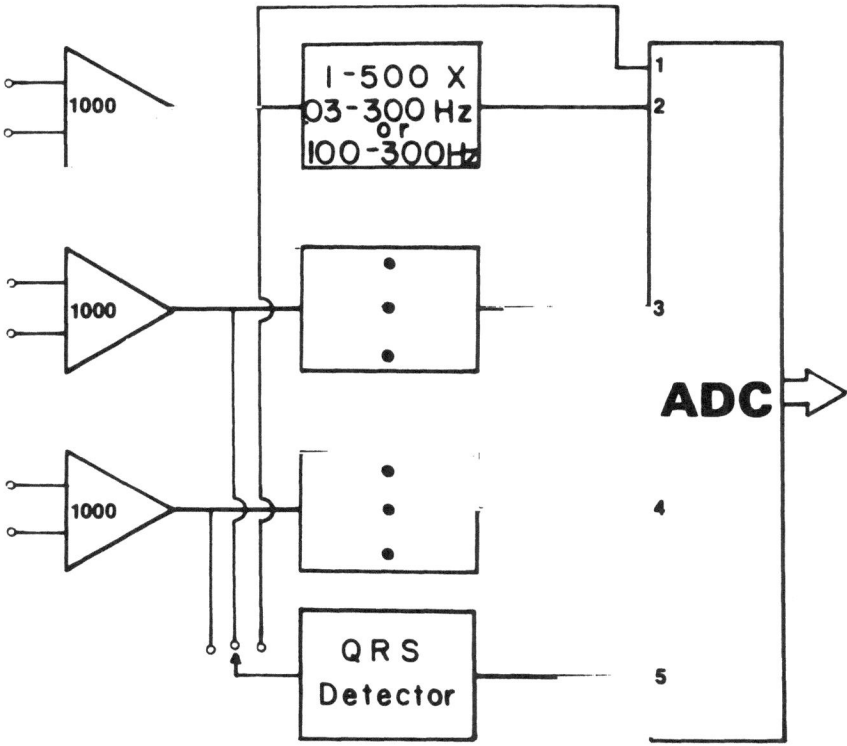

Figure 1. A block diagram of the system front end. Each lead is preamplified with gain of 1000. This amplifier is battery powered. A variable gain stage and bandpass filter follows. High pass filters of .03 or 100 Hz may be selected. The low pass filter was 300 Hz. All were first order (20 db/decade) filters. The 12 bit A/D converter sampled each of the five signals at rates as high as 2000 Hz.

rate on the late potentials. In a group of 18 patients undergoing electrophysiological testing for the evaluation of ventricular tachycardia signal averaged recordings were obtained during sinus rhythm and at several atrial paced rates. In all cases at least two and usually three repeated 100 beat averages were performed. Patients with bundle branch block were excluded. In 14 cases the patients were in the drug free state while the remaining were studied while medicated with Quinidine (2) or Procainamide (2). This study did not attempt to determine the efficacy of the antiarrhythmic drugs from late potential analysis.

Results

One key aspect of this study was to observe the reproducibility of sequential 100 beat averages. If the late potentials were not reproducible, and at this time reproducibility is determined by the observer, then it would be impossible to

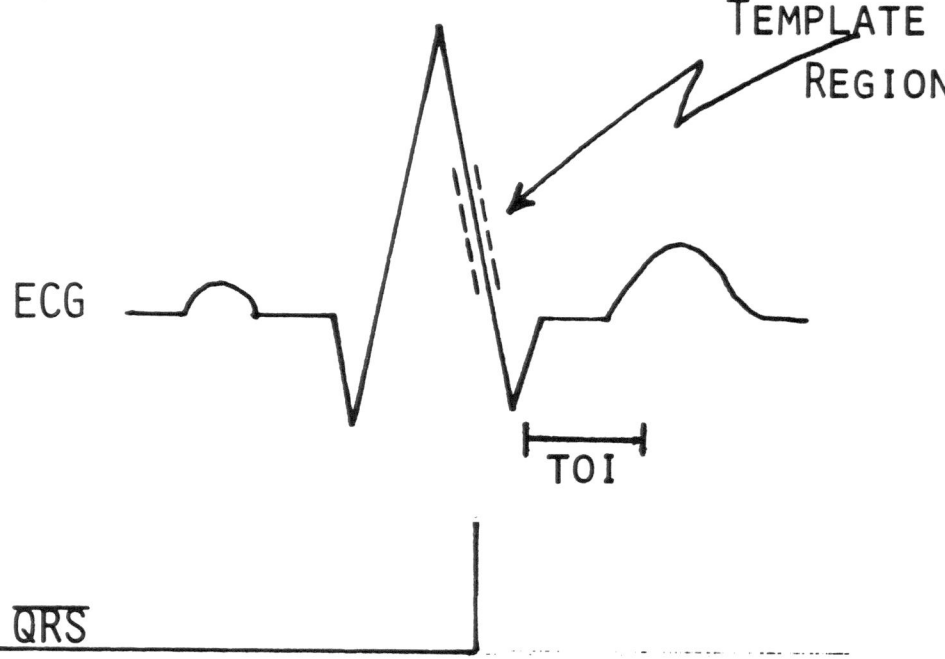

Figure 2. A schematic representation of the ECG and QRS detector output demonstrating the template region surrounding the trigger point and the time of interest (TOI) of the signal averaging window.

measure any heart rate or drug induced changes which would be independent of the averaging process itself. Figure 3 is from a patient in the drug free state during normal sinus rhythm. Traces A-D are four repeated 100 beat averages. Looking at the terminal region of the QRS and ST segment, one observes a low level signal lasting almost 100 msec with an average amplitude of roughly 10 microvolts. These four traces demonstrate by visual inspection a highly reproducible waveform. One can also observe the main QRS and also observe reproducibility in the entire QRS. In trace A some of the signal is not seen due to clipping of the display unit.

One of the most formidable problems we faced was trying to quantify the changes observed in the late potentials due to heart rate. Figure 4 shows three traces. The top trace is from normal sinus rhythm (NSR). Traces 2 and 3 were obtained during atrial pacing at cycle lengths of 600 and 500 msec, respectively. Concentrating on the terminal late potential segment of the waveforms there are only slight changes at the 600 msec cycle length compared to NSR. However, at the 500 msec cycle length the character of the late potential is markedly changed. Note that the main QRS portion does not seem to have changed ruling out the possibility of an averaging induced change, e.g., trigger jitter. (The waveform to

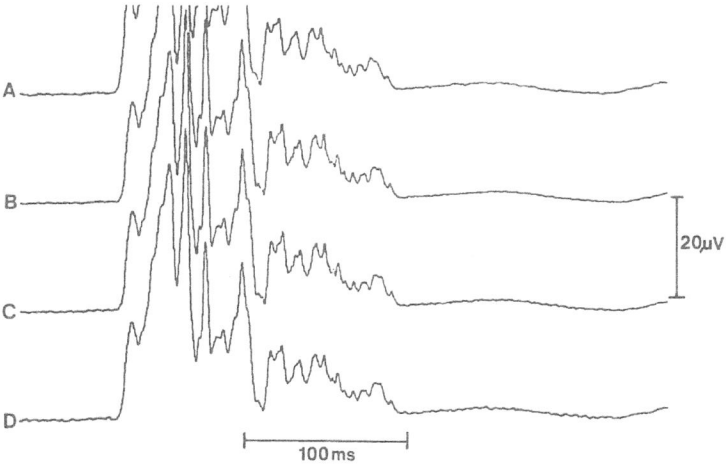

Figure 3. Demonstration of reproducibility of the signal averaged recordings of the filtered vector magnitude. Each trace was obtained after averaging 100 cardiac cycles. The low level potentials (<20 microvolts) extend the QRS duration to about 170 msec.

the extreme right of the 500 msec trace is the stimulus artifact). The total QRS duration and mean amplitude of the late potential do not appear to be markedly changed.

An example of minimal change in the late potentials as a function of heart rate

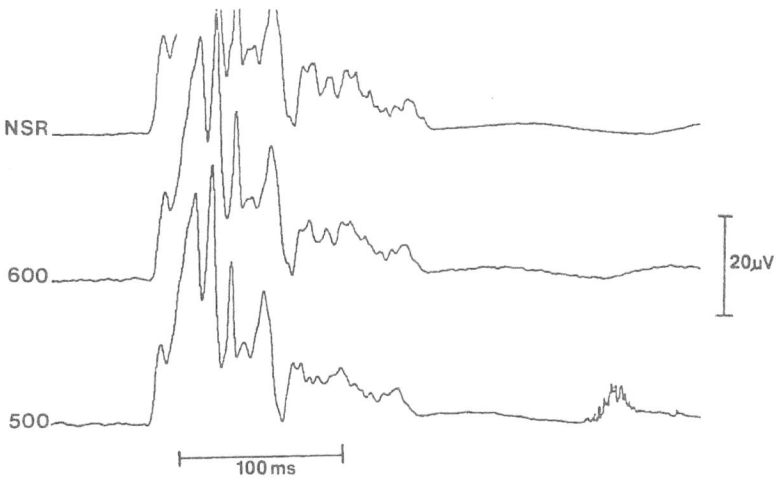

Figure 4. Effects of atrial pacing on late potentials is shown in this figure. The waveforms are from the same patient depicted in figure 3. The top trace was during normal sinus rhythm (NSR) and traces 2 and 3 were at cycle lengths of 600 and 500 msec, respectively. Note the change in the terminal potentials while the large amplitude signals were not affected by heart rate. The wavefore at the right in trace 3 is due to the stimulus artefact.

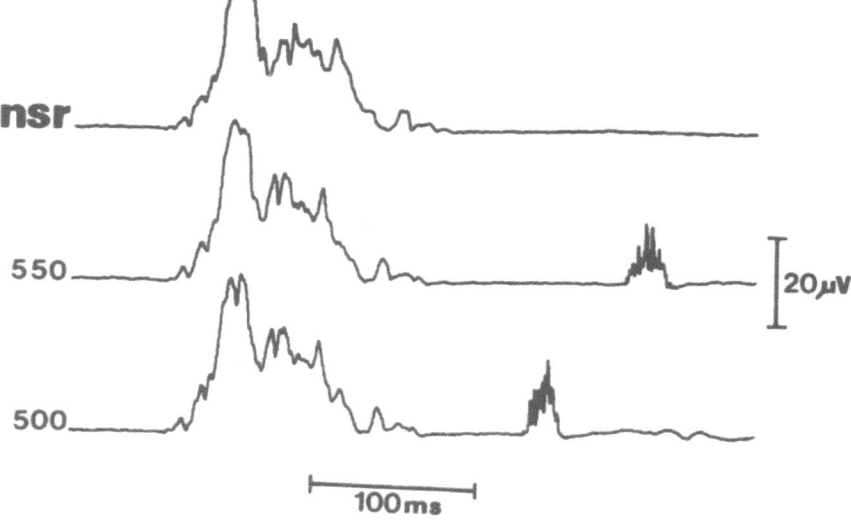

Figure 5. Demonstration of minimal late potential changes as a function of heart rate. The format is similar to that in figure 4.

is shown in Figure 5. The top trace was obtained during normal sinus rhythm and traces 2 and 3 were obtained at cycle lengths of 550 and 500 msec, respectively. While some changes may be observed it is difficult to consider these significant from a subjective viewpoint.

There were eight patients with inducible ventricular tachycardia that showed changes in the late potentials as a function of heart rate. There were five patients that had no inducible ventricular tachycardia and no pacing induced changes in the late potentials. There were four noninducible patients that showed pacing changes and only one that was inducible with but had no rate induced changes. A chi square test did not find these results significant for using the pacing changes as a means of predicting VT inducibility. However, there are too few patients to make a definitive statement.

Drugs were also found to change the late potentials as well as the QRS. Figure 6, shows four traces all obtained during sinus rhythm. The top trace was obtained in the drug free, control state. The 2 and 3 trace were obtained after sequential 800 mg injections of quinidine. There is an expected widening of the QRS and change in late potential appearance. After the second injection to a total of 1600 mg there was a further QRS widening and late potential changes. There is an obvious diminution of the late potential amplitude. However, 45 min after the second injection, another average (trace 4) shows the return of the QRS-late potential characteristics to the 800 mg level.

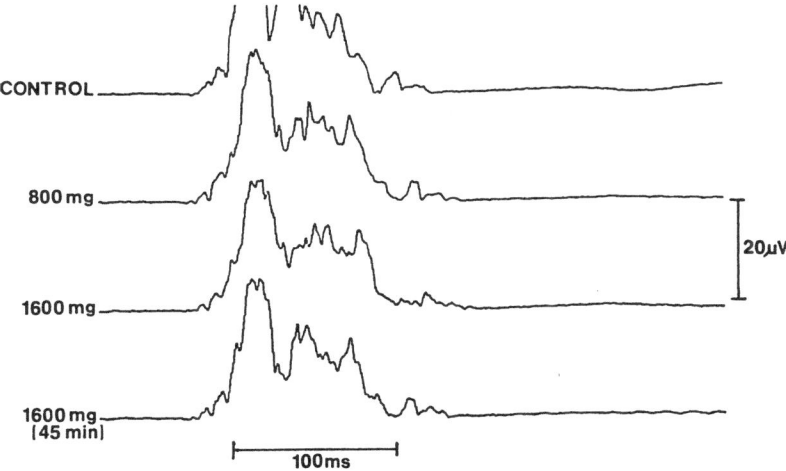

Figure 6. Changes in late potentials as a function of Quinidine. An average after the initial 800 mg dose is shown in the second trace. After another 800 mg dose the average in trace 3 was obtained. Forty five minutes after this second dose another average was obtained and is shown in trace 4. See text for discussion.

Discussion

The types of changes observed in the late potentials as a function of heart rate did not lend themselves to traditional time and amplitude measurement changes. The use of a subjective determination of change also has many pitfalls. More quantitative descriptors are necessary. Frequency analysis is one method which has been deonstrated to show changes when the analysis window includes the late potential region [29, 30]. However, such measurements also include other regions and it may not be possible to ascribe the observed change to the late potential 'generator' alone.

Changes in late potential characteristics due to drugs present the same problems as those described for heart rate induced changes. It is usually further complicated in that drugs may also produce global changes, e.g., QRS widening. Again, the traditional measures fall short in relating the changes to the underlying late potential generator. The fundamental bases of late potentials must be determined and studied independent of other cardiac events. This should allow the more precise quantification of the functional characteristics of the late potentials.

Acknowledgements

Thanks are given to Pamela Tomey for her help in typing and preparing the

254

manuscript. This work was supported by NIH Grant, HL 27646, and funds from the Veterans Administration.

References

1. Boineau JP, Cox JL. 1973. A slow ventricular activation in acute myocardial infarction. A source of reentrant ventricular contractions. Circ 48: 702–713.
2. Waldo AL, Kaiser GA. 1973. A study of ventricular arrhythmias associated with acute myocardial infarction in the canine heart. Circ 47: 1220–1228.
3. Scherlag BJ, El-Sherif N, Hope RR, Lazzara R. 1974. Characterization and localization of ventricular arrhythmias due to myocardial ischemia and infarction. Circ Res 35: 372–383.
4. Hope RR, Williams DO, El-Sherif N, Lazzara R. 1974. The efficacy of antiarrhythmic agents during acute myocardial ischemia and the role of heart rate. Circ 50: 507–514.
5. Williams DO, Scherlag BJ, Hope RR, Lazzara R. 1974. The pathophysiology of malignant ventricular arrhythmias during acute myocardial ischemia. Circ 50: 1163–1172.
6. El-Sherif N, Scherlag BJ, Lazzara R, Hope RR. 1977. Reentrant ventricular arrhythmias in the late myocardial infarction period. I. Conduction characteristics in the infarction zone. Circ 55: 686–702.
7. El-Sherif N, Hope RR, Scherlag BJ, Lazzara R. 1977. Reentrant ventricular arrhythmias in the late myocardial infarction period. Circ 55: 702–719.
8. Hope RR, Williams DO, El-Sherif N, Lazzara R, Scherlag BJ. 1974. The efficacy of antiarrhythmic agents during acute myocardial ischemia and the role of heart rate. Circ 50: 507–514.
9. El-Sherif N, Scherlag BJ, Lazzara R, Hope RR. 1977. Reentrant ventricular arrhythmias in the late myocardial infarction period. 4. Mechanism of action of lidocaine. Circ 56: 396–402.
10. Patterson E, Gibson JK, Lucchesi BR. 1982. Electrophysiologic actions of lidocaine in a canine model of chronic myocardial ischemic damage-Arrhythmogenic actions of lidocaine. J Cardiovasc Pharmacol 4: 925–934.
11. El-Sherif N, Smith A, Evans K. 1981. Canine ventricular arrhythmias in the late myocardial infarction period: Epicardial mapping of reentrant circuits. Circ Res 49: 255.
12. Wit AL, Allessie MA, Bonke FIM, Lammas W, Smeets J, Fenoflio JJ, Jr. 1982. Electrophysiologic mapping to determine the mechanism of experimental ventricular tachycardia initiated by premature impulses: Experimental approach – Initial results demonstrating reentrant excitation. Am J Cardiol 49: 166.
13. Josephson ME, Wit AL. 1984. Fractionated electrical activity and continuous electrical activity: Fact or Artifact? Circ 70: 529–532.
14. Josephson ME, Horowitz LN, Farshidi A. 1978. Continuous local electrical activity: A mechanism of recurrent ventricular tachycardia. Circ 57: 658.
15. Fontaine G, Guiraudon G, Frank R, Vedel J, Grossgogent Y, Cabrol C. 1978. Modern concepts of ventricular tachycardia. Eur J Cardiol 8: 565.
16. Berbari EJ, Scherlag BJ, Hope RR, Lazzara R. 1978. Recording from the body surface of arrhythmogenic ventricular activity during the ST segment. Am J Cardiol 41: 697.
17. Berbari EJ, Brachmann J, Scherlag BJ, Lazzara R. 1981. Recording late depolarization potentials in dogs: Correlation with ventricular arrhythmias. In: Signal Averaging Technique in Clinical Cardiology, V Hombach and HH Hilger, eds., FK Schattauer Verlag, Stuttgart: pp. 109–119.
18. Berbari EJ, Brachmann J, Harrison LA, Lazzara R, Scherlag BJ. 1983. Changes in late ventricular activity due to epinephrine, lidocaine and atrial pacing. Circ 68: III–218.
19. Berbari EJ, Brachmann J, Scherlag BJ, Lazzara R. The response of late ventricular activity to lidocaine and epinephrine in conjunction with atrial pacing, under revision.
21. Simson MB, Euler D, Michelson EL, Falcone RA, Spear JF, Moore EN. 1981. Detection of

delayed ventricular activation on the body surface in dogs. Am J Physiol 241: H363.

22. Blake GJ, Spear JR, Richards DA, Moore EN. 184. Delayed epicardial conduction in dogs with late potentials identified by signal averaging. Circ 70: II–220.

23. Rozanski JJ, Mortara D, Myerburg RJ, Castellanos A. 1981. Body surface detection of delayed depolarizations in patients with recurrent ventricular tachycardia and left ventricular aneurysm. Circ 63: 1172–1178.

24. Marcus NH, Falcone RA, Harken AH, Josephson ME, Simson MB. 1984. Body surface late potentials with ventricula tachycardia. Circ 70: 632–637.

25. Simson MB. 1981. Use of signals in the terminal QRS complex to identify patients with ventricular tachycardia after myocardial infarction. Circ 64: 235–242.

26. Breithardt G, Becker R, Seipel L, Abendroth RR, Ostermeyer J. 1981. Noninvasive detection of late potentials in man: A new marker for ventricular tachycardia. Eur Heart J 2: 1–11.

27. Breithardt G, Schwarzmaier J, Boygrefe M, Haerten K, Seipel L. 1983. Prognostic significance of late ventricular potentials after acute myocardial infarction. Eu Heart J 4: 487–495.

28. Denes P, Santarelli P, Hauser RG, Uretz EF. 1983. Quantitative analysis of the high frequency components of the terminal portion of the body surface QRS in normal subjects and in patients with ventricular tachycardia. Circ 67: 1129.

9. Cain ME, Ambos HD, Witkowski FX, Sobel BE. 1984. Fast-Fourier transform analysis of signal-averaged electrocardiograms for identification of patients prone to sustained ventricular tachycardia. Circ 69: 711–720.

30. Cain ME, Ambos HD, Fischer AE, Markham J, Schechtam KB. 184. Noninvasive prediction of antiarrhythmic drug efficacy in patients with sustained ventricular tachycardia from frequency analysis of signal averaged ECG's. Circ 70: II–252.

31. Simson MB, Waxman HL, Falcone R, Marcus NH, Josephson ME. 1983. Effects of antiarrhythmic drugs on noninvasively recorded late potentials. In: New Aspects in the Medical Treatment of Tachyarrhythmias: Role of Amiodarone, G Breithardt and F Loogen, eds., Urban and Schwarzenberg, Munich, Germany: p. 80.

32. Kanosky MS, Falcon RA, Dresden CA, Josephson ME, Simson MB. 1984. Identification of patients with ventricular tachycardia after myocardial infarction: Signal averaged electrocardiogram, Holter monitoring, and cardiac catheterization. Circ 70: 264–270.

19. Role of ventricular late potentials for identification of patients at risk of ventricular tachycardia

GÜNTER BREITHARDT, MARTIN BORGGREFE, KLAUS HAERTEN,
JOACHIM SCHWARZMAIER, ULRICH KARBENN,
and ANDREA PODCZECK
*Hospital of the University of Düsseldorf, Department of Cardiology,
Pneumology, and Angiology, Düsseldorf, Germany, F.R.*

Recent interest in the field of non-invasive clinical electrophysiology has focused on the use of signal averaging for detection of abnormal, low-amplitude electrical activity at the end of or after the QRS-complex on the body surface in patients with documented ventricular tachycardia [1–7]. These signals have been called ventricular late potentials ('potential tardif') [7]. They probably originate from areas of regional slow conduction in the border zone of old myocardial infarction. There is convincing evidence that their presence is closely correlated with the propensity to ventricular tachycardia [2–5, 9–11]. With conventional methods of ECG recording, these signals can normally not be registered on the body surface. Berbari et al. [1] in the experimental animal and Fontaine et al. [7] in man were the first to report that these signals could be recorded from the body surface by the use of high-gain amplification, appropriate filtering and computer averaging techniques.

Since then, a great number of reports has been published showing the positive correlation between the presence of ventricular late potentials in the signal-averaged surface ECG and the presence of ventricular tachycardia in patients after myocardial infarction [2–6, 8–25]. Further studies attempted to correlate changes in various characteristics of late potentials under the influence of antiarrhythmic drugs to antiarrhythmic drug efficacy [26–32]. This issue is still controversial as none of the presently available studies has shown a clear correlation [26]. In contrast, several authors were able to establish a positive correlation between the efficacy of map-guided antitachycardic surgery in patients with documented ventricular tachycardia and either the disappearance or a reduction in duration of ventricular late potentials [4, 33–36].

Though the detection of a late potential on the body surface may be of importance for the characterization of patients with documented ventricular tachycardia and/or for the control of efficacy of antitachycardic surgery, these applications obviously are of limited significance in the vast majority of patients with coronary artery disease. However, previous work has shown that ventricular late potentials cannot only be detected in patients with documented ventricular tachycardia after myocardial infarction, but also in about one third of patients after myocardial infarction who, up to the time of the study, have been free of sustained ventricular arrhythmias [9]. On the basis of these findings, prospective studies seemed to be warranted to assess whether the detection of ventricular late potentials may be able to predict the subsequent occurrence of either sustained ventricular tachycardia or sudden cardiac death after myocardial infarction.

For this purpose, a prospective trial was initiated at Düsseldorf University in 1980. This study can be divided into two parts. First, a prospective study using the methodology for recording of signal-averaged ECGs which was developed in our department between 1978 and 1979. This system is primarily based on a hard-wired signal averager [2, 9–11] which has also been used by other groups [30, 37, 38]. It consists of analogue unidirectional filtering and visual analysis of the highly amplified signals. This study included patients either after recent myocardial infarction studied within the first 6 weeks, mostly within week 2 to 3, or patients who were referred with a clinical indication for coronary angiography to establish or exclude the diagnosis of coronary artery disease. None of these patients had a history of syncope. Patients with complete bundle branch were excluded. The second study, started in January 1983, included only male patients after recent Q-wave infarction. All patients were studied within the first 3 weeks after onset of myocardial infarction. The upper age limit was 65 years. Signal-averaging was performed using the software program by M. Simson [5] which includes bidirectional digital filtering and automated analysis of signal-averaged ECGs. In addition to the original analysis of the voltage-time-relation in the terminal portion of the QRS-complex, an additional algorithm for identification of ventricular late potentials was included [39]. This multi-center study (PILP: Post Infarction Late Potential-Study) has recently been completed after inclusion of 800 male patients. Data analysis has not yet been completed.

The purpose of this chapter is to review our presently available information in the first group of patients in whom our initially developed system for signal-averaging had been used.

Patient selection

Two groups of patients were studied. First, patients referred for coronary angiography. These patients were eligible if they had no history of sustained ventricular tachycardia, of cardiac arrest unrelated to an acute myocardial infarction, or of syncope. Patients referred for documented complex ventricular arrhythmias or unstable angina not responding to medical therapy were excluded. Second, patients drawn from survivors of acute myocardial infarction who were admitted from the emergency area covered by the participating 2 departments (University of Düsseldorf and Marienhospital Wesel).

Methods

Besides the clinically indicated studies, signal-averaging was performed using our previously described system [2]. Late potentials were visually identified in the high-gain averaged recordings as low amplitude activity appearing at the end of the QRS complex. The criteria used for identification of a late potential and the method used for the measurement of its duration have previously been described [2, 9–11].

All patients were followed either in the out-patient clinic or by mail or telephone contact with the patient and/or the referring physician. Arrhythmic events were defined as spontaneous symptomatic sustained ventricular tachycardia requiring emergency intervention or sudden cardiac death (within less than 1 hour of onset of symptoms) without accompanying acute cardiac failure and occurring during a period of stable state. When unwitnessed, death was considered arrhythmic when it occurred unexpectedly and without previous clinical deterioration (i.e. during sleep). Events that occurred in conjuction with another episode of myocardial infarction were not considered as primary arrhythmic events. Follow-up was terminated in case of reinfarction or at the time of cardiac surgery. The events occurring during follow-up were classified without knowledge of the results of signal-averaging. In the following, data of only those patients in whom prolonged follow-up has been obtained were included.

Patients' characteristics

628 patients were studied. Mean age ($\pm$ standard deviation) was 54 ± 7.6 years. 578 patients were male. 159 patients (25.3%) had no history of myocardial infarction. In the remaining patients, anterior (n = 224, 35.7%) or inferior wall myocardial infarction (n = 230; 36.6%) antedated the study. In an additional 15 patients, both anterior and inferior wall myocardial infarction had occurred. Thus, a total of 469 patients had a history of myocardial infarction. Coronary angiography was performed in 415 of 628 patients. In 93 patients (22.4%), there was no coronary artery disease detectable. In 104 patients (25.1%), there was 1-vessel disease, in 101 patients (24.3%) there was 2-vessel disease, and in 117 (28.2%), there was 3-vessel disease.

Prevalence of late potentials

A ventricular late potential was considered to be present if its duration exceeded at least 10 msec. On the basis of this definition, 379 patients (60.4%) had no late potential detectable on the body surface whereas the remaining patients had late potentials of either less than 40 msec duration (n = 191; 30.4%) or of 40 msec duration or more (n = 58; 9.2%).

Clinical events during follow-up

The mean duration of follow-up has now been extended to 39 ± 15.0 months (mean $\pm$ standard deviation). At the end of follow-up, 554 patients (88.2%) were alive. 21 patients (3.3%) suffered sudden cardiac death (within 1 h), almost all either instantaneously or during sleep. Another 3 patients (0.5%) died within 1 to 24 hours. 14 patients (2.2%) died from other cardiac causes such as reinfarction or cardiac failure. Non-cardiac causes of death were present in 10 cases (1.6%). In another 14 patients (2.2%), spontaneous symptomatic sustained ventricular tachycardia requiring emergency admission to a hospital and immediate intervention was documented.

Correlation between late potentials and follow-up

The prevalence of sudden cardiac death (within 1 h) increased from 1.6% in patients without late potentials to 5.2% in those with late potentials of less than 40 msec duration, and to 8.6% in those with a duration of 40 msec or greater (Figure 1). The risk of subsequent sustained symptomatic ventricular tachycardia increased from 0.8% in those without late potentials to 1.6% in those with late potentials of less than 40 msec duration and to 13.8% in those with potentials of greater duration. Considering the occurrence of sudden cardiac death and sustained symptomatic ventricular tachycardia together as arrhythmic events, their incidence increased from 2.4% to 6.8% and to finally 22.4% in those with late potentials of 40 msec duration or more (Figure 1). Thus, the risk ratio of developing sudden death (within 1 h) in a patient with late potentials was 3.3 and 5.4 times greater depending on the duration of late potentials (less than 40 msec and 40 msec or greater). Similarly, the risk ratio for sustained symptomatic ventricular tachycardia increased from 2.0 (less than 40 msec duration) to 17.3 (40 msec duration or more) compared to those patients without late potentials.

Correlation to total cardiac mortality

There were 38 cardiac deaths. The prevalence of total cardiac mortality increased from 4.5% in patients without to 7.3% with late potentials of less than 40 msec duration and 12.1% with a duration of 40 msec or greater. This is in accordance to data by von Leitner et al [40] who studied 518 patients that participated in a cardiac rehabilitation program after myocardial infarction. Cardiac mortality was 1.5% in those without and 7.3% in those with ventricular late potentials.

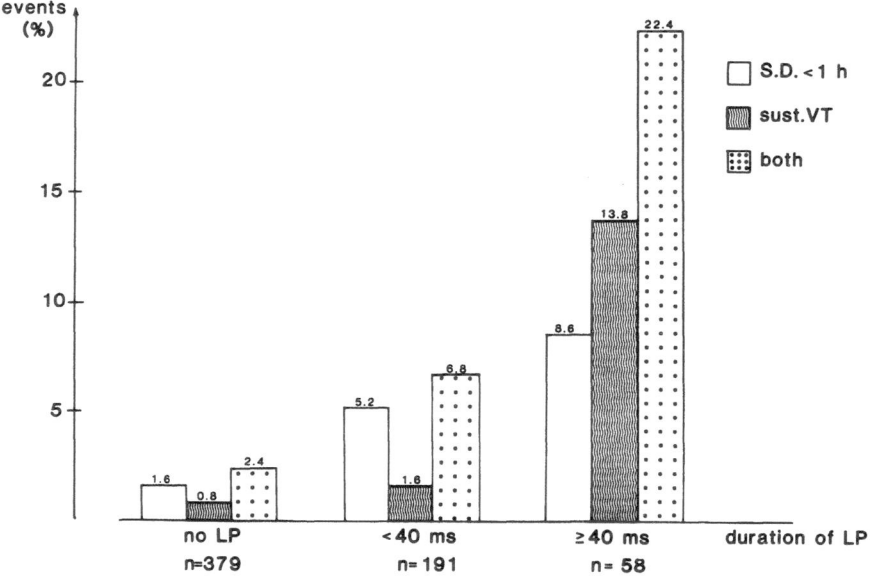

Figure 1. Prevalence of sudden death (within 1 hour) or sustained symptomatic ventricular tachycardia during follow-up of 628 patients as a function of absence or presence of late potentials and their duration.

Significance of the site of myocardial infarction

454 patients had a history of either anterior wall or inferior wall myocardial infarction. Sudden cardiac death within 1 hour occurred more frequently in patients with anterior wall myocardial infarction than in those with inferior wall myocardial infarction (Figure 2). Similarly, the prevalence of sustained symptomatic ventricular tachycardia during follow-up was markedly higher in those patients with anterior versus inferior wall myocardial infarction (Figure 3).

Significance of the degree of left ventricular dysfunction

In 314 patients, a relation between the presence and duration of late potentials and mean pulmonary artery pressure during exercise could be established. In 87 patients, mean pulmonary artery pressure at the end of symptom-limited exercise was 30 mm Hg or less whereas in the remaining patients, it exceeded 30 mm Hg (Figure 4).

The prevalence of sudden cardiac death (within 1 h) or sustained symptomatic ventricular tachycardia was low and unrelated to the presence or duration of late potentials in those with a mean pulmonary artery pressure at the end of exercise of 30 mm Hg or less. In contrast, those patients with an increase beyond

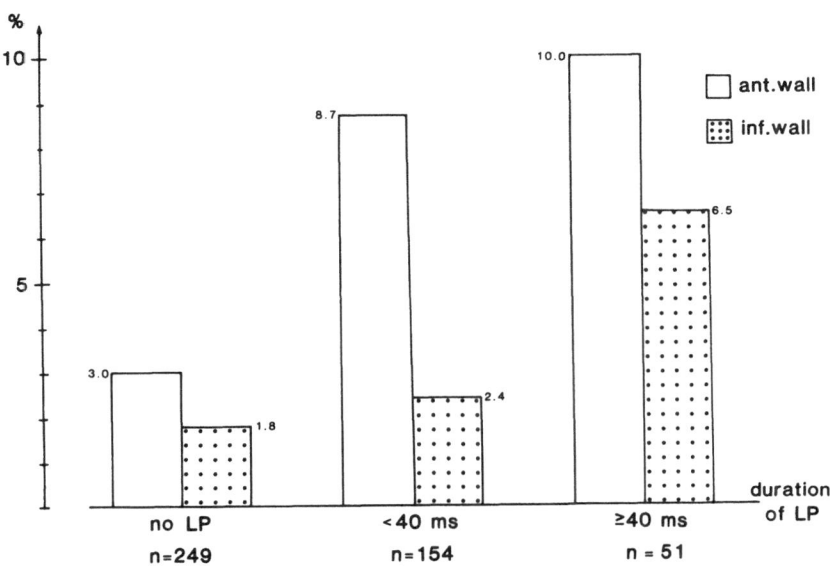

Figure 2. Prevalence of sudden death (within 1 hour) during follow-up in 454 of 628 patients who had a previous myocardial infarction as a function of the site of myocardial infarction (anterior versus inferior wall infarction) and the absence or presence and duration of late potentials.

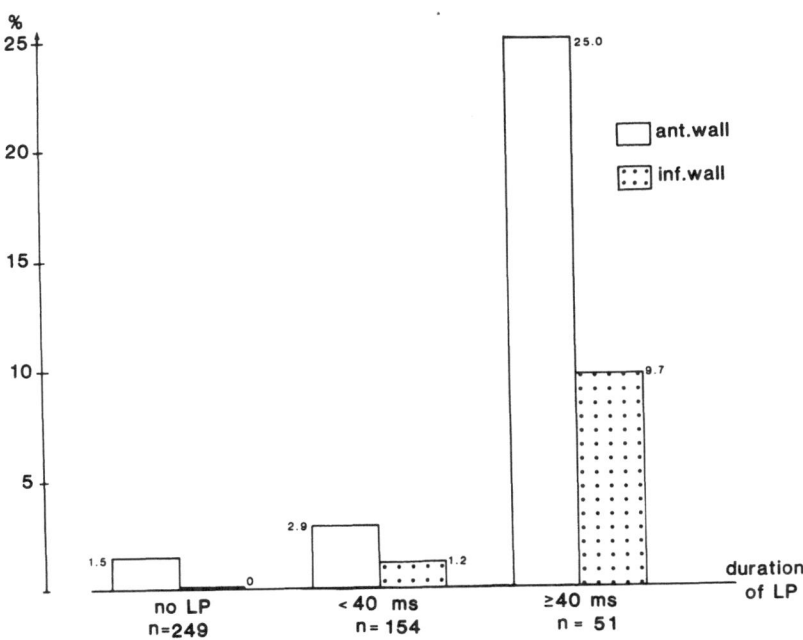

Figure 3. Prevalence of sustained symptomatic ventricular tachycardia during follow-up in 454 of 628 patients who had a previous myocardial infarction as a function of the site of myocardial infarction (anterior versus inferior wall infarction) and the absence or presence and duration of late potentials.

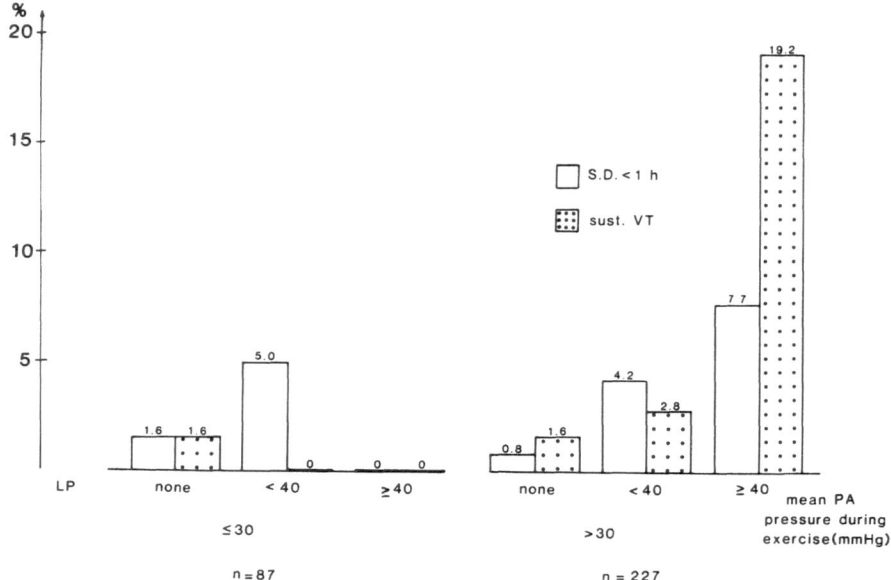

Figure 4. Prevalence of subsequent sudden death (within 1 hour) or sustained symptomatic ventricular tachycardia in 314 of 628 patients in whom exercise testing with measurement of mean pulmonary artery pressure was performed. Patients were sub-divided on the basis of their mean pulmonary artery pressure at end-exercise.

30 mm Hg exhibited a significant increase in the prevalence of subsequent sudden cardiac death or sustained symptomatic ventricular tachycardia as a function of the absence or presence (and duration) of ventricular late potentials.

Sensitivity and specificity of late potentials

Data on sensitivity and specificity of late potentials for predicting sudden death (within 1 h) or sustained symptomatic ventricular tachycardia are presented in table 1.

The absence or presence of late potentials had a moderate sensitivity and specificity for predicting either sudden death or sustained symptomatic ventricular tachycardia. Furthermore, the predictive value of a positive test was low (6.0% and 4.4%). In contrast, a negative test (absence of late potentials) predicted with a very high probability that a given patient will be free of subsequent occurrence of sudden death or sustained ventricular tachycardia. One of the major limitations was the great number of false-positive results which means that despite the presence of late potentials, the majority of patients is not going to develop either of both arrhythmic events.

The predictive value of a positive test could be increased by considering only late potentials of 40 msec duration or more (Table 1). It increased to 8.6% for sudden death, to 13.8% for sustained symptomatic ventricular tachycardia, and to 31.0% for both events combined.

Influence of therapy

There was no significant difference in the percentage of patients receiving antiarrhythmic drugs, beta-blockers, and/or digitalis in the subgroup of patients with and without late potentials.

Significance of programmed ventricular stimultion

In a subset of 132 patients after recent myocardial infarction, programmed ventricular stimulation was performed [41]. By combining the results of signal-averaging and of programmed stimulation (number of induced repetitive beats or of sustained ventricular tachycardia; rate of induced tachyarrhythmia), subsets of patients could be identified in whom the risk of subsequent development of a sustained symptomatic ventricular tachycardia was markedly increased in comparison to the remaining patients (Figure 5). The subset of patients with the greatest risk of development of ventricular tachycardia was characterized by late potentials of 40 mm duration or more and the induction of sustained ventricular tachycardia at rates below 270 b.p.m.. In this subgroup, the risk of subsequent sustained symptomatic ventricular tachycardia was 50% (i.e. 4 of 8 patients).

Table 1. Sensitivity and specificity of late potentials for predicting sudden death (<1 h) or sustained symptomatic ventricular tachycardia.

Type of event Sudden death	Sustained VT		Any type of death or sustained VT			
Late potential	Absent vs. present	Absent or <40 ms vs. ≥40 ms	Absent vs. present	Absent or <40 ms vs. ≥40 ms	Absent vs. present	Absent or <40 ms vs. ≥40 ms
Sensitivity (%)	71.4	23.8	<78.6	57.1	54.1	24.3
Specificity (%)	61.4	91.3	<61.2	91.9	62.3	92.8
False-positive (%)	94.0	91.4	<95.6	86.2	83.9	69.0
False-negative (%)	1.6	2.8	0.8	1.0	9.0	9.8
Predictive value positive test (%)	6.0	8.6	4.4	13.8	16.1	31.0
Negative test (%)	98.4	97.2	99.2	98.9	91.0	90.2

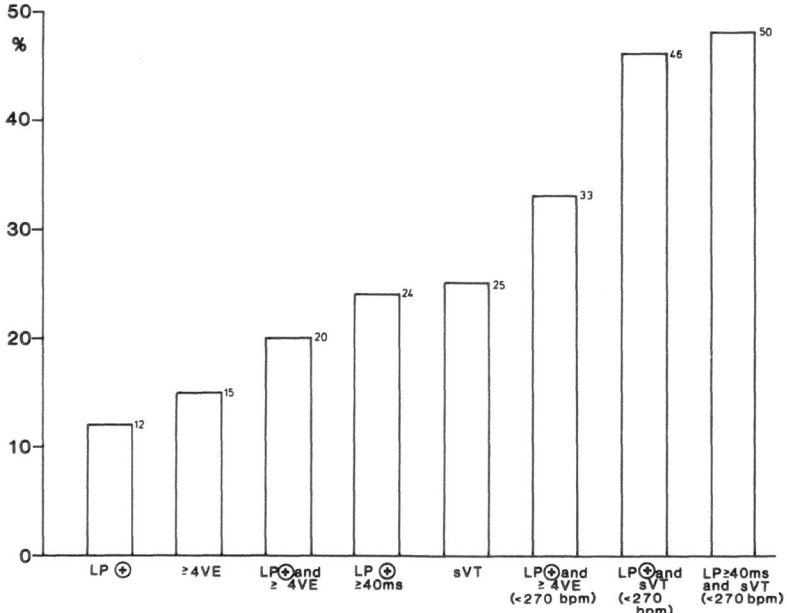

Figure 5. Predictive value of a positive test using signal averaging for detection of late potentials (LP) and programmed ventricular stimulatin for induction of ventricular echo beats (VE) or sustained ventricular tachycardia (sVT) in 132patients after recent myocardial infarction. Using various combinations of parameters (presence and duration of LP; induction of ≥4 E or sVT; rate of induced ventricular arrhythmia below 270 bpm), subgroups of patients can be identified at high risk of subsequently devloping symptomatic sustained ventricular tachycardia.

Further studies will be necessary to confirm these preliminary results in larger groups of patients.

Conclusions

In patients with coronary artery disease, ventricular late potentials can predominantly be found in those with regional akinesia or aneurysms after prior myocardial infarction [9]. This is also the case in patients with documented ventricular tachycardia in whom late potentials were more frequent in those with left ventricular akinesia or aneurysms [9]. Similarly, a greater incidence of abnormal electrical activity has been found during open-heart surgery using epicardial and endocardial mapping or during endocardial catheter mapping in patients with documented ventricular tachycardia [42–44]. The greater prevalence of late potentials in patients with regional or diffuse ventricular contraction abnormalities, both in patients with and without a history of ventricular tachycardia, suggests that the anatomic substrate for late potentials is diseased tissue. Obviously, a transmural infarction may show no abnormal activation pattern because such tissue is electrically silent. However, tissue immediately adjacent to the infarction contains viable myocardium interspersed with fibrotic tissue [45, 46]. Such tissue may result in fragmentation of the propagating electro-motive forces with the consequent development of high-frequency components [46, 47].

Though data on the presence, duration and/or frequency content of late potentials in patients with documented sustained ventricular tachycardia are of value for characterization of these patients, the most essential question that may lead to a more wide-spread use of signal-averaging is whether the prognosis of patients with coronary artery disease can be predicted. Thus, only prospective studies in well-defined populations at risk of ventricular tachyarrhythmias can give the ultimate answer. Our inital experience in 160 patients who were studied prospectively after recent myocardial infarction (medium day of study 24.5) suggested that averaging might indeed be a promising non-invasive technique for the identification of patients prone to ventricular tachycardia or possibly even sudden death [10].

The present prospective sudy of 628 patients using high-gain amplification, appropriate filtering, and visual analysis of surface ECGs is an extension of this previous study. It has shown that the presence of ventricular late potentials at the end of the QRS-complex or within the ST-segment can be considered as an indicator for subsequent occurrence of sudden cardiac death or sustained symptomatic ventricular tachycardia in patients with coronary artery disease. Not only the mere presence of late potentials, but also their duration was of prognostic significance. Furthermore, the site of myocardial infarction was a determining factor whether a patient with late potentials will subsequently develop arrhythmic events. Other factors such as the degree of left ventricular dysfunction and the inducibility of ventricular arrhythmias using programmed ventricular stimulation played an additional role.

The correlation between the presence of late potentials and their duration and the subsequent occurrence of sudden death or sustained ventricular tachycardia, as demonstrated in the present study, suggests a causal relationship between late potentials and these arrhythmic events. The fact that ventricular late potentials within a given range of duration had a higher predictive value in patients with anterior versus inferior myocardial infarction is of significant clinical importance. This difference may be explained by the larger extent of most anterior wall myocardial infarctions, and the greater degree of subsequent left ventricular dysfunction. This is also suggested by the findings in patients in whom pulmonary artery pressure was measured during exercise. Those with an abnormal increase in mean pulmonary artery pressure during exercise reflecting a greater extent of left ventricular dysfunction, had the greatest chance for subsequently developing sudden death or sustained symptomatic ventricular tachycardia.

Only few other prospective studies on the significance of late potentials exist. A total of 1483 patients has been included in 5 prospective studies (including our

266

Table 2. Signal averaging in postmyocardial infarction patients – prognostic significance.

Authors	n	interval after MI	follow-up duration	prognostic value of late potentials (LP)			
Düsseldorf (1986)	628		39 ± 15.0 months (mean ± S.D.)	*cardiac mortality*		*sudden death*	*sust. VT*
	n = 258	≤1 month		no LP	4.5%	1.6%	0.8%
	n = 52	2 months		<40 ms	7.3%	5.2%	1.6%
	n = 60	3–12 months		≥40 ms	12.1%	8.6%	13.8%
	n = 99	≥12 months					
	n = 159	no MI 6 to 8 weeks (rehabilitation group)					
von Leitner et al., (1983)	518		10 months (mean)	*LP*	*cardiac mortality*	*sudden death*	*sust. VT*
				absent	1.5%	0.9%	no
				present	7.3%	3.6%	event
Denniss et al., (1983)	110	7–28 days (mean 11)	2–12 months (means 5)	*LP*			
				absent	no		1.1%
				present	inf.		17.4%
Kacet et al., (1986)	104	no inf.	8.5 ± 4 months 6–15	*LP*			
				absent	no	0%	4.5%
				present	inf.	13%	28.9%
Kucher et al., (1985)	123	10 days	3–12 months	*LP*	*arrhythmic event* (sudden death or symptomatic VT)		
				absent	1.4%		
				present	20.5%		
total	1483						

own study), the results of which have not yet been completely published (Table 2). Patients in the early and late post-myocardial infarction period as well as patients without previous myocardial infarction were included. In one study [40], only patients who were referred to a rehabilitation program were included. The duration of follow-up ranged from 2 months to 39 months (mean). The end points in these studies differed. As far as the data were reported, the presence (and duration) of late potentials showed a positive correlation to cardiac mortality, sudden death mortality and to the subsequent occurrence of sustained symptomatic ventricular tachycardia. Sustained ventricular tachycardia and sudden death occurred more frequently in patients with anterior versus inferior wall myocardial infarction (Figures 2 and 3).

One of the apparent limitations of ventricular late potentials is the great number of false-positive results. That means that even if patients have ventricular late potentials, their chance for subsequently developing an arrhythmic event is still relatively small, although several times greater than in those without late potentials. In contrast, the lack of late potentials predicts an uneventful course during follow-up. A similar problem exists with long-term ECG recording which, though sensitive, also has a large proportion of false-positive results [48–50]. Therefore, there is a need for further parameters that may help to increase the predictive value of late potentials, and reduce the number of false-positive findings. One such parameter may be the use of programmed ventricular stimulation as has been suggested recently [41]. By combining various parameters, such as the duration of the induced ventricular tachyarrhythmia and its rate, the predictive value of late potentials can be increased. Thus, risk stratification of patients with coronary artery disease, mainly those after myocardial infarction, should include several parameters such as the size and location of the myocardial infarction, the interval after infarction, spontaneous ventricular arrhythmias during long-term ECG recording, the absence or presence of ventricular late potentials, and the results of programmed ventricular stimulation.

Acknowledgements

We acknowledge technical assistance by Petra Helmig (MTA), stud. med. Sven Kielgas, stud. rer. nat. Eugen Keim, and Ing. grad. K. Balkenhoff.

This work was supported by a grant from the Sonderforschungsbereich 30 (Kardiologie), and the Sonderforschungsbereich 242 (Koronare Herzkrankheit – Prophylaxe und Therapie akuter Komplikationen) of the Deutsche Forschungsgemeinschaft, Bonn-Bad Godesberg, (Germany, F.R.), the Johann A. Wülfing-Stiftung (Düsseldorf, Germany), and the Ernst und Berta-Grimmke-Stiftung (Düsseldorf, Germany).

268

References

1. Berbari EJ, Scherlag BJ, Hope RR, Lazzara R. 1978. Recording from the body surface of arrhythmogenic ventricular activity during ST segment. Am J Cardiol 41: 697–702.
2. Breithardt G, Becker R, Seipel L, Abendroth R-R, Ostermeyer J. 1981. Noninvasive detection of late potentials in man – a new marker for ventricular tachycardia. Eur Heart J 2: 1–11.
3. Hombach V, Höpp H-W, Braun V, Behrenbeck DW, Tauchert M, Hilger HH. 1980. Die Bedeutung von Nachpotentialen innerhalb des ST-Segmentes im Oberflächen-EKG bei Patienten mit koronarer Herzkrankheit. Dtsch med Wschr 195: 1457–62.
4. Rozanski JJ, Mortara D, Myerburg RJ, Castellanos A. 1981. Body surface detection of delayed depolarizations in patients with recurrent ventricular tachycardia and left ventricular aneurysm. Circulation 63: 1172–8.
5. Simson MB. 1981. Identification of patients with ventricular tachycardia after myocardial infarction from signals in the terminal QRS complex. Circulation 64: 235–42.
6. Uther JB, Dennett CJ, Tan A. 1978. The detection of delayed activation signals of low amplitude in the vectorcardiogram of patients with recurrent ventricular tachycardia by signal averaging. In: Sandoe E, Julian DG, Dell JW, eds. Management of ventricular tachycardia – role of mexiletine. Amsterdam: Excerpta Medica: 80–2.
7. Fontaine G, Frank R, GallaisHamonno F, Allali I, Phan-Tuc H, Grosgogeat. 1978. Electrocardiographie des potentiels tradifs du syndrome de post-excitation. Arch Mal Coeur 71: 854–64.
9. Simson MB, Untereker WJ, Spielman SR et al. 1983. Relation between late potentials on the body surface and directly recorded fragmented electrocardiograms in patients with ventricular tachycardia. Am J Cardiol 51: 105.
9. Breithardt G, Borggrefe M, Karbenn U, Abendroth R-R, Yeh HL, Seipel L. 1982. Prevalence of late potentials in patients with and without ventricular tachycardia: Correlation with angiographic findings. Am J Cardiol 49: 1932–7.
10. Breithardt G, Schwarzmaier J, Borggrefe M, Haerten K, Seipel L. 1983. Prognostic significance of ventricular late potentials after acute myocardial infarction. Eur Heart J 4: 487–95.
11. Breithardt G, Borggrefe M, Quantius B, Karbenn U, Seipel L. 1983. Ventricular vulnerability assessed by programmed ventricular stimulation in patients with and without late potentials. Circulation 68: 275–81.
12. Höpp HW, Hombach V, Braun V, Behrenbeck DW, Tauchert M, Hilger HH. 1981. Kammerarrhythmien und ventrikuläre Spätdepolarisationen bei akutem Myokardinfarkt. Z Kardiol 70: 319 (Abstr.).
13. Simson M, Spielman S, Horowitz L, Josephson M, Harken A, Kastor J. 1981. Slow ventricular activation detected on the body surface in patients with ventricular tachycardia after myocardial infarction. Am J Cardiol 47: 498 (Abstr.).
14. Denes P, Santarelli P, Hauser RG, Uretz EF. 1983. Quantitative analysis of the high frequency components of the terminal portion of the body surface QRS in normal subjects and in patients with ventricular tachycardia. Circulation 67: 1129–38.
15. Poll DS, Marchlinski FE, Falcone RA, Simson MB. 1984. Abnormal signal averaged ECG in nonischemic congestive cardiomyopathy: Relationship to sustained ventricular tachyarrhythmias. Circulation 70 (Suppl II): II—253.
16. Kertes PJ, Glabus M, Murray A, Julian DG, Campbell RWF. 1984. Delayed ventricular depolarization – correlation with ventricular activation and relevance to ventricular fibrillation in acute myocardial infarction. Eur Heart J 5: 974–83.
17. Haberl R, Hoffmann E, Steinbeck G. 1985. Low-frequency components in patients with delayed ventricular activation. Circulation 72: Suppl III–6.
17a. Freedman RA, Gillis AM, Kern A, Sonderholm-Difatte V, Mason JW. 1985. Signal-averaged electrocardiographic late potentials in patients with ventricular fibrillation or ventricular tachycardia: correlation with clinical arrhythmia and electrophysiologic study. Am J Cardiol 55: 1350–53.

18. Kanovsky MS, Falcone RA, Dresden CA, Josephson ME, Simson MB. 1984. Identification of patients with ventricular tachycardia after myocardial infarction: Signal averaged electrocardiogram. Holter monitoring, and cardiac catheterization. Circulation 70: 264–70.

19. Buxton AE, Simson MB, Falcone R et al. 1984. Signal averaged ECG in patients with nonsustained ventricular tachycardia: Identification of patients with potential for sustained ventricular arrhythmias. JACC 3: 495 (Abstr.).

20. Cain ME, Ambos HO, Witowski FX, Sobel BE. 1984. Fast-Fourier transform analysis of signal-averaged electrocardiograms for identification of patients prone to sustained ventricular tachycardia. Circulation 69: 711–20.

21. Cain ME, Ambos HD, Markham J, Fisher AE, Sobel BE. 1985. Quantification of differences in frequency content of signal-averaged electrocardiograms in patients with compared to those without sustained ventricular tachycardia. Am J Cardiol 55: 1500–05.

22. Denniss AR, Holley LK, Cody DV et al. 1983. Ventricular tachycardia and fibrillation: Differences in ventricular activation times and ventricular function. J Am Coll Cardiol 1: 606 (Abstr.).

23. Borggrefe M, Karbenn U, Breithardt G. 1982. Spätpotentiale und elektrophysiologische Befunde bei ventrikulären Tachykardien. Z Kardiol 71: 627 (Abstr.).

24. Edvardsson N, Hirsch I, Pettersson A-S, Olsson SB. 1984. Noninvasive recording of continuous diastolic electrical activity during ventricular tachycardia. Circulation 4: 487–95 (Abstr.).

25. Simson MB, Falcone RA, Dresden CA, Josephson ME. 1984. Late potentials in anterior versus inferior myocardial infarction: J Am Coll Cardiol 3: 624 (Abstr.).

26. Breithardt G, Borggrefe M, Karbenn U, Schwarzmaier J. 1986. Effects of pharmacological and non-pharmacological interventions on ventricular late potentials. Eur Heart J (in press).

27. Simson MB, Spielman SR, Horowitz LN et al. 1982. Effects of antiarrhythmic drugs on body surface late potentials in patients with ventricular tachycardia. Am J Cardiol 49: 1030 (Abstr.).

28. Denniss AR, Ross DL, Cody DV, Ho B, Russell PA, Young AA. 1984. Effect of antiarrhythmic therapy on delayed potentials in patients with ventricular tachycardia (Abstr.) JACC 3: 495.

29. Höpp HW, Deutsch H, Hombach V, Braun V, Hilger HH. 1982. Medikamentöse Beeinflußbarkeit ventrikulärer Spätpotentiale. H Z Kardiol 71: 206 (Abstr.).

30. Jauerning RA, Senges J, Langfelder W et al. 1983. Effect of antiarrhythmic drugs on ventricular late potentials at sinus rhythm and at constant heart rate. In: Cardiac pacing. Eds.: Steinbach K, Glogar D, Laszkovics A. Scheiblhofer W, Weber H. Steinkopff Verlag: 767–72.

31. Cain ME, Ambos HD, Fischer AE, Markham J, Schechtmann KB. 1984. Noninvasive prediction of antiarrhythmic drug efficacy in patients with sustained ventricular tachycardia from frequency analysis of signal averaged ECGs. Circulation 70 (Suppl II): II—252.

32. Simson MB, Falcone R, Kindwall E. 1985. The signal averaged electrocardiogram does not predict antiarrhythmic drug success. Circulation 72: Suppl III-7.

33. Breithardt G, Borggrefe M, Karbenn U et al. 1982. Verhalten ventrikulärer Spätpotentiale nach operativer Therapie ventrikulärer Tachykardien. Z Kardiol 71: 381–6.

34. Breithardt G, Seipel L, Ostermeyer J et al. 1982. Effects of antiarrhythmic surgery on late ventricular potentials recorded by precordial signal averaging in patients with ventricular tachycardia. Am Heart J 104: 996–1003.

35. Simson MB, Spielman SR, Horowitz LN, Falcone RA, Harken AH, Josephson ME. 1981. Effects of surgery for control of ventricular tachycardia on late potentials. Circulation 64 (Suppl IV): IV–88.

36. Marcus NH, Falcone RA, Harken AL, Josephson ME, Simson MB. 1984. Body surface late potentials: effects of endocardial resection in patients with ventricular tachycardia. Circulation 70: 632–7.

37. Oeff M, von Leitner E-R, Brüggemann T, Andresen D, Sthapit R, Schröder R. 1982 Methodische Probleme bei der Registrierung ventrikulärer Spätpotentiale. Z Kardiol 71: 204 (Abstr.).

38. Oeff M, von Leitner ER, Sthapit R et al. 1983. Methods for noninvasive detection of ventricular late potentials – a comparative multicenter study. In: Steinbach K, Glogar D, Laszkovics A,

Scheiblhofer W, Weber H eds. Cardiac Pacing. Darmstadt: Steinkopff Verlag: 641–7.

39. Karbenn U, Breithardt G, Borggrefe M, Simson MB. 1985. Automatic identification of late potentials. J Electrocardiol 18: 123–34.

40. von Leitner ER, Oeff M, Loock D, Jahns B, Schröder R. 1983. Value of noninvasively detected delayed ventricular dpolarization to predict prognosis in post myocardial infarction patients. Circulation 68 (Suppl III): III—83.

41. Breithardt G, Borggrefe M, Haerten K. 1985. Role of programmed ventricular stimulation and noninvasive recording of ventricular late potentials for the identification of patients at risk of ventricular tachyarrhythmias after acute myocardial infarction. In: Zipes DP, Jalife J. Cardiac electrophysiology and arrhythmias. Grune and Stratton: 553–61.

42. Spielman SR, Untereker WJ, Horowitz LN et al. 1981. Fragmented electrical activity – relationship to ventricular tachycardia. Am J Cardiol 47: 448 (Abstr.).

43. Klein H, Karp RB, Kouchoukos NT, James TN, Waldo AL. 1979. Ventricular mapping of abnormal myocardiun in patients with and without arrhythmias. Circulation (Suppl): II–24 (Abstr.).

44. Wiener I, Mindich B, Pitchon R. 1984. Endocardial activation in patients with coronary artery disease: Effects of regional contraction abnormalities. Am Heart J 107: 1146.

45. Daniel T, Boineau J, Sabiston D. 1971. Comparision of human ventricular activation with canine model in myocardial infarction. Circulation 44: 74–89.

46. Gardner PI, Ursell PC, Fenoglio JJ, Wit AL. 1985. Electrophysiologic and anatomic basis for fractionated eectrograms recorded from healed myocardial infarcts. Circulation 72: 596–611.

47. Ideker RE, Mirvis DM, Smith WM. 1985. Late fractionated potentials. Am J Cardiol 55: 1614–21.

48. Moss AJ. 1980. Clinical significance of ventricular arrhythmias in patients with and without artery disease. Prog Cardiovasc Dis 23: 33–52.

49. Cats VM, Lie KI, van Capelle FJL, Durrer D. 1979. Limitations of 24 hour ambulatory electrocardiographic recording in predicting coronary events after acute myocardial infarction. Am J Cardiol 44: 1257–62.

50. van Durme JP, Pannier RH. 1976. Prognostic significance of ventricular dysrhythmias 1 year after myocardial infarction. Am J Cardiol 37: 178 (Abstr.).

51. Kuchar D, Thorburn C, Sammel N. 1985. Natural history and clinical significance of late potentials after myocardial infarction. Circulation 72: Suppl. III–477.

52. Denniss AR, Cody DV, Fenton SM et al. Significance of delayed activation potentials in survivors of myocardial infarction. J Am Coll Cardiol 1983; 1: 582 (Abstr)

53. Kacet S, Libersa C, Caron J, Boudoux B, d'Haute Feuille X, Marchand J, Dagano J, Lekieffre J. The prognostic value of averaged late potentials inpatients suffering from coronary artery disease. Abstracts of the international symposium 'Ventricular Techycardies' May 1986.

20. The contribution of electrophysiologic techniques to the diagnosis of ventricular tachycardia

P. TOUBOUL*, G. KIRKORIAN, P. LAVAUD, G. ATALLAH,
and J.R. KIENY
* *Hôpital Cardiovasculaire et Pneumologique Louis Pradel, BP Lyon Montchat,
69394 Lyon Cedex 03, France*

Clinical electrophysiology has greatly developed over the past twenty years. Various techniques have been proposed to explore the electrical phenomena of the human heart. Catheter recording of the electrical activity of the His bundle was a decisive step in this evolution [1]. At the same time electrical stimulation of the heart began to be routinely performed in patients with cardiac arrhythmias. Initially, these techniques were applied almost exclusively to supraventricular tachycardias. Re-entrant junctional tachycardias have been the subject of numerous publications. The ability to initiate and terminate such tachycardias by electrical cardiac stimulation was considered evidence of the intervention of a circus movement. The possible role of atrioventricular accessory pathways in the formation of the excitation circuit was demonstrated. A few years later, electrophysiologic studies annexed the field of ventricular tachycardias. Admittedly, intracardiac techniques had occasionally been utilized to identify the origin of wide QRS complexes [2]. Wellens et al. in 1972 were the first to report observations of ventricular arrhythmias in man which could be initiated and terminated by electrical stimulation of the heart [3]. In most cases the patients had a history of myocardial infarction. From then on electrophysiologic investigation of ventricular tachycardias steadily gained ground. Research programs on sudden death created renewed interest in ventricular arrhythmias. Simultaneously new treatments, antiarrhythmic drugs and various surgical procedures, made their appearance. The utilization of clinical electrophysiology to guide therapy has become increasingly popular.

We shall only consider the contribution of these techniques to the diagnosis of ventricular tachycardia. This field covers: 1) the differentiation of ventricular tachycardia from supraventricular tachycardia with wide QRS complexes: 2) the identification of patients with previous ventricular tachyarrhythmias: 3) the elucidation of the underlying mechanism of the tachycardia: 4) the localization of the site of the origin.

Identification of ventricular tachycardia from supraventricular tachycardia with wide QRS complexes

During regular tachycardias, wide QRS complexes should first of all suggest a ventricular origin. However, a supraventricular arrhythmia may be involved as various mechanisms are able to produce aberrant QRS complexes. Thus, a preexisting bundle branch block will persist during a supraventricular tachycardia accounting for the QRS anomaly. An intraventricular conduction disorder occasionnally results from the rapid rhythm. The cardiac impulse, on arriving in the ventricles, is blocked in some portions of the His-Purkinje system which have not recovered (phase 3 block). The maintenance of the bundle branch block can be related to concealed retrograde conduction in the blocked branch. Moreover, in some tachyarrhythmias associated with the Wolff-Parkinson-White syndrome, conduction to the ventricles occurs via the atrioventricular accessory pathway. QRS enlargement demonstrates ventricular preexcitation. Mahaim fibers have also been invoked in the genesis of aberrant tachycardia complexes.

Two electrocardographic criteria may clinch the diagnosis of a ventricular tachycardia: 1) slower and/or dissociated atrial activity; 2) fusion or capture beats. Unfortunately these signs are not always manifest. The utilization of electrophysiologic techniques is indispensable when doubt subsists as therapy is based on a correct diagnosis of the arrhythmia.

Catheter recording of atrial activity

This can be achieved by the utilization of esophageal leads [4]. An electrode catheter is advanced 35 to 40 mm into the esophagus so that its extremity is positioned just behind the left atrium. Although this procedure is poorly tolerated, it is still utilized as it is easy to carry out, and does not require any sophisticated equipment. In intensive care units right heart catheterization is generally performed. The catheter is introduced percutaneously into the internal jugular, sub-clavian, basilic or femoral vein. Its progression is verified by fluoroscopy. At its distal tip there can be one electrode or several with a 1 cm inter-electrode distance. Esophageal or intraatrial recordings are either uni or bipolar. Atrial and ventricular deflections can be detected. The tallest generally correspond to atrial activity. The utilization of multiple electrode catheters permits comparison of activation times in upper, middle or lower atrium and the identification of the mode of atrial depolarization. Thus, sinus or retrograde activation and all atrial tachyarrhythmias can be recognized. Synchronous recordings from surface leads are required to analyse the relationship between the atriograms and the QRS complexes.

Ventricular tachycardia is frequently associated with slower atrial rhythm. This can be composed of sinus P waves, ectopic P waves or P waves related to

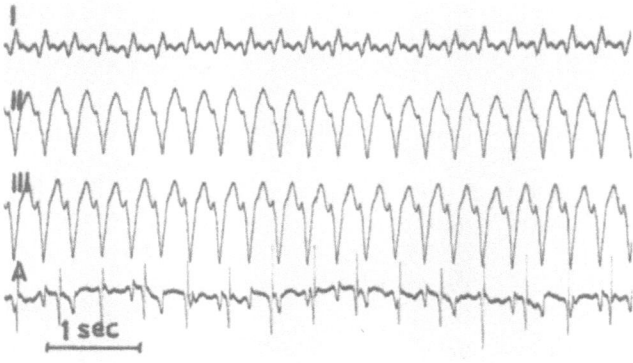

Figure 1. Ventricular tachycardia at a rate of 185 beats/min. The right atrial lead (A) shows atrioventricular dissociation.

ventriculoatrial conduction with intermittent retrograde block (Fig. 1). Occasionally, an atrial tachyarrhythmia is revealed whose rate exceeds that of the ventricles. The absence of a simple arithmetical ratio (2 : 1, for example) between atrial and ventricular beats would exclude a supraventricular origin of the QRS complexes. During regular tachycardia, atrial fibrillation is usually a reliable index of atrioventricular dissociation (Fig. 2). Nonetheless, in this case the ventricular activity can exceptionally emerge from an atrial zone isolated by an intraatrial block. Figure 3 shows a regular tachycardia during a Wolff-Parkinson-White syndrome due to a 2 : 1 flutter in the left atrium with simultaneous fibrillation in the right atrium. Lastly, the recording of atrial and ventricular activities with similar rates is always perplexing. When this is observed it can just as well correspond to a supraventricular mechanism (atrial or junctional) as to as ventricular tachycardia with 1 : 1 retrograde conduction to the atria. The purpose of the diagnostic tests is to demonstrate the independence of the tachycardia as regards the atrial activation. Carotid sinus massage or intravenous administration of ATP can suppress atrial activation temporarily (by retrograde nodal block) without any modification of the ventricular rate (Fig. 4). Occasionally, the use of antiarrhythmic drugs can also produce an intermittent retrograde block during the tachycardia or even complete atrioventricular dissociation.

Therefore, a tachycardia with wide QRS complexes independent of the atria will almost certainly be ventricular. The exceptions are rare. Tachycardias arising in the His bundle and dissociated from the atria by a retrograde nodal block must be mentioned in this respect. If they are associated with an intraventricular conduction disturbance, they can mimic ventricular arrhythmias. Another exception concerns infranodal reciprocating tachycardia with participating Mahaim fibers. According to the direction of the circus movement, the enlargement of the QRS complexes can be related to ventricular preexcitation or to a bundle branch

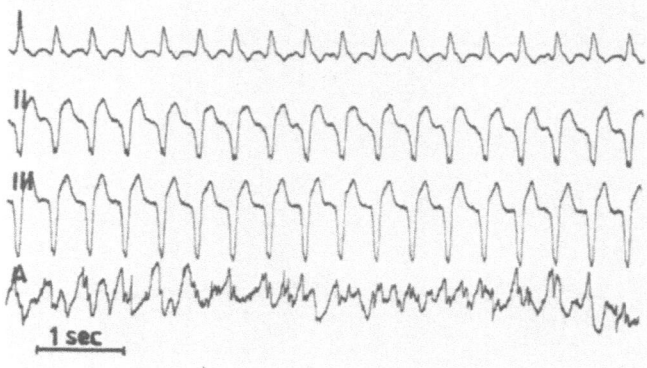

Figure 2. Ventricular tachycardia at 145 beats/min. The right atrial lead shows the coexistence of atrial fibrillation.

block. The atrioventricular node located between the excitation loop and the atria might be the cause of retrograde block.

The effect of competitive atrial pacing

The technique consists of electrically pacing the atria at a rate superior to that of the spontaneous tachycardia [5]. Stimulation of the right atrium is generally performed. The utilization of esophageal pacing has also been reported [6].

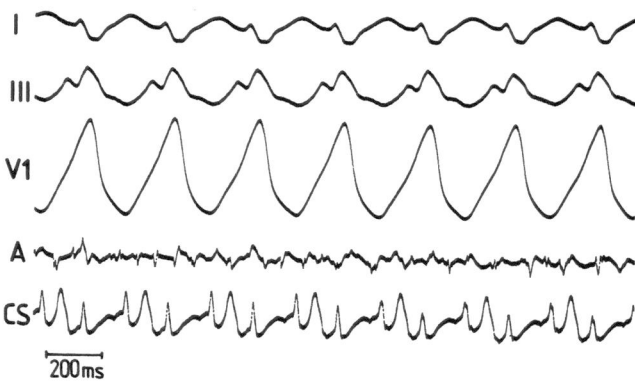

Figure 3. Atrial tachyarrythmia during a type A Wolf-Parkinson-White syndrome. Atrial fibrillation is recorded within the right atrium. The ventricular response is regular at 200 beats/min. Left atrial recordings obtained by catheterizing the coronary sinus provide an explanation. A regular tachyarrhythmia at 400/min is present in the left atrium. There is an atrial dissociation. The ventricular response is dependent on the left atrium where the accessory pathway is inserted. The left atrial tachycardia is associated with a 2 : 1 atrioventricular block. Abbreviation: CS : coronary sinus lead.

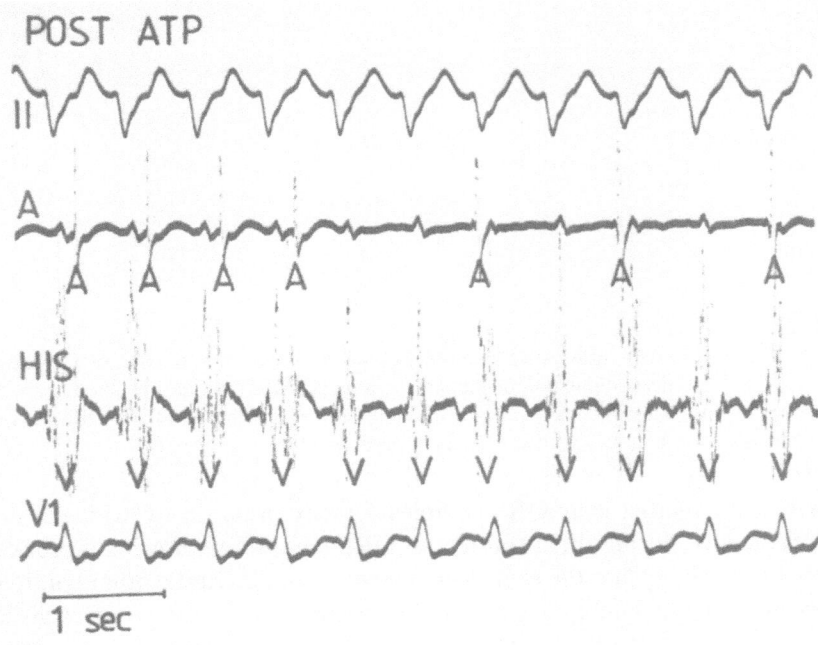

Figure 4. Ventricular tachycardia with a 1:1 atrial activity related to retrograde conduction. Intravenous administration of ATP results in a ventriculo-atrial block. The ventricular rate remains unchanged. Abbreviation: HIS: His bundle lead.

During ventricular tachycardia the wide QRS complexes are replaced by more rapid beats with a supraventricular pattern (Fig. 5). Thus the aberrant morphology of the tachycardia QRS complexes can no longer be attributed to a bundle branch block accompanying a supraventricular rhythm. Rapid atrial pacing artificially provokes ventricular captures. It is utilized in addition to atrial recordings and is essential in tachycardias with wide QRS complexes associated with 1:1 atrial activity. However, the normalization of QRS following atrial pacing can be interpreted in more than one way. Such response could be related to the suppression of ventricular prexcitation. The pacing rate would induce conduction block within accessory pathways (Fig. 6). It can also be surmised that during supraventricular tachyarrhythmias with bundle branch block the increase in cardiac frequency normalizes the QRS complexes by producing supernormal conduction in the blocked branch or by delaying the transmission of the impulse in the contralateral branch. Another explanation implies the concept of ventricular aberrancy due to asynchonous impulse transmission from a hisian focus. The conduction of atrial impulses could normalize the QRS complexes by homogenizing the His bundle depolarization. Despite these restrictions the appearance of normal QRS complexes identical to sinus beats during competitive atrial pacing

276

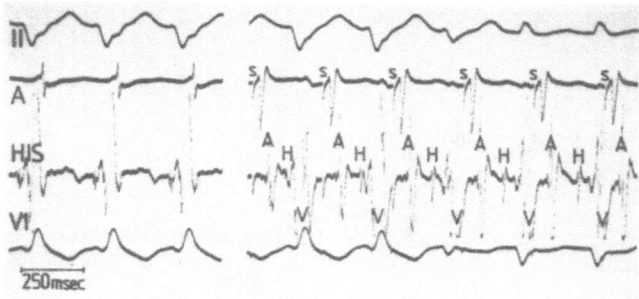

Figure 5. Ventricular tachycardia with a 1 : 1 retrograde conduction to the atria. The tachycardia rate is 200 beats/min. Electrical stimulation of the atria at a higher rate (250/min) is able to capture the ventricular activity. This phenomenon is associated with normalization of the QRS complexes. Simultaneously a His bundle potential appears 50 ms befre QRS.

strongly suggests that wide QRS complexes tachycardia is of ventricular origin. The occurrence during the atrial test of QRS complexes showing a preexisting bundle branch block has the same significance (Fig. 7). On the other hand, in the absence of any QRS anomaly, wide paced complexes differing from tachycardia beats are more difficult to interpret. The diagnosis of capture with aberrant conduction is the most feasible. However, when a pattern suggestive of alternating bundle branch block is observed one cannot exclude the possibility of a supraventricular tachycardia with abnormal QRS complexes due to slow con-

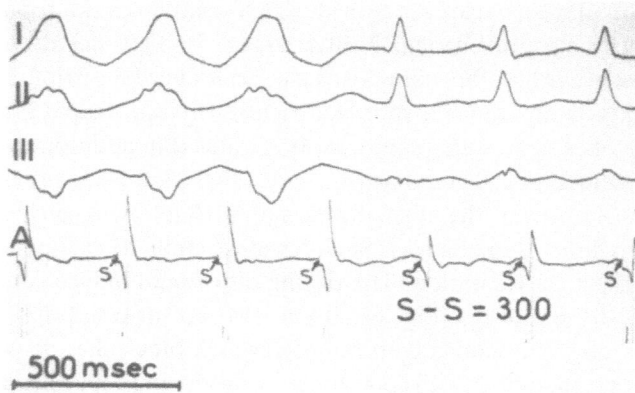

Figure 6. Junctional reentrant tachycardia with aberrant conduction. The cardiac impulse is conducted to the ventricles by nodo-ventricular accessory fibers and then travels retrogradly along the A-V node-His pathway (same patient as in figure 14). The tachycardia rate is 175 beats/min. Electrical stimulation of the atria at 200/min is followed by an early preexcited beat. Then there is normalization of the QRS complexes. A conduction block has occurred within the Mahaim fibers. The paced atrial impulses are conducted to the ventricles through the normal pathways only.

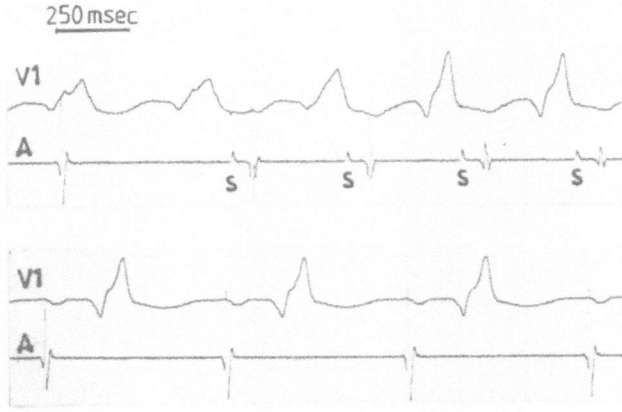

Figure 7. Ventricular tachycardia with atrioventricular dissociation. Rapid atrial pacing at 150 beats/min is followed by ventricular captures. The paced QRS complexes are aberrant because of a preexisting right bundle branch block (see lower recording during sinus rhythm).

duction in a bundle branch during which the atrial overdrive produces a more marked blockade in the opposite branch.

Atrial stimulation during tachycardia can also increase ventricular rate without altering QRS morphology. Supraventricular arrhythmia should be involved since tachycardia beats are reproduced by atrial impulses conducted to the ventricles (Fig. 8). But a ventricular mechanism is still possible (Fig. 9). This is the case when the abnormal excitation is propagated exclusively from a bundle branch. Thus, in bundle branch reentry the cardiac impulse reaches the ventricular myocardium through a bundle branch and returns to the common bundle via the other. Paced atrial beats could very well take the same route resulting in identical QRS complexes but at a more rapid rate. A similar response can occur when the tachycardia arises from a focus at the origin of a bundle branch and there is a conduction block in the other.

Finally, there are some cases in which competitive atrial pacing has no effect. Infranodal tachycardia can be postulated, the absence of ventricular capture being related to block within the atrioventricular junction. Electrical stimulation of the His bundle can then be envisaged [7]. This procedure circumvents the atrioventricular nodal obstacle. It can also be utilized in cases of rapid atrial rhythm making stimulation of the atria ineffective. Hisian overdrive is generally difficult to perform. Interpretation of the results is the same as that following atrial pacing. Nonetheless, it has been demonstrated that His bundle stimulation could normalize intraventricular conduction in patients with bundle branch block, which somewhat reduces the significance of the test [8].

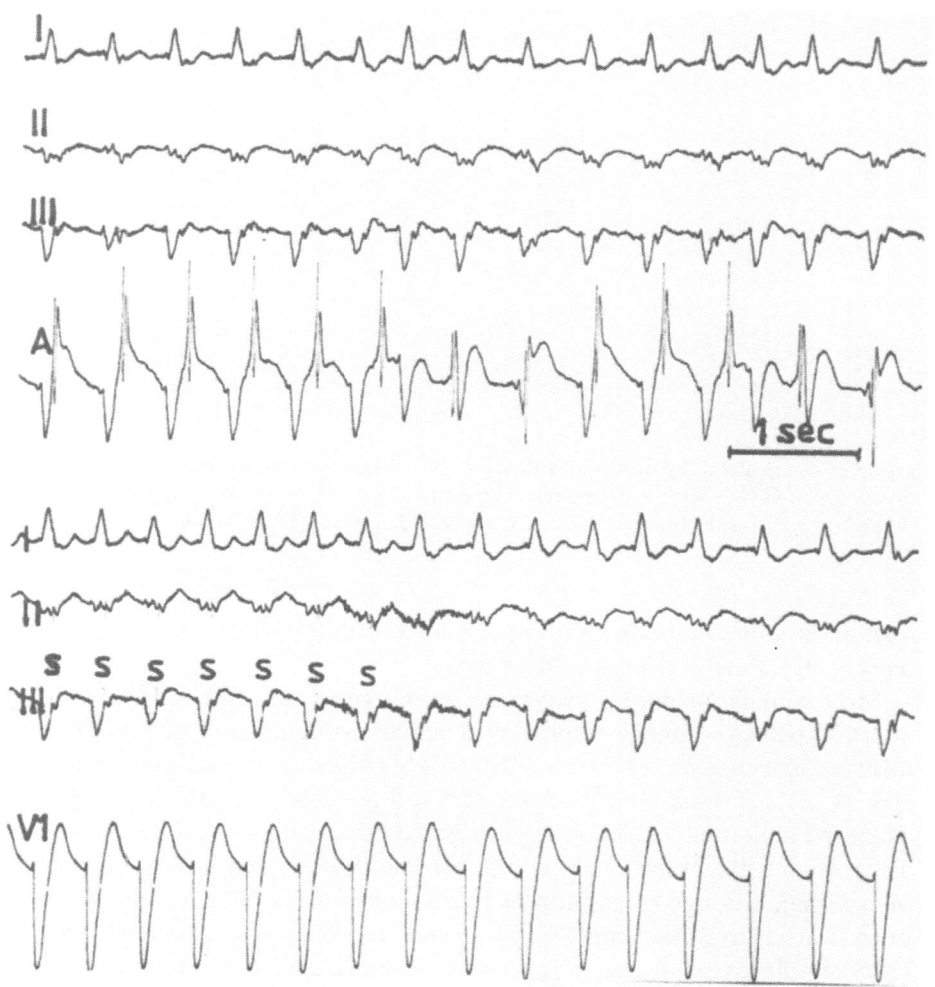

Figure 8. Irregular tachycardia with left bundle branch block pattern. The heart rate ranges from 120 to 150 beats/min. Recordings within the right atrium show a rather regular activity between 110 and 120/min Atricventricular dissociation is present. Electrical pacing of the atria at 150/min results in a regular ventricular response of the same rate. The pattern of the paced QRS complexes is unchanged (lower panel). Following cessation of pacing, the spontaneous arrhythmia resumes. A juntional tachycardia with atrioventricular dissociation and left bundle branch block is likely to be present. Digitalis toxicity could account for the irregular ventricular response.

His bundle recordings

His bundle recordings have greatly contributed to the diagnosis of tachyar-rhythmias with wide QRS complexes. Whenever a tachycardia has its origin

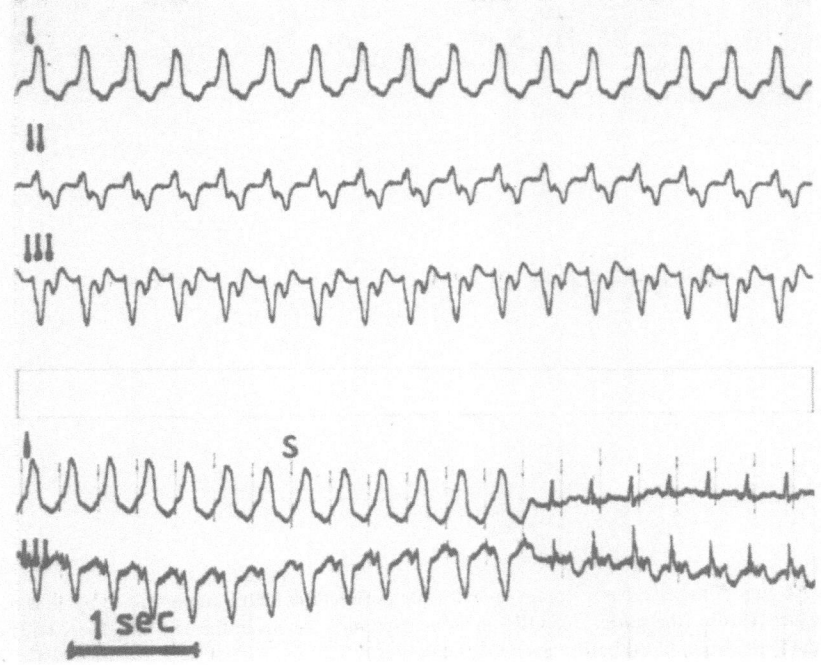

Figure 9. Ventricular tachycardia at 165 beats/min with retrograde conduction to the atria. In leads II and III inverted P waves are superimposed on the ST segment of the ventricular complexes. Electrical stimulation of the atria at 200/min results in transient entrainment of the tachycardia (lower panel). After a few seconds, the QRS complexes become normal. The interval between the stimulus artefact and the QRS complex is 0.24 s (for more details, see text).

above the His bundle bifurcation, and is therefore supraventricular, the impulse necessarily progresses via the common bundle to reach the ventricles. A His bundle deflection (H) precedes each QRS by at least 35 msec which is the minimum time required for conduction in the bundle branches (Fig. 10). Conversely, the excitation propagated from an abnormal ventricular zone spreads firstly into the surrounding myocardium before entering the atrioventricular junction retrogradely. The H potential is inscribed after the beginning of the QRS complex [9] (Fig. 11). It is often impossible to discern as it is buried in the ventriculogram. Should this problem arise the accurate positioning of the recording atheter must be verified. This can be done by fluoroscopy but correct placement is, above all, clearly demonstrated by the reappearance of the His potential during capture beats or following resumption of the sinus rhythm. During tachycardia the H potential may also reveal its presence intermittently following certain P waves wich occur late after the preceding QRS. In this case the effects of the concealed retrograde conduction resulting from ventricular depolarization have had time to fade permitting the atrioventricular node-His

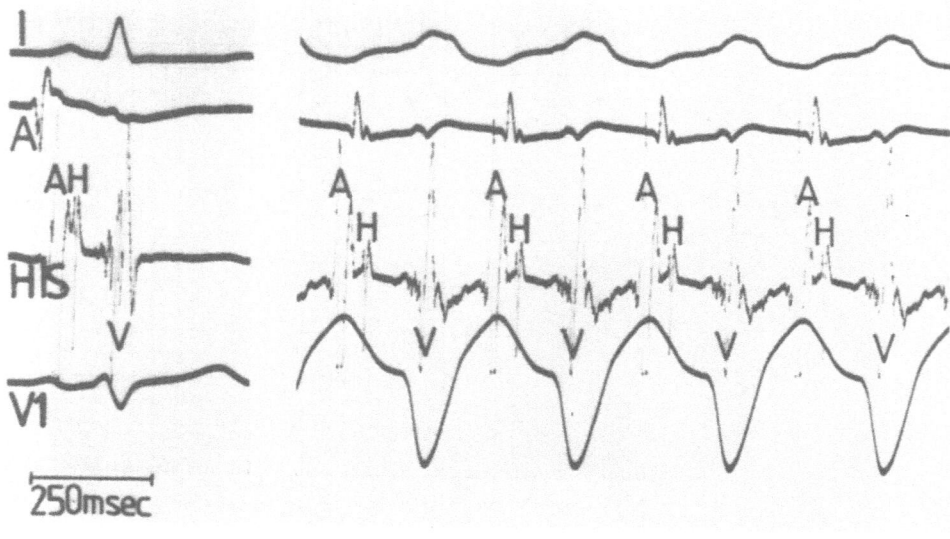

Figure 10. Junctional circus movement tachycardia. A functional left bundle branch block is present during tachycardia (the pattern of QRS in sinus rhythm is shown in the left panel). A His bundle potential is recorded 65 ms before each QRS complex.

pathway to popagate the atrial impulses. Exceptionally a retrograde block appears between the zone of tachycardia and the His bundle. Then the His bundle potential can be seen after the QRS complex, disappearing occasionally (second degree ventriculohisian block), or it remains linked to the dissociated atrial activity (complete retrograde block) (Fig. 12).

In fact, this mode of differentiating supraventricular arrhythmias from ventricular arrhythmias deserves further discussion. During supraventricular tachycardias the His bundle potential can be inscribed within the ventricular electrogram. This happens in atrial tachyarrhythmias associated with the Wolff-Parkinson-White syndrome during which conduction to the ventricles proceeds preferentially along the accessory pathway (Fig. 13). His bundle activity is also concealed in reciprocating tachycardias utilizing a circuit with antegrade impulse conduction through an accessory pathway (Kent or Mahaim bundle) and retrograde conduction via the atrioventricular node His pathway [10] (Fig. 14).

Recording of a His bundle potential prior to the QRS complex does not eliminate the possibility of a ventricular tachycardia. Abnormal activity arising close to the origin of the bundle branches can reach te common bundle before spreading to the ventricular myocardium. However, the H-V interval should be shorter than that seen in sinus rhythm. Irrespective of the site of origin of the tachycardia in the conduction tissue the presence of a block distal to the arrhythmogenic focus will have similar consequences. A ventricular tachycardia

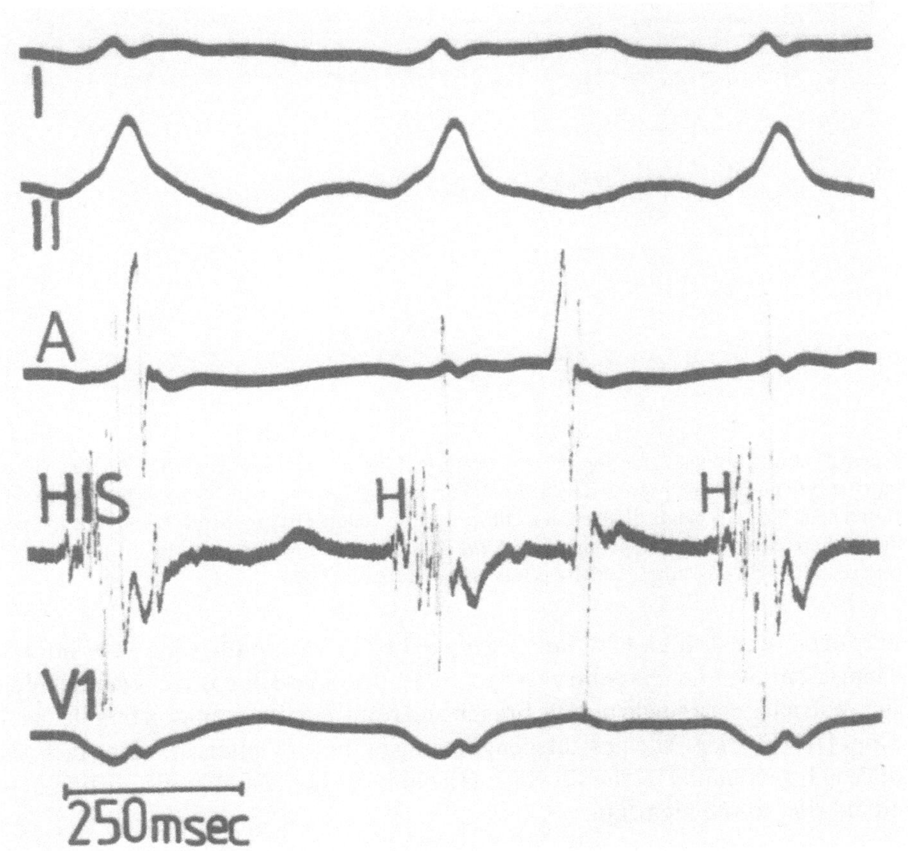

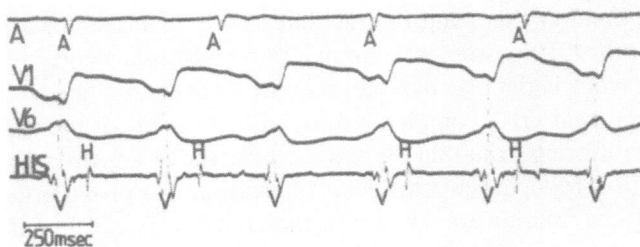

Figure 11. Ventricular tachycardia at 130 beats/min. The atrial activity is dissociated. The His bundle activity is recorded at the beginning of the QRS complex.

Figure 12. Ventricular tachycardia with atrioventricular dissociation. The His bundle recordings reveal a retrograde H deflection. This activity is not seen after the third and sixth beats. There is a second degree ventriculo-hisian block.

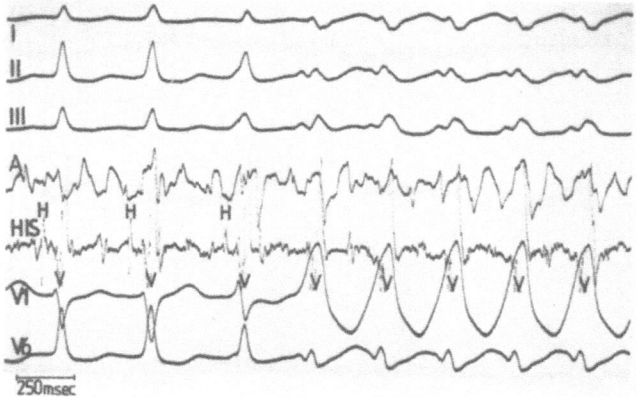

Figure 13. Atrial fibrillation during a type A Wolff-Parkinson-White syndrome. The first two vetricular beats are normal and preceded by a His bundle activity. (HV interval: 50 ms). The third beat is a fusion beat. The His bundle deflection is still visible, preceding QRS by 20 ms. During the following beats, there is exclusive conduction through the accessory pathway giving rise to a pattern of major preexcitation. No His bundle activity is then apparent before QRS.

may even occur with a H-V interval equal or superior to the sinus H-V interval. Thus in bundle branch reentry tachycardias, the circulating wave is conducted to the ventricles via a single bundle branch and returns to the common bundle via the other [11] (Fig. 15). The possible lengthening of the H-V interval during tachycardia can be explained by the slowing of the impulse in the antegrade portion of the circuit due to the high rate.

Identification of patients with previous ventricular tachycardia

We may have to identify ventricular arrhythmia from various symptoms (palpitation, dizziness or syncope), or from a previous history of tachycardia. Electrophysiologic studies are then carried out during sinus rhythm. Thus rapid atrial pacing performed at the same rate as that of the spontaneous arrhythmia can induce aberrant QRS complexes similar to tachycardia beats. A positive test favors a supraventricular origin of the tachycardia beats (Fig. 16). Conversely, the absence of aberrant QRS complexes during atrial pacing or the appearance of a deformation differing from that observed during the attack does not exclude this eventuality. Reproducing a ventricular aberration can prove arduous as it depends on critical relationships between the coupling interval of the first paced beat and the length of the preceding sinus cycles. Furthermore, a functional bundle branch block during tachycardia may only appear some time later (fatigue phenomenon). In other cases a second degree atrioventricular nodal block develops in response to atrial pacing and the ventricular frequency that is sought

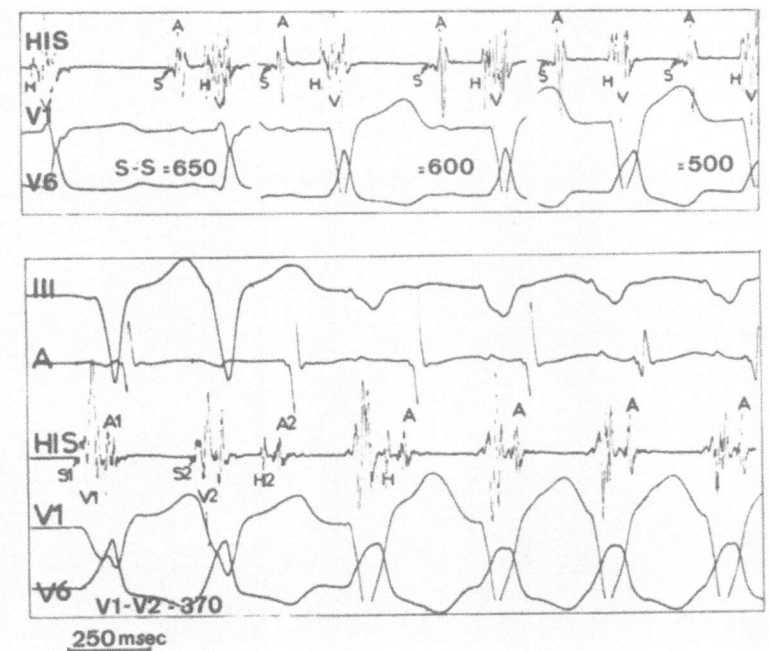

Figure 14. Ventricular preexcitation due to Mahaim fibers. The upper panel shows the response to rapid atrial pacing. The PR and AH intervals are increased. The His bundle activity is progressively included within the ventricular electrogram. Simultaneously the QRS complex is increasingly broadened. Premature ventricular stimulation (lower panel) results in a tachycardia with wide QRS complexes identical to those induced by atrial pacing. A retrograde His bundle activity can be seen after the first tachycardia beat. A 1 : 1 retrograde atrial response is present. A circus movement within the atroventricular junction is likely to occur. The circulating wave is conducted to the ventricles through the Mahaim fibers, then retrogradely travels along the His bundle. There is no His bundle activity before QRS. (Reproduced from Touboul et al. Br Heart J 40: 806, 1978.)

cannot be reached. Anyway, this result would make the hypothesis of a suprahisian arrhythmia most unlikely. His bundle stimulation would be then justified. We have aready mentioned its limitations.

Most important is the use of electrophysiologic testing to induce tachycardia. There are several modes of cardiac stimulation. Programmed stimulation of the atria is mainly used in the study of supraventricular arrhythmias. Only in rare cases it can provoke ventricular tachycardias [12]. Figure 17 shows a paroxysm of ventricular tachycardia elicited by premature atrial stimulation. Electrical stimulation of the ventricles is the usual way of inducing ventricular tachycardia. The production of premature ventricular depolarization is preferred to rapid pacing which is less effective (Fig. 18). The procedure consists of introducing a ventricular extrastimulus of increasing prematurity during sinus rhythm or regular ventricular pacing, the scanning of the cardiac cycle being limited by the ventricular

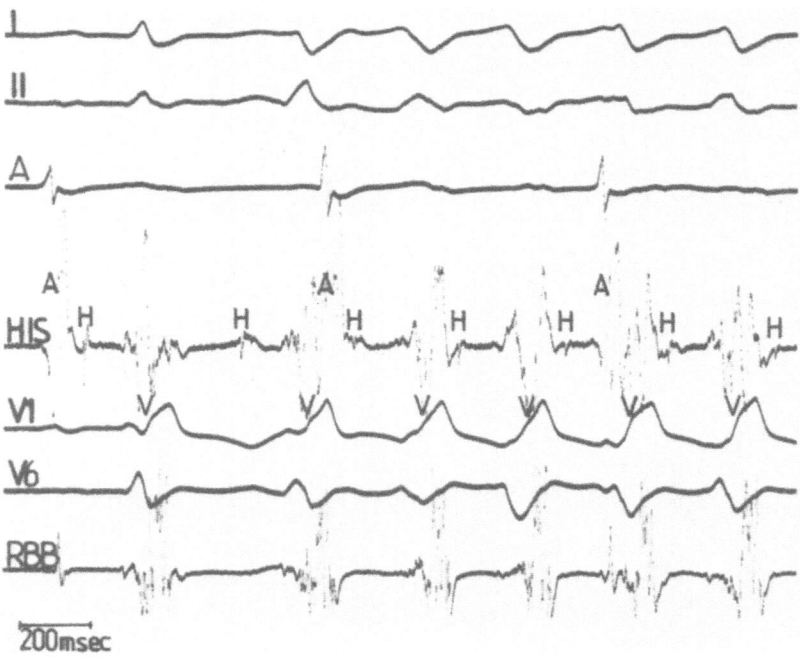

Figure 15. Bundle branch reentrant tachycardia. The tachycardia beats show a right bundle branch block pattern identical to that of the sinus beats. A His bundle potential precedes each QRS by 110 ms (same value as in sinus rhythm). The atrial activity is dissociated. Actually a His bundle tachycardia cannot be excluded. In this patient the evidence for bundle branch reentry was provided by the tachycardia suppression following electrical ablation of the right bundle branch. (Reproduced from Touboul et al. J Am Coll Cardiol 7, 1986.)

effective refractory period. Should this fail, the effect of two premature ventricular responses is studied. Then more rapid basic rates and three successive ventricular extrastimuli can be used. The apex of the right ventricle is the first stimulation site. In this way almost all inducible ventricular tachycardias can be reproduced. One rarely has to transfer the site of stimulation to the pulmonary infundibulum or to the left ventricle. If unsuccessful the electrophysiologic testing can be continued during isoprenaline infusion. Using this procedure, ventricular tachycardia can be induced in 80–90 per cent of patients with spontaneous episodes of sustained ventricular tachycardia. Conversely, when there is no history of ventricular arrhythmia, the testing is usually ineffective.

Elucidation of the tachycardia mechanism

A certain number of ventricular tachycardias can be initiated by electrical stim-

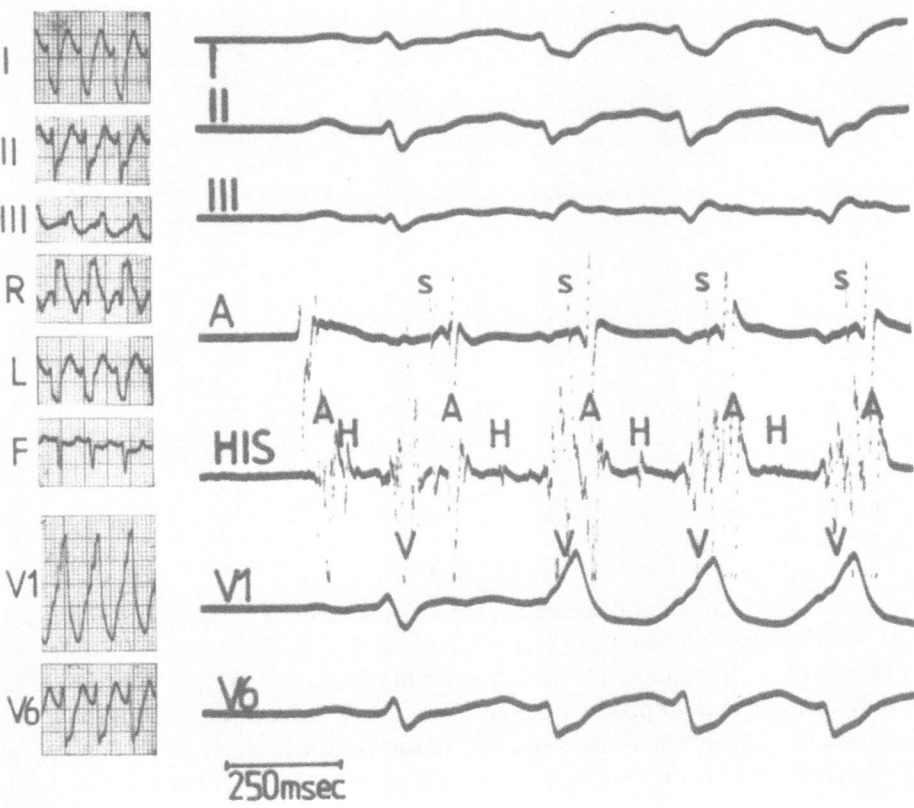

Figure 16. Regular tachycardia at 210 beats/min with wide QRS complexes exhibiting a right bundle branch block pattern (left panel). In this patient, the tachycardia could not be reproduced by the techniques of programmed cardiac stimulation. Rapid atrial pacing during sinus rhythm resulted in QRS complexes identical to those of the spontaneous arrhythmia (right panel). This result strongly suggests that the tachycardia is of supraventricular origin.

ulation of the heart. This response suggests a reentry mechanism. Such hypothesis is all the more likely as a majority of cases involve ischemic ventricular tachycardias associated with an old myocardial infarction [13]. The initiation of the arrhythmia is supposedly related to a critical slowing of conduction within the reentry circuit. This delay would allow the impulse, on return to its point of departure via a unidirectional block zone, to reach the tissues after recovery and to reexcite the heart. The inverse relationship between the V1-V2 coupling interval and the V2-V3 interval separating the premature response from the first tachycardia beat has been invoked in favor of a reentry mechanism [14]. It is postulated that the increased prematurity of the ventricular responses is accompanied by progressively slower conduction in the reentry zone with a corre-

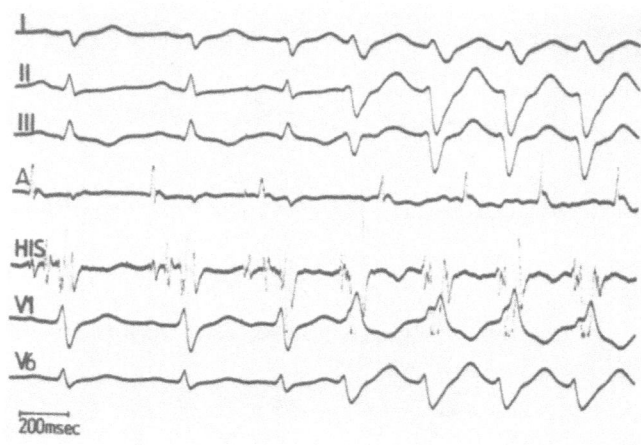

Figure 17. Ventricular tachycardia induced by premature stimulation of the right atrium. For more details see text.

sponding delay in the appearance of the ectopic beats. Transient entrainment of the tachycardia in response to rapid atrial stimulation also suggests the intervention of a reentry mechanim [15]. Atrial stimulation at higher rates than that of the tachycardia is able to produce stable fusion beats. It is assumed that the supraventricular impulses not only take part in the ventricular activation but also, by penetrating the reentry zone, reinitiate the circus movement and accelerate the emergence of the abnormal wave. This response is, however, exceptional. Endocardial mapping of the ventricles also supplies data in favor of a reentry mechanism. The technique, popularized by Josephson et al consists of recording local electrograms by catheter from various endocardial sites in the right and left ventricles [16]. The detection in an endocardial zone of a continuous electrical activity throughout the interval between two electrograms would indicate the presence of an underlying reentry circuit permanently traversed by the abnormal impulse [17] (Fig. 19). Termination of the tachycardia by premature or rapid ventricular stimulation provides further evidence for reentry (Fig. 18). Electrically induced activation is supposed to penetrate the circuit prematurely. Preceding the circulating wave, with which it collides, it meets a refractory state in the antegrade pathway, hence the cessation of reentry.

However, the effects of electrical stimulation of the heart can be interpreted differently. It has been demonstrated in isolated cardiac tissues showing diastolic oscillations of the membrane potential (oscillatory potentials) that an extrastimulus could initiate repetitive response [18]. Automatic activity then stops spontaneously or following premature electrical stimulation. Some ventricular arrhythmias in man would be related to trigered automatic activity. They exhibit the following charatetistics [19]: 1) the tachycardia is initiated following a critical

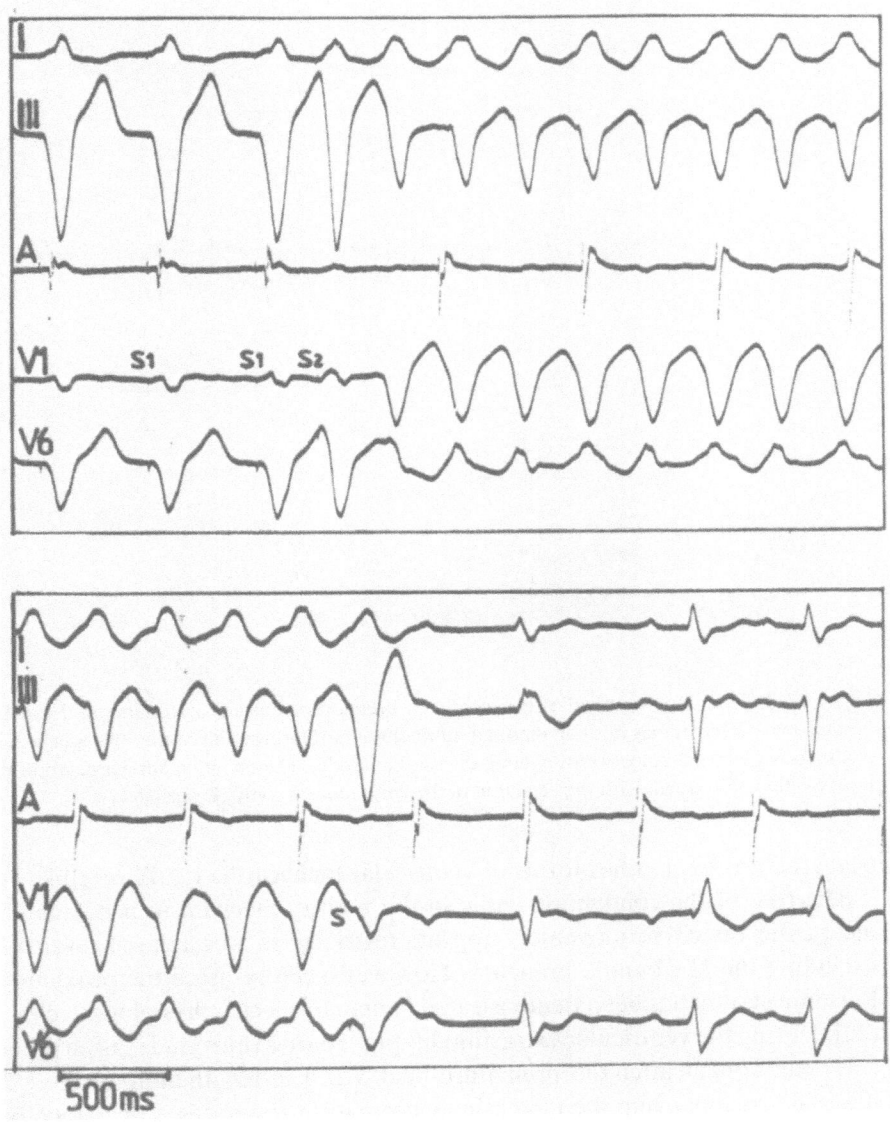

Figure 18. Induction of ventricular tachycardia by premature electrical stimulation of the right ventricle (upper panel). The tachycardia can also be interrupted by a ventricular premature depolarization (lower panel).

increase in heart rate (induced by atrial or ventricular stimulation); 2) the QRS complexes during arhythmia have a pattern of right bundle branch block and left anterior hemiblock; 3) the arrhythmia can be suppressed by intravenous administration of verapamil. Such a case is shown in figure 17. However the role of

288

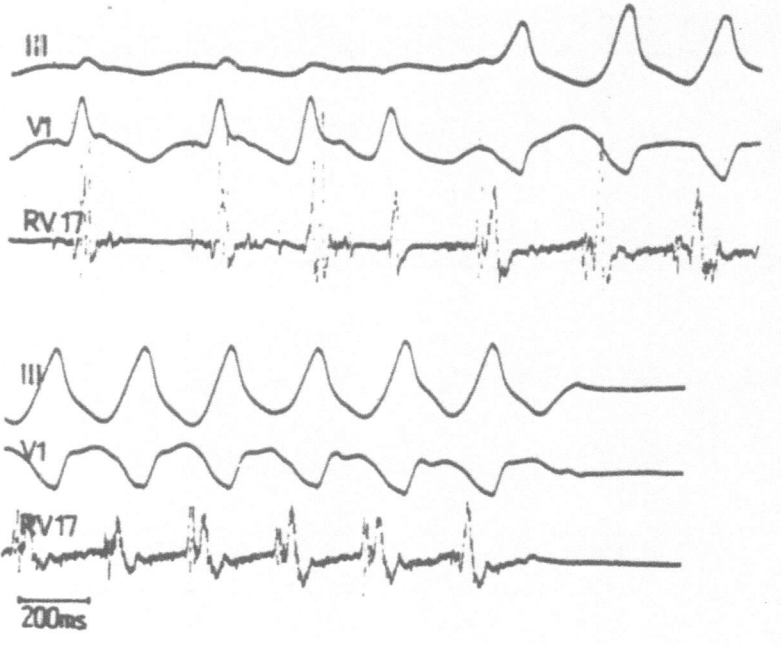

Figure 19. Induction of ventricular tachycardia by premature ventricular stimulation. Lead RV 17 corresponds to recordings in the pulmonary infundibulum. During tachycardia, this area exhibits a continuous electrical activity throughout the cardiac cycle. The spontaneous termination of the tachycardia is coincident with the cessation of the continuous activity (lower panel).

triggered acivity in other forms of ventricular tachycardia is still possible.

The role of the conducting tissue in the reentry mechanism is debatable. In most cases the circus movement appears restricted to a peripheral cardiac zone excluding the His bundle branches. However, reentry using the proximal His-Purkinje system has been demonstrated in man by electrophysiologic techniques [20]. During the ventricular extrastimulus procedure a retrograde hisian potential (H2) can appear after the premature beat V2. The lengthening of the V2-H2 interval accompanying the increasingly premature responses is occasionally followed by the recording of a supplementary beat V3, the H2-V3 interval being equal or superior to the HV interval in sinus rhythm (Fig. 20). It is postulated that the depolarization wave resulting from the premature stimulation of the right ventricle meets a refractory state in the ramifications of the right bundle branch. Crossing the septum it proceeds along the left bundle branch and reaches the His bundle. Then the reentrant impulse returns to the ventricle via the right bundle branch which has recovered. This phenomenon can exceptionally give rise to a repetitive ventricular response. Several clinical reports have evoked the role of bundle branch reentry in the genesis of ventricular tachycardias in man [11, 21,

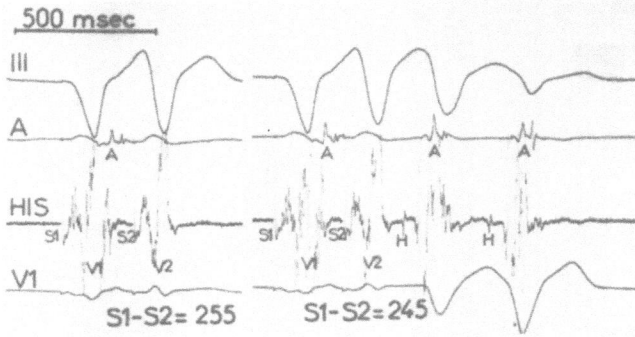

Figure 20. Premature stimulation of the right ventricle during a regular ventricular drive. In the left panel, following the premature ventricular response, there is no apparent retrograde activity. At shorter coupling interval (right panel) the premature ventricular response is accompanied by retrograde His bundle and atrial electrograms. The main retrograde delay takes place within the His-Purkinje system. These changes are associated with the occurrence of two successive ventricular complexes, each of them being preceded by a His bundle deflection with a H-V interval at 50 ms. Such phenomena are attributed to intraventricular reentry involving the bundle branch system (for more details, see text).

22]. The criteria in favor of this mechanism offer convincing evidence when associated. 1) In all cases a His bundle potential is visible between two tachycardia complexes. It is separated from the following beat by an interval at least equal to the sinus HV interval. 2) In the same patient the QRS complexes during tachycardia have the morphology of supraventricular beats with bundle branch block. 3) Atrial activation is unrelated to the arrhythmia as proven by the atrioventricular dissociation or the occurrence of intermittent retrograde block. 4) Premature ventricular stimulation elicited at the time when the His bundle potential is recorded, is capable of advancing the next H wave evidencing functional dissociation within the intraventricular conduction pathways. 5) The onset of the tachycardia is associated with the occurrence of a complete block of one of the His bundle branches. 6) The arrhythmia can be terminated by premature ventricular depolarization which is not propagated to the His bundle. However, although the role of the His-Purkinje system in the reentry mechanism seems evident the possible participation of Mahaim fibers in retrograde conduction cannot be excluded. Recording of the right bundle branch activity permits a more accurate approach in some cases. Finally, the ability to control tachycardia presumably due to bundle branch reentry using electrical ablation of a bundle branch, brings further proof for this mechanism [23].

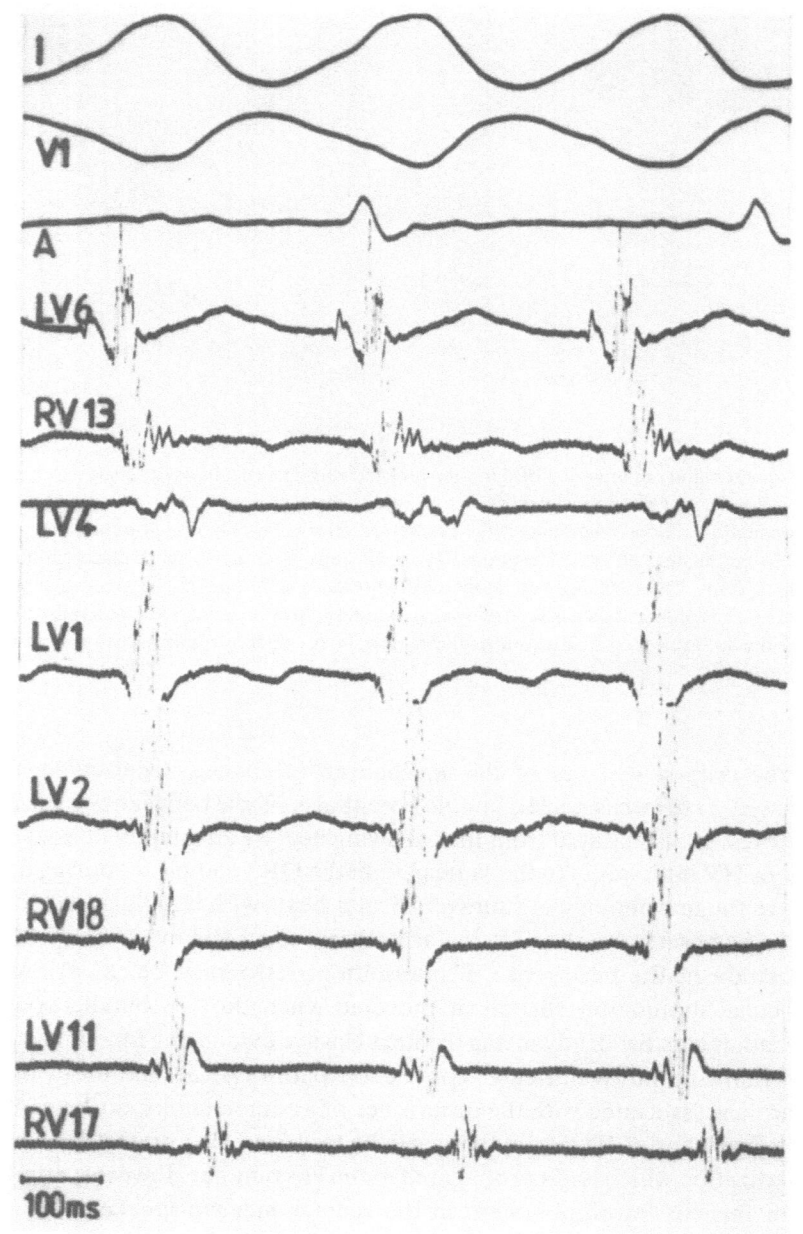

Figure 21. Catheter endocardial mapping of the ventricules during an episode of ventricular tachycardia. Simultaneous recordings made at various sites of the right and left ventricules are shown. During tachycardia, the site of earliest depolarization is located in the postero-inferior area of the left ventricle (lead LV 6). Then the activation wave spreads towards the septum and reaches the anterior wall of the ventricules. Leads LV1, LV2, LV4, LV6, LV11 are left ventricular endocardial sites corresponding to the apex, the anterior septum, the posterior septum, the inferior wall and the anterior wall respectively. Leads RV13, RV17 and RV18 are right ventricular endocardial sites located in the posterior septum, the pulmonary infundibulum and the anterior wall respectively.

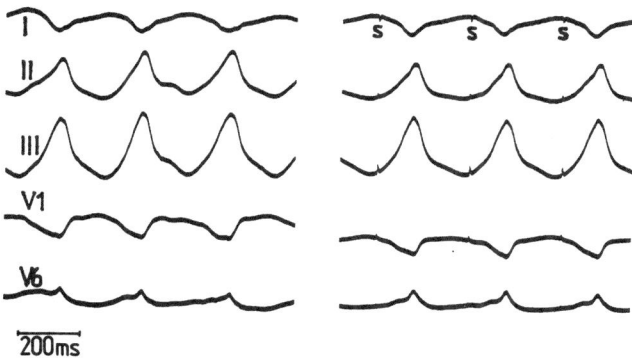

Figure 22. Ventricular tachycardia (left panel). In this patient electrical stimulation of the right ventricular outflow tract produced QRS complexes identical to those of the spontaneous arrhythmia (right panel).

Localisation of the site of origin

Endocardial mapping is utilized to determine the site of origin of the ventricular tachycardia. Local bipolar electrograms are recorded after amplification and filtering [16]. The explored sites (18 or more) involve the septum and the right and left free walls. During the tachycardia the site of the earliest depolarization is considered to be the site of origin of the abnormal activity (Fig. 21). Moreover, the relevant electrogram must precede the onset of the QRS complex in the surface ECG by at least 20 msec. A zone of continuous electrical activity can occasionally be detected. It would localize the reentry circuit and consequently the origin of the tachycardia. However, endocardial mapping may not provide an accurate diagnosis particularly when the number of endocardial sites reached by the catheter is too limited. Besides, endocardial mapping cannot be performed if the arrhythmia is poorly tolerated and necessitates electrical cardioversion. Under these circumstances indirect methods can be utilized during sinus rhythm. Abnormal electrograms of low voltage, fractionated, or extending beyond the QRS complex are of little interest when identifying the site of origin of the tachycardia. On the other hand, the pace-mapping technique is commonly utilized. It consists of electrical stimulation of the endocardial sites. The morphology of the paced QRS complexes is compared with that of the tachycardia beats in 8 to 12 surface leads. When similar the stimulated zone is assumed to be the site of the tachycardia (fig. 22). The results of pace-mapping and tachycardia mapping are often concordant. However, in patients with coronary heart disease discrepancies have been observed which could indicate that the site of earliest depolarization and the site from which the endocardial invasion wave emerges are distinct in some cases. Results obtained by catheterization techniques generally concord with data supplied during surgery in patients undergoing endocardial resection.

Localization of the site of origin of ventricular tachycardias has become of the utmost significance since the introduction of catheter ablation techniques [24]. Successful electrical ablation is greatly dependent on precise endocardial mapping.

References

1. Scherlag BJ, Lau SH, Helfant RH, Berkowitz WD, Stein E, Damato AN. 1969. Catheter technique for recording His bundle activity in man. Circulation 39: 13.
2. Puech P, Grolleau R, Fijac E, Posner J. 1970. The diagnosis of supraventrcular arrhythmias and the differentiation between supraventricular tachycardias wih aberrant conduction and ventricular tachycardias. In: Symposium on Cardiac Arrhythmias edited by Sandoe E, Flensted, Jensen E, and Olesen KH, Södestälje, Astra, p. 199.
3. Wellens HJJ, Schuilenburg RM, Durrer D. 1972. Electrical stimulation of the heart in patients with ventricular tachycardia. Circulation 46: 216.
4. Kistin AD. 1966. Ventricular tachycardia and esophageal leads. In: Mechanisms and Theapy of cardiac arrhythmias, edited by Dreifus LS and Likoff W. 14th Hahnemann Symposium, New York, Grune and Stratton, p. 274.
5. Easley RM Jr, Goldstein S. 1968. Differentiation of ventricular tachycardia from junctional tachycardia with aberrant conduction. The use of competitive atrial pacing. Circulation 37: 1015.
6. Gallagher JJ, Smith WM, Kerr CR, Kasell J, Cook L, Reiter M, Sterva R, Harte M. 1982. Esophageal pacing: A diagnostic and therapeutic tool. Circulation 65: 336.
7. Narula OS, Scherlag BJ, Samet P. 1970. Pervenous pacing of the specialized conducting system in man: His bundle and A-V nodal stimulation. Circulation 41: 77.
8. Narula DS. 1977. Longitudinal dissociation in the His bundle. Bundle branch block due to asynchronous conduction within the His bundle in man. Circulation 56: 996.
9. Puech P. 1975. Ectopic ventricular rhythms: ventricular tachycardia and His bundle recordings. In: His Bundle Electrocardiography and Clinical Electophysiology, edited by Narula OS, Philadelphia, Davis, p. 65.
10. Gallagher JJ, Pritchett ELC, Sealy WC, Kasell J, Wallace AG. 1978. The preexcitation syndromes. Prog Cardiovasc Dis 20: 285.
11. Touboul P, Kirkorian G, Atallah G, Moleur P. 1983. Bundle branch reentry: A possible mechanism of ventricular tachycardia. Circulation 67: 674.
12. Touboul P, Claveyrolas R, Huerta F, Porte J, Delahaye JP. 1975. Tachycardie ventriculaire induite par des battements supraventriculaires prématurés à complexe QRS normal. Arch Mal Coeur 68: 969.
13. Wellens HJJ, Lie KI, Durrer D. 1974. Further observations on ventricular tachycardia as studied by electrical stimulation of the heart. Chronic recurrent ventricular tachycardia and tachycardia during acute myocardial infarction. Circulation 49: 647.
14. Wellens HJJ, Duren DR, Lie KI. 1976. Observations on mechanism of ventricular tachycardia in man. Circulation 54: 237.
15. Waldo AL, Henthorn RW, Plumb VJ, MacLean WAH. 1984. Demonstration of the mechanism of transient entrainment and interruption of ventricular tachycardia with rapid atrial pacing. J Am Coll Cardiol 3: 422.
16. Josephson ME, Horowitz LN, Farshidi A, Spear JF, Kastor JA, Moore NE. 1978. Recurrent sustained ventricular tachycardia. 2. Endocardial mapping. Circulation 57: 440.
17. Josephson ME, Horowitz LN, Farshidi A. 1978. Continuous local electrical activity. A mechanism of recurrent ventricular tachycardia. Circulation 57: 659.
18. Wit AL, Cranefield PF, Gadsby DC. 1980. Triggered activity. In: The Slow Inward Current and

Cardiac Arrhythmias, edited by Zipes DP, Bailey JC and Elharrar V. The Hague, Martinus Nijhoff, p. 437.

19. Zipes DP, Foster PR, Troup PJ,Peterson DH. 1979. Atrial induction of ventricular tachycardia. Reentry vs triggered automaticity. Am J Cardiol 44: 1.
20. Akhtar M, Damato AN, Batsford WP, Ruskin JN, Ogunkelu JB, Vargas G. 1974. Demonstration of re-entry within the His-Purkinje system in man. Circulation 50: 1150.
21. Guerot C, Valere PE, Castillo-Fenoy A, Tricot R. 1973. Tachycardie par rentrée de branche à branche. Arch Mal Coeur 66: 1045.
22. Brechenmacher C, Mossard JM, Voegtlin R. 1977. Rentrée ventriculaire permanente cachée et tachycardie ventriculaire paroxystique par mouvement circulaire. Arch Mal Coeur 70: 61.
23. Touboul P, Kirkorian G, Atallah G, Lavaud P, Moleur P, Lamaud M, Mathieu MP. 1986. Bundle branch rentrant tachycardia treated by electrical ablation of the right bundle branch. J Am Coll Cardiol 7: 1404.
24. Hartzler GO. 1983. Elecrode catheter ablation of refractory focal ventricular tachycardia. J Am Coll Cardiol 2: 1107.

21. Mechanisms of ventricular tachycardia: re-entry versus triggered activity in man

HEIN J.J. WELLENS, ANTON P.M. GORGELS, and PEDRO BRUGADA
Department of Cardiology, Academic Hospital Maastricht, University of Limburg, Maastricht, The Netherlands

In 1972 it could be demonstrated in patients suffering from recurrent sustained monomorphic ventricular tachycardia that their clinically occurring arrhythmia could reproducibly be initiated and terminated by programmed stimulation [1].

The similarity between these observations and those previously made during programmed stimulation of the heart in patients with supraventricular tachycardia [2] suggested that re-entry was the mechanism of the sustained monomorphic ventricular tahycardia of these patients.

Shortly thereafter, however, observations in the experimental laboratory indicated that sustained rhythmic activity could be based upon delayed afterdepolarizations reaching threshold [3–14]. The arrhythmias based on delayed afterdepolarizations, like those based on re-entry, could reproducibly be initiated and terminated during programmed stimulation of the heart and have therefore been called triggered activity. This raised the question of a possible role of such a mechanism in human arrhythmias. Because direct recordings of the cellular events in the intact human heart are not possible the question about a possible role of triggered activity in clinical human arrhythmias has to be approached indirectly.

The experiments in the tissue bath and the intact animal led to a description of criteria considered to be typical for triggered activity based upon delayed afterdepolarizations. Table 1 lists the different phenomena one may observe at the time of initiation, termination and during tachycardia using programmed stimulation of the heart and the value of these findings to distinguish between re-entry and triggered activity as the mechanism of a tachycardia. As we have discussed elsewhere [15] our initial enthusiasm that findings like overdrive acceleration or a concordant relation between the premature beat interval initiating tachycardia and the interval between the premature beat and the first beat of the tachycardia were specific for triggered activity disappeared when we critically analysed findings in patients with the Wolff-Parkinson-White syndrome where intracardiac recordings proved re-entry to be the arrhythmia mechanism [15]. In some of the patients with the Wolff-Parkinson-White syndrome we observed findings considered to be typical for triggered activity. We also found that in patients with ventricular tachycardia a concordant relation between the premature beat interval and the interval from premature beat to first tachycardia complex could be present at one basic pacing cycle length and an inverse relation at a different basic pacing cycle length [15]. In a series of 161 consecutive patients with sustained monomorphic ventricular tachycardia of different etiologies, we had only one patient who consistently showed a concordant relation between the premature beat interval and the interval to the first beat of the tachycardia. Table 1 therefore indicates the problem one encounters if one tries to use the listed criteria to differentiate between the two tachycardia mechanisms. It also suggests that triggered activity is probably rare as a causal mechanism in the patient suffering from a sustained monomorphic ventricular tachycardia coming to the electrophysiologic laboratory for study.

One might argue that if all criteria listed in table 1 could be tested more patients could be identified having triggered activity as their tachycardia mechanism. This would lengthen the study to such an extent however, that it would become impossible to impose this upon a patient. Programmed stimulation therefore, does not seem to be the direction to go to make the distinction between re-entry and triggered activity. What about the use of specific drugs? Ten years ago [16] we introduced the use of drugs to study mechanisms of recurrent sustained monomorphic ventricular tachycardia in man. At that time we found that in the patients studied neither propanolol nor verapamil had any effect on tachycardia induction or tachycardia rate. Triggered activity in the tissue bath is facilitated by catecholamines [17] and suppressed by calciumantagonists like verapamil [18]. This suggests that these drugs might be helpful in elucidating tachycardia mechanisms. Our previous observations [16] with verapamil and propanolol indicate that triggered activity is not the causal mechanism in the commonly encountered clinical types of sustained monomorphic ventricular tachycardia in man. There are ventricular tachycardias, however, who are sensitive to verapamil [19, 20] vagal maneuvers [21] and adenosine [22]. Most of these cases fall in the category of idiopathic ventricular tachycardia or exercise related ventricular tachycardia. Triggered activity might be their mechanism.

Another type of ventricular arrhythmia occurring in the human heart and probably based upon triggered activity is the ventricular tachycardia occurring during digitalis intoxication [23]. This is of course supported by the observations during digitalis intoxication in the animal heart [3, 7, 14]. It is likely that the mechanism of delayed afterdepolarizations is not the same under different circumstances, as for example in digitalis intoxication [18] or the adenosine sensitive ventricular tachycardia [22].

For diagnostic and therapeutic purposes it would be extremely important to develop specific drugs that provoke or counteract a specific mechanism of production of delayed afterdepolarizations. To be able to use such an approach more work has to be done in the experimental laboratory. Ultimately, the development

Table 1. Criteria used to differentiate between re-entry and triggered activity as mechanisms of chronic recurrent sustained monomorphic ventricular tachycardia.

At the time of inititation of tachycardia	Re-entry	T.A.
Initiation by critically time stimuli	+	+
Initiation related to rate of preceding spontaneous or paced cycle length	+	+
Initiation related to number of preceding paced beats (<50)	−/?	+
Concordant relation between pacing rate and rate of induced tachycardia	−	+
Concordant relation between premature beat interval initiating tachycardia and echo-interval (interval between premature beat and first complex of tachycardia)	−/+	+/−
Inverse relation between premature beat interval initiating tachycardia and echointerval	+/−	−/+
Increase in rate of tachycardia after its initiation ('warming-up')	+	+
At the time of termination of tachycardia		
Termination by critically timed stimuli	+	+
Termination by overdriving	+	+
Termination by a premature beat followed by one or more tachycardia cycles before termination	+	+
Overdrive termination related to paced cycle length	+	+
Slowing of tachycardia rate before termination	+	+
Acceleration of tachycardia rate before termination	+	+
Effect of timed premature beats and overdriving during regular sustained ventricular tachycardia		
Overt perpetuation	+	+
Concealed perpetuation	+	?
Suppression	−	−
Acceleration	+	+
Entrainment	+	?
Termination with re-initiation by an even or odd number of impulses	+	−/?
Change to another tachycardia	+	+
Termination	+	+
Biphasic response curve	−	+/?
Effect of changes in autonomic tone and effect of drugs in ventricular tachycardia		
Enhanced sympathetic activity		
Acceleration	+	+
Deceleration	−	−
Termination	+/−	?
Facilitation	+/−	+
Enhanced parasympathetic activity		
Acceleration	−/+	?/+
Deceleration	+/−	?/+
Termination	+/−	?
Facilitation	−/+	+/?

Table 1. Continued.

At the time of inititation of tachycardia	Re-entry	T.A.
Drugs		
digitalis	?	+
verapamil	−	+
adenosine	−	+

+ = positive; − = negative; ? = unknown; t.a. = triggered activity.

of these drugs should be accompanied by the development of catheter techniques allowing the reliable recording of cellular membrane action potentials in the intact human heart.

References

1. Wellens HJJ, Schuilenburg RM, Durrer D. 1972. Electrical stimulation of the heart in patients with ventricular tachycardias. Circulation 46: 216–226.
2. Wellens HJJ. 1971. Electrical stimulation of the heart in the study and treatment of tachycardias. Baltimore, University Park Press.
3. Rosen MR, Reder RF. 1981. Does triggered activity have a role in the genesis of cardiac arrhythmias? Ann Intern Med 94: 794–801.
4. Davis LD. 1973. Effect of changes in cycle length on diastolic depolarization produced by ouabain in canine Purkinje fibers. Circ Res 32: 206–214.
5. Ferrier GR, Saunders JH, Mendez C. 1973. A cellular mechanism for the generation of ventricular arrhythmias by acetylstrophantidin. Circ Res 32: 600–609.
6. Hoshimoto K, Moe GK. 1973. Transient depolarizations induced by acetylstrophantidin in specialized tissue of dog atrium and ventricle. Circ Res 32: 618–624.
7. Ferrier GR. 1977. Digitalis arrhythmias. Role of oscillatory afterpotentials. Prog Cardiovasc Dis 19: 459–474.
8. Rosen MR, Gelband H, Hoffman BF. 1973. Correlation between effects of ouabain on the canine electrocardiogram and transmembrane potentials of isolated Purkinje fibers. Circulation 47: 65–72.
9. Wit AL, Fenoglio JJ, Wagner BM, Basset AL. 1973. Electrophysiologic properties of cadiac muscle in the anterior mitral valve leaflet and the adjacent atrium in the dog. Circ Res 32: 731–745.
10. Wit AL, Cranefield PF. 1976. Triggered activity in cardiac muscle fibers of the simian mitral valve. Circ Res 38: 85–98.
11. Wit AL, Boyden PA, Gadsby DC, Cranefield PF. 1979. Triggered activity as a cause of atrial arrhythmias. In: Cardiac Arrhythmias. Narula O, Ed. Baltimore: Williams and Wilkins, pp. 14–31.
12. Hiraoka M, Okamoto Y, Sano T. 1981. Oscillatory afterpotentials in dog ventricular muscle fibers. Circ Res 48: 510–518.
13. Wald RW, Waxman MB. 1981. Pacing-induced automaticity in sheep Purkinje fibers. Circ Res 48: 531–538.

298

14. Gorgels APM, Beekman HDM, Brugada P, Dassen WRM, Richards DAB, Wellens HJJ. 1983. Extrastimulus related shortening of the first postpacing interval in digitalis induced ventricular tachycardia. Observations during programmed stimulation in the conscious dog. JACC 1: 840–857.

15. Brugada P, Wellens HJJ. 1984. The role of triggered activity in clinical ventricular arrhythmias. PACE 7: 260–271.

16. Wellens HJJ, Bär FWHM, Lie KI, Düren DR, Dohmen HJ. 1977. Effect of procainamide, propanolol and verapamil on mechanism of tachycardia in patients with chronic recurrent ventricular tachycardia. Am J Cardiol 40: 579–585.

17. Wit AL, Cranefield PF, Gadsby DC. 1982. Electrogenic sodium extrusion can stop triggered activity in the canine coronary sinus. Circ Res 49: 1029–1042.

18. Rosen MR, Danilo P Jr. 1980. Effects of tetrodotoxin, lidocaine, verapamil and AHR-2666 on ouabain-induced delayed afterdepolarizations in canine Purkinje fibers. Circ Res 46: 117–124.

19. Wellens HJJ, Brugada P, Vanagt EJDM, Ross DL, Bär FW. 1981. New studies with triggered automaticity. In: Cardiac arrhythmias, a decade of progress. Harrison DC (ed). Boston, GK Hall Medical: pp. 601—610.

20. Zipes DP, Foster PR, Troup PF, Pedersen DH. 1979. Atrial induction of ventricular tachycardia; re-entry vs triggered automaticity. Am J Cardiol 44: 1–8.

21. Waxman MB, Wald RW. 1984. Effect of autonomic tone on tachycardias. In: Tachycardias. Surawicz B, Pratap Reddy C, Prystowski EN (eds). Martinus Nijhoff, Boston: 67–102.

22. Lerman BB, Belardinelli L, DiMarco JP. 1986. Adenosine sensitive ventricular tachycardia: Evidence suggesting cyclic AMP mediated triggered activity. JACC 7: 155A.

23. Vanagt EJ, Wellens JHH. 1981. The electrocardiogram in digitalis intoxication. In: What's new in electrocardiography? Wellens HJJ, Kulbertus HE (eds). Martinus Nijhoff, The Hague: pp. 315–343.

22. Is there an ideal ventricular stimulation protocol?

JAY W. MASON

Cardiology Division, University of Utah School of Medicine

Interest in defining the correct protocol to use to initiate and evaluate ventricular tachyarrhythmias has recently grown because of expanding clinical use of cardiac electrophysiologic study. Investigators have been aware of the large influence which seemingly small details of the stimulation technique have upon the results of ventricular stimulation. For example, Swerdlow and colleagues [1] found that a third extrastimulus produced far more false-negative predictions of drug efficacy than a maximum of two extrastimuli. Though uniformity of protocols has increased with each new publication on the topic, there remains considerable divergence from laboratory to laboratory. Furthermore, the rationale for many 'standard,' uniformly applied features of existing protocols is not developed.

While details of the stimulation protocol influence the results of stimulation, criteria applied to interpret those results have an equally profound influence upon the final result: use of the clinical electrophysiologic study to guide therapy. For example, Swerdlow and associates [2] found that their arbitrary criterion of drug inefficacy, induction of more than five consecutive beats, was incorrect and had falsely predicted drug failure; a criterion of 15 beats would have been more accurate.

The problem of defining the ideal protocol becomes even more complex with recognition that different clinical subgroups of patients respond differently to a given stimulation protocol. For example, patients with cardiomyopathy are more susceptible to induction of unsustained ventricular tachycardia than subjects without cardiac disease [3].

The magnitude of the problem is further enlarged by the multiple interactions between protocol, criteria and disease subgroups. The purpose of this manuscript is to review these interactions. The inevitable conclusion of this review is that an ideal stimulation protocol for study of ventricular tachyarrhythmias does not and will never exist.

Stimulation protocol

There are innumerable features of a stimulation protocol which can be varied. Some of these features are listed in Table 1. Although the influence upon study results of many of these variables has not been examined, the clinical significance of some of them is now recorded is the literature: Stimulus amplitude [4–6], stimulus polarity [7, 8], catheter location [9–11], isoproterenol infusion [12], drive rate and number of drive rates [13–15], number of extrastimuli [1, 6, 16–20] and order of steps [13, 21].

For purposes of illustration, let us examine this latter variable. Morady and coworkers [21] compared stimulation protocols in which the major difference was the order in which certain stimulation features were applied. They found a marked difference in the ratio of specific to nonspecific induced rhythms at each step in the differently-ordered protocols. The specific modes of stimulation included in a given protocol will also influence sensitivity and specificity. Brugada and colleagues [13] found that use of three extrastimuli at multiple drives had a better yield of inducibility than use of multiple current strengths at a single drive, and high currents are known to increase the yield of nonspecific rhythms.

Thus, both the specific techniques and the order in which they are applied influence the result of stimulation. The potential number of combinations of techniques and orders of stimulation approaches infinity, and, therefore, so do the potential results of stimulation.

Interpretive criteria

There are two primary sets of criteria which must be used to interpret the results of stimulation. The first determines the endpoint (that is, an induced arrhythmia which signals that no more pacing attempts are needed) during the baseline study, when the patient's vulnerability to arrhythmia induction in the absence of antiarrhythmic drug therapy is being measured. The second determines the significance which one attaches to various characteristics of arrhythmia induced during the

Table 1. Features of a ventricular stimulation Protocol.

Stimulus amplitude	Isoproterenol infusion
Stimulus duration	Drive duration
Stimulus shape	Number of drive cycles
Stimulus polarity	Drive rate
Electrode size	Number of drive rates
Electrode metal	Number of extrastimuli
Interelectrode distance	Prematurity of extrastimuli
Catheter location	Order of steps

subsequent drug efficacy assessment studies. These characteristics include the rate, duration, morphology, and reproducibility of the arrhythmia. Additional important characteristics are the cardiovascular response to the arrhythmia and the ease of induction of the arrhythmia compared to that in the baseline study.

Brugada and coworkers [22] have produced data relevant to the first set of criteria. They have shown that sustained, monomorphic ventricular tachycardia is rarely, if ever, induced in a subject who has not experienced sustained ventricular tachyarrhythmias, while unsustained ventricular tachycardia, polymorphic ventricular tachycardia and ventricular fibrillation can be induced in such patients. One might conclude that the only reliable endpoint at baseline study, therefore, is sustained, monomorphic ventricular tachycardia. The validity of that conclusion has not been adequately tested, but this endpoint is undoubtedly the correct one in certain circumstances.

Reproducibility of arrhythmia inducibility is an interesting facet of both the first and second sets of criteria. For the first set of criteria, one wonders how many times the selected arrhythmia endpoint must be reached during baseline study. One also wonders if the endpoint must be reproducible over a period of time, such as days or weeks, to be truly reliable. For the second set, one wonders if arrhythmia non-inducibility, however defined, must be reproducible on separate days to render a valid prediction of drug efficacy. Four recent publications [23–26] concerning reproducibility of arrhythmia inducibility have demonstrated the marked dependence of reproducibility upon the stimulation protocol in use, the arrhythmia endpoint at baseline study and the patient subgroup under examination. These publications further the theme that interactions between protocol, criteria and patient subgroup are complex. This is the topic of the remainder of this manuscript.

Interactions

Figure 1 summarizes interactions between the major variables which influence the clinical meaning of a ventricular stimulation protocol. Although the total number of variables which interact is much greater we will limit our attention to those diagrammed in the figure, as they are the most important and interesting ones.

Protocol:criteria

The most extensive interactions occur between the pacing protocol and the criteria applied to interpretation of the results of stimulation. The interaction is bidirectional.

Stated most simply, the aggressiveness of the stimulation protocol alters the

302

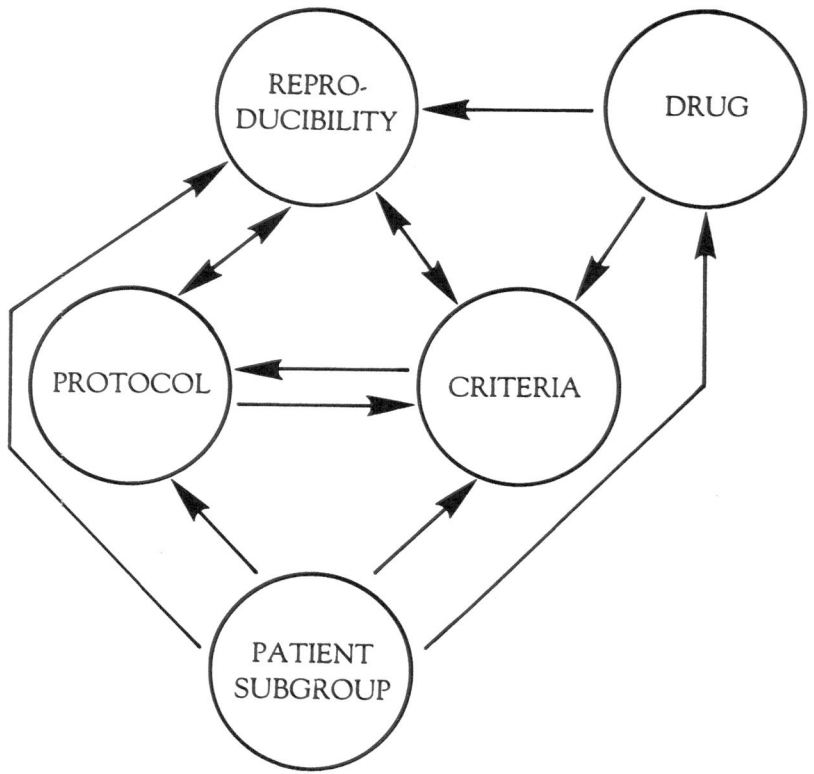

Figure 1. Interactions. The diagram illustrates many of the categories of interaction known to influence the end result of electrophysiologic study in patients with ventricular arrhythmias. Each variable is known to affect more than one other variable, and many of the variables affect one another bidirectionally.

extent of clinical relevance of the resultant induced arrhythmia; therefore, interpretation of the significance of an induced arrhythmia is directly linked to the means by which it was induced. There are some obvious examples. It is possible to induce ventricular fibrillation in an entirely normal heart by application of alternating current of sufficient magnitude. Thus, the clinical relevance or induced ventricular fibrillation by a protocol including a large AC current would be nil. On the other hand, ventricular fibrillation induced by a single extrastimulus would have great clinical relevance, since this is not a normal result of unaggressive stimulation [22].

Somewhat more subtle interactions have greater practical importance. It has now been shown repeatedly that use of a greater number of extrastimuli yields a higher rate of tachyarrhythmia induction, but the rate of non-clinical arrhythmia induction also increases [1, 6, 16–20]. Ideally, a balance would be struck in which the stimulation protocol was precisely aggressive enough to produce only clinically relevant tachyarrhythmias only in truly vulnerable patients. Or, alternately, the interpretive criteria used with a protocol which did not invariably induce the desired arrhythmia would make up for the protocol's deficiencies by successfully detecting all true positive and negative responses. The practical difficulties of discerning such a protocol or set of criteria are obvious. Any change in protocol would require a concomitant change in criteria, and visa versa; but the potential number of variations is enormous.

Patient subgroup:protocol, criteria

There is published literature concerning results of ventricular stimulation in several distinct subgroups of patients, categorized according to underlying cardiac disease or type of ventricular arrhythmia. Table 2 is a partial list.

Different cardiac diseases, in and of themselves, produce varying degrees of vulnerability to arrhythmia induction, independent of the patient's spontaneous arrhythmia history. For example, Anderson and colleagues have shown that hypertrophic cardiomyopathy predisposes to induction of polymorphic ventricular tachycardia or fibrillation in nearly all patients without spontaneous ventricular tachyarrhythmias [42]. It is also likely that the extent of disease influences vulnerability and the nature of the induced arrhythmia.

Patients with different types of documented spontaneous ventricular arrhythmias have varying susceptibilities to arrhythmia induction, and the nature of the induced arrhythmias varies in these subgroups [3, 4, 37–44]. Patients with documented, sustained ventricular tachycardia are likely to have sustained, monomorphic ventricular tachycardia induced, while patients with no more than simple ventricular ectopy rarely do [36].

One can see that the complex interplay between protocol and criteria is made even more complicated by the added effect upon it of disease or arrhythmia category. A given protocol with its specific criteria for interpretation can be applied most accurately to only a single patient subgroup.

Table 2. Patient subgroups undergoing ventricular stimulation.

Subgroup	References
Sustained VT	27–30
Aborted sudden death or VF	31
Unexplained syncope	32, 33
Unsustained VT	34, 35
Ventricular premature beats	36
Post-myocardial infarction	4, 37–39
Dilated cardiomyopathy	3, 40, 41
Hypertrophic cardiomyopathy	42
Coronary artery disease	43, 44

Patient subgroup:drug

A patient's disease and clinical arrhythmia may influence the efficacy of a drug and the accuracy of assessment of that drug's efficacy by electrophysiologic study. One example is the patient with ventricular premature beats which trigger ventricular tachycardia. A drug may be capable of suppressing 100% of the premature beats, thereby eliminating the possibility of a tachycardia recurrence, but the tachycardia may remain inducible. In this example, the drug suppresses spontaneous ectopy but does not impair the function of a putative reentry circuit. Essentially no research has been directed to this area.

Patient subgroup:reproducibility

Disease category clearly influence the reproducibility of arrhythmia inducibility. Schoenfeld and colleagues have demonstrated that the baseline tachyarrhythmia is highly reproducibly inducible over months and years in patients with coronary artery disease, but not in subjects with other forms of cardiac disease [24]. There are undoubtedly disease:reproducibility interactions which have not yet been investigated.

Reproducibility:protocol, criteria

The protocol employed to induce the tachyarrhythmia has an effect upon the reproducibility of induction. McPherson and colleagues showed that reproducibility of tachycardia by a protocol using only one or two extrastimuli was 95%. Use of a third extrastimulus increased overall inducibility, but markedly reduced its reproducibility [23].

Interpretive criteria also influence reproducibility. Lombardi and colleagues [25] showed very poor reproducibility, much lower than others have found. However, they accepted an initial endpoint of only three repetitive beats. This incorrect criterion undoubtedly reduced reproducibility; a sustained tachycardia endpoint would have been more reproducible.

Drug:criteria

Amiodarone provides a good example of the influence of a specific drug upon interpretive criteria. Conventionally, any induced arrhythmia, as long as it is sustained, has been considered evidence of drug inefficacy. In the case of amiodarone, however, other features of the induced arrhythmia, aside from its duration, have been found to contain predictive value [45, 46]. Patients treated with amiodarone whose arrhythmia becomes harder to induce or less hemo-dynamically unstable are less likely to have an arrhythmia recurrence.

Drug:reproducibility

It is likely that certain drugs, by virtue of their pharmacokinetic and other characteristics, will affect reproducibility of inducibility differently than others. For example, a drug with very low bioavailability, especially if its half life is relatively short, may provide more unpredictable plasma levels than one with high bioavailability and a long half life. The probability that its concentration will be the same during serial electrophysiologic studies will be much greater for the latter drug. Likewise, some drugs may take substantial lengths of time to achieve a full electrophysiologic effect even after steady state is reached. In this situation, serial studies will have differing results despite stable plasma levels.

Conclusions

The implications of the interactions illustrated in Figure 1 and discussed above lead to the inevitable conclusion that the concept of an ideal ventricular stimulation protocol is an empty one. Not only is the number of potential combinations of techniques and interpretive criteria mind-boggling, but in every clinical circumstance the ideal combination is likely to be unique. Thus, the answer to the question posed in the title is 'No, there is no ideal stimulation protocol.'

Where does this conclusion leave the clinical electrophysiologist, who must select patient and protocol and interpret the results of study on a daily basis? In a difficult but not hopeless situation. Fortunately, many of the influences of variations in protocol and criteria are small, and many of the important ones are adequately understood. I believe that our current state of knowledge calls for the following actions. First, current and future attempts to discover the ideal stimulation protocol should be abandoned. Second, worldwide, or at least nationwide agreement among clinical electrophysiologists to utilize a few rational protocols and accompanying well-reasoned interpretive criteria, and to apply only one of them to each of a few carefully delineated constellations of clinical situations, should be arrived at. This latter objective could be met by a series of meetings by experts, followed by pilot use of the developed algorithm by them and culminating in dissemination of the final recommendations of these experts through the medical literature.

References

1. Swerdlow CD, Blum J, Winkle RA, Griffin JC, Ross DL, Mason JW. 1982. Decreased incidence of antiarrhythmic drug efficacy at electrophysiologic study associated with the use of a third extrastimulus. Am Heart J 104: 1004–1011.
2. Swerdlow CD, Winkle RA, Mason JW. 1983. Prognostic significance of the number of induced ventricular complexes during assessment of therapy for ventricular tachyarrhythmias. Circulation 68: 400–405.
3. Poll DS, Marchlinski FE, Buxton AE, Doherty JU, Waxman HL, Josephson ME. 1984. Sustained ventricular tachycardia in patients with idiopathic dilated cardiomyopathy: Electrophysiologic testing and lack of response to antiarrhythmic drug therapy. Circulation 70: 451–456.
4. Richard DA, Cody DV, Denniss AR, Russell PA, Young AA, Uther JB. 1983. Ventricular electrical instability: A predictor of death after myocardial infarction. Am J Cardiol 51: 75–80.
5. Morady F, DiCarlo LA, Liem LB, Krol RB, Baerman JM. 1985. Effects of high stimulation current on the induction of ventricular tachycardia. Am J Cardiol 56: 73–78.
6. Herre JM, Mann DE, Luck JC, Magro SA, Figali S, Breen T, Wyndham CRC. 1986. Effect of increased current, multiple pacing sites and number of extrastimuli on induction of ventricular tachycardia. Am J Cardiol 57: 102–107.
7. Mitamura H, Ohm OJ, Michelson EL, Sauermelch C, Dreifus LS. 1985. Importance of the pacing mode in the initiation of ventricular tachyarrhythmia in a canine model of chronic myocardial infarction. J Am Coll Cardiol 6: 99–103.
8. Stevenson WG, Wiener I, Weiss JN. 1986. Comparison of bipolar and unipolar programmed electrical stimulation for the initiation of ventricular arrhythmias: Significance of anodal excitation during bipolar stimulation. Circulation 73: 693–700.
9. Michelson EL, Spear JF, Moore EN. 1981. Initiation of sustained ventricular tachyarrhythmias in a canine model of chronic myocardial infarction: Importance of the site of stimulation. Circulation 63: 776–784.
10. Doherty JU, Kienzle MG, Waxman HL, Buxton AE, Marchlinski FE, Josephson ME. 1983. Programmed ventricular stimulation at a second right ventricular site: An analysis of 100 patients, with special reference to sensitivity, specificity and characteristics of patients with induced ventricular tachycardia. Am J Cardiol 52: 1184–1189.
11. Morady F, Hess D, Scheinman MM. 1982. Electrophysiologic drug testing in patients with malignant ventricular arrhythmias: Importance of stimulation at more than one ventricular site. Am J Cardiol 50: 1055–1060.
12. Freedman RA, Swerdlow CD, Echt DS, Winkle RA, Soderholm-Difatte V, Mason JW. 1984. Facilitation of ventricular tachyarrhythmia induction by isoproterenol. Am J Cardiol 54: 765–770.
13. Brugada P, Wellens HJJ. 1985. Comparison in the same patient of two programmed ventricular stimulation protocols to induce ventricular tachycardia. Am J Cardiol 55: 380–383.
14. Echt D, Swerdlow C, Anderson K, Mitchell L, Mason J, Winkle R. 1983. Value of adding extrastimuli vs. shortening drive cycle length in ventricular tachycardia induction. PACE 6: A-141.
15. Estes NAM, III, Garan H, McGovern B, Ruskin JN. 1986. Influence of drive cycle length during programmed stimulation on induction of ventricular arrhythmias: Analysis of 403 patients. Am J Cardiol 57: 108–112.
16. Breithardt G, Abendroth RR, Borggrefe M, Yeh HL, Haerten K, Seipel L. 1984. Prevalence of clinical significance of the repetitive ventricular response during sinus rhythm in coronary disease patients. Am Heart J 107: 229–236.
17. Denker S, Lehmann M, Mahmud R, Gilbert C, Akhtar M. 1984. Facilitation of ventricular tachycardia induction with abrupt changes in ventricular cycle length. Am J Cardiol 53: 508–515.
18. Morady F, Shapiro W, Shen E, Sung RJ, Scheinman MM. 1984. Programmed ventricular stimulation in patients without spontaneous ventricular tachycardia. Am Heart J 107: 875–882.

19. Mann DE, Luck JC, Griffin JC, Herre JM, Limacher MC, Magro SA, Robertson NW, Wyndham CRC. 1983. Induction of clinical ventricular tachycardia using programmed stimulation: Value of third and fourth extrastimuli. Am J Cardiol 52: 501–506.

20. Waspe LE, Seinfeld D, Ferrick A, Kim SG, Matos JA, Fisher JD. 1985. Prediction of sudden death and spontaneous ventricular tachycardia in survivors of complicated myocardial infarction: Value of the response to programmed stimulation using a maximum of three ventricular extrastimuli. J Am Coll Cardiol 5: 1292–1301.

21. Morady F, DiCarlo L, Winston S, Davis JC, Scheinman MM. 1984. A prospective comparison of triple extrastimuli and left ventricular stimulation in studies of ventricular tachycardia induction. Circulation 10: 52–57.

22. Brugada P, Abdollah H, Heddle B, Wellens HJJ. 1983. Results of a ventricular stimulation protocol using a maximum of 4 premature stimuli in patients without documented or suspected ventricular arrhythmias. Am J Cardiol 52: 1214–1218.

23. McPherson CA, Rosenfeld LE, Batsford WP. 1985. Day-to-day reproducibility of responses to right ventricular programmed electrical stimulation: Implications for serial drug testing. Am J Cardiol 55: 689–695.

24. Schoenfeld MH, McGovern B, Garan H, Ruskin JN. 1984. Long-term reproducibility of responses to programmed cardiac stimulation in spontaneous ventricular tachyarrhythmias. Am J Cardiol 54: 564–568.

25. Lombardi F, Stein J, Podrid PJ, Graboys TB, Lown B. 1986. Daily reproducibility of electrophysiologic test results in malignant ventricular arrhythmia. Am J Cardiol 57: 96–101.

26. Kudenchuk PJ, Kron J, Walance CG, Murphy ES, Morris CD, Griffith KK, McAnulty JH. 1986. Reproducibility of arrhythmia induction with intracardiac electrophysiologic testing: Patients with clinical sustained ventricular tachyarrhythmias. J Am Coll Cardiol 7: 819–828.

27. Mason JW, Winkle RA. 1978. Electrode-catheter arrhythmia induction in the selection and assessment of antiarrhythmic drug therapy for recurrent ventricular tachycardia. Circulation 58: 971–985.

28. Horowitz LN, Josephson ME, Farshidi A, Kastor JA. 1978. Recurrent sustained ventricular tachycardia 3. Role of the electrophysiologic study in selection of antiarrhythmic regimens. Circulation 58: 986–997.

29. Swerdlow CD, Winkle RA, Mason JW. 1983. Determinants of survival in patients with ventricular tachyarrhythmias. New Engl J Med 308: 1436–1442.

30. Swerdlow CD, Gong G, Echt DS, Winkle RA, Griffin JC, Ross DL, Mason JW. 1983. Clinical factors predicting successful electrophysiologic-pharmacologic study in patients with ventricular tachycardia. J Am Coll Cardiol 1: 409–416.

31. Ruskin JN, DiMarco JP, Garan H. 1980. Out-of-hospital cardiac arrest. N Engl J Med 303: 607–613.

32. Hess DS, Morady F, Scheinman MM. 1982. Electrophysiologic testing in the evaluation of patients with syncope of undetermined origin. Am J Cardiol 50: 1309–1315.

33. Olshanski B, Mazuz M, Martins JB. 1985. Significance of inducible tachycardia in patients with syncope of unknown origin: A long-term follow-up. J Am Coll Cardiol 5: 216–223.

34. Buxton AE, Marchlinski FE, Waxman HL, Flores BT, Cassidy DM, Josephson ME. 1984. Prognostic factors in nonsustained ventricular tachycardia. Am J Cardiol 53: 1275–1279.

35. Spielman SR, Greenspan AM, Kay HR, Discigil KF, Webb CR, Sokoloff NM, Rae AP, Morganroth J, Horowitz LN. 1985. Electrophysiologic testing in patients at high risk for sudden cardiac death. I. Nonsustained ventricular tachycardia and normal ventricular function. J Am Coll Cardiol 6: 31–39.

36. Gomes JAC, Hariman RI, Kang PS, El-Sherif N, Chowdhry I, Lyons J. 1984. Programmed electrical stimulation in patients with high-grade ventricular ectopy: Electrophysiologic findings and prognosis for survival. Circulation 70: 43–51.

37. Hamer A, Vohra J, Hunt D, Sloman G. 1982. Prediction of sudden death by electrophysiologic

studies in high risk patients surviving acute myocardial infarction. Am J Cardiol 50: 223–229.

38. Roy D, Marchand E, Theroux P, Waters DD, Pelletier GB, Bourassa MG. 1985. Programmed ventricular stimulation in survivors of an acute myocardial infarction. Circulation 72: 487–494.

39. Denniss AR, Baaijens H, Cody DV, Richards DA, Russell PA, Young AA, Ross DL, Uther JB. 1985. Value of programmed stimulation and exercise testing in predicting one-year mortality after acute myocardial infarction. Am J Cardiol 56: 213–220.

40. Naccarelli G, Prystowsky EN, Jackman WM, Heger JJ, Rahilly GT, Zipes DP. 1982. Role of electrophysiologic testing in managing patients who have ventricular tachycardia unrelated to coronary artery disease. Am J Cardiol 50: 165–171.

41. Meinertz T, Treese N, Kasper W, Geibel A, Hoffman T, Zehender M, Bohn D, Pop T, Just H. 1985. Determinants of prognosis in idiopathic dilated cardiomyopathy as determined by programmed electrical stimulation. Am J Cardiol 56: 337–341.

42. Anderson KP, Stinson EB, Derby GC, Oyer PE, Mason JW. 1983. Vulnerability of patients with obstructive hypertrophic cardiomyopathy to ventricular arrhythmia induction in the operating room: Analysis of 17 patients. Am J Cardiol 55: 811–816.

43. Greene HL, Reid PR, Schaeffer AH. 1978. The repetitive ventricular response in man: A predictor of sudden death in man. N Engl J Med 299: 729–734.

44. Kowey PR, Folland ED, Parisi AF, Lown B. 1983. Programmed electrical stimulation of the heart in coronary artery disease. Am J Cardiol 51: 531–536.

45. Horowitz LN, Greenspan AM, Spielman SR, Webb CR, Morganroth J, Rotmensch H, Sokoloff NM, Rae AP, Segal BL, Kay HR. 1985. Usefulness of electrophysiologic testing in evaluation of amiodarone therapy for sustained ventricular tachyarrhythmias associated with coronary heart disease. Am J Cardiol 55: 367–71.

46. Naccarelli GV, Fineberg NS, Zipes DP, Heger JJ, Duncan G, Prystowsky EN. 1985. Amiodarone: Risk factors for recurrence of symptomatic ventricular tachycardia identified at electrophysiologic study. J Am Coll Cardiol 6: 814–821.

23. The role of electrophysiological studies in the management and therapy of recurrent ventricular tachycardias in patients with ischemic heart disease

MARK E. JOSEPHSON, JOHN M. MILLER, JOSEPH A. VASSALLO,
JESUS M. ALMENDRAL, FRANCIS E. MARCHLINSKI,
and ALFRED E. BUXTON
*Clinical Electrophysiology Laboratory, Hospital of the University of
Pennsylvania, Cardiovascular Section, Department of Medicine, University of
Pennsylvania School of Medicine, Philadelphia, Pennsylvania, USA*

Programmed electrical stimulation and endocardial catheter mapping have been widely employed over the last ten years to establish the diagnosis and mechanism of ventricular tachycardia (VT) as well as to determine the potential role of pharmacologic, electric or surgical therapy. The present manuscript will concentrate on the role of electrophysiologic studies for the management of VT.

VT in the setting of coronary artery disease is accepted by most workers to be due to reentry [1–5]. The reentrant circuit is probably at least partially anatomically determined by prior myocardial infarction. The infarction isolates viable myocardial cells in areas of fibrosis in the presence or absence of Purkinje fibers. The disorder in anatomy results in non-uniform anisotropy which, together with alterations in conduction and refractoriness, set up a pathophysiologic substrate for the tachycardia [6]. The substrate, however, requires some form of triggering mechanism to establish the sustained VT. This may be ventricular premature complexes but may also include changes in autonomic tone, heart rate, hemodynamics, or ischemia, all or some of which may be totally inapparent.

In order for programmed stimulation to be of value in the management of VT, certain prerequisites are necessary: (1) tachycardias that occur spontaneously can be replicated by programmed stimulation, (2) laboratory responses to pharmacologic agents predict clinical responsiveness to clinical therapy, (3) termination of VT by programmed stimulation allows one to test the safety and efficacy of electrical forms of therapy, and (4) mapping of VT can localize the arrhythmogenic substrate to an area which can be obliterated.

Programmed stimulation for induction of ventricular tachycardia

Many different programmed stimulation protocols have been employed in an attempt to induce sustained VT. Determination of the optimal protocol is not the subject of this manuscript and will be discussed elsewhere in this symposium. It is, however, known that paced cycle length, number of extrastimuli, site of stimlation and delivered current can all affect the inducibility of ventricular arrhythmias. In our laboratory we use one to three extrastimuli at twice diastolic threshold using 1 msec pulse widths. We initiate stimulation with one ventricular extrastimulus delivered during sinus rhythm and paced cycle lengths of 600 and 400 msec first from the right ventricular apex and then from a second catheter at the right ventricular outflow tract. If this fails to induce VT, two extrastimuli are given in a similar manner. Following this, rapid pacing is used from 300 msec down to cycle lengths resulting in loss of capture. Since we have not found rapid ventricular pacing to be an effective method of inducing VT, in recent studies it has been used only after other methods have failed. Three ventricular extrastimuli are then delivered during sinus rhythm and at paced cycle lengths of 600 and 400 msec alternately from the right ventricular apex and the outflow tract. If three extrastimuli fail to induce the tachycardia, then stimulation at other paced cycle lengths and/or right ventricular sites is employed. If this fails to induce a tachycardia, the entire protocol is repeated from one or two left ventricular sites. Using this protocol, we have been able to replicate clinical uniform sustained VT in approximately 95% of patients with coronary artery disease. As shown in Table 1, VT can be induced in the majority of patients with right ventricular stimulation and with up to three right ventricular extrastimuli delivered from either the right ventricular outflow tract or apex. Rapid pacing has a much lower yield of inducing the tachycardia and of the patients who required right ventricular pacing, at least half occurred early in our experience when only two extrastimuli were routinely used. The need for left ventricular stimulation for VT induction has been reduced from 10% when 2 right ventricular extrastimuli were utilized [7] to less than 5% now that three ventricular extrastimuli, or sometimes more, are utilized. Although Brugada et al suggest that three extrastimuli from

Table 1. Sustained ventricular tachycardia. 461 patients; inducible – 433 (94%).

Minimum stimulation required to induce VT			
RV	406	LV	27
1 VES	110	1 VES	6
2 VES	194	2 VES	16
3 VES	87	3 VES	2
4 VES	5	4 VES	2
RVP	10	RVP	2

LV = left ventricle.
VES = ventricular extrastimuli.
RV = right ventricle.
RVP = right ventricular pacing.

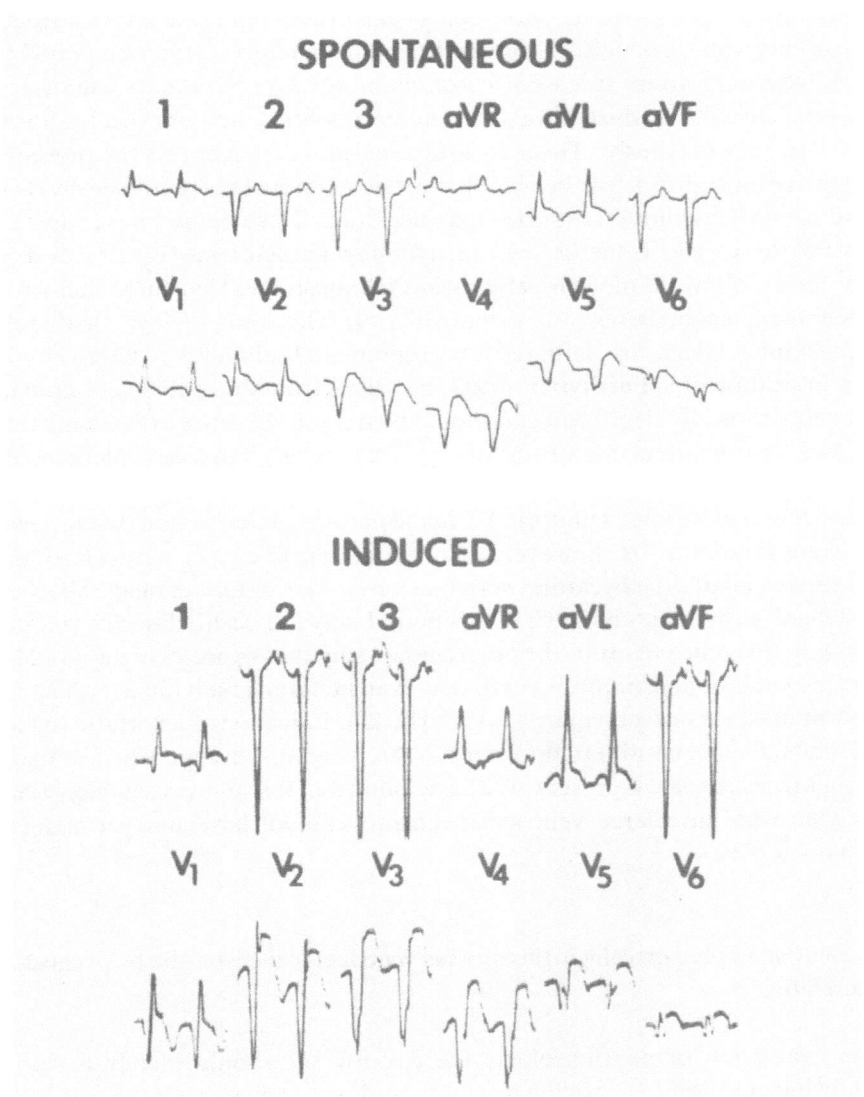

Figure 1. Spontaneous and induced ventricular tachycardia. The 12-lead ECG of the spontaneous and the induced ventricular tachycardia are shown. It is readily apparent that the induced tachycardia closely mimics that of the spontaneous tachycardia both in rate and morphology.

the right ventricular apex at three drive cycle lengths is adequate [8], our data suggest use of the right ventricular outflow tract can increase the yield of inducible VT by up to 25% [9, 10]. The use of multiple extrastimuli during sinus rhythm may be reserved for late in the study since induction of VT during sinus rhythm alone occurs in less than 5% of patients. Similar inducibility rates have been found by several groups [11–13].

A tachycardia with similar morphology and cycle length can always be induced in patients with sustained VT outside the immediate peri-infarction period (Fig. 1). In coronary artery disease it is common, however, to induce uniform, sustained tachycardias which have different morphologies and/or cycle lengths than are seen spontaneously. This becomes even more frequent in the presence of antiarrhythmic drugs. We believe that these additional morphologically distinct sustained VT are important since mapping studies (see below) have shown that most of these come from the same arrhythmogenic substrate [14, 15]. Moreover, long term follow-up of such patients has demonstrated that these tachycardias often recur spontaneously if drugs fail [15]. Thus, we believe that uniform tachycardias which are initiated by programmed stimulation before or after administration of antiarrhytmic drugs, but differ from the initial tachycardia, are probably clinically significant and should be treated. Because of these indings we believe that the induction of sustained VT can be used to assess pharmacologic therapy.

Induction of sustained uniform VT in the peri-infarction period (within 6 weeks of acute infarction) is, however, of uncertain significance, particularly in the absence of similar tachycardias spontaneously. We and others have shown that sustained arrhythmias induced in this period may not occur clinically [16–18]. In addition, the more vigorous the programmed stimulation protocol the more likely one is to induce nonspecific arrhythmias even in normal individuals, which in the bulk of instances are polymorphic VT's [19, 20]. Induction of a uniform sustained VT outside the peri-infarction period rarely occurs except when a fixed or permanent substrate is present. We have found that this may occasionally occur in patients who have large ventricular anneurysms but have not yet manifested sustained VT.

Evaluation of pharmacologic therapy for ventricular tachycardia by programmed stimulation

The evaluation of pharmacologic therapy for VT should ideally answer the following questions: (1) can the drug slow and/or terminate spontaneous VT? (2) can the drug prevent initiation of VT after VT is terminated by programmed stimulation and/or drugs? and (3) can long term oral therapy of the agent prevent induction and spontaneus recurrence of the tachycardia?. The first objective; i.e., the ability to slow and terminate the tachycardia, can only be answered if the tachycardia is hemodynamically tolerated long enough for the agent to be administered. Because this is relatively infrequent it is not answerable in the overall population of patients with VT secondary to coronary artery disease. It has been noted, however, that all standard Type IA agents of the quinidine class can, if delivered intravenously, slow VT [21] (Fig. 2). On the other hand, the administration of lidocaine-like drugs intravenously has not in our experience had any

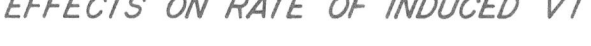

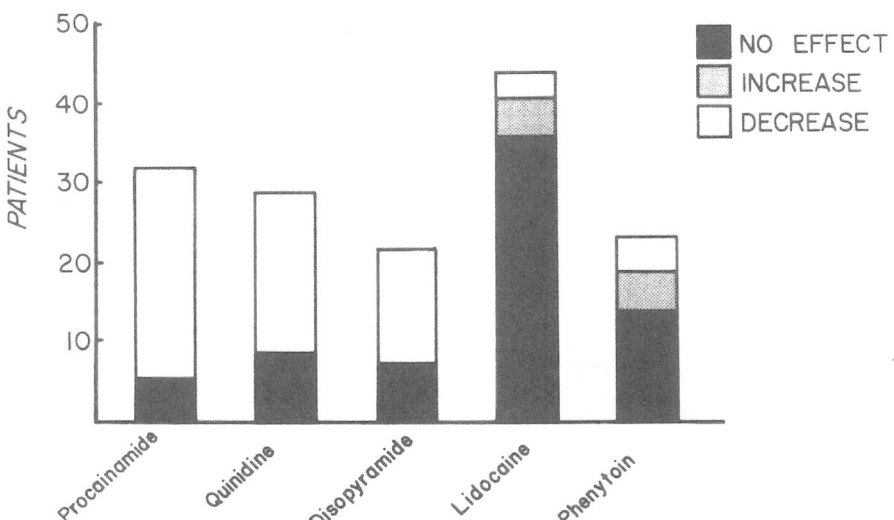

Figure 2. Effects of Type I agents on rate of induced ventricular tachycardia. Thenumber of patients is shown on the vertical axis and each of the individual agents are shown underneath bars along the horizontal axis. The filled, dark area represents no effect on tachycardia rate, stippled area represents increase in tachycardia rate, and open area reprsents a decrease in tachycardia rate. It is readily apparent that procainamide, quinidine, and disopyramide tend to slow tachycardia rates, while lidocaine and phenytoin either have no effect or may actually accelerate the tachycardia. (From Horowitz et al., with permission.) [21]

significant effect on tachycardia cycle lengths except in occasional patients where it may even shorten the tachycardia cycle length [21].

Most of the available data relate to the ability of a drug to affect initiation of VT acutely and/or on oral (>72 hours) therapy. Several criteria have been proposed to assess a drug efficacy in the prevention of sustained VT [24, 25]. These include: (1) narrowing of the zone of tachycardia induction; (2) increased difficulty in initiation of the tachycardia (i.e., greater number of extrastimuli or shorter drive cycle length); (3) prevention of induction of any tachycardia, even nonsustained tachycardia; and (4) prevention of inducible sustained VT; i.e., the clinical arrhythmia. We believe that only the prevention of the sustained arrhythmia is necessary as a successful endpoint. If the patient has sustained VT spontaneously, then induction of a nonsustained tachycardia, which almost invariably is less than ten beats in duration, would be considered a successful endpoint. An example of drug testing in a patient is shown in Figure 3. Dose response curves can also be evaluated (Fig. 4).

In order to abbreviate the number of studies using Type I agents in a given patient we sought to determine if the response to high-dose procainamide could

CONTROL

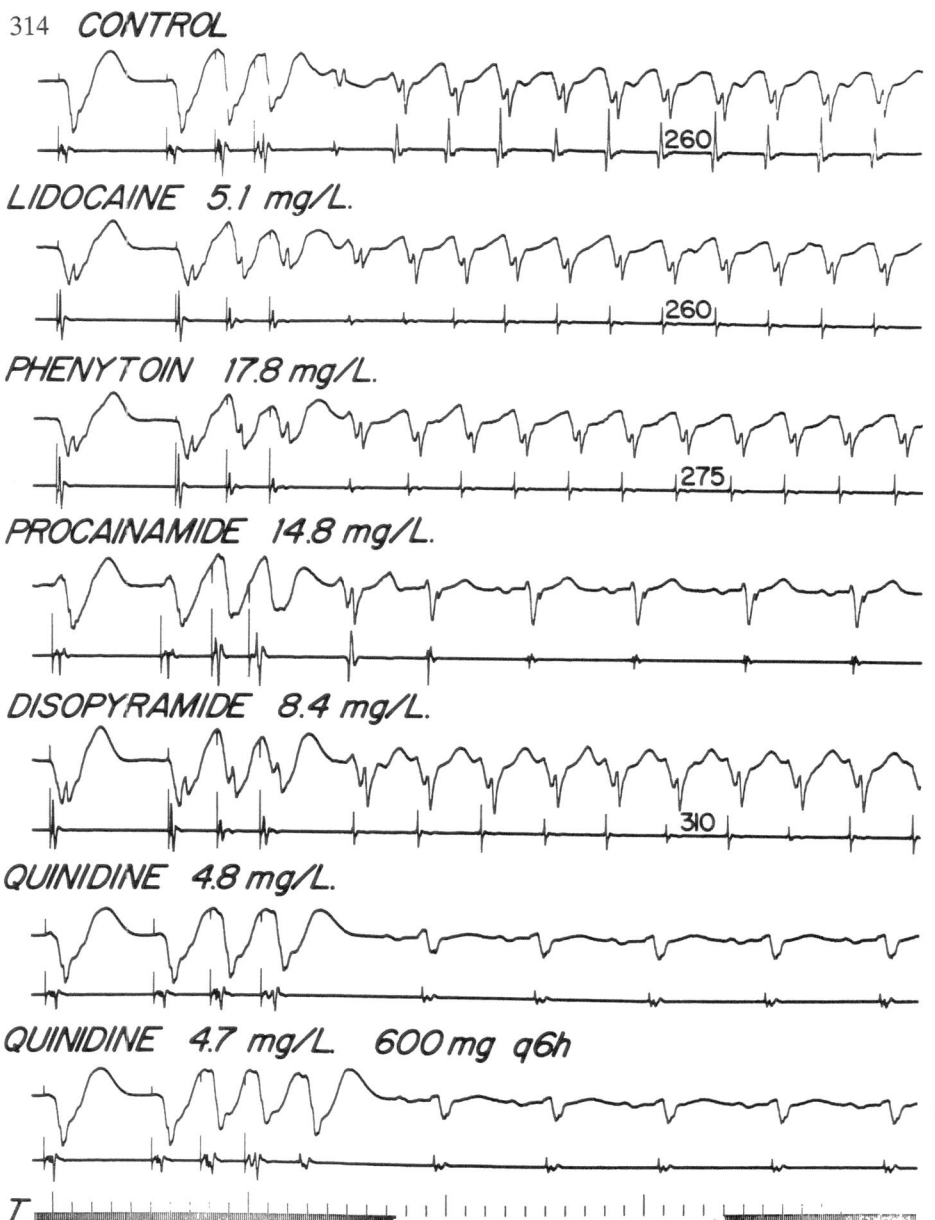

LIDOCAINE 5.1 mg/L.

PHENYTOIN 17.8 mg/L.

PROCAINAMIDE 14.8 mg/L.

DISOPYRAMIDE 8.4 mg/L.

QUINIDINE 4.8 mg/L.

QUINIDINE 4.7 mg/L. 600 mg q6h

Figure 3. Chronic drug study for ventricular tachycardia. In each panel is shown surface lead V_1 and an intracardiac recording from the right ventricular apex during ventricular stimulation. On the top is shown the control induction where two extrastimuli induced a sustained, uniform tachycardia with a left bundle branch block configuration having a cycle length of 260 msec. On different days lidocaine, phenytoin, procainamide, disopyramide, and quinidine are tested. The effects of these agents on inducibility is shown. Lidocaine, phenytoin, and disopyramide at the plasma levels shown failed to prevent initiration of the tachycardia and only disopyramide significantly slows this tachycardia. Both procainamide and quinidine at their respective plasma levels prevent initiation of the tachycardia. Quinidine was chosen for chronic therapy and was administered at 600 mg q6h to produce a plasma level comparable to that noted in the laboratory which prevented induction of the tachycardia. The patient has remained free of tachycardia on this regimen.

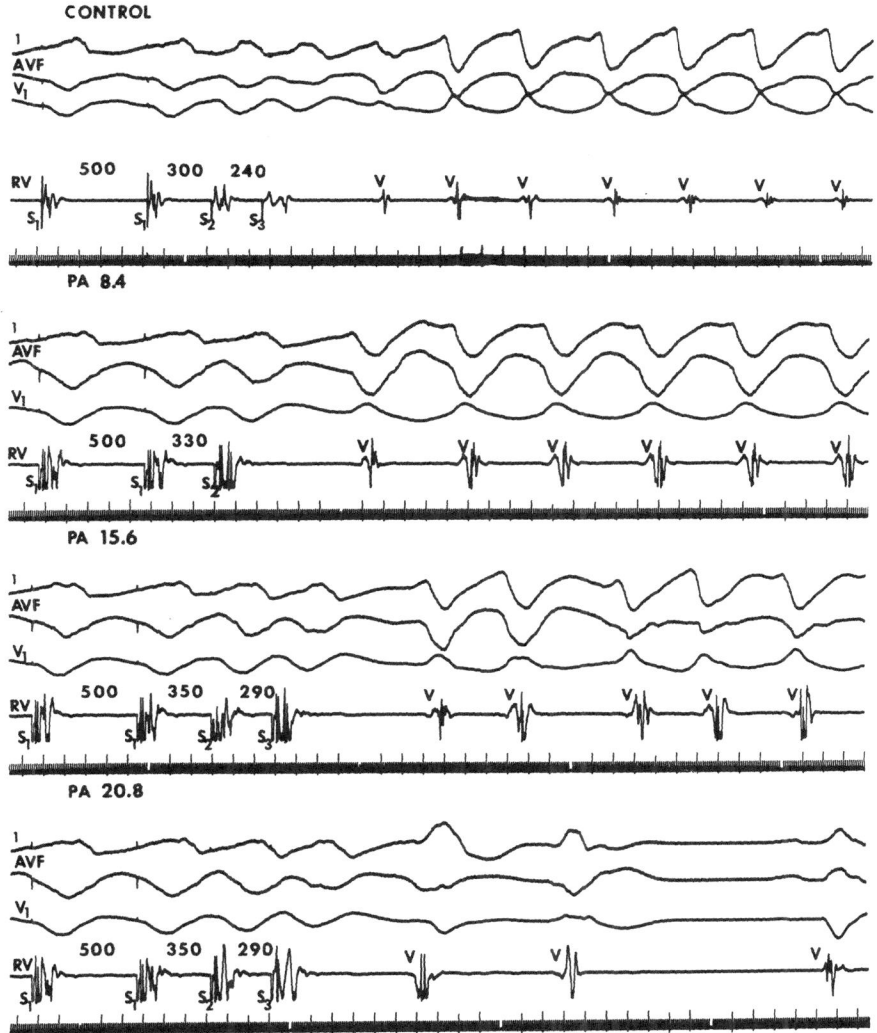

Figure 4. Effects of increasing dose of procainamide on ventricular tachycardia induction. In all four panels leads 1, AVF and V₁ are shown along with a right ventricular apical electrogram (RV) and time lines. During the control study two ventricular extrastimuli (S₂, S₃) delivered during a drive cycle length of 500 msec induced ventricular tachycardia with a right bundle branch block, right superior axis. Following 1 gram of procainamide producing a plasma level of 8.4 mg/ml the tachycardia is more easily induced (only a single extrastimulus is required). In addition the tachycardia is slower and the interval from the initiating impulse to the onset of the tachycardia is increased. Following an additional 500 mg the tachycardia once again requires two extrastimuli to induce and is relatively unstable with marked oscillations in cycle length. Note that th interval from the initiating impulse to the first beat of the tachycardia is even further prolonged. Finally, after an additional 500 mg the tachycardia is no longer inducible althouh two intraventricular responses are. (From Greenspan et al. Am J Cardiol 46: 453, 1980, with permission.)

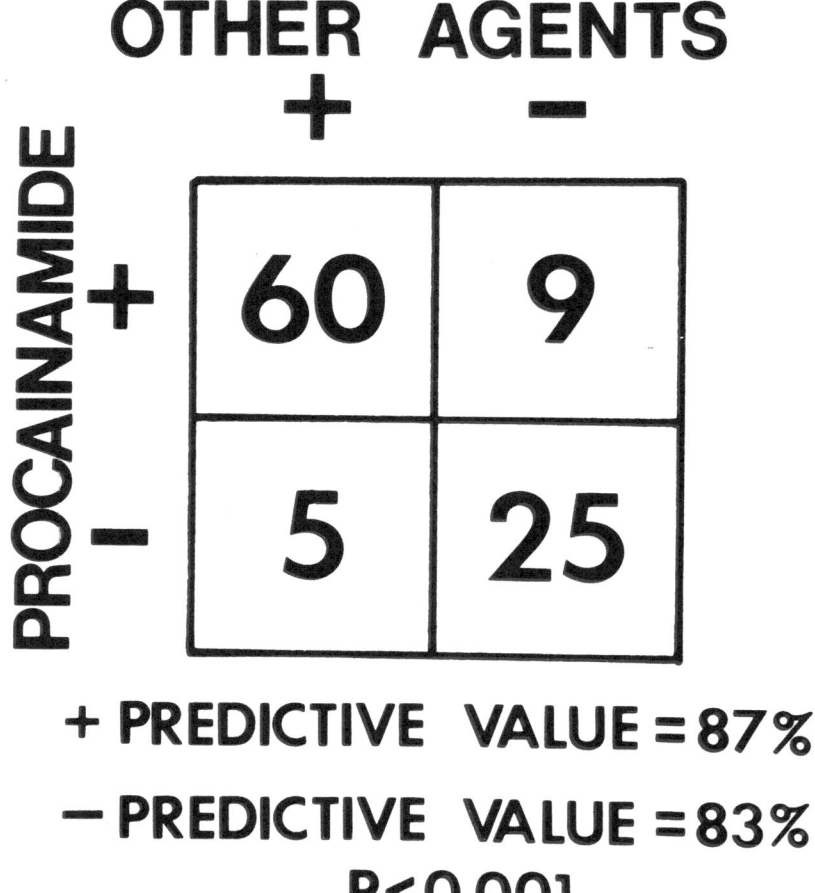

OTHER AGENTS

	+	**−**
+	60	9
−	5	25

(vertical axis label: **PROCAINAMIDE**)

+ PREDICTIVE VALUE = 87%
− PREDICTIVE VALUE = 83%
P < 0.001

Figure 5. Patient response during serial electrophysiologic testing compared with response to procainamide. The response to programmed stimulation following procainamide (vertical axis) is compared to that following other Type I agents singly and/or in combination. The plus sign refers to inducibility and the minus sign to non-inducibility of ventricular tachycardia. It can be seen that if a tachycardia is inducible after procainamide it is likely to be inducible on other Type I agents (positive predictive value of 87%). Conversely, failure to have a tachycardia inducible on procainamide corresponds to failure of inducibility on other Type I agents with a predictive value of 83%. (From Waxman et al., with permission.) [22]

predict the outcome for other agents. In a report of 126 patients, Waxman et al [22] have shown that the response to procainamide can correctly predict a positive or negative response to other Type I agents singly and/or in combination of approximately 85% of patients (Fig. 5). Thus, it is our current policy to administer 15 mg/kg of procainamide initially and assess the induction of VT at this dosage. If this fails to prevent induction of VT, incremental doses up to 30 mg/kg are administered. If procainamide fails to prevent induction of the tachycardia, then experimental drugs, usually amiodarone, are employed. In patients who are intolerant of amiodarone or who demonstrate proarrhythmic effects to other antiarrhythmic agents we will return to the Type I agents and try the other agents singly and/or in combination, hoping that they will be among the 15% of patients who will respond favorably despite failing a procainamide trial.

Using the methodology outlined above, several laboratories have shown a good predictive accuracy of electrophysiologic testing for Type I agents [13, 21, 23–25]. Patients whose tachycardias are rendered noninducible have approximately an 85% chance of remaining free of arrhythmias while maintaining adequate drug levels over an approximate two-year period. More variable, however, is the prediction of failure of an agent. The range of negative predictive accuracy ranges from 40 to 100%; however, on the average approximately 70% of patients in whom induction of VT is not prevented by programmed stimulation will have a recurrence [13, 21, 23–25]. Our current data showing a 90% positive predictive value and 70% negative predictive value for Type I agents, is similar to that presented by Mason et al and others [23]. Swerdlow et al [26] have shown that failure to respond to a Type I agent based on programmed extrastimulation is an independent predictor of sudden cardiac death in patients with recurrent VT.

We have found amiodarone to be the single most effective drug in those patients failing Type I agents. Amiodarone, however, differs from the Type I agents in that we do not feel that programmed stimulation can accurately predict clinical success. Approximately 11% of patients given amiodarone will have their tachycardia rendered noninducible, yet the clinical success may be 60 to 70% [27–32]. In addition, we have not found either the absolute number of extrastimuli required for induction or the relative ease or difficulty in induction of the arrhythmia to predict recurrence [28]. Others do not agree and feel that a decrease in the ease of inducibility predicts recurrence and an increase in difficulty predicts success [31–33]. We, however, have not found this to be the case in treating 200 patients who have sustained VT using amiodarone.

In sum, programmed stimulation remains the most successful and reproducible method of replicating and studying clinical arrhythmias. In the selected population with ischemic heart disease and VT studied to date, effective drug therapy can be identified in less than 50% of patients. Response to conventional drugs (Type I) assessed by programmed stimulation predicts clinical outcome. Programmed stimulation appears to have limited value in predicting the efficacy (particularly a negative predictive of value; i.e., failure rate) of amiodarone. A similar problem may exist in other experimental drugs which have active metabolites. There needs to be a clarification of what the endpoints of the stimulation study are and these will be discussed elsewhere in this symposium. There are problems generic to pharmacologic therapy that are independent of how the drug is chosen. These include the fact that: (1) there is no uniformly successful drug, (2) all drugs are potentially arrhythmogenic, (3) there is a narrow toxic/therapeutic ratio to currently available drugs, and (4) patient compliance is variable.

Electrical therapy of ventricular tachycardia

Electrical therapy currently involves the use of pacemakers, automatic implantable defibrillators, low energy cardioverters, and catheter ablation. All of these topics will be discussed in detail subsequently in this symposium; however, some comments concerning termination of VT by stimulation are required to better understand the potential for and limitations of electrical therapy. Our protocol for stimulation during VT is similar to that used for inducing VT. Thus, one, two, and three ventricular extrastimuli are sequentially given during VT from one or more right ventricular sites. Synchronized bursts are then given which may include additional ventricular extrastimuli. It is important that bursts be synchronized for reproducibility and safety of termination sequences. Factors influencing the ability to terminate VT include cycle length of the VT, distance from the stimulation site to the VT site of origin, the refractory period of the stimulation site, the conduction time from the stimulation site to the VT site, and the duration of the excitable gap in the reentrant circuit. These all assume a reentrant circuit which is responsible for VT. The tachycardia cycle length is probably the most important factor because it secondarily will determine whether the stimulation site is too distant and the coupling interval of stimuli too long to conduct to and terminate the tachycardia. The size of the excitable gap is also critical. Circuits which have in essence no fully excitable gap; i.e., leading circuit type VT's, are unlikely to be terminated by programmed stimulation, while those with fully and/or partially excitable gaps are most likely to be terminated. The exact role of the excitable gap in the termination of VT has not been evaluated in detail. Preliminary data from our laboratory suggest that resetting of a VT is a requisite to termination by one or more extrastimuli. This is probably just an indication that an excitable gap is present and can be penetated by the stimulated impulse.

We have evaluated the role of cycle length and number of extrastimuli on the ability to terminate tachycardia [34]. We have found that single extrastimuli rarely terminated VT with cycle lengths less than 300 msec. Most commonly, if a tachycardia can be terminated by a single extrastimulus, the VT rate will be ≤150 beats/minute. Termination by two extrastimuli similarly usually require relatively slow tachycardias. Rapid ventricular pacing is usually required for tachycardias with cycle lengths 300 msec or less. It is the same rapid tachycardias in which cardioversion is often necessary, either primarily or secondary to acceleration of the tachycardia by burst pacing. We hve found that rapid ventricular pacing with synchronized bursts is the most effective way to terminate VT, being successful in approximately 76% of patients. Single extrastimuli succeed in perhaps only 25% of patients where double extrastimuli are effective in approximately 50 to 60% of those patients in whom they can be delivered. Acceleration of VT bears a direct relationship to efficacy; while only 1 to 2% of tachycardias are accelerated with single extrastimuli, up to 35% of tachycardias may be accelerated with bursts of rapid pacing. Fisher et al. have reviewed this subject in detail and gave similar data on acceleration [35, 36]. Thus, the most effective pacing modality is also the most dangerous and potentially lethal. Despite the many technological advances inpacing, we therefore believe that pacing remains a low priority in the management of VT in the absence of a defibrillator backup. In the rare cases in which pacing is offered as a therapeutic modality, hundreds of attempts of the pacing modality should be utilized to show that it is reproducible, and safe; a single instance of acceleration could result in death. It is our impression that if pacemakers are used they should have scanning and adaptive capability in order to adjust for changes in cycle lengths of tachycardia.

The major advance in electrical therapy has been the development of the automatic internal cardioverter/defibrillator [37, 38]. This device, which was developed by Dr. Mirowski, will be discussed later in this symposium. Basically, the device is able to sense VT and/or fibrillation and deliver 25 to 35 joules of energy to terminate the tachycardia or fibrillation (Fig. 6). The device has clearly been shown to decrease the incidence of sudden death in patients withlife-threatening arrhythmias and is an absolute necessity to accompany any anti-tachycardia pacing modality. There are, however, important limitations and problems with this device [39]. Sensing of rates in excess of the trigger rate due to sinus tachycardia or atrial fibrillation remains a problem and may result in multiple shocks in conscious patients. Similarly, paroxysms of nonsustained VT can result in a mean rate exceeding that of the trigger rate and the automatic implantable cardioverter/defibrillator will discharge during sinus rhythm in a conscious patient. These problems may be resolved through the use of antiar-rhyhmic drugs and/or beta-blockers. The limited longevity of the device (100 shock capacity) makes it unwise to use in someone with multiple recurrent episodes of VT/fibrillation. Antiarrhythmic therapy to decrease the number of episodes is necessary. It is hoped that advances in technology over the next ten years will miniaturize this device, improve its sensing capabilities, include adaptive pacing modalities and backup demand pacemaker support. With these developments, this device will have a more widespread application in the management of ventricular tachyarrhythmias. Electrophysiologic testing must be done to determine whether the device works in situ and as well as to assess the potential effects of drugs on the defibrillation capability. While the use of alternate current has been suggested to accomplish this end, we do not believe this is a useful way to induce tachycardia. More often ventricular fibrillation is induced and not the clinical tachycardia.

Localization of the site of origin of the tachycardia

VT arises near the subendocardium of the ventricle [4, 40, 41]. It does so in areas of prior infarction which are usually, but not always, visible to the naked eye as scar tissue. Studies using activation mapping both preoperatively and intra-

320

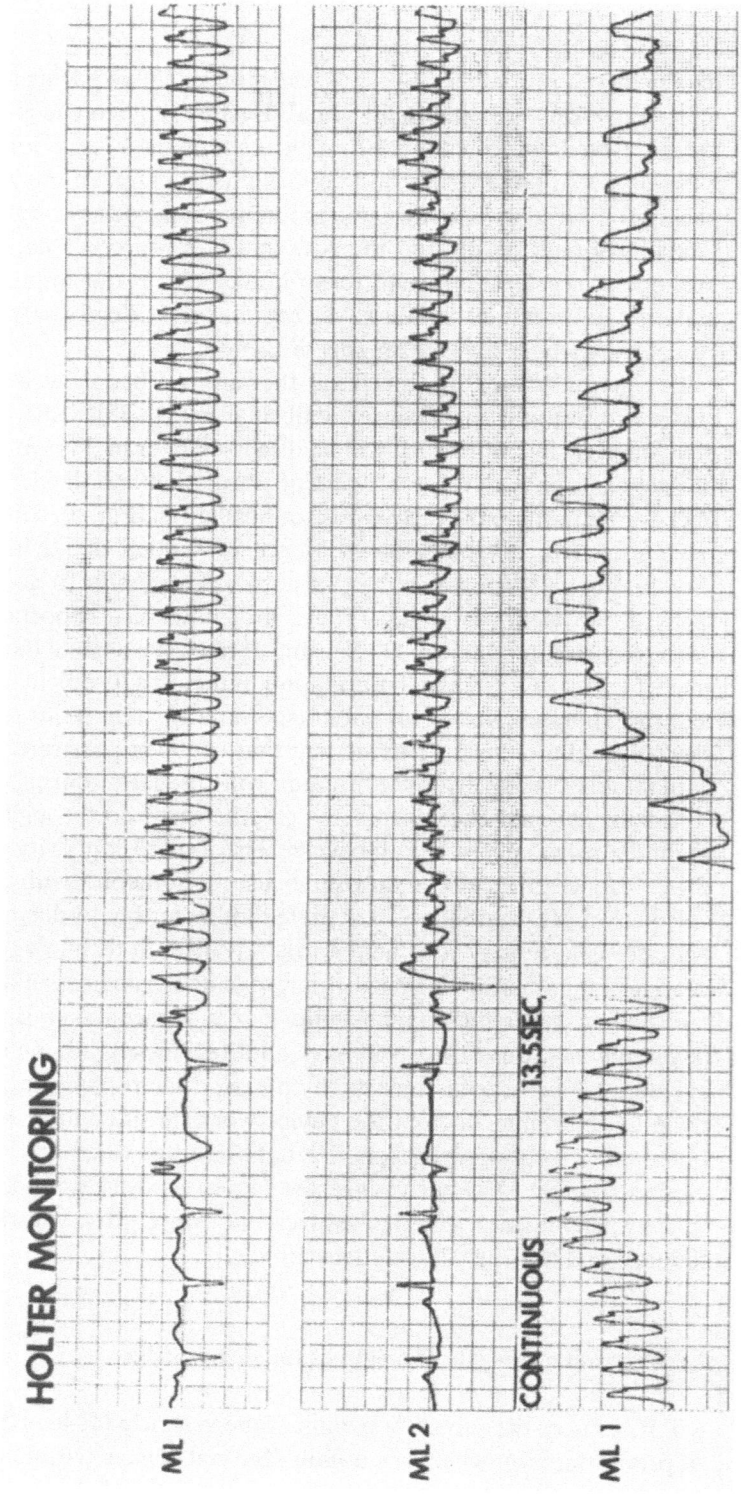

HOLTER MONITORING

ML 1

ML 2

CONTINUOUS   13.5 SEC.

ML 1

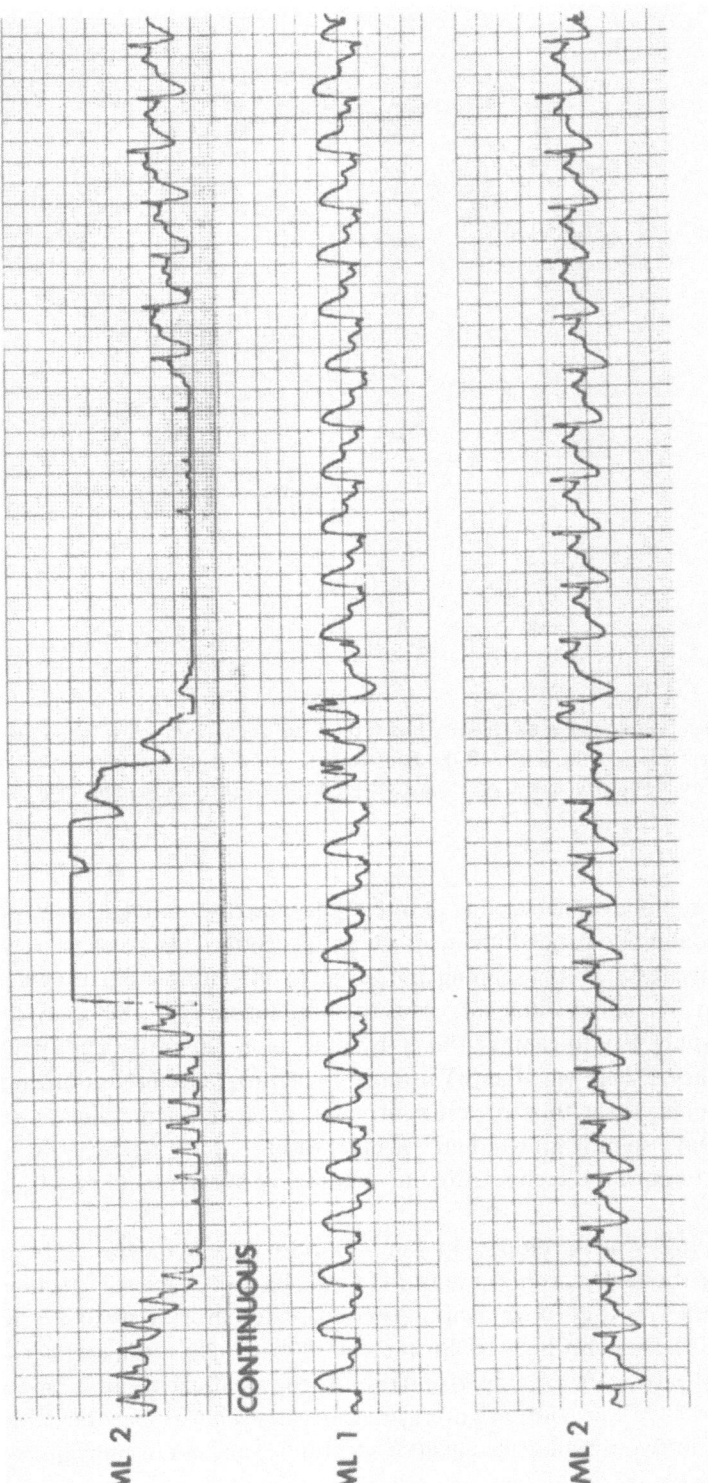

Figure 6. Successful function of the automatic implantable cardioverter/defibrillator (AICD) during Holter monitoring. Simultaneous two-lead Holter monitor is shown. In the top tracing sustained ventricular tachycardia spontaneously occurs at a rate of approximately 210 beats per minute after 13.5 seconds of the tachycardia the AICD discharges at 25 joules and converts the tachycardia to sinus rhythm. Note the persistence of ST elevation in the ML 1 lead which resolved within 1 minute of monitoring.

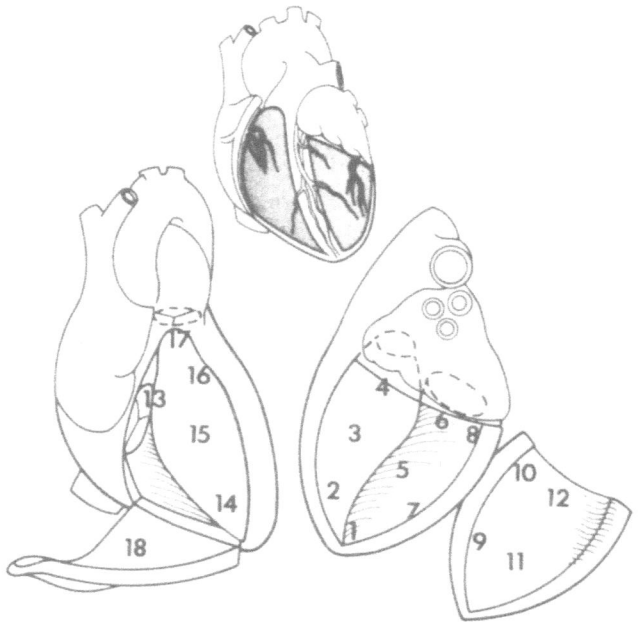

Figure 7. Mapping schema of the heart. The heart, which is shown on top, is opened up to allow one to visualize the right ventricle (on the left) and the left ventricle (on the right). There are 12 left ventricular sites and 6 right ventricular sites which are used for mapping. (From Josephson et al., with permission.) [42]

operatively can, we believe, accurately define areas of arrhythmogenicity which can be altered by ablative procedures or isolation procedures to prevent recurrences of the tachycardia. Both mapping and surgery will be discussed elsewhere in this symposium. We believe that surgery is the only sure way to cure tachycardia since it is the only way to remove the arrhythmogenic substrate. The typical ptient with coronary disease who has VT usually has a prior large infarction and a left ventricular aneurysm with poor left ventricular function. Many have heart failure and 80% have significant residual coronary disease; thus, surgery offers a method not only to cure the tachycardia but to improve survival and functional capacity.

Catheter mapping was developed in our laboratory as a means to better understand where the tachycardia came from [4, 40, 42, 43]. A mapping schema as shown in Figure 7 is used in our laboratory to regionalize areas of the left ventricle which can be reliably located. Sustained uniform tachycardias which are hemodynamically stable can be mapped and usually show a focal origin, as shown in Figure 8. Of note, VT in coronary artery disease arises at or near the subendocardium of the left ventricular free wall or septum regardless of morphology. Multiple tachycardia morphologies are often present and they, too, can be

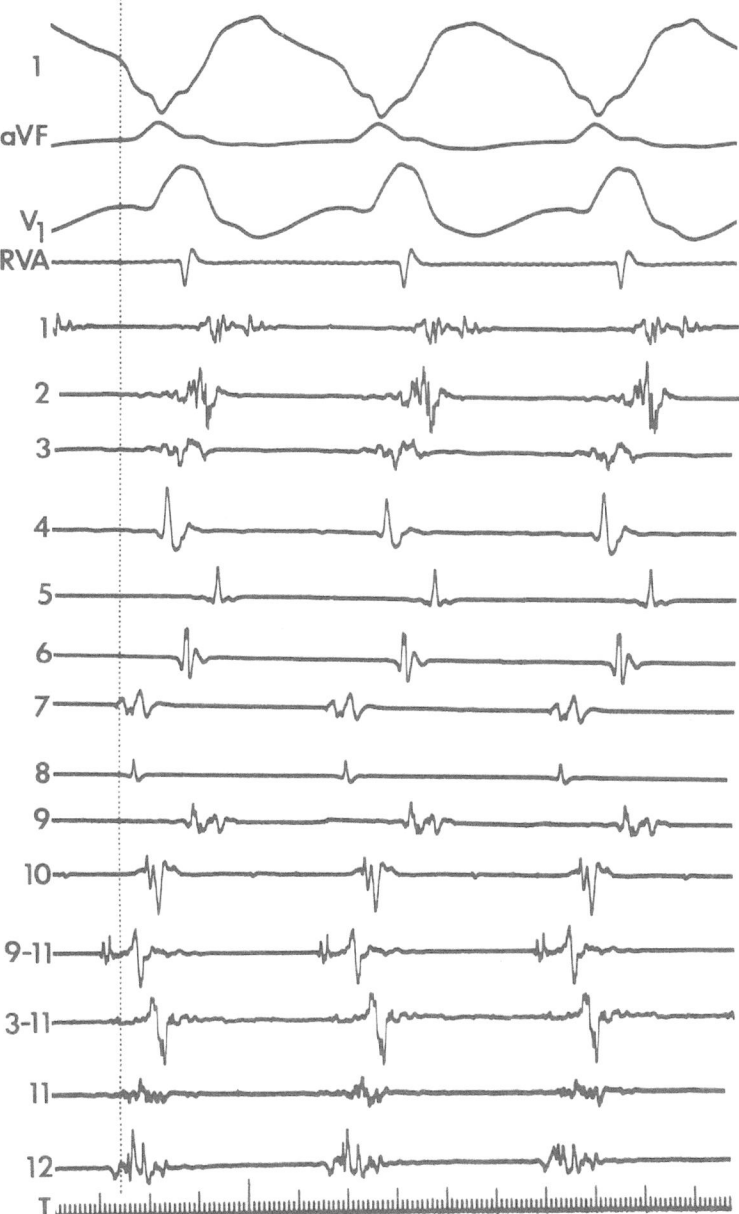

Figure 8. Catheter map of ventricular tachycardia. ECG leads 1, aVF, and V₁ are shown with a reference electrogram from the right ventricular apex (RVA) and electrograms from various left ventricular sites. The tachycardia has a right bundle, right inferior axis. The dotted line marks the onset of the QRS. The earliest site of activation is noted at site 9–11 which is on the anterolateral wall of the left ventricle. Note that activation precedes next to the adjacent sites 11 and 12. Block is evident toward site 9 since its activation is markedly delayed relative to the adjacent site of origin of 9–11. Note the abnormalities in the local electrograms at the site of origin of the tachycardia and elsewhere in the left ventricle.

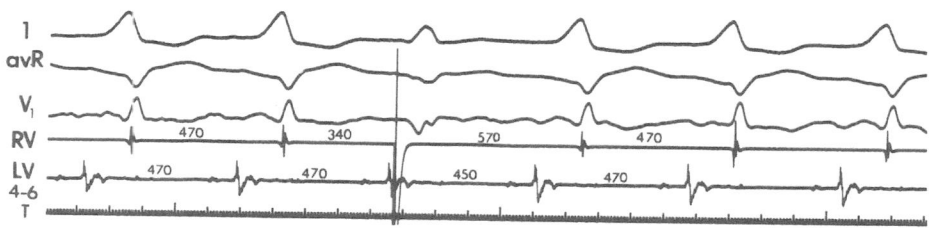

Figure 9. Use of resetting to distinguish a diastolic electrogram as being related to the site of origin. Shown is ventricular tachycardia. Leads 1, avR and V₁ are shown along with a reference electrogram from the right ventricular apex and the assumed early site of origin at the left ventricular site 4–6. Time lines are shown in addition (T). A presystolic electrogram is seen in mid-diastole 130 msec prior to the onset of the QRS. Following the second beat of the tachycardia, a right ventricular extrastimulus is delivered. This resets the tachycardia which is advanced in the next complex. Note that presystolic activity remains in a fixed relationship to the subsequent QRS although it is brought in by the prior premature impulse. This fixed relationship to the QRS makes this presystolic electrogram 'early', at the likely site of origin of the tachycardia.

mapped. Approximately 60% of all VT can be mapped in the catheterization laboratory. The remainder cannot be mapped due to hemodynamic intolerance or transient appearance and must undergo activation mapping intraoperatively. We have shown that most of these tachycardias also originate in the same general area, although 15 to 20% may arise from disparate sites [14, 15]. Occasionally multicomponent electrograms are present which are observed throughout diastole. It is extremely important to prove that mid-diastolic signals are in fact a necessary and early part of the tachycardia circuit rather than representing extremely slow conduction to areas not involved in the circuit. This requires stimulation during the tachycardia to demonstrate that these diastolic components bear a fixed relationship to the onset of the QRS and are not independent, late sites (Fig. 9).

Pace-mapping is another procedure which has been employed as a means of corroborating our mapping data [44, 45]. When certain tachycardias cannot be mapped due to lack of inducibility or hemodynamic instability, pacing multiple sites within the left ventricle, trying to find the site from which stimulation replicates the tachycardia morphology on 12-lead ECG, may occasionally be useful (Fig. 10). In addition, mapping during sinus rhythm to localize abnormal electrograms can be used to define the anatomic substrate of VT. Recent data from our laboratory has shown that abnormal and fractionated electrograms are more a reflection of infarction than a reflection of the site of origin of the tachycardia [46]. We therefore define a potential anatomic or pathophysiologic substrate but not necessarily the precise regions responsible for the VT. If used as the basis for surgery, a more widespread resection than absolutely necessary will be performed. The use of catheter mapping, which will be discussed later in this symposium, and intraoperative mapping has markedly improved our understanding of the mechanism of VT and has led to the development of surgical techniques which have been successful in curing VT.

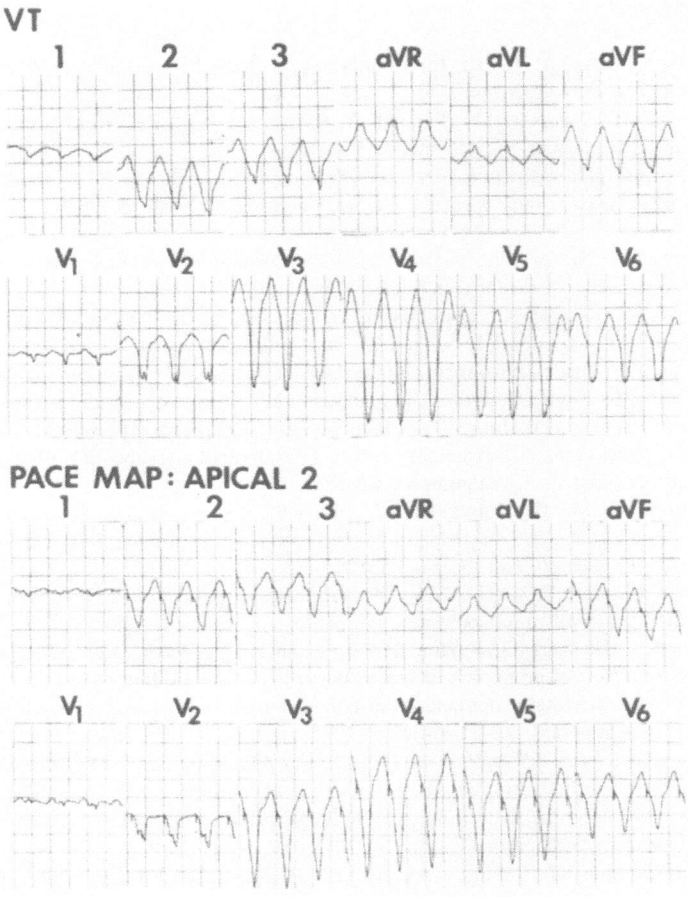

Figure 10. Pace-mapping of ventricular tachycardia. Ventricular tachycardia with a left bundle branch block, right superior axis morphology is shown on top. Pacing the inferoapical left ventricular septum at a cycle length approximating that of the tachycardia replicates a QRS morphology of the tachycardia. This suggests that this site is at or near the site of origin of the tachycardia. See text for further discussion.

Summary

The evolution of programmed stimulation and activation mapping has allowed for a rational and reproducible approach to the management of VT associated with coronary artery disease. Effective selection of pharmacologic, electrical or surgical therapy can be made. The limitations of these techniques as well as the various forms of therapy will be discussed elsewhere in this symposium.

References

1. Wellens JJ, Duren DR, Lie KI. 1976. Observations on mechanisms of ventricular tachycardia in man. Circulation 54: 237–244.
2. Josephson ME, Horowitz LN, Farshidi A, Kastor JA. 1978. Recurrent sustained ventricular tachycardia. 1. Mechanisms. Circulation 57: 431–440.
3. Josephson ME, Horowitz LN, Farshidi A, Spielman SR, Michelson EL, Greenspan AM. 1978. Sustained ventricular tachycardia: Evidence for protected localized reentry. Am J Cardiol 42: 416–424.
4. Josephson ME, Horowitz LN, Farshidi A. 1978. Continuous local electrical activity. A mechanism of recurrent ventricular tachycardia. Circulation 57: 659–665.
5. Josephson ME, Buxton AE, Marchlinski FE, Doherty JU, Cassidy DM, Kienzle MG, Vassallo JA, Miller JM, Almendral J, Grogan W. 1985. Sustained ventricular tachycardia in coronary artery disease – Evidence for reentrant mechanism. In: *Cardiac Electrophysiology and Arrhythmias*. Edited by Zipes DP, Jalife J, Orlando, Florida, Grune & Stratton, pp. 409–418.
6. Fenoglio JJ, Pham TD, Harken AH, Horowitz LN, Josephson ME, Wit AL. 1983. Recurrent sustained ventricular tachycardia: Structure and ultrastructure of subendocardial regions in which tachycardia originates. Circulation 68: 518–533.
7. Robertson JF, Cain ME, Horowitz LN, Spielman SR, Greenspan AM, Waxman HL, Josephson ME. 1981. Anatomic and electrophysiologic correlates of ventricular tachycardia requiring left ventricular stimulation. Am J Cardiol 48: 263–268.
8. Brugada P, Wellens HJJ. 1985. Comparison in the same patient of two programmed ventricular stimulation protocols to induce ventricular tachycardia. Am J Cardiol 55: 380–383.
9. Doherty JU, Kienzle MG, Buxton AE, Marchlinski FE, Waxman HL, Josepson ME. 1984. Discordant results of programmed ventricular stimulation at different right ventricular sites in patients with and without spontaneous sustained ventricular tachycardia: A prospective study of 56 patients. Am J Cardiol 54: 336–342.
10. Doherty JU, Kienzle MG, Waxman HL, Buxton AE, Marchlinski FE, Josephson ME. 1983. Programmed ventricular stimulation at a second right ventricular site: An analysis of 100 patients, with special references to sensitivity, specificity and characteristics of patients with induced ventricular tachycardia. Am J Cardiol 52: 1184–1189.
11. Fisher JD, Cohen ML, Mehra R, Altschuler M, Escher DJW, Furman S. 1977. Cardiac pacing and pacemakers. II. Serial electrophysiologic-pharmacologic testing for control of recurrent tachyarrhythmias. Am Heart J 93: 658–668.
12. Mason JW, Winkle RA. 1978. Electrode-catheter arrhythmia induction in the selection and assessment of antiarrhythmic drug therapy for recurrent ventricular tachycardia. Circulation 58: 971–985.
13. Ruskin JN, Garan H. 1979. Chronic electrophysiologic testing in patients with recurrent sustained ventricular tachycardia. Am J Cardiol 43: 400.
14. Josephson ME, Horowitz LN, Farshidi A, Spielman SR, Michelson EL, Greenspan AM. 1979. Recurrent sustained ventricular tachycardia. 4. Pleomorphism. Circulation 59: 459–468.
15. Miller JM, Kienzle MG, Harken AH, Josephson ME. 1984. Morphologically distinct sustained ventricular tachycardia in coronary artery disease: Significance and surgical results. JACC 4: 1073–1079.
16. Marchlinski FE, Buxton AE, Waxman HL, Josephson ME. 1983. Identifying patients at risk of sudden death after myocardial infarction: Value of the response to programmed stimulation, degree of ventricular ectopic activity and severity of left ventricular dysfunction. Am J Cardiol 52: 1190–1196.
17. Roy D, Marchand E, Theroux P, Waaters DD, Pelletier GB, Bourassa MG. 1985. Programmed ventricular stimulation in survivors of an acute myocardial infarction. Circulation 72: 487–494.
18. Santarelli P, Bellocci F, Loperfido F, Mazzari M, Mongiardo R, Montenero AS, Manzoli U,

Denes P. 1985. Ventricular arrhythmia by programmed ventricular stimulation after acute myocardial infarction. Am J Cardiol 55: 391–394.

19. Brugada P, Abdollah H, Heddle B, Wellens HJJ. 1983. Results of a ventricular stimulation protocol using a maximum of 4 premature stimuli in patients without documented or suspected ventricular arrhythmias. Am J Cardiol 52: 1214–1218.

20. Brugada P, Green M, Abdollah H, Wellens HJJ. 1984. Significance of ventricular arrhythmias initiated by programmed ventricular stimulation: The importance of the type of ventricular arrhythmia induced and the number of premature stimuli required. Circulation 69: 87–92.

21. Horowitz LN, Josephson ME, Kastor JA. 1980. Intracardiac electrophysiologic studies as a method for the optimization of drug therapy in chronic ventricular arrhythmia. Prog Cardiovasc Dis 23; 81–98.

22. Waxman HL, Buxton AE, Sadowski LM, Josephson ME. 1983. The response to procainamide during electrophysiologic study for sustained ventricular tachyarrhythmias predicts the response to other medications. Circulation 67: 30–37.

23. Mason JW, Winkle RA. 1980. Accuracy of the ventricular tachycardia-induction study for predicting long-term efficacy and inefficacy of antiarrhythmic drugs. N Engl J Med 303: 1973–1977.

24. Horowitz LN, Spielman SR, Greenspan AM, Webb CR, Kay HR. 1983. Ventricular arrhythmias: use of electrophysiologic studies. Am Heart J 106: 881–886.

25. Naccarelli GV, Prystowsky EN, Jackman WM, Heger JJ, Rahilly GT, Zipes DP. 1982. Role of electrophysiologic testing in managing patients who have ventricular tachycardia unrelated to coronary artery disease. Am J Cardiol 50: 165–171.

26. Swerdlow CD, Winkle RA, Mason JW. 1983. Determinants of survival in patients with ventricular tachyarrhythmias. N Engl J Med 308: 1436–1442.

27. Heger JJ, Prystowsky EN, Zipes DP. 1983. Clinical efficacy of amiodarone in treatment of recurrent ventricular tachycardia and ventricular fibrillation. Am Heart J 106: 887–894.

28. Waxman HL, Groh WC, Marchlinski FE, Buxton AE, Sadowski LM, Horowitz LN, Josephson ME, Kastor JA. 1982. Amiodarone for control of sustained ventricular tachyarrhythmias: clinical and electrophysiologic effects in 51 patients. Am J Cardiol 50: 1066–1074.

29. Nademanee K, Hendrickson J, Kannan R, Singh BN. 1982. Antiarrhythmic efficacy and electrophysiologic actions of amiodarone in patients with life-threatening ventricular arrhythmias: potent suppression of spontaneously occurring tachyarrhythmias versus inconsistent abolition of induced ventricular tachycardia. Am Heart J 103: 950–959.

30. Heger JJ, Prystowsky EN, Jackman WM, Naccarelli GV, Warfel KA, Rinkenberger RL, Zipes DP. 1981. Amiodarone: clinical efficacy and electrophysiologic effects during long-term therapy for recurrent ventricular tachycardia or ventricular fibrillation. N Engl J Med 305: 539–545.

31. Borggrefe M, Breithardt G, Seipel L. 1983. Value of serial electrophysiological testing in the treatment of ventricular tachyarrhythmias with amiodarone. Circulation 68 (suppl III): III-381.

32. McGovern B, Garan H, Malacoff RF, DiMarco JP, Selleres TD, Ruskin JN. 1982. Predictive accuracy of electrophysiologic testing in the treatment of ventricular arrhythmias with amiodarone. Circulation 66 (Suppl III): III-280.

33. Naccarelli GV, Fineberg N, Zipes DP, Heger JJ, Duncan G, Prystowsky EN. 1982. Amiodarone: discriminant analysis successfully predicts clinical outcome in patients who have ventricular tachycardia induced by programmed stimulation. Circulation 66 (Suppl II): II-223.

34. Roy D, Waxman HL, Buxton AE, Marchlinski FE, Cain ME, Gardner MJ, Josephson ME. 1982. Termination of ventricular tachycardia: Role of tachycardia cycle length. Am J Cardiol 50: 1346–1350.

35. Fisher JD, Kim SG, Matos JA, Ostrow E. 1983. Comparative effectiveness of pacing techniques for termination of well-tolerated sustained ventricular tachycardia. PACE 6: 915–922.

36. Fisher JD, Kim SG, Waspe LE, Matos JA. 1983. Mechanisms for the success and failure of pacing for termination of ventricular tachycardia: Clinical and hypothetical considerations. PACE 6: 1094–1105.

37. Mirowski M, Reid PR, Mower MM, Watkins L, Gott VL, Schauble JF, Langer A, Heilman MS, Kolenik SA, Fischell RE, Weisfeldt ML. 1980. Termination of malignant ventricular arrhythmias with an implanted automatic defibrillator in human beings. N Engl J Med 303: 322–324.
38. Reid PR, Mirowski M, Mowere MM, Platia EV, Griffith LSC, Watkins L Jr, Bach SM Jr, Imran M, Thomas A. 1983. Clinical evaluation of the internal automatic cardioverter-defibrillator in survivors of sudden cardiac death. Am J Cardiol 51: 1608–1613.
39. Marchlinski FE, Flores BT, Buxton AE, Hargrove WC Jr, Addonizio VP, Stephenson LW, Harken AH, Doherty JU, Grogan EW, Josephson ME. 1986. The automatic implantable cardioverter-defibrillator: Efficacy, complications, and device failures. Ann Int Med 104: 481–488.
40. Josephson ME, Horowitz LN, Farshidi A, Spear JF, Kastor JA, Moore EN. 1978. Recurrent sustained ventricular tachycardia. 2. Endocardial mapping. Circulation 57: 440–447.
41. Josephson ME, Harken AH, Horowitz LN. 1979. Endocardial excision: A new surgical technique for the treatment of recurrent ventricular tachycardia. Circulation 60: 1430–1439.
42. Josephson ME, Horowitz LN, Spielman SR, Waxman HL, Greenspan AM. 1982. The role of catheter mapping in the preoperative evaluation of ventricular tachycardia. Am J Cardiol 49: 207–221.
43. Josephson ME, Horowitz LN, Spielman SR, Greenspan AM, VandePol C, Harken AH. 1980. Comparison of endocardial catheter mapping with intraoperative mapping of ventricular tachycardia. Circulation 61: 395–404.
44. Josephson ME, Waxman HL, Cain ME, Gardner MJ, Buxton AE. 1982. Ventricular activation during ventricular endocardial pacing. II. Role of pace-mapping to localize origin of ventricular tachycardia. Am J Cardiol 50: 11–22.
45. Waxman HL, Josephson ME. 1982. Ventricular activation during ventricular endocardial pacing. I. Electrocardiographic patterns related to the site of pacing. Am J Cardiol 50: 1–10.
46. Cassidy DM, Vassallo JA, Buxton AE, Doherty JU, Marchlinski FE, Josephson ME. 1985. Catheter mapping during sinus rhythm: Relation of local electrogram duration to ventricular tachycardia cycle length. Am J Cardiol 55: 713–716.

24. Pharmacokinetics of antiarrhythmic drugs

PATRICE JAILLON

Unité de Pharmacologie Clinique Hôpital Saint-Antoine, Paris

A knowledge of the pharmacokinetics of antiarrhythmic drugs is most useful for cardiologists dealing with this group of drugs, which have relatively narrow therapeutic ratio. The complex processes of drug disposition in the body, including absorption, distribution and elimination, are the determinants of the drug plasma concentration. These determinants should be systematically considered in order to allow a better therapeutic efficacy, with less risk of toxicity, in patients with heart disease.

The objectives of this review are to show how the pharmacokinetics of antiarrhythmic drugs determines their plasma concentration and in what circumstances therapeutic drug monitoring may be a useful tool for the management of antiarrhythmmic therapy.

Principles of pharmacokinetics

When a drug is introduced into the blood either directly by an IV injection or after an absorption process (oral administration or intramuscular or subcutaneous injection), it will distribute to the tissues and will be eliminated from the body. Most transfers of the drug from one part of the body to another will follow a diffusion process controlled by the concentration gradient across cellular membranes. Similarly, drug elimination from the body will correspond to a first order process and the rate of elimination will be proportional to the concentration of the drug in the blood.

One open compartment model

When the distribution phase of the drug between blood and tissues is fast and uniform, one can consider that there is only one distribution volume, which is the volume of the compartment into which the dose of the drug in the body must be diluted to result in a given plasma concentration [1]. In this case, the evolution of plasma concentration against time can best be described by an exponential curve. Elimination half-life ($t\frac{1}{2}$el) of the drug (i.e. the time necesary for plasma concentration to decrease by half) is then unique and equal to: $t\frac{1}{2}$el = 0.693/K el; where K el is the first order rate constant for elimination. The plasma clearance of the drug corresponds to the volume of plasma which is cleared per unit of time and represents a constant fraction of the volume of distribution. In this model, $t\frac{1}{2}$el will be proportional to the volume of distribution (Vd) and inversely proportional to the plasma or systemic clearance (Cl syst): $t\frac{1}{2}$el = 0.693 × Vd/Cl syst.

Systemic clearance is equal to the sum of excretion and metabolic clearances since an antiarrhythmic drug can be either excreted unchanged by the kidneys, or metabolised by the tissue (mainly the liver). Considering $t\frac{1}{2}$el of a given antiarrhythmic drug, one may calculate the time necessary for the almost complete elimination of the drug from the body. Practically, we must consider that 97% of the drug will be eliminated from the body after 5 elimination half-lives.

Two open compartments model

In fact the distribution phase of the drug into the body is often more complex and corresponds to a 2 open compartments model: 1) the central compartment includes blood and tissues in fast equilibrium with blood, 2) the peripheral compartment corresponds to the tissues in which the drug is diffusing more slowly. In this case, the evolution of drug plasma concentration versus time can be described as a sum of two exponentials (Fig. 1). During the first phase (so-called 'distribution phase'), the drug distributes to the peripheral compartment and begins to be eliminated from the central compartment. During the second phase (so-called 'elimination phase'), the drug is eliminated from the tissues via the central compartment. The passage from the first to the second exponential curve corresponds approximately to the time of equilibrium diffusion between plasma and tissues. In this model, the volume of distribution of the drug at equilibrium is the sum of the volumes of central and peripheral compartments.

Steady-state plasma level
When a drug is administered by IV infusion at a constant rate, its plasma concentration increases progressively to a plasma level which then remains constant (steady-state level). This means that at the beginning of the infusion, the plasma concentration of the drug is low and the amount of the drug eliminated from the body per unit of time is low. When plasma concentration increases drug elimination increases, and at steady-state the amount of the drug introduced by IV infusion per unit of time is equal to the excreted amount over the same period.

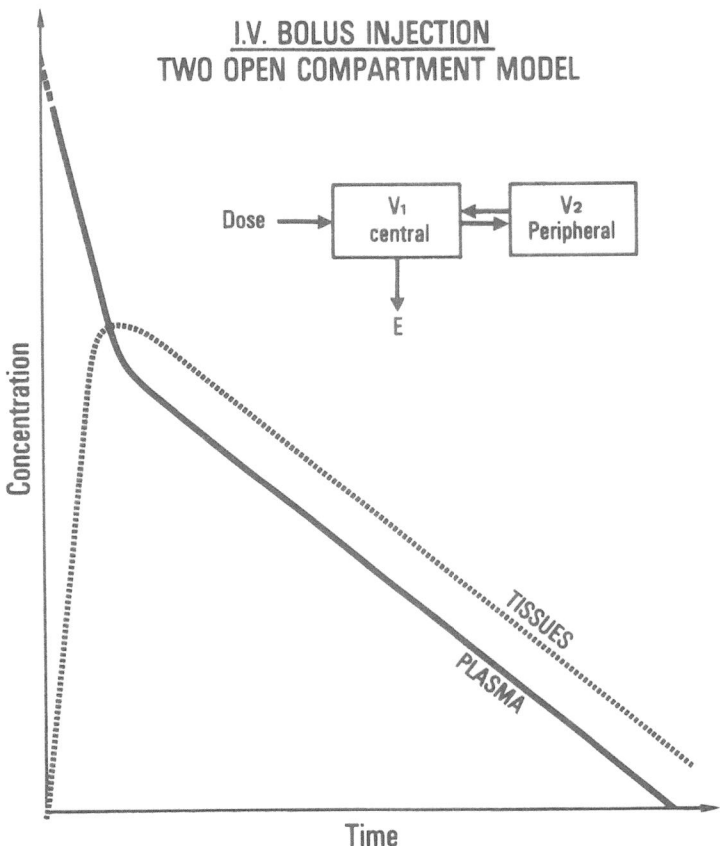

Figure 1. Evolution of drug concentration versus time in plasma (central compartment) and tissues (peripheral compartment).

Approximately 97% of the plasma steady-state level will be reached after a period of IV infusion equal to $5 \times t_{1/2}$ el. At this time, the drug infusion rate (R) and the systemic clearance of the drug will determine the steady-state plasma concentration (Cp ss), according to the formula: Cp ss = R/Cl syst. Therefore, knowledge of the drug systemic clearance will allow the cardiologist to choose R in order to maintain Cp ss in the therapeutic plasma range.

Similarly, when a drug is administered by oral or IV route at constant time intervals, there is a progressive accumulation of the drug in the body until the time when the amount of drug removed during the dosing interval is equal to the administered dose. At this time (steady-state), plasma concentrations will vary uniformly between a maximum (peak) following drug administration and a minimum (trough) before the next dosage.

Oral administration and bio-availability

When a drug is administered orally, a certain amount of the ingested dose can either stay in the digestive tract or be metabolised when passing through the digestive membranes or the liver. This initial metabolism is called the first-pass phenomenon and is the major determinant of drug absolute bio-availability. The only way to measure absolute bio-availability (F) of a drug in a patient is to compare the areas under the plasma concentration-time curves when the same dose is injected intravenously and administered per os. If these areas are equal, we may consider that 100% of the oral dose has reached systemic circulation and F = 1. If there is a first-pass phenomenon, the area under the plasma concentration-time curve after oral administration will be less than the area after IV administration and F<1.

Antiarrhythmic drugs, which are mainly eliminated from the body by hepatic metabolism, will have a low oral bio-availability because of the first pass phenomenon. However, since the hepatic clearance of a drug may vary with changes in hepatic blood flow and hepatocyte clearing functions, these drugs will show important interindividual variability in absolute bio-availability.

Pharmacokinetics of antiarrhythmic drugs

Extensive reviews of the pharmacokinetics of antiarrhythmic drugs are available in the literature [2–5]. However, when one considers the practical use of pharmacokinetic information, it must be recognised that the most interesting data concern drug elimination from the body. According to this practical point of view, the 10 most commonly used antiarrhythmc drugs have been classified by their major route of elimination from the body (Fig. 2). Considering the two major routes of elimination (renal excretion and hepatic metabolism), 3 groups of antiarrhythmic drugs can be distinguished: *group A:* (amiodarone, propafenone, lidocaine, verapamil, mexiletine) with extensive hepatic metabolism and more than 90% of the drug being metabolised; *group B:* (quinidine, flecainide, tocainide, procainamide) with mixed renal and hepatic elimination; *group C:* (disopyramide, cibenzoline, sotalol) with predominantly renal elimination and more than 50% of the drug being excreted unchanged in urine.

Group A – hepatic metabolism

Table 1 summarises the pharmacokinetic parameters of antiarrhythmic drugs which are mainly eliminated by hepatic metabolism with a high hepatic extraction ratio. This group of drugs includes amiodarone [6], propafenone [7], lidocaine [8], verapamil [9] and mexiletine [10]. Most of these drugs show a low and highly

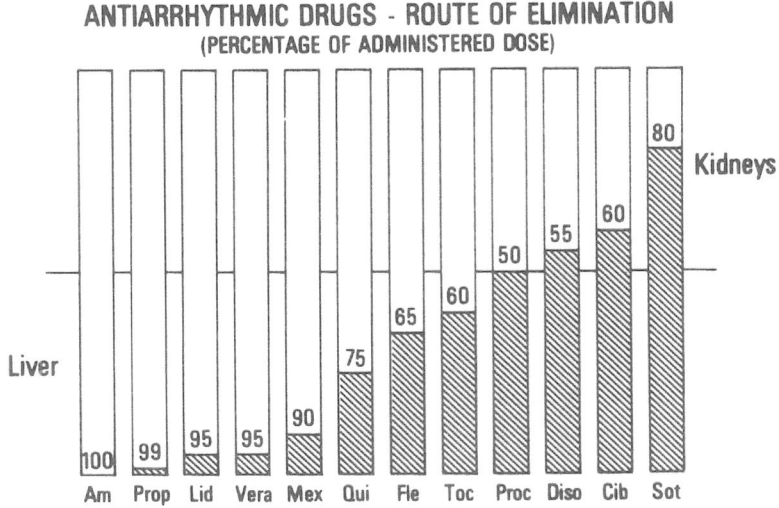

Figure 2. Pharmacokinetics of antiarrhythmic drugs.

variable oral bio-availability because of first-pass metabolism. They are highly bound to plasma proteins and their pharmacokinetics may be variable with the dose and duration of treatment. Hepatic clearance of these drugs may decrease in hepatic insufficiency or during liver cirrhosis [11]. On the other hand, a decrease in hepatic blood flow during congestive heart failure may result in a decrease in hepatic clearance [12].

Table 1. Pharmacokinetics of Antiarrhythmic drugs – Group A: Hepatic Metabolism.

	Amiodarone	Propafenone	Lidocaine	Verapamil	Mexiletine
F (%)	20–90 variable	3–50 variable	<30	10–20	90
t max (h)	2–12	2–4	–	2	0.5–2
Plasma protein binding (%)	95	95	40–80	90	70
$t\,{}^{1}\!/_{2}$ el (h)	variable 24h–24d	variable 2–32	2	2–5	8–12
Vd_{ss} (l/kg)	12–65 variable	2–4	1.3	3–6	6–10
Cl syst (ml/mn/kg)	7 variable	10 variable	10	8–20	5–7
% dose excreted unchanged in urine	<1	<1	<5	<5	10

Group B – mixed hepatic and renal elimination

Table 2 summarises the pharmacokinetic parameters of antiarrhythmic drugs which are eliminated by hepatic metabolism and renal excretion. This group of drugs includes quinidine [13], flecainide [14], tocainide [15] and procainamide [16]. Their absolute bio-availability is high and fairly constant and their pharmacokinetics seem to be linear with increasing doses.

Group C – renal elimination

Table 3 summarises the pharmacokinetic parameters of antiarrhythmic drugs which are mainly eliminated by the kidneys. This group of drugs includes disopyramide [17], cibenzoline [18] and sotalol [19]. Oral bio-availability of these drugs is high and constant and their renal clearance is correlated with creatinine

Table 2. Pharmacokinetics of Antiarrhythmic drugs – Group B: mixed hepatic and renal elimination.

	Quinidine	Flecainide	Tocainide	Procainamide
F (%)	70–80	>90	100	75–80
t max (h)	1.5–5	3	0.5–2	1
Plasma protein binding (%)	75 variable	40	50	15
$t_{1/2}$ el (h)	6	13	13	2.5–4
Vd_{ss} (l/kg)	2–3	8–10	1.6	1.5–2.5
Cl syst (ml/mn/kg)	4	7.6	2.2	12
% dose excreted unchanged in urine	<25	35	40	50

Table 3. Pharmacokinetics of Antiarrhythmic drugs – Group C: renal elimination.

	Disopyramide	Cibenzoline	Sotalol
F(%)	80–85	98–100	75–100
t max (h)	0.5–2	1.5	3–4
Plasma protein binding (%)	20–80 variable	60	50
$t_{1/2}$ el (h)	4–7	5–10	7
Vd_{ss} (l/kg)	1–1.3	5	1–1.3
Cl syst (ml/mn/kg)	3.4 variable	7	2
% dose excreted unchanged in urine	55	60	80

clearance. However, while cienzoline and sotalol show linear pharmacokinetics with increasing doses, renal clearance of disopyramide may vary because of changes in plasma protein bindin. It is known that the binding of disopyramide to plasma acid alpha-1-glycoprotein may vary among individuals, with the total plasma concentration of the drug and with the plasma concentration of the binding protein [20]. These changes in plasma protein binding will result in changes in the free fraction of disopyramide which in turn will result in changes in its renal clearance.

Factors influencing pharmacokinetics

Four major factors will influence the pharmacokinetics of antiarrhythmic drugs: 1) genetic polymorphism of metabolism; 2) linear or non-linear pharmacokinetics; 3) age and pathology; 4) drug interactions. This latter factor will not be discussed in this review.

Genetic polymorphism of metabolism

Genetic polymorphism of the metabolism of antiarrhythmic drugs may play an important role in interindividual variations in drug disposition. For instance [21], approximately 45% of the white caucasian population are slow acetylors of procainamide with a mean $t\frac{1}{2}$ el equal to 4 h. This group of individuals forms smaller amounts of the N-acetyl metabolite of procainamide (NAPA), and the NAPA/procainamide concentration ratio is low in plasma (0.6) and urine (0.4). Inversely, fast acetylors of procainamide have a shorter mean $t\frac{1}{2}$ el (2.5 h) and their NAPA/procainamide concentration ratio is higher in plasma (1.8) and urine (3.0). A very recent antiarrhythmic drug, encainide, which is not yet marketed in France, shows a genetic polymorphism of metabolism [22]. Non-extensive metabolisers of encainide show a long $t\frac{1}{2}$ el (8 h) and a high bio-availability (F = 0.88) of the drug, while extensive metabolisers show a shorter $t\frac{1}{2}$ el (2.5 h) and a lower bio-availability (F = 0.26). Only the extensive metabolisers are able to form the methoxy-0-demethyl metabolite of encainide which has a long $t\frac{1}{2}$ el. Wang et al. [22] have shown that the genetic polymorphism of metabolism of an antihypertensive drug, debrisoquin, follows the same pattern of metabolism as encainide and a debrisoquin test would yield a good forecast of encainide disposition in patents.

Genetic polymorphism of the metabolism of antiarrhythmic drugs may be more important than previously expected. For instance, propafenone metabolism may vary among individuals [23]. In a recent unpublished study, we have observed that among 10 patients treated during 3 consecutive days with propafenone for supraventricular arrhythmias, two showed different pharmacokinetics when

336

compared with the eight remaing subjects (Poirier J.M., personal communication). In these 2 patients, bio-availability of propafenone was relatively low, with a short t$\frac{1}{2}$ el (2–6 h) which did not increase during treatment. In the 8 remaining patients, bio-availability was higher and the drug accumulated with considerably higher plasma levels and increasing t$\frac{1}{2}$ el, from 6 to 13 h after the first dose to 9 to 28 h after 3 days of treatment. We postulated that these differences could be related to a genetic polymorphism of the metabolism of propafenone in man. Further investigations will be needed to confirm this hypothesis, but from a practical point of view, it could be of great importance to know in what patients propafenone accumulation is more likely to occur during chronic treatment.

Linearity of pharmacokinetics

Drug disposition in the body is linear when t$\frac{1}{2}$ el and systemic clearance remain stable when increasing the dose. In this case, plasma concentrations of the drug at steady state are proportional to the dose. It is of great interest for cardiologists to know if any change in drug dosage will result in a proportional change in plasma levels. Antiarrhythmic drugs show either linear or non-linear pharmacokinetics (Table 4). Non-linear pharmacokinetics may result from changes in either volume of distribution or clearance, or bio-availability, during drug administration. On the other hand, we have seen that changes in disopyramide plasma protein binding could account for changes in renal clearance of the drug. In any cases, cardiologists should be aware of these pharmacokinetic characteristics since for instance Connolly et al. [7] have shown that a two-fold increase in the oral dose of propafenone could result in a four-fold increase in the steady-state plasma concentration of the drug.

Age and pathology

The pharmacokinetic parameters of antiarrhythmic drugs as shown in Tables 1–3

Table 4. Antiarrhythmic drugs: linearity of pharmacokinetics.

Linear	Non-linear	Uncertain
Procainamide	Lidocaine	Quinidine
Tocainide	Disopyramide	Mexiletine
Flecainide	Amiodarone	
Cibenzoline	Propafenone	
Sotalol	Verapamil PO	
Verapamil IV		

have been observed in young healthy volunteers. Cardiologists know that age and pathology can influence pharmacokinetics. In elderly patients, the elimination rate of procainamide, quinidine and cibenzoline will decrease, resulting in a longer elimination half-life. These changes seem to be related to a decrease in the glomerular filtration rate. In renal insufficiency, systemic clearance of the following drugs will be decreased: procainamide, quinidine, cibenzoline, tocainide, flecainide, disopyramide, sotalol. Changes in drug plasma clearance will most often be correlated with changes in creatinine clearance.

During hepatic disease, the elimination rate of verapamil, lidocaine and mexiletine may decrease, resulting in longer $t\frac{1}{2}$ el. The consequences of congestive heart failure for drug pharmacokinetics are morecomplex, since this pathology may result in a decrease in glomerular flow and hepatic blood flow, as well as changes in volume of distribution [12]. Plasma concentrations of procainamide, quinidine, lidocaine [8, 24], mexiletine and flecainide may be much higher in patients with congestive heart failure than in patients with normal left ventricular function. Different mechanisms may account for these important modifications.

Therapeutic drug monitoring

Therapeutic monitoring of antiarrhythmic drugs may be a useful tool for cardiologists when they are using drugs with a high interindividual variability in disposition. However, we must recognise that either practical or more theoretical reasons have precluded a wide utilisation of plasma level measurements during antiarrhythmic treatment. Specific and reproducible assays of drugs and of their

Table 5. Antiarrhythmic drugs – therapeutic plasma range and active metabolites.

	Therapeutic plasma range (μg/ml)	Active metabolites
Amiodarone	0.5–5 (?)	N-desethyl-A (?)
Propafenone	0.5–1.5	5-OH-P
Lidocaine	1.5–6	GX
		MEGX
Verapamil	0.2–0.5	Nor-V (?)
Mexiletine	0.75–2	–
Quinidine	1.5–5	3-OH-Q
Flecainide	0.5 (0.3–1.2)	–
Tocainide	4–10	–
Procainamide	4–8	NAPA
Cibenzoline	2–3 (0.4–3.5)	–
Disopyramide	3.5 (3–8)	mono-N-dealkyl D
Sotalol	0.5–4	–

active metabolites are not always available at low cost for patients. The relationships between the plasma concentrations and the effects of antiarrhythmic drugs are not always documented and may vary according to the type of arrhythmias. Previous determinationsof 'therapeutic' and 'toxic' ranges of plasma levels vary in the literature and the existence of active metabolites may greatly interfere with drug efficacy and/or toxicity.

For practical reasons, we have tried to summarise in Table 5 the most commonly observed therapeutic plasma ranges for antiarrhythmic drugs [2–4]. The presence of active metabolites must be taken into account when a cardiologist is dealing with unexpected drug toxicity. The most interesting situations where therapeutic drug monitoring can help the physician are the following:

1. Prevention of repetitive life-threatening arrhythmias (ventricular tachycardia or fibrillation);
2. Lack of efficacy of standard administered doses (in order to differentiate non-compliance, low plasma concentrations, poor bio-availability and true inefficacy);
3. Suspicion of intoxication;
4. Drug monitoring in congestive heart failure, renal insufficiency and hepatic disease;
5. Drug interactions resulting in loss of efficacy or intoxication.

In these precise situations, the management of the treatment can be improved by following the evolution of drug plasma concentrations in patients.

Conclusions

A large amount of work remains to be done in order to successfully use pharmacokinetic parameters to optimise an antiarrhythmic treatment. To date we can conclude that:

1. The pharmacokinetic parameters of antiarrhythmic drugs have to be used as tools to improve therapeutic efficacy and to decrease drug toxicity.
2. The major route of drug elimination and the factors influencing drug disposition are the most useful pharmacokinetic data for cardiologists.
3. Therapeutic drug monitoring may be helpful in specific indications when plasma concentrations/effects relationships have been documented.

Acknowledgements

We gratefully aknowledge the technical assistance of Mrs A. Cros in preparing the manuscript.

References

1. Woosley RL, Shand DG. 1978. Pharmacokinetics of antiarrhythmic drugs. Am J Cardiol 41: 986.
2. Winkle R. 1983. Antiarrhythmic therapy. p. 46. In: Cardiac Arrhythmias. Current Diagnosis and Practical Management. Roger Winkle Edit. Addison-Wesley Pub. Co. Menlo Park.
3. Siddoway LA, Roden DM, Woosley RL. 1985. Clinical pharmacology of old and new antiarrhythmic drugs. p. 199. In: Sudden Cardiac Death. Mark E. Josephson Edit. Davis Co, Philadelphia.
4. Gillis AM, Kates RE. 1985. Clinical pharmacokinetics of the newer antiarrhythmic agents. Clin Pharmacokin 9: 375.
5. Anderson JL, Harrison DC, Meffn PJ et al. 1978. Antiarrhythmic drugs: Clinical pharmacology and therapeutic uses. Drugs 15: 271.
6. Holt DW, Tucker GT, Jackson PS et al. 1983. Amiodarone Pharmacokinetics. Am Heart J 106: 840.
7. Connolly SJ, Kates RE, Lebsack CS et al. 1983. Clinical pharmacology of propafenone. Circulation 68: 589.
8. Thompson PD, Melmon KL, Richardson JA et al. 1973. Lidocaine pharmacokinetics in advanced heart failure, liver disease and renal failure in humans. Ann Intern Med 78: 499.
9. Kates RE. 1983. Calcium antagonists: Pharmacokinetic properties. Drugs 25: 113.
10. Campbell NPS, Kelly JG, Adjee AAG et al. 1978. The clinical pharmacology of mexiletine. Br J Pharmacol 6: 103.
11. Williams RL. 1983. Drug administration in hepatic disease. New Engl J Med 309: 1616.
12. Benowitz NL, Meister W. 1976. Pharmacokinetics in patients with cardiac failure. Clin Pharmacokinet 1: 389.
13. Ochs HR, Greenblatt DJ, Woo E. 1980. Clinical pharmacokinetics of quinidine. Clin Pharmacokinet 5: 150.
14. Conard GJ, Ober RE. 1984. Metabolism of flecainide. Am J Cardiol 53: 41B.
15. Lalka D, Meyer NB, Duce BR et al. 1976. Kinetics of the oral antiarrhythmic lidocaine congener tocainide. Clin Pharmacol Ther 19: 757.
16. Giardina EGV, Dreyfuss J, Bigger JT Jr et al. 1976. Metabolism of procainamide in normal and cardiac subjects. Clin Pharmacol Ther 19: 339.
17. Giacomini KM, Swezey SE, Turner-Tamiyasu K et al. 1982. The effect of saturable protein binding to plasma proteins on the pharmacokinetic properties of disopyramide. J Pharmacokinet Biopharm 10: 1.
18. Brazzell RK, Colburn WA, Aogaichi K et al. 1985. Pharmacokinetics of oral cibenzoline in arrhythmia patients. Clin Pharmacokin 10: 178.
19. Poirier JM, Aubry JP, Cheymol G, Jaillon P. 1981. Etude pharmacocinetique du sotalol administré par voie intraveineuse chez l'homme sain. Thérapie 36: 465.
20. Meffin PJ, Roberts GW, Winkle RA et al. 1979. Role of concentration-dependent plasma protein binding in dysopyramide disposition. J Pharmacokinet Biopharm 7: 29.
21. Reidenberg MM, Drayer DE, Levy M et al. 1975. Polymorphic acetylation of procainamide in man. Clin Pharmacol Ther 17: 722.
22. Wang T, Roden DM, Wolfenden HT, Woosley RL et al. 1984. Influence of genetic polymorphism on the metabolism and disposition of encainide in man. J Pharmacol Experim Therap 228: 605.
23. Siddoway LA, Mc Allister CB, Wang T et al. 1983. Polymorphic oxidative metabolism of propafenone in man. Circulation 68: III, 64.
24. Stenson RE, Constantino RT, Harrison DC. 1971. Interrelationship of hepatic blood flow, cardiac output and blood levels of lignocaine in man. Circulation 43: 205.

25. Invasive electrophysiological tests in the choice of class I antiarrhythmic drugs

R.W.F. CAMPBELL

Academic Department of Cardiology, Freeman Hospital, Newcastle upon Tyne, England

The clinical value of electrophysiological studies

Management of arrhythmias

Electrophysiological studies have rapidly established their place for the investigation and management of a variety of arrhythmias, particularly for the accurate diagnosis of a wide range of narrow QRS tachycardias. The value of invasive electrophysiology in managing ventricular arrhythmias is largely limited to monomorphic and multimorphic (multiple discrete patterns) ventricular tachycardia. Polymorphic ventricular tachycardia, ventricular flutter and ventricular fibrillation are less amenable to electrophysiological investigation particularly as these arrhythmias may occur as 'non-specific' responses to aggressive stimulation protocols. It is unlikely that stable monomorphic ventricular tachycardia is ever a 'non-specific' response. The value of electrophysiological investigation of ventricular tachycardia is the facility to induce and terminate the clinically relevant arrhythmia in conditions of relative safety. This permits investigation of the tachycardias haemodynamic consequences, its site of origin and its response to a variety of antiarrhythmic strategies.

Prognostication

There is substantial interest in the value of electrophysiological stimulation for the prediction of individuals at high risk of sudden death or serious ventricular tachyarrhythmias. Survivors of acute myocardial infarction have received most attention. Initial reports of provocative stimulation detailed that ventricular responses additional to the stimulated beats – the repetitive ventricular response (RVR) – were associated with a poor prognosis [1]. Subsequent studies failed to confirm this relationship [2] but recent reports have reopened the controversy. Using a high energy stimulation protocol, clinically useful specificity and sensitivity has been achieved for electrophysiological tests in predicting prognosis of AMI survivors [3]. Risk prediction by electrophysiological tests in patients with other clinical conditions associated with sudden arrhythmic death has proved disappointing.

Limitations of electrophysiology studies – non inducibility

If the ventricular tachyarrhythmia cannot be reliably provoked by programmed stimulation then little or no value can be gleaned from the investigation. This situation may indicate that the ventricular tachyarrhythmia has an automatic rather than a re-entrant mechanism, but another explanation is that the triggering stimulation was too far removed from the re-entrant circuit to precipitate the arrhythmia. At least two right ventricular stimulation sites should be tested and in some circumstances left ventricular stimulation may be necessary [4]. Another cause of non-inducibility of an arrhythmia by programmed stimulation is impermanence of the arrhythmia substrate. In survivors of myocardial infarction who develop late recurrent ventricular tachycardia, the arrhythmogenic substrate probably is present permanently. This is reflected in the high success rates for arrhythmia induction at electrophysiological studies [5]. In other circumstances the arrhythmia substrate may not be so stable. This situation is exemplified by the ventricular tachyarrhythmias associated with exercise induced myocardial ischaemia and the ventricular arrhythmias complicating conditions such as the long QT syndrome and mitral valve prolapse in which critical autonomic conditions may create the arrhythmia substrate.

Electrophysiological studies are of value in selecting antiarrhythmic therapy only when arrhythmia induction is reliable. Thus it is a selected group of ventricular arrhythmias for which programmed stimulation procedures will yield information of therapeutic relevance. Electrophysiologically non-inducible ventricular arrhythmias commonly, but not exclusively, are poorly responsive to Vaughan Wiliams Class I antiarrhythmic therapies. The role for beta blockers and or revascularisation procedures in their management is important to consider.

Drug testing and electrophysiology

Reliable initiation and termination of a clinically relevant ventricular tachyarrhythmia is the goal of electrophysiological investigation and, if achieved, permits evaluation of administered antiarrhythmic therapy. Drugs of all four Vaughan Williams classes have been tested intravenously during electrophysiological procedures, but agents of classes II, III and IV are either of marginal efficacy against ventricular tachyarrhythmias or are difficult to test. Intravenous beta blockers (Class II) and calcium antagonists (Class IV) have a low success rate in abolishing stimulus provokable ventricular tachyarrhythmias. Intravenous amiodarone (Class III) has proved more effective but there is still substantial controversy as to whether the intravenous effects of this agent reliably predict the value of long term oral therapy. The Vaughan Williams Class I drugs are those most easily tested for efficacy and those which offer particular potency against stimulus inducible ventricular tachyarrhythmias.

Methodology, definitions and drug effects during electrophysiological testing

Methodology and definitions are of crucial importance if reliable conclusions are to be made from drug testing during electrophysiological studies.

It is questionable whether definitions of drug efficacy other than complete abolition (e.g. slower, more difficult to provoke, more easily terminated) have any clinical relevance.

Rendering a previously inducible ventricular tachyarrhythmia non-inducible by drug therapy is generally considered as reflecting efficacy of that agent. Whether it is sufficient to test the drug by repeating only the control (pre-drug) protocol or whether more aggressive stimulation procedures should be adopted before declaring drug success, is much debated. In one study [6], efficacy of therapy was based on arrhythmia abolition as identified by repetition of the pre-drug protocol. This entailed ventricular driving stimuli with S2/3 extra stimuli. However, with the addition of S4 stimulation, drug efficacy based on non-inducibility of the ventricular arrhythmia fell from 100% to only 47%.

Prevention of ventricular tachyarrhythmia induction by therapy at electro-physiological study may occur for reasons other than direct modification of the arrhythmogenic substrate. The drug might operate by modifying the triggering action of the delivered stimuli. An example would be of a Class IC drug slowing conduction of premature stimuli to such an extent that they never reached the re-entrant circuit during the initiation window. The drug might be evaluated as effective in preventing the stimulus induced ventricular tachyarrhythmia, but prove of little value against its spontaneous recurrence.

Non-inducibility of a ventricular tachyarrhythmia post therapy is not as accurately predictive of long term efficacy as has been believed. In drug responders defined at electrophysiological study (100% efficacy), a 20% arrhythmia recurrence had occurred by six months and the success rate of the initially identified therapy continued to fall on subsequent follow-up [7].

Arrhythmogenicity is a topical and important issue. Two forms should be recognised. Clinical arrhythmogenicity is when arrhythmia aggravation is of clinical importance, as when ventricular tachycardia accelerates, previously stable VT degenerates to ventricular fibrillation, a new ventricular tachyarrhythmia occurs, and when previously reliable spontaneous termination of a tachyarrhythmia fails to happen. Technical arrhythmogenesis is of debatable relevance and includes when the tachycardia is easier to induce, more difficult to terminate and when it is marginally faster. Repeated electrophysiological inductions of the ventricular tachyarrhythmia would be required to establish the biological variability in induction, termination and expression of the patient's ventricular arrhythmia before any of these features could be accepted as reliable.

Differences in class I drugs

All Vaughan Williams Class I drugs share the common feature of reducing the maximal rates of depolarisation of the action potential [8]. Subdivisions of the class reflect additional distinguishing features. Drugs of Class IA increase and those of Class IB decrease action potential duration in His Purkinje tissue. Class IC drugs prolong conduction in the myocardium. These different features are explicable on the basis of the drug receptor time constants which in turn have some relation to molecular weight of the compounds [9]. Some Class I agents have unique properties as for instance disopyramide's anticholinergic actions. The common electrophysiological actions of all these compounds has prompted consideration as to whether one drug could be used as a representative of Class I action, avoiding the tedious testing of each individual compound.

Procainamide has been suggested for this role and it has the benefit of extensive use in intravenous drug testing during electrophysiological studies. Sixty four per ent of ventricular tachyarrhythmias responsive to intravenous procainamide responded to other Class IA or IB drugs. Only 7% of tachyarrhythmias unresponsive to procainamide were controlled by other Class IA and IB drugs [10]. There is thus some systematic responsiveness of arrhythmias to Class I drugs in general but this relationship is not strong enough to recommend rejection of all Class I therapies on the basis of inefficacy of procainamide. As yet little account has been taken of the relatively recently introduced Class IC agents which appear to have a much better efficacy profile against ventricular tachyarrhythmias than Class IA and IB drugs.

Conclusions

Programmed stimulation supplies trigger stimuli to test for a latent arrhythmogenic substrate. Drug administration during the procedure examines the action of the agent on that substrate. Any beneficial drug action on natural trigger phenomena would not be identified by the procedure. This may be an important deficiency, as near complete abolition of ventricular ectopic activity, which is possible with Class IC drugs, could theoretically be important in the management of some ventricular tachyarrhythmias.

Efficacy and arrhythmogenicity of antiarrhythmic drugs can be determined by electrophysiological study, but the end points must be rigorously defined and the methodology of the test should be standardised.

Drug abolition of a ventricular tachyarrhythmia during electrophysiological study is a useful clinical goal which identifies a drug as likely to have reasonable long term efficacy. However, there is an important incidence of antiarrhythmic drug failure during follow-up. Whether this reflects progression of the disease, patient non-compliance, drug tachyphylaxis or whether the frequency of critical conjunction of triggers and substrates has been reduced but not abolished by therapy, is unknown.

Evidence suggests that the basic electrophysiology and pharmacokinetic differences of the various Class I agents do have clinical relevance and, as most are available in intravenous forms, invasive electrophysiological testing is a useful method for comparing actions and selecting the most appropriate for further patient management. Invasive electrophysiology is appropriate for only selected ventricular tachyarrhythmias and has little or no role to play in selecting Class I therapy for managing ventricular tachyarrhythmias which are electrically non-inducible.

Acknowledgement

I should like to acknowledge the invaluable assistance of Miss Sue Murray in the preparation of this manuscript.

References

1. Greene HL, Reid PR, Schaeffer AH. 1978. The repetitive ventricular response in man. A predictor of sudden death. N Engl J Med 299: 729–734.
2. Ruskin JN, DiMarco JP, Garan H. 1981. Repetitive responses to single ventricular extrastimuli in patients with serious ventricular arrhythmias: Incidence and clinical significance. Circulation 63: 767–772.
3. Richards DA, Cosy DV, Denniss AR, Russell PA, Young AA, Uther JB. 1983. A new protocol of programmed stimulation for assessment of predisposition to spontaneous ventricular arrhythmias. Eur Heart J 4: 376–382.
4. Robertson JF, Cain ME, Horowitz LN, Spielman Sr, Greenspan AM, Waxman HL, Josephson ME. 1981. Anatomic and electrophysiologic correlates of ventricular tachycardia requiring left ventricular stimulation. Am J Cardiol 48: 263–268.
5. Wellens HJJ, Schnilenberg RM, Durrer D. 1972. Electrical stimulation of the heart in patients with ventricular tachycardia. Circulation 46: 216–226.
6. Mason JW, Winkle RA. 1978. Electrode catheter arrhythmia induction in the selection and assessment of antiarrhythmic drug therapy for recurrent ventricular tachycardia. Circulation 58:971.
7. Mason JW, Winkle RA. 1980. Accuracy of the ventricular tachycardia induction study for predicting long-term efficacy and inefficacy of antiarrhythmic drugs. N Engl M Med 303: 1073.
8. Vaughan Williams EM. 1978. Some factors that influence the activity of antiarrhythmic drugs. Br Heart J 40 (suppl): 52–61.

9. Campbell TJ. 1983. Kinetics of onset of rate-dependent effects of Class I antiarrhythmic drugs are important in determining their effects on refractoriness in guinea-pig ventricle, and provide a theoretical basis for their subclassification. Cardiovasc Res 17: 344–352.

10. Waxman HL, Buxton AE, Sadowski LM, Josephson ME. 1983. The response to procainamide during the electrophysiology study for sustained ventricular tachycardia predicts the response to other medications. Circulation 67 (1): 30–37.

26. New drugs for the treatment of ventricular tachycardia

F. ZANNAD, E. ALIOT, K. KHALIFE, and J.M. GILGENKRANTZ

Département de Cardiologie, C.H.R.U. de Nancy, Hôpital Central, C.O. no. 34, 54037 Nancy Cedex, France

There is a manifest need for more effective and better tolerated therapy in patients with ventricular tachycardia (VT). Electrical and surgical treatments of VT remain to be used in very special circumstances (see elsewhere in this book) and cannot be employed as a large scale preventive therapy. At the moment, they are only indicated in the case of failure of drug therapy.

New antiarrhythmic drugs are now available, many of them still being investigated, and more are coming. The latest class Ic new antiarrhythmic drugs (AAD) have shown unusual efficacy in suppressing chronic stable ventricular arrhythmias in oral-dosing trials, and have been dubbed the 'VPC killers'! But despite these highly favourable results, reponses to these agents generally differ in patients with malignant VT.

In this review, we examine the available evidence of efficacy of, and tolerance to Flecainide, Propafenone, Encainide and Cibenzoline. Amiodarone, while being available for use in angina and arrhythmias in Europe since the last decade, was extensively investigated in VT only recently. We decided to include it in our review.

In order to reach any conclusion, reliable clinical trials are needed including randomised comparative trials versus placebo or versus other 'older' AAD. Patients study groups must be representative of the average population requiring treatment for VT. The number of patients in each trial should be sufficient to allow reliable statistical analysis, etc. .... Very few clinical studies satisfy these requirements. Moreover the criteria upon which one could state whether an AAD is effective or not are very controversial. Variability in the spontaneous occurrence of VT attacks make Holter monitoring obsolete in judging the efficacy of AAD. The value of programmed ventricular electrical stimulation (PES) in predicting the long term efficacy of AAD is still debated [1] (see elsewhere in this book).

Obviously the major goal of treating VT is to reduce the high mortality rate related to these life-threatening arrhythmias. Thus survival must be the major endpoint and is actually a reliable criterion to judge the efficacy of AAD. At present there is no long term randomised study of mortality with the newer AAD.

Bearing in mind these limitations, we decided to review the published clinical trials of the AAD listed above. We did not review abstract published data and company unpublished data. We focused on papers dealing specifically with the prevention of VT recurrence. Therefore, we did not report studies dealing more generally with the treatment of ventricular ectopic beats (VEB), although suppressing VEB may be relevant to the prophylactic treatment of VT.

Except for some studies comparing the new drug to other AAD, all the published trials reported here were open studies, therefore it is difficult to have a fair estimate of the efficacy of the drug tested, since the spontaneous outcome of the patients was largely unknown. Moreover, methods for assessing the efficacy of the drugs varied widely with different PES programs, different Holter recordings timings and largely variable follow-up periods. Thus one should not be surprised by the large variability of the results. Long term studies were conducted usually in patients who responded favourably to short-term evaluations with PES. This is undoubtedly a major bias which has to be kept in mind.

Flecainide

Seventy-three percent of electrically induced, sustained VT could be reverted to sinus rhythm after a 2 mg/kg injection of Flecainide [2]. The effect of Flecainide on the rate of initiation of VT using PES in patients with electrically inducible VT is extremely variable. The worst results were obtained by Reid et al. [3] who obtained one success out of 17 patients. Ten of these patients died very shortly after the start of the treatment, with sustained VT, resistant to electric cardioversion in five patients. Other authors reported more favourable results with success rates ranging from 12 to 60%. If partial successes were accounted for, including increase in the tachycardia cycle length or reversion to non sustained VT this rate increased to 29–100% [2–7]. In long term studies [2–7], Flecainide prevented the recurrence of VT on occasional Holter recordings in 40 to 94% of patients. But these figures may not necessarily reflect the true success rates. Reid et al. [3] reported complete elimination of VT from Holter monitoring in 32 out of 36 patients (89%). Actually the drug was subsequently discontinued in a total of 29 of 36 (81%) for drug ineffectiveness, side effects or death. Only 7 patients (19%) still receiving the drug ended up with favourable results (Table 1).

It is difficult to define any baseline criteria predicting the success or the failure of Flecainide in the prophylactic treatment of VT. Acute results with PES did not necessarily predict long term results. Poor left ventricular function (ejection fraction inferior to 30%) seems to be responsible for lower success rates.

Three comparative trials with other AAD were conducted with Flecainide (Table 2). In an open randomised crossover study, Stern [8] compared Flecainide to Propranolol in 10 patients with ventricular arrhythmias. Flecainide totally suppressed VT from Holter recordings while Propranolol had no effect on VT periods. The combination of Flecainide with Propranolol was better than Flecainide given alone. In a large multicenter double blind study, Flecainide was compared to Quinidine [9] in 280 patients of whom 139 had VT runs on their Holter recordings. VT runs were suppressed totally in 79% of the patients with Flecainide and in 55% with Quinidine. Another trial [10] included 25 patients with more than 10 VT episodes per week. These patients received randomly and double-blind Flecainide or Disopyramide. Flecainide decreased the number of VT episodes to 5 and then to 3/week while Disopyramide had no effect. There was a 92% suppression of VEB with Flecainide compared to 39% with Disopyramide.

Tolerance

Table 3 summarises the most frequent side effects reported in clinical trials with Flecainide in patients with VT. The arrhythmogenecity of this drug is now well established. Aggravation of ventricular arrhythmias occurred in 0 to 23% of the patients, mainly in patients with poor left ventricular function and ischemic heart disease [11]. No clear relationship with the dosage and plasma concentrations of

Table 1. Prophylactic use of Flecainide in VT: clinical trial.

Reference	No of patients	Study design	Patient history	Daily dosage	Duration of trial (m)	Method of monitoring (n)	Percentage of success
Anderson 1984 1983	15	o	9C 2M 4N 4C 2M 4N	300–400 mg 200–500 mg	4–6d 0.5–14.5m (13)	Pes (15) Pes (10) + Holt	60 (72a) 53 (30a) 40 (53b)
Lal 1985	38	o	33C 3M 2N	200–400 mg	in hospital 2–21m (11)	Pes (28) Clin (18) + Holt	36 (82a) 39b
Leclercq 1983	20	o	8C 6M 6N	250–500 mg	2d–15m	Holt	? (score)
Platia 1985	22	o	22C	200–600 mg	8–11d 3–4d 14m	Pes (17) Holt (16) Holt (2)	12 (29a) 94 –
Reid 1984	36	o	22C 14M	200–400 mg	(101d) 5d	Holter Pes (17)	89 6
Ward 1986	15	o	12C 1M 2N	200–300 mg	1–3d ?	Pes (10) Clin (10)	20 (100) 50

o: open label. C: coronary artery disease. M: cardiomyopathy and other cardiac disease. N: normal heart. m: months; d: days. (m): mean follow-up period. Pes: programmed electrical stimulation. Holt: Holter monitoring. Clin: clinical observation. a: including improved response (= reduction in ventricular rate or reversion to non sustained VT). b: including success with concommitant therapy.

the drug could be found. Sellers [12] described 3 cases of sinusoidal VT with Flecainide, but usually the induced arrhythmias were similar in nature to the preexisting ones in the same patient, although sometimes more resistant to treatment, and particulary to electric conversion [3]. Aggravation of heart failure and/or conduction disturbances were uncommon. Heart failure occurred in 4.3% of 373 patients with ventricular arrhythmias [13]. Podrid [14] reported an inci-

Table 2. Flecainide clinical trials – side effects.

Reference	No of pts	Study design	Daily dosage	Duration of trial (m)	Side effects Nature	N (%)
Anderson 1984	15	o	300–400 mg	4–6d (15) 0.5m (10)	Proarrhythmic Blurred vision Light headedness Dizziness	1 (7%) 10 (70%)
Lal 1984	38	o	200–400 mg	in hospital	Proarrhythmic Heart failure LBBB Weakness Headache Anorexia Nausea Visual blurring	4 (10%) 1 (3%) 1 (3%) 3 (8%) 2 (6%)
Platia 1985	22	o	200–600 mg	4–10d	Proarrhythmic Heart failure Bradycardia Blurred vision Diplopia Light headedness Nausea Numbness	5 (23%) 1 (3.5%) 1 (3.5%) 8 (36%) 2 (7%) 7 (32%) 1 (3.5%) 1 (3.5%)
Ward 1986	10	o	200–300 mg	?	Proarrhythmic Skin rash	1 (10%) 1
Flecainide Quinidine Research group 1983	280	db (Q) multi-center	400–600 mg	15d	Dizziness Blurred vision Nausea Headache Heart failure Proarrhythmic	30% 28% 9% 9% 0.7% 0
Reid 1984	36	o	200–400 mg	101d	Proarrhythmic Conduction disturbances Numbness Blurred vision Ataxia	2 (5.5%) 3 (8%) 2 (5.5%)

o: open label; db: double blind. (m): mean follow-up duration; m: month; d: day.

dence of heart failure of 16% with Disopyramide compared to 4.3% with Flecainide in patients not specifically treated for life threatening VT.

Other extracardiac side effects, usually dominated by blurred vision, were not serious enough to require treatment discontinuation. They appeared at the beginning of the treatment and usually abated or disappeared spontaneously or when doses were lowered [15].

From the available data with Flecainide in VT, the following recommendations could be made: Treatment should be started in hospitalised patients with a dose of 100 mg bid to be increased progressively to a maintenance dosage of 200 to 400 mg/day in 2 to 3 doses/day. The maximum recommended dosage is 600 mg/day. Patients should be monitored and PES performed in order to test the efficacy and detect any proarrhythmic effect. Dosage should be reduced in case of renal failure, heart failure or conduction disturbances. Plasma levels of the drug could be helpful if doses of more than 400 mg/day are required and in any case they should be kept under 1 000 ng/ml.

Table 3. Flecainide – Comparative trials with other antiarrhythmic agents.

Reference	Other drugs	Study design	N of pts	Daily dosage	Dosage of other drugs	Duration of trial (m)	Method of monitoring	Results
Flecainide Quinidine Research group 1983	Quinidine	d.b multicenter	139	400–600 mg	1200–1600mg	week 1: P week 2–3: F or Q week 4: P	Holt	F>Q
Kjeskus 1984	Disopyramide	d.b, c.o	25	400 mg	600 mg	week 1: P week 2: D or F week 4: P week 5–6: D or F week 7: P	Holt	F>D
Stern 1985	Propranolol	o. co	7	150 mg	60 mg	week 1: control week 2: PR week 3: F week 6: PR + F	Holt	F>P F = F + P

P: placebo. db: double blind. o: open. co: cross over. (m): mean follow-up period. Holt: Holter monitoring.

Propafenone

To our knowledge, there are no published reports of the effects of IV Propafenone on the termination of VT episodes. Acute testing of the drug with PES showed rates of prevention of the reinitiation of VT from 7 to 36% [16, 17].

Table 4. Prophylactic use of Propafenone in ventricular tachycardia clinical trials.

Reference	No of patients	Study design	Patient history	Daily dosage	Duration of trial (m)	Method of monitoring (n)	Percentage of success
Brodsky 1985	12d	o	10C 2M	900 mg	?	Pes (6) Ext (5b)	83 100
Chilson 1985	25	o	17C 4M 2N	600–900 mg 600–900 mg	4d ? (11m)	Pes (15b) Clin (10c) + Holt	20 (67a) 80
Cointe 1985	11	o	10C 1N	900 mg	2–3d	Pes	18 (72a)
Connoly 1985	16	o	14C 2M	900 mg	6–8d	Pes	6 (12a)
Heger 1984	29	o	20C 4M 5N	450– 900 mg	4–6d 4–6d 2–26m (15m)	Pes (29) Holt (29) Holt + Clin (16c)	21 (62a) 96 56
Podrid 1984a	30	o	19C 7M 4N	450 mg 450–900 mg 450–900 mg 900 mg	2d 4d 2–4d 3–13m (10m)	Holt (22) Holt (30) Pes (9) Clin (10c)	50 57 77 100
Podrid 1984b	60	o	37C 14M 9N	450 mg 450– 900 mg	4d 4d 4d 4d 1–24m (16)	Pes (31) Ext (53) Holt (57) Holt + Ext (53) Clin (20b)	61a 63 60 53 52
Prystowsky 1984	26	o	18C 4M 4N	450–900 mg 450– 900 mg	4d 1–26m (11)	Pes (26) Clin (17b)	19 65
Naccarella 1984	10 11	o o	8C 1M 1N 7C 2M 2N	900 mg 450 mg	90–270d (154) 40–150d (96)	Holt Holt	70 64

Ext: exercise testing. a: including improved response (reduction of ventricular rate or reversion to non sustained VT). b: selected patients with satisfactory clinical response and no adverse reaction. c: selected patients with satisfactory electrophysiologic response. d: patients with heart failure, ejection fraction <40%. o: open label; C: coronary artery disease; M: cardiomyopathy and other cardiac disease; N: normal heart; m: months; d: days; (m): mean follow-up period. Pes: programmed electrical stimulation. Holt: Holter monitoring. Clin: clinical observation.

Prevention of sustained VT reinduction using PES (Table 4) was obtained at rates ranging from 6 to 83% in short term open studies.

The drug is effective in the prophylactic treatment of VT in long term studies in 50 to 96% of the patients, as judged from occasional Holter recordings. Induction of VT with PES did not necessarily predict recurrence of spontaneous VT [18, 19]. Nevertheless, Heger et al. [20] have shown that short term success of Propafenone as judged from PES, Holter recordings and stress tests performed together within four days from the beginning of the treatment could predict long-term efficacy in 84% of the cases.

Propafenone was compared to Disopyramide in two studies (Table 5). In an open cross-over study including 34 patients with recurrent VT, Palmieri et al. [21] observed, in the same patients, 27 VT episodes within 8 months on Disopyramide

Table 5. Propafenone – Comparative trials with other antiarrhythmic agents.

Reference	Other drugs	Study design	N of pts	Daily dosage	Dosage of other drugs	Duration of trial (m)	Method of monitoring	Results
Dinh 1985	Quinidine	d.b parallel	19b	600–900 mg	800–1,600 mg	W1: Pcb W2: Prop/Q dose 1 W2: Prop/Q dose 2	Holt	Prop = Q
Palmieri 1984	Disopyramide	o. co	34	900 mg	600 mg	Months 1 to 4 Prop or Dis Months 5 to 8	Holt + Clin	Prop >Dis[a]
Rehnquist 1984[c]	Lidocaine	o. random parallel	b.c 20	1 mg/kg IV + 4× 150 mg p.o	75 mg IV + 2–3 mg/ min IV	24 hours Lid or Prop	Holt	Prop = Lid
Naccarella 1985	Disopyramide	d.b c.o	6	900 mg	600 mg	W1: Pcb/ Prop W2: Prop/Pcb W3: Pcb/ Dis W4: Dis/ Pcb W5: P	Holt	Prop >Dis

[a]: comparable antiarrhythmic activity on PVC, slightly better activity for propafenone in VT. [b]: short runs, non sustained VT. [c]: patients with acute myocardial infarction. d.b: double blind. o: open. co: cross over.

versus 14 VT episodes within 8 months on Propafenone. Naccarella et al. [22] compared the efficacy of both drugs in 16 patients. Six had sustained VT episodes. The trial was double-blind randomised with cross-over periods of one week each. Propafenone suppressed VT episodes in 6/6 patients and Disopyramide in 3/5. In another double-blind parallel study, Propafenone was compared to Quinidine in 19 patients with VT runs. Both drugs were equally effective. Finally, a comparative trial versus Lidocaine was performed openly in 20 patients with acute myocardial infarction and various ventricular arrhythmias [23]. No difference was found between the two drugs.

Tolerance

Aggravation of ventricular arrhythmias was reported in 0 to 40% of the treated patients including cases of torsades de pointe in patients with acute myocardial infarction [23]. This occurred in an unpredictable manner usually in the first few days of treatment. No clear relationship was found with changes in the ECG intervals or plasma levels of the drug. There are some indications of a greater risk of arrhythmogenecity in patients with severe ventricular dysfunction and prior serious sustained VT (Table 6).

Exacerbation of heart failure could occur in 0 to 16% of the patients treated with Propafenone. This should not preclude the use of the drug in patients with heart failure since Brodsky et al. [24] gave the drug to 12 such patients with ejection fraction lower than 40% and did not observe major side effects while results were favourable in 9/12 after a mean follow-up period of 14 months. However Podrid et al. [25] reported a decrease of 34 to 29% in ejection fraction values in 21 patients with basal ejection fractions lower than 50%.

Other side effects included conduction disturbances which were uncommon, and extra-cardiac side effects dominted by taste disturbances, unspecific neurologic symptoms and minor gastro-intestinal intolerance.

As compared to other AAD, Propafenone was better tolerated than Disopyramide [22] and produced the same incidence of side effects as Quinidine [26].

Recommendations for the use of Propafenone in VT should be the same as for Flecainide regarding cautions to be taken in severe ventricular dysfunction and stepwise increments of doses. Initial dose should be 100 mg t.i.d. and maintenance doses 150 to 300 mg t.i.d. Treatment should be started in hospital and short term efficacy tested with PES, Holter monitoring and stress test if possible, with special attention for the detection of proarrhythmic effects. Plasma levels of the drug although being somehow related to drug efficacy [27], have no established value for routine monitoring, largely because of complex pharmacokinetics with the generation of an active metabolite and probably genetic variations in the rate of metabolisation.

Table 6. Propafenone – Clinical trials – Side effects.

Reference	No of pts	Study design	Daily dosage	Duration of trial (m)	Side effects	
					Nature	N (%)
Brodsky 1985	12[a]	o	900 mg	?	Heart failure	2 (16%)
					Dizziness	1 (9%)
					Proarrhythmic	1 (9%)
Chilson 1985	25	o	900 mg	2–4d	Nausea	3 (12%)
					Paresthesia	2 (8%)
					Chest pain	2 (8%)
Cointe 1985	11	o	900 mg	2–3d	*Proarrhythmic*	3 (27%)
					Sinoatrial block	2 (18%)
Connoly 1985					*Proarrhythmic*	4 (25%)
					Nausea	1 (6%)
Dinh 1985	15[b]	d.b	450 to 900 mg	4 to 8m	Conduction disturbances	1 (7%)
					Bitter taste	6 (40%)
					Dry mouth	2 (13%)
					Dizziness	2 (13%)
					Gastrointestinal	3 (20%)
					Blurred vision	1 (7%)
Heger 1984	29	o	450 to 900 mg	6d–26m	Pleuritis	1 (3.5%)
					Bitter taste	4 (14%)
					Rash	1 (3.5%)
					Anaphylactic	1 (3.5%)
					Tremor, Weakness	2 (7%)
Naccarella 1984	21	o	450 to 900 mg	40–270d	Gastric intolerance and vomiting	3 (14%)
					Hypotension	1 (5%)
					Bitter taste	5 (24%)
Naccarella 1985	16[b]	d.b.c.o	900 mg	14d	Nausea, bitter taste, hypotension	2 (12%)
					Dizziness	1 (6%)
					Conduction disturbances	1 (6%)
Podrid 1984	30	o	450 to 900 mg	2–4d	Heart failure	2 (6.6%)
					Conduction disturbances	2 (6.6%)
					Proarrhythmic	2 (6.6%)
Podrid 1984	60	o	450 to 900 mg	4d–24m	*Proarrhythmic*	6 (10%)
					Conduction disturbances	2 (3.3%)
					Heart failure	3 (5%)
					Gastro-intestinal	7 (12%)
					Bitter taste	3 (5%)
Rehnqnist 1984	10[b, c]	o	1 mg/kg IV 4 × 150 mg po	24 h	*Torsade de pointe*	1 (10%)
					Proarrhythmic	4 (40%)
					Perspiration	2 (20%)

a: patients with heart failure, ejection fraction <40%. b: patients with ventricular arrhythmia including short runs of VT. c: patients with acute myocardial infarction. o: open-label. d.b: double blind. c.o: cross over.

Encainide

Encainide is a very powerful AAD in suppressing VEB [28, 29]. Experience with this drug in VT is still relatively limited. Acute testing of the drug with PES showed rates of prevention of the reinitiation of VT from 30 to 44% [30, 31]. Short term studies with Holter monitoring and/or exercise testing showed rates of success ranging from 27 to 59% in patients with sustained VT [30–32]. In non-sustained VT, Encainide prevented new VT episodes in 81% of patients [32]. Long-term studies, usually performed in patients having responded favourably to short-term titration phase, showed rates of 58 to 81% prevention of VT recurrence.

The value of acute testing with PES, exercise testing and/or Holter monitoring in predicting long term efficacy of Encainide is presently unknown. We have no knowledge of randomised trials comparing Encainide to other AA in VT.

Table 7. Prophylactic use of Encainide in VT clinical trials.

Reference	No of patients	Study design	Patient history	Daily dosage	Duration of trial (m)	Method of monitoring (n)	Percentage of success
Anderson 1982	22	o	17C 3M 2N	individual individual 125–240 mg	few days few days 0.3–25.5m (135m)	Holt + Ext Pes (10) Clin (24) + Holt	59 (86d) 30 (80d) 50
Chesnie 1983	80	o	45C 19M 16N	(day 1: 75 mg) Adjusted from 150 to 300 mg	2–6d 12–44m (21m)	Pes (16) Holt (63) Ext (51) Holt + Ext (63) Clin (27c)	44 (88d) 57 69 54 81
Duff 1985	11[a] 26[b] 24[c]	o o o	8C 3N 7C 9M 10N –	individual individual 180–400 mg	few days few days 21.5m	ECG ECG Clin + Holt (24c)	27 81 58
Mascn 1981	38	o	26C 6M 6N	150–250 mg	6m 18–30m	Clin + Holt Clin + Holt	54 29

Ext: Exercise testing. [a]: patients with sustained VT. [b]: patients with non-sustained VT. c: responders to encainide in dose-titration-phase. d: including improved response i.e. slowing VT cycle length. o: open label. c: coronary artery disease. M: cardiomyopathy and other cardiac disease. N: normal heart. m: months; d: days. (m): mean follow-up period. Pes: programmed electrical stimulation. Holt: Holter monitoring. Clin: clinical observation.

Tolerance

The major pitfall in the use of Encainide is its arrhythmogenecity which is reported consistently at rates as high as 36%. Compared to other AA, including the newer ones, Encainide has the highest proarrhythmic effects. More disturbing is the total unpredictability of these effects which appear to be rather idiosyncratic, unrelated to QRS or QT lengthening, not necessarily initiated by R on T PVC. Induced arrhythmias can be different with Encainide compared to other AA, and usually did not self-terminate [33]. Relationship with the plasma concentrations of the drug or of its active metabolite, O-demethyl Encainide, is rarely found [29]. Actually, there is a wide ratio of toxic to therapeutic concentrations and the drug's pharmacokinetic properties are extremely variable [34]. As a consequence, monitoring plasma concentrations of the drug and/or its active metabolite seems of little help. Luckily, aggravation of arrhythmias with Encainide is more likely to occur in the first 48 hours after the initiation of oral maintenance therapy or within two hours after a single large dose [33]. Thus, it is strongly recommended to start treatment in the hospital with continuous ECG monitoring, starting with low doses (25 to 50 mg) increased progressively from 25 mg t.i.d. to 75 mg t.i.d. which should be the maximum dosage.

Table 8. Side effects of Encainide in patients with VT clinical trials.

Reference	No of pts	Study design	Daily dosage	Duration of trial (m)	Side effects	
					Nature	N (%)
Anderson 1982	22	o	125–240 mg	few days to 255m	*Proarrhythmic*	8 (36%)
					Neurologic	5 (23%)
Chesnie 1983	80	o	80–300 mg	few days	*Proarrhythmic*	18 (23%)
					AV block	1 (1.2%)
					Neurologic	3 (4%)
					Nausea	1 (1.2%)
Duff 1985	37	o	180–400 mg	few days to 40 months	BBB	4 (11%)
					Proarrhythmic	7 (19%)
					Sinus pause	1 (3%)
					AV 11° block	1 (3%)
					Diplopia	2 (5%)
					Skin exanthema	1 (3%)
Mason 1981	38	o	150–250 mg	(4–2m)	*Proarrhythmic*	4 (10%)
					Neurologic	18 (47%)
					Gastro-intestinal	2 (5%)

o: open label.

Table 9. Prophylactic use of Cibenzoline in VT clinical trials.

Reference	No of patients	Study design	Patient history	Daily dosage	Duration of trial (m)	Method of monitoring (n)	Percentage of success
Browne 1983	26[a]	o	16C 6M 4N	200–300 mg	1–4d / 4d	Holt (16d) / Pes (9d)	50 / 22
Cocco 1984	28[d]	o	20C 8M	560–700 mg	30d	ECG + Holt (28)	18
Klein 1986	49[a]	s-b Pcb-c	37C 9M 3N	week 1: Pcb / week 2: 260 mg / week 3: 320 mg / week 4: 330 mg / MD = 260–330 mg	30d / 3–12m	Holt (27)[b] Ext / Holt (29)[a]	78 / 73 to 100[c]
Kostics 1984	24[a]	d-b Pcb-c c-o	18C 6M	260–320 mg	7d	ECG + Holt (10[b, c])	90

o: open label. S-b: single blind; Pcb-c: placebo-controlld; MD: maintenance dose. Ext: exercise testing; d-b: double blind; c-o: cross over. C: coronary artery disease. M: cardiomyopathy and other cardiac disease. N: normal heart. m: months; d: days. (m): mean follow-up period. [a]: patients with ventricular arrhythmias including short runs of non-sustained VT. [b]: patients with non-sustained VT. [c]: according to the time of evaluation. d: patients with sustained VT. [e]: patients preselected to be responders to Cibenzoline. Holt: Holter monitoring. Pes: programmed electrical stimulation.

Cibenzoline

Cibenzoline is a more recent new AA with class Ic and class III electrophysiologic properties. Few studies have yet been performed in VT. Except the study of Cocco et al. [35], other trials reported in Table 9 included only patients with PVC some of them having short runs of non sustained VT. Cocco et al. [35] reported a weak efficacy of Cibenzoline in patients with sustained VT. In less severe arrhythmias VT suppression on Holter recordings could be obtained in 73 to 100% of the patients. Data with PES are still very preliminary [36]. Cibenzoline had been compared to Procainamide [37] and to Quinidine [38] in patients with VT and was found with no better efficacy than that of both drugs (Table 10), but tolerance was much better with Cibenzoline. Indeed, although few trials are available, good tolerance of the drug seems to be one of its advantages. Very occasional and non specific side effects have been reported (Table 11) in clinical trials in patients with VT. Arrhythmogenecity was reported by Cocco [35] in 3 of 28 treated patients. Aggravation of heart failure or conduction disturbance were uncommon. Rigaud et al. [39] reported a dose-related cardiac depressant effect of cibenzoline. Plasma concentrations of less than 300 ng/ml had no significant hemodynamic effect. Care must be taken in patients with severe left ventricular dysfunction and patients with conduction disturbances.

The recommended dosage is 260 to 300 mg daily. The relatively long elimination half life could permit a twice daily regimen. Therapeutic plasma concentrations are in the range of 0.3 to 0.6 μg/ml; relationship between plasma concentrations and antiarrhythmic effects is not well established.

Table 10. Comparative trials of Cibenzoline with other antiarrhythmic agents.

Refer- ence	Other drugs	Study design	N of pts	Dosage	Dosage of other drugs	Duration of trial (m)	Method of moni- toring	Results
Miura 1985	Proca- inamide	o-r	33	1–3 mg/ kg[a] IV	100– 1500 mg[a] IV	acute	Pes	P = 68 C = 48
Wasty 1985	Quini- dine	o-r c-o	13[b]	260– 320 mg/d	1200– 1600 mg/ d	2 × 2 weeks	Holt	Q = C

o-r: open-randomised. c-o: cross-over. [a]: cumulative doses, infusion by intermittent IV bolus/5 min. [b]: patients with ventricular arrhythmias including short runs of non-sustained VT. Pes: programmed electrical stimulation. Holt: Holter monitoring.

Amiodarone

Amiodarone is an anti-anginal drug whose antiarrhythmic properties were described since the 1970s. Thanks to modern evaluation tools such as Holter monitoring and PES, its electrophysiologic properties and antiarrhythmic potential are better established.

In VT numerous studies have been performed with Amiodarone [40, 41, 43–53]. Acutely, intravenous Amiodarone reverted VT to sinus rhythm in 6/7 cases [49]. Results with PES were very inconsistent with rates of prevention of VT reinitiation ranging from 8% [52] to 67% [48]. But dosages and routes of administration varied widely among investigators. Loading doses were always used but were very variable. Inconsistent and sometimes poor short-term results with PES contrast with better long term efficacy as judged from clinical follow-up and Holter recordings (Table 12). The value of PES in predicting long-term clinical efficacy of Amiodarone was questioned by many authors. Nevertheless, Mc Govern et al. [46] were able to show a very good predictive value of PES (67%) with an excellent specificity (91%) while sensitivity was lower (58%). Veltri et al. [53] tested the predictive value of Holter recordings, performed within two weeks

Table 11. Cibenzoline clinical trials – side effects.

Reference	No of pts	Study design	Daily dosage	Duration of trial (m)	Side effects	
					Nature	N (%)
Cocco 1984	28	o	560–700 mg	30d	*Proarrhythmic*	3 (11%)
					BBB	3 (11%)
					1st ȩ AV block	5 (18%)
					2nd AV block	2 (7%)
					Neurologic	4 (14%)
					Gastro-intestinal	4 (14%)
					Dry mouth	1 (4%)
Klein 1986	49[a]	s-b Pcb-c	260–330 mg	1–12m	Nervousness	5 (10%)
					Nausea	2 (4%)
					Heart failure	3 (6%)
					Lethargy	1 (2%)
					Fatigue	1 (2%)
					LBBB	1 (2%)
					↗Transaminases	2 (4%)
					↗White cells	1 (2%)
					Proteinuria	1 (2%)
Wasty 1985	13[a]	o-r c-o	260–320 mg	15d	↗Alk-phos.	2 (15%)
					↗LDH	1 (7%)
					Weakness	1 (7%)

o-r: open-randomized. c-o: cross-over. s-b: single blind. Pcb-c: placebo controlled. a: patients with ventricular arrhythmias including short runs of non-sustained VT.

Table 12. Prophylactic use of Amiodarone in VT – clinical trials.

Reference	No of patients	Study design	Patient history	Daily dosage	Duration of trial (m)	Method of monitoring (n)	Percentage of success
Cassagneau 1984	18	o	10C 7M 1N	L = 400–600 mg M = 400–600 mg	21d 6–27m (14m)	Pes Holt + Clin	28 (61)[a] 67
Flaker 1985	17	o	15C 2M	L = 1000 mg 10 days M = 200–600 mg	(9m)	Clin	76
Heger 1983	196	o	129C 56M 9N	L = 800–1600 mg 2 to 4 weeks M = 200–600 mg	15d 1–57m (16–2m)	Pes (101) Clin (177)	15 78
Horowitz 1985	100	o	100C	L = 1000 mg week 1 800 mg week 2 or 10 mg/kg/IV + 600 mg day 1 to 3 800 mg day 4 to 10 M = 600 mg 4 months 400 mg later	9–15d 4–31m (18m) 2–32m (12m)	Pes (100) Holt + Clin (20b) Holt + Clin (80c)	20 100 52
Kaski 1981	23	o	14C 9M	L = 600–2000 mg M = 200–1200 mg	8d–59m (30 m)	Holt + Clin	65 (87)[a]
McGovern 1984	42	o	36C 4M 2N	L = 950–260 mg 6 days M >400 mg	0.3–45m (10m)	Pes (42) Holt + Clin (42)	45 74

			Dose	Duration	Method	%
Nademanee 1981	22	13C 6M 3N	o	600–1200 mg	2–12m	Holt + Clin (19)	100
Nademanee 1982	13	11C 2N	o	L = 1000–1800 mg M = 200–400 mg	14–56d (28) 7–18m (12m)	Pes (12) Holt	67 100
Rasmussen 1982	33	22C 8M 3N	o	L = 800–1000 mg week 1 M = 290–800 mg	10–30d 0–16m (6.1m)	Pes (20) Holt (33)	20 61
Reddy 1984	17	16C 1N	o	L = 1000– 1400 mg 10 to 14 days M = 600–1000 mg	2–18m (5–3m) 4–53m (18–6m)	Pes Holt + Clin	60 82
Saksena 1984	17	12C 3M	o	L = 10–20 mg/ kg/d week 1 M = 400–800 mg	24–53d	Clin + Holt	53
Veltri 1985[a]	13	9C 4M	o	L = 1200 mg week 1 + 2 M = 200–800 mg	6–15m (6m)	Pes (13)	8
Veltri 1985[b]	42	31C 9M 2N	o	L = 1000– 1600 mg week 1 + 2 M = 400–600 mg	2w 1–42m (22m)	Holt Holt + Clin	69–81 57

L = loading; M = maintenance doses. [a] = including improved response i.e. = isolated recurrences of VT. [b] = selected patients with satisfactory electrophysiologic response. [c] = patients with negative electrophysiologic response to amiodarone. o: open label. C: coronary artery disease. M: cardiomyopathy and other cardiac disease. d: day; m: month; w: week. Pes: programmed electrical stimulation. Holt: Holter monitoring. Clin: clinical observation. (m): mean follow-up period. N: normal heart.

of the start of treatment, for long term efficacy. 72 hours continuous Holter recordings were best suited since they predicted efficacy in 79% of the cases with a 10% specificity and 62% sensitivity.

No comparative trials with other AA drugs were performed in VT, probably because of the peculiar pharmacokinetics of Amiodarone requiring special dosing conditions difficult to match in double-blind controlled trials.

Table 13. Amiodarone clinical trials – side effects.

Reference	No of pts	Study design	Daily dosage	Duration of trial (m)	Side effects	
					Nature	N (%)
Rasmussen 1982	33	o	L = 800–1000 M = 290–800 mg	0–16m (6.1m)	Sinus node depression Skin Thyroid Gastro-intestinal Visual disturbances	5 (15) 6 (18) 2 (6) 3 (9) 1 (3)
McGovern 1984	42	o	L = 950–260 mg 6d M = 491–205 mg	0.3–45m (10m)	Proarrhythmic Sinus node depression Pneumonitis Hepatitis	4 (10) 3 (7) 1 (2) 1 (2)
Flake 1985	17	o	L = 1000 mg 10d M = 200–600 mg	(9m)	Sinus bradycardia Nausea Liver function test Weakness	1 (6) 2 (11) 1 (6) 1 (6)
Kaski 1981	23	o	L = 600–2000 mg M = 200–1200 mg	8d–59m (30m)	Skin coloration	2 (8)
Reddy 1984	17	o	L = 1000–1400 mg 10 to 14d M = 600–1000 mg	4–53m (18.6m)	AV block Skin coloration Mild elevation of transaminase	1 (6) 4 (23) 12 (70)
Heger 1983	196	o	L = 800–1600 mg 2 to 14 weeks M = 200–600 mg	1–57m (16.2m)	*Proarrhythmic* Sinus node depression + bradyarrhythmias Pneumonitis Skin coloration Other mild side effects Thyroid	9 (4.5) 4 (2) 7 (3.5) 19 (9.7) 76 (39) 2 (1)
Nademanee 1981	22	o	600–1200 mg	2–12m	Photosensibility Nausea Weakness	2 (9) 2 (9) 1 (4.5)

o: open label. L: loading dose. M: maintenance dose. (m): mean follow-up duration. m: months; d: days.

Tolerance

A large number of side effects was reported with Amiodarone. In trials including patients with VT and life-threatening ventricular arrhythmias (Table 14) proarrhythmic activity was reported very occasionnally 4.5 to 10% [43, 46]. Conduction disturbances, mainly sinus depression, were more common. Other benign, but frequent, side effects were photosensibilisation and visual disturbances. Thyroid dysfunction, pneumonitis and hepatitis were the most severe undesirable effects, but their incidence was fortunately relatively low. However, pneumonitis is reported very frequently in some studies using very high doses. Undoubtedly, these numerous and sometimes serious side effects are the major hindrance to the larger use of this very efficient drug. Of notice is the remarquable efficacy of Amiodarone in improving survival in hypertrophic cardiomyopathy with VT [54]. Although uncontrolled, the trial performed by Mc Kenna et al. [54] showed, indeed, a 20% reduction in the sudden death rate with Amiodarone, over conventional AA treatment.

Recommendations for use of Amiodarone in VT are the following: treatment should always be initiated with a loading dose from 800 to 1200 mg orally, or 10 mg/kg IV in one hour followed by 600 mg/24 h continuous infusion. Maintenance doses are 100 to 800 mg/24 h. A once daily regimen is recommended, and the true necessity for the week-end discontinuation of the drug is not established, but strongly supported, by the extremely long elimination half-life of the drug. Side effects are dose-related and it is not surprising that the incidence of undesirable effects seems much lower in Europe where the usual dose does not exceed 400 mg/day. Clinical trials with such lower doses are obviously needed in order to test the real benefit/risk ratio with this drug. Monitoring the plasma concentrations of Amiodarone and of its major metabolite, N-desethylamiodarone, had no definite proven value, since tissue levels seem to be better related to electrophysiologic activity and to clinical tolerance than plasma levels of the drug.

As for predicting long term efficacy from short term data, Dicarlo et al. [55] and Horowitz et al. [44] suggest the following recommendations. PES should be performed within 15 days from te start of the treatment and Amiodarone should be continued if PES was negative. If positive, Amiodarone is still recommended if the VT is non-sustained and/or with a slow ventricular rate, when ejection fraction is higher than 40% and when 24 h Holter recording does not show VT episodes. If these conditions were not present and VT reinitiation still possible with PES, the addition of another AA is recommended.

References

1. Lombardi F, Stein J, Podrid PJ, Graboys TB, Lown B. 1986. Daily reproducibility of electrophysiologic test results in malignant ventricular arrhythmia. Am J Cardiol 57: 96–101.

2. Ward DE, Cheesman M, Dancy M. 1986. Effect of intravenous and oral flecainide on ventricular tachycardia. Int J Cardiol 10: 1–12.

3. Reid PR, Griffith LSC, Platia EV, Ord SE. 1984. Evaluation of flecainide acetate in the management of patients at high risk of sudden cardiac death. Am J Cardiol 53: 108B–111B.

4. Anderson JL, Lutz JR, Allison SB. 1983. Electrophysiologic and antiarrhythmic effects of oral flecainide in patients with inducible ventricular tachycardia. J Am Coll Cardiol 2: 105–114.

5. Anderson JL. 1984. Experience with electrophysiologically guided therapy of ventricular tachycardia with flecainide: summary of long-term follow-up. Am J Cardiol 53: 79B–86B.

6. Lal R, Chapman PD, Naccarrellig V, Troup PJ, Rinkenberger RL, Dougherty AH, Ruffy R. 1985. Short- and long-term experience with flecainide acetate in the management of refractory life-threatening ventricular arrhythmias. J Am Coll Cardiol 6: 772–779.

7. Platia E, Estes M, Heine DL, Griffith SC, Garan H, Ruskin J, Reid PR. 1985. Flecainide: electrophysiologic and antiarrhythmic properties in refractory ventricular tachycardia. Am J Cardiol 55: 956–962.

8. Stern H, Scheininger M, Theisen F, Theisen K. 1985. Antiarrhythmic therapy with flecainide in combination and comparison with propranolol. Drugs 29 (suppl. 4): 77–85.

9. Flecainide-Quinidine research group. 1983. Flecainide versus quinidine for treatment of chronic ventricular arrhythmias. A multicenter clinical trial. Circulation 67: 1117–1123.

10. Kjeskus J, Bathen J, Orning O, Storstein L. 1984. A double-blind crossover comparison of flecainide acetate and disopyramide phosphate in the treatment of ventricular premature complexes. Am J Cardiol 53: 72B–78B.

11. Morganroth J, Horowitz LN. 1984. Flecainide: its proarrhythmic effect and expected changes on the surface electrocardiogram. Am J Cardiol 53: 89B–94B.

12. Sellers TD, Di Marco JP. 1985. Sinusoidal ventricular tachycardia associated with flecainide acetate. Chest 5: 647–649.

13. Josephson MA, Ikeda N, Singh B. 1984. Effect of flecainide on ventricular function: clinical and experimental correlation. Am J Cardiol 53: 95B–100B.

14. Podri DPJ, Schoenberger A, Lown B. 1980. Congestive heart failure caused by oral disopyramide. N Engl J Med 302: 189–192.

15. Warnowicz MA, Denes P. 1980. Chronic ventricular arrhythmias: comparative drug effectiveness and toxicity. Prog Cardiovasc Dis 23: 225–236.

16. Shen EN, Sung RJ, Morady F, Schwartz AB, Scheinman MM, Dicarlo L, Shapiro W. 1984. Electrophysiologic and hemodynamic effects of intravenous propafenone in patints with recurrent ventricular tachycardia. J Am Coll Cardiol 3: 1291–1297.

17. Doherty JH, Waxman HL, Kienzle MG, Cassidy DM, Marchlinski FE, Bruxton AE, Josephson ME. 1984. Limited role of intravenous propafenone hydrochloride in the treatment of sustained ventricular tachycardia: electrophysiologic effects and results of programmed ventricular stimulation. J Am Coll Cardiol 4: 378–381.

18. Chilson DA, Heger JJ, Zipes DP, Browne KF, Prystowsky EN. 1985. Electrophysiologic effects and clinical efficacy of oral propafenone therapy in patients with ventricular tachycardia. J Am Coll Cardiol 5: 1407–1413.

19. Prystowsky EN, Heger JJ, Chilson DD, Miles WM, Hubbard J, Zipes DP. 1984. Antiarrhythmic and electrophysiologic effects of oral propafenone. Am J Cardiol 54: 26D–28D.

20. Heger JJ, Hubbard J, Zipes D, Miles WM, Prystowsky EN. 1986. Propafenone treatment of recurrent ventricular tachycardia: comparison of continuous electrocardiographic recording and electrophysiologic study in predicting drug efficacy. Am J Cardiol 54: 40D–44D.

21. Palmieri M, Capucci A, Lombardi G, Naccarella F, Bomba E, Bracchetti D. 1984. Studio comparativo sull'eficacia della disopiramide e del propafenone nella prevenzione delle recidive di tachicardia ventricolare. G Ital Cardiol 14: 52–54.

22. Naccarella F, Bracchetti D, Palmieri M, Cantelli I, Bertaccini P, Ambrosioni E. 1985. Comparison of propafenone and disopyramide for treatment of chronic ventricular arrhythmias: placebo-

controlled, doubleblind, randomized crossover study. Am Heart J 109: 833–840.

23. Rehnqvist N, Ericsson CG, Eriksson S, Olsson G, Svensson G. 1984. Comparative investigation of the antiarrhythmic effect of propafenone (Rythmonorm) and lidocaine in patients with ventricular arrhythmias during acute myocardial infarction. Acta Med Scand 216: 525–530.

24. Brodsky MA, Allen BJ, Abate D, Henry WL. 1985. Propafenone therapy for ventricular tachycardia in the setting of congestive heart failure. Am Heart J 110: 794–799.

25. Podrid PJ, Cytryn R, Lown B. 1984. Propafenone: non invasive evaluation of efficacy. Am J Cardiol 54: 53D–59D.

26. Dinh H, Murphy ML, Baker BJ, De Soyza N, Franciosa JA. 1985. Efficacy of propafenone compared with quinidine in chronic ventricular arrhythmias. Am J Cardiol 55: 1520–1524.

27. Podrid PJ, Lown B. 1984. Propafenone: a new agent for ventricular arrhythmia. J Am Coll Cardiol 4: 117–125.

28. Di Bianco R, Fletcher RD, Cohen AI, Gottdiener JS, Singh SN, Katz RJ, Bates HR, Sauberbrunn B. 1982. Treatment of frequent ventricular arrhythmia with encainide: assessment using serial ambulatory electrocardiograms intracardiac electrophysiology studies, treadmill exercise tests and radionuclide cineangiographic studies. Circulation 65: 1134–1147.

29. Morganroth J, Poul P, iller R, Hsu PH, Lee I, Clark DM for the Encainide research group. 1986. Dose-response range of encainide for benign and potentially lethal ventricular arrhythmias. Am J Cardiol 57: 769–774.

30. Anderson JL, Stewart JR, Johnson TA, Lutz JR, Pitt B. 1982. Response to encainide of refractory ventricular tachycardia: clinical application of assays for parent drug and metabolites. J Cardiovasc Pharmacol 4: 812–819.

31. Chesnie B, Podrid P, Lown B, Reader E. 1983. Encainide for refractory ventricular tachyarrhythmia. Am J Cardiol 52: 495–500.

32. Duff HJ, Roden DM, Garey EL, Wang T, Primm K, Woosley RL. 1985. Spectrum of antiarrhythmic response to encainide. Am J Cardiol 56: 887–891.

33. Winkle RA, Peters F, Kates RE, Tucker C, Harrison DC. 1981. Clinical pharmacology and antiarrhythmic efficacy of encainide in patients with chronic ventricular arrhythmias. Circulation 64: 290–296.

34. Winkle RA, Mason JW, Griffin JC, Ross D. 1981. Malignant ventricular arrhythmias associated with the use of encainide. Am Heart J 102: 857–864.

35. Cocco G, Strozzi C, Pansini R, Rochat N, Bulgarelli L, Padvla A, Sfirsi C, Kamal AL, Yassini A. 1984. Antiarrhythmic use of cibenzoline, a new class I antiarrhythmic agent with class 3 and 4 properties in patients with recurrent ventricular tachycardia. Eur Heart J 5: 108.

36. Browne KF, Prystowsky EN, Zipes DP, Chilson DA, Heger JJ. 1984. Clinical efficacy and electrophysiologic effects of Cibenzoline therapy in patients with ventricular arrhythmias. J Am Coll Cardiol 3: 857–864.

37. Miura DS, Keren G, Torres V, Butler B, Aogaichi K, Somberg JC. 1985. Antiarrhythmic effects of Cibenzoline. Am Heart J 109: 827–833.

38. Wasty N, Saksena S, Barr MJ. 1985. Comparative efficacy and safety of oral Cibenzolne and quinidine in ventricular arrhythmias: a randomized crossover study. Am Heart J 110: 1181–1188.

39. Rigaud M, Jouret G, Canal M, Bardet J, Flouvat B, Bourdarias JP. 1985. Hemodynamic effects of a new antiarrhythmic agent: Cibenzoline. J Pharmacol (Paris) 16: 247–257.

40. Cassagneau B, Calazel J, Puel J, Mashbuau P, Tournadre P, Fauvel JM, Bounhoure JP, Marin T, Narula OS. 1984. Intérêt des tests de provocation dans l'appréciation du traitement des tachycardies ventriculaires par l'amiodarone. Arch Mal Coeur 77: 766–772.

41. Flaker GC, Alpert MA, Webel RR, Ruder MA, Sanfelipo JF, Tsvtakawa RK. 1985. Amiodarone and sustained ventricular arrhythmias: statistical evidence of drug effeciveness. Am Heart J 110: 371–375.

42. Hariman RJ, Gomes JAC, Kang PS, El-Sherif N. 1984. Effects of intravenous amiodarone in patients with inducible repetitive ventricular response and ventricular tachycardia. Am Heart J 107: 1109–1117.

43. Heger JJ, Prystowsky EN, Zipes DP. 1983. Clinical efficacy of amiodarone in treatment of recurrent ventricular tachycardia and ventricular fibrillation. Am Heart J 106: 887–894.
44. Horowitz LN, Greenspan AM, Spielman SR, Webb CR, Morganroth J, Rotmensch H, Sokoloff NM, Rae AP, Segal BL, Kay HR. 1985. Usefulness of electrophysiologic testing in evaluation of amiodarone therapy for sustained ventricular tachyarrhythmias associated with coronary heart disease. Am J Cardiol 55: 367–371.
45. Kaski JC, Girotti LA, Messuti H, Rutitzky B, Rosenbaum MB. 1981. Long-term management of sustained, recurrent, symptomatic ventricular tachycardia with amiodarone. Circulation 64: 273–279.
46. Mc Govern, Garan H, Malakoff RF, Dimarco JP, Grant G, Sellers D, Ruskin JN. 1984. Long term clinical outcome of ventricular tachycardia or fibrillation treated with amiodarone. Am J Cardiol 53: 1558–1563.
47. Nademanee K, Hendrickson JA, Cannom DS, Goldreyer BN, Singh BN. 1981. Control of refractory life-threatening ventricular tachyarrhythmias by amiodarone. Am Heart J 101: 759–768.
48. Nademanee K, Hendrickson J, Kannan R, Singh BN. 1982. Antiarrhythmic efficacy and electrophysiologic actions of amiodarone in patients with life-threatening ventricular arrhythmias: potent suppression of spontaneously occurring tachyarrhythmias versus inconsistent abolition of induced ventricular tachycardia. Am Heart J 103: 950–953.
49. Leak D. 1986. Intravenous amiodarone in the treatment of refractory lifethreatening cardiac arrhythmias in the critically ill patient. Am Heart J 111: 456–462.
50. Rasmussen K, Winkle R, Ross D, Griffin J, Peters F, Mason J. 1982. Antiarrhythmic efficacy of amiodarone in recurrent ventricular tachycardia evaluated by multiple electrophysiological and ambulatory ECG recordings. Acta Med Scand 212: 367–374.
51. Jaksena S, Rothbart ST, Shah Y, Cappello G. 1984. Clinical efficacy and electropharmacology of continuous intravenous amiodarone infusion and chronic oral amiodarone in refractory ventricular tachycardia. Am J Cardiol 54: 347–352.
52. Veltri EP, Reid PR, Platia EV, Griffith L. 1985. Results of late programmed electrical stimulation and long-term electrophysiologic effects of amiodarone therapy in patients with refractory ventricular tachycardia. Am J Cardiol 55: 375–379.
53. Veltri EP, Reid PR, Platia EV, Griffith LS. 1985. Amiodarone in the treatment of life-threatening ventricular tachycardia: role of Holter monitoring in predicting long-term clinical efficacy. J Am Coll Cardiol 6: 806–813.
54. Mc Kenna W, Oakley CM, Krikler DM, Goodwin JF. 1985. Improved survival with amiodarone in patients with hypertrophic cardiomyopathy and ventricular tachycardia. Br Heart J 53: 412–416.
55. Dicarlo LA, Morady F, Sauve MJ, Malone P, Davis JC, Evans-Becc T, Winston SA, Scheinman MM. 1985. Cardiac arrest and sudden death in patients treated with amiodarone for sustained ventricular tachycardia or ventricular fibrillation: risk stratification based on clinical variables. Am J Cardiol 55: 372–374.

27. Permanent pacemakers for ventricular tachycardia control: current status

SAMUEL LÉVY* and PIERRE LACOMBE* *
* Professor of Cardiology, University of Marseille, School of Medicine, Director of Clinical Electrophysiology and Pacing Department, Marseille, France
* * Fellow in Cardiology. Supported by Notre Dame Foundation, Montréal, Canada

Permanent pacing has been considered for the last two decades as an alternative therapy for the treatment of tachycardias [1–5]. Recent advances in pacemaker technology, the advent of new treatments for ventricular tachycardias such as surgery, automatic implantable cardioverter-defibrillator and electrical ablation, make it necessary to evaluate the role of permanent pacing for ventricular tachycardia control.

The indication of an implantable pacemaker in a patient with ventricular tachycardia may be discussed in order to achieve one or several of the following goals: 1) rate support in a patient with associated bradycardia; 2) ventricular tachycardia prevention; 3) tachycardia termination in a patient refractory to drug therapy.

Pacing for rate-support

Pacemaker implantation in a patient with ventricular tachycardia may be indicated for associated bradycardia. The latter may be part of the so-called bradycardia-ventricular tachycardia syndrome usually associated with an ominous prognosis [6, 7]. The bradycardia may be related to sick sinus node syndrome or to advanced atrioventricular block.

In a significant number of patients bradycardia may be a side-effect of antiarrhythmic therapy in patients with pre-existing disorder in impulse formation or conduction. We have observed this unwanted effect in some patients particularly on amiodarone at daily doses above 400 mg or propafenone above 900 mg. Implantation of a demand pacemaker for rate support allows also the use of antiarrhythmic drugs at adequate doses necessary for tachycardia control.

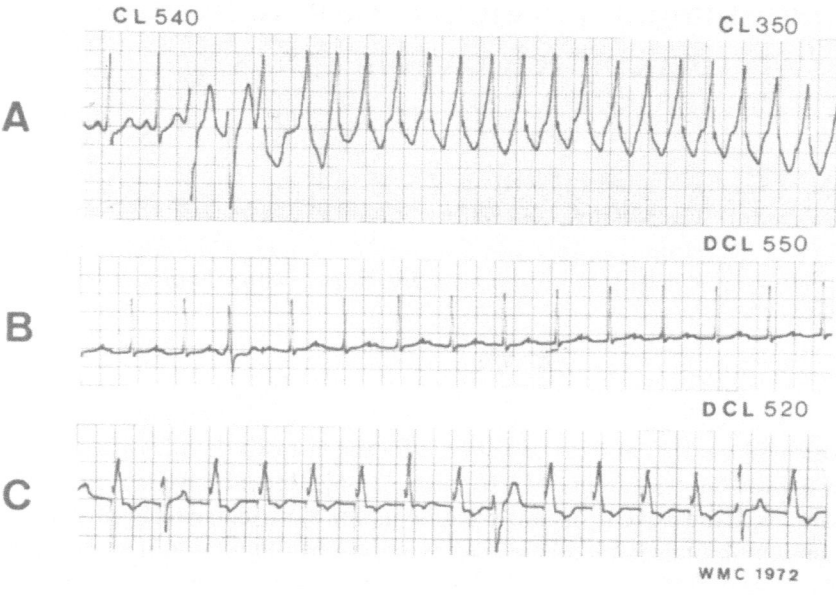

Figure 1. Electrocardiographic recording of lead X in a 21 year old woman with ventricular tachycardia (VT) related to cardiac sarcoïdosis. On panel A spontaneous VT is shown. On panel B atrial pacing at a rate of 110 beats per minute (driven cycle length (DCL) of 550 ms) prevents successfully the VT. Panel C shows ventricular pacing at a DCL of 520 ms through an implantable pacemaker (see text).

Pacing for ventricular tachycardia prevention

Cardiac pacing may be needed to prevent the ventricular tachycardia or/and to suppress ventricular premature beats which may trigger the arrhythmia. These goals may be achieved by pacing the atrium, the ventricle or both cavities using atrioventricular pacing at rates within the physiologic range (below 100 beats/minute) or above. The rate selected is the slowest capable of tachycardia or/and premature beats prevention and which is functionally and hemodynamically well tolerated. This is best achieved in patients with spontaneous slow rates. Atrial or ventricular pacing at a rate higher than spontaneous rate and slower than the rate of tachycardia (overdrive suppression) is effective although the mechanism is not completely understood. Overdrive suppression may be particularly effective in bradycardia related ventricular arrhythmias. The mechanism of the arrhythmia may be enhanced automaticity, triggered automaticity or reentry. An example of prevention of ventricular tachycardia in a patient with cardiac sarcoidosis is shown in figure 1. In panel B, temporary atrial pacing at a rate slower than the rate of tachycardia and in panel C, permanent ventricular pacing at a rate of 115 beats/minute were able to prevent drug refractory ventricular tachycardia.

Temporary pacing is widely used in preventing drug-induced torsades de

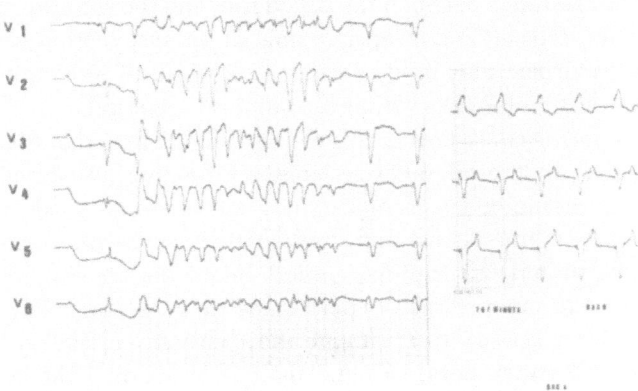

Figure 2. Prevention of torsade de pointes using ventricular pacing. On the left hand panel ventricular tachycardia with the features of torsades de pointes occurred on an underlying paced rate of 50 beats/minute. The right hand side panel shows leads I, II, III and a paced rate of 70 beats per minute which prevented successfully the arrhythmia.

pointes and ventricular arrhythmias occurring in the setting of bradycardia during acute myocardial infarction, hypokalemia or digitalis toxicity. In contrast, permanent pacing is rarely used for ventricular arrhythmia prevention. The use of ventricular pacing to prevent 'torsades de pointes' related to congenital or idiopathic long QT syndrome has been proposed. However, this indication need to bevalidated. Prevention of iatrogenic torsade de pointe is shown in figure 2. The rate of pacing is emphasized. Torsades de pointe were not prevented by ventricular pacing at a rate of 50 beats per minute in this patient with a previously implanted pacemaker. Programming the pacemaker at a rate of 70 beats/minute was able to suppress the arrhythmia.

Pacing for tachycardia termination

Temporary pacing is currently used in the electrophysiologic laboratory to terminate ventricular tachycardia. It seemed therefore logical to apply this technique in a chronic fashion using an antitachycardia device.

Pacing modes

Termination of ventricular tachycardia may be achieved by different techniques.
Underdrive pacing designates pacing at a rate slower than that of the tachycardia rate. This mode is also referred to as competitive or asynchronous pacing as

there is an interference between the paced rate and the spontaneous tachycardia until a stimulus falls at he appropriate time of the tachycardia cycle and terminates the tachycardia. This mode carries a high risk of induction of ventricular fibrillation if a stimulus falls within the vulnerable period.

Overdrive pacing consists of pacing at a rate higher than that of the tachycardia. A burst with a predetermined cycle length and number of stimuli, is delivered. The first beat should be synchronized in order to avoid ventricular fibrillation.

Extrastimulus method consist on scanning the tachycardia during diastole. The extrastimulus should fall within a period called the termination zone located between the ventricular refractory period and the reset zone. Two, three or more stimuli may be necessary to terminate the tachycardia. The first stimulus may shorten the refractory period of the tissue surrounding the reentrant circuit allowing the second stimulus to supervene in the termination zone. Another explanation has been recently proposed by El Sherif et al. [9]: the tachycardia is terminated if the stimulated wavefront arrives at a strategically located area and at a critical time.

Combination or variants of the above: other modes of stimulation have been proposed which are basically a combination or variants of the three essential modes of stimulation. Combination of overdrive with scanning on the last stimulus has been found to be successful when extrastimulus method or overdrive failed when used separately [10]. Delivering a series of burst which have a cycle length shorter and shorter has been referred to as 'adaptive mode, scanning burst or concertina pacing' [11]. Orthorhythmic pacing consists of delivering an extrastimulus at a determined percentage of the cardiac cycle. Recently Charos et al. [12] reported another modality of pacing that they described as autodecremental overdrive pacing. A number of stimuli which a varying cycle shorter by a predetermined decrement up to a minimum, are delivered during tachycardia. Train stimulation [13] is an attempt to cover the cardiac cycle by a burst with a short cycle length (2 ms per example). The number of stimuli is programmed in such fashion that only one capture occurs and terminate the tachycardia. Although, these recent techniques have been used with good results on a temporary basis, there is not to our knowledge and at the time of this writing a permanent unit using this mode.

Factors influencing the results

Whatever the technique used a number of factors may influence the results. The location of the tachycardia circuit as opposed to the pacing site (usually the apex of the right ventricle) is of paramount importance [14, 15]. If the reentrant circuit is far from the pacing site, the time necessary for the stimulated wavefront to depolarize the intermediate myocardium may be too long and it may not reach the reentrant circuit. The size of the reentrant circuit, therefore the cycle length of the

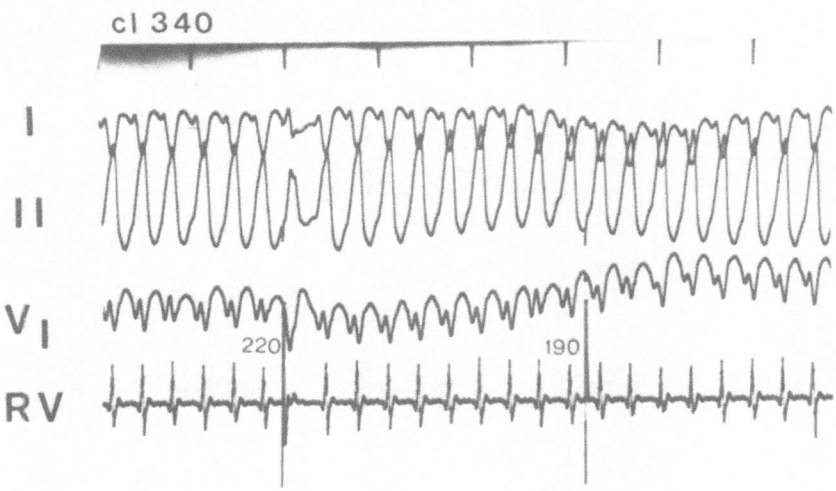

Figure 3. From top to bottom, electrocardiographic leads I, II and VI and endocavitary right ventricular (RV) lead. A premature paced beat with a coupling interval of 220 ms or longer captures the tachycardia without terminating it. At shorter intervals the effective refractory period of the ventricle is reached.

tachycardia will determine the duration of the tachycardia termination zone, therefore the success rate in the termination of the tachycardia. The energy delivered is an important parameter as it has been stressed recently by Waxman et al. [16], the percentage of success being higher with higher energy.

Patient selection

Not all ventricular tachycardias are obviously successfully terminated using ventricular pacing, as shown by the attempts performed in the electrophysiologic laboratory. Therefore in order to be elligible for an antitachycarda device, the patient with ventricular tachycardia should fulfill two prerequisites which are mandatory (but not sufficient): 1) The tachycardia should be reproducibly terminated by the selected pacing technique; 2) The safety of the pacing technique should be demonstrated in the matter of acceleration or degeneration of the tachycardia into ventricular fibrillation.

There is only little information in the literature regarding termination of ventricular tachycardia using programmed electrical stimulation [17, 18]. All the reported series state the percentage of successful attempts for each technique modality. However, data regarding the reproducibility of each technique in an individual patient is lacking.

Table 1.

Authors	Years	Patients	Pacing techniques	Observation time (months)	Malfunction or unwanted effects	Remarks
Friday et al.	1981	2	Patient activated synchronised burst	11	0	1 death. Device not activated
Rotheman et al.	1984	5	Automatic, tachylog single or multiple extrastimulus	6	3 deaths	2 unrelated deaths 2 Pts controlled
Saksena et al.	1984	4	Patient activated Cordis omni orthocor	17	0	Used successfully in 2
Djordjevic et al.	1984	2	Patient activated Siemens Elema PZY, extrastimulus	13		
		2	Siemens-Elema tachylog Extrastimulus, automatic	43		
Griffin et Sweeney	1984	52 (in USA)	Automatic, burst, Cyberback 60	13	0	14 deaths unrelated 4
Rothman et Keefe	1984	53	Patient activated, burst extrastimuli (synchronized) Cordis omni-Orthocor	52	sensin (1) failure to terminate 10/105 épisodes	23 deaths 6 sudden (3 documented VT/VF)
Sowton	1984	9 (GB)	Automatic multifunctiuns Siemens Elema tachylog Extrastimuli (scanning) Burst overdrive, combination	12	0	4 deaths unrelated
Peters et al.	1985	6	Medtronic 5998, automatic burst	3–36	Acceleration VF (2 patients 1 death	3 proved unsuccessful 1 patient controlled
Aonecma et al.	1985	6	Omni-Orthocor 234A Patient activated Overdrive burst atrium in	22		2 deaths unrelated
Tanabe et al.	1985	1	Patient activated Medtronic 9701 Overdrive atrial pacing	17	1 episode of atrial fibrillation	
Higgens et al.	1985	1	Automatic Telectronics PASAR 4151	16	0	

In order to determine the percentage of patients in whom termination of ventricular tachycardia using pacing techniques would be a suitable technique, we have analysed the data of 33 consecutive patients. All patients had pacing-induced sustained ventricular tachycardia requiring intervention in order to be terminated. The pacing-induced ventricular tachycardia was comparable in electrocardiographic configuration to the documented spontaneous episode. Whenever tolerance of the arrhythmia was acceptable we delivered single or double extrastimuli and overdrive pacing in that sequence. In case of failure or acceleration, DC cardioversion was applied. The goal was to define the simplest pacing method which would terminate the arrhythmia in a reproducible fashion. Of the 33 patients, 6 required immediate DC cardioversion because of hemodynamic compromise. Pacing techniques were applied to the remaining 27 patients. The percentage of successful attempts for each technique single, double or overdrive pacing was 11, 43 and 67%. Overdrive pacing is the most successful technique for ventricular tachycardia termination and this is consistent with the literature (Table 1). The mode of pacing which terminates reproducibility the tachycardia in a given patient (and not by attempts) shows that one extrastimulus is only successful in 3%, 2 extrastimuli in 14% and overdrive in 34%. It appears that pacing for tachycardia termination could be applied to approximatly half of the patients, which would be satisfactory in the absence of the risk of acceleration of the tachycardia or its degeneration into ventricular fibrillation. Acceleration was observed in 8 patients (29.6%) using 1 extrastimulus in 2 patients, 2 extrastimuli in 1 patient and overdrive pacing in 5 patients. Following acceleration, DC cardioversion was needed in 6 patients and spontaneous termination was observed in 2. The occurrence of such phenomenon is a contra-indication in a given patient to the use of an implantable pacing-device for tachycardia termination without back-up defibrillator. The absence of this phenomenon despite a large number of attempts for tachycardia termination does not exclude this potential hazard which may be facilitated by a number of factors (Autonomous nervous system, myocardial ischemia, electrolyte imbalance, exercise and other possibly unknown factors) which may not be present at the time of testing. The incidence of acceleration of ventricular tachycardia found in ours series is within the range (5–35%) of the litterature.

Implantable devices for tachycardia termination

Pacing devices for ventricular tachycardia termination may be subdivided into patient or physician-activated devices and automatic pacemakers which are capable of automatic tachycardia detection and termination.

374

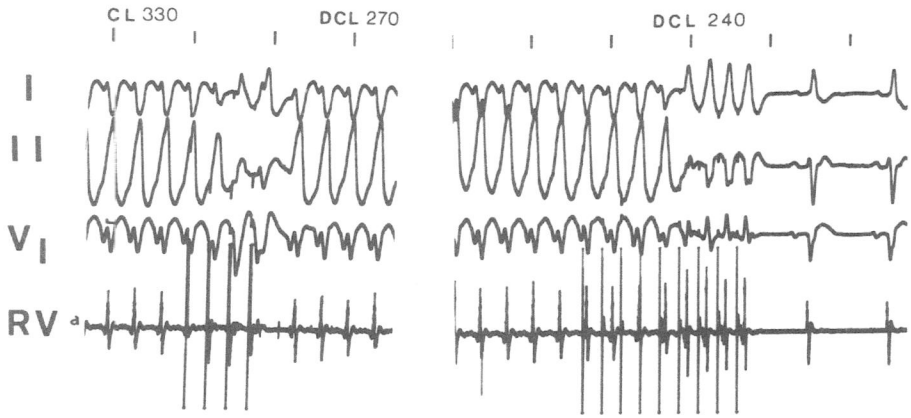

Figure 4. (Same patient as figure 2). Four paced beats are unsuccessful in terminating the ventricular tachycardia. A larger number of stimuli with a shorter cycle length (right panel) is necessary in order to terminate the tachycardia.

Patient or physician activated devices [19–23]

Manually-activated devices were the first systems to be introduced for tachycardia termination. They can be applied only to those patients with symptomatic and well tolerated arrhythmia. If the arrhythmia is associated with syncope, such systems are not obviously suitable.

The first and the simplest manually-activated system consists of applying a magnet over the pacemaker pocket, therefore producing asynchronous pacing. Such pacing mode carries a high risk of acceleration or ventricular fibrillation.

Radiofrequency systems consist of a subcutaneous receptor connected to epicardial electrodes and an external adaptator connected to pulse-generator. The generator is actived by the patient during tachycardia.

More sophisticated devices have been recently available as they are capable of two-way communication. The therapeutic programme will be administered only after the tachycardia has been confirmed by the internal system. Three such systems are, to our knowledge, available: Cordis Omni-Orthocor 230A [19], Siemens-Elema P24 and the Medtronic SP503 [23]. We have had clinical experience with the Medtronic SP503. This system is capable of rate support at a rate of 50 beats/minute. The patient or the physician may use an activator which applied over the pacemaker pocket will deliver a pre-determined therapeutic programme if the tachycardia is recognised. The rate of detection of the tachycardia and the pacing programme (number of stimuli and their coupling intervals, number of treatments to be delivered and time-interval between two treatments) are selected and transmitted to the activator using a programmer. It is possible, using the programmer, to perform a non-invasive electrophysiologic study and this type of system is sometimes referred to as implantable electrophysiologic laboratory.

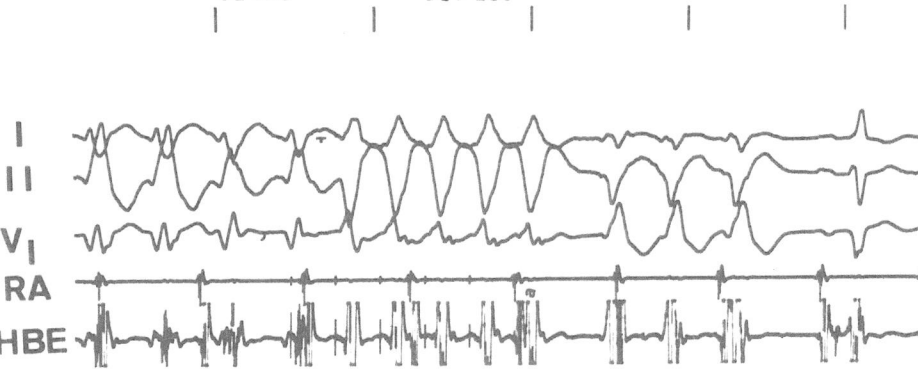

Figure 5. (Same patient as figures 2 and 3). The patient has been on amiodarone therapy. Endocavitary right atrium (RA) and His Bundle electrogram (HBE) are displayed. The tachycardia is easier to terminate. Note few beats of a different type of self-terminating tachycardia.

Automatic pacemakers [25–30]

These devices are capable of automatic tachycardia detection and termination. The tachycardia is defined as a number of QRS complexes shorter than a pre-established cycle length. When the tachycardia is detected the pacing treatment, consisting of a rapid burst or a scanning stimulus, is delivered. The Medtronic 2404 or 5998 [25] the Intermedics Cybertach [26], and the Biotronik Phylax all utilise overdrive pacing for tachycardia termination. The Telectronics 4151 (PASAR) [28] or the Siemens Tachylog 451B [27] utilise the scanning technique. Recently the Medtronic Symbios 7007-7008 [29], which uses different pacing modes for rate support (VVI, DVT, DDD), has been available for tachycardia termination as it functions on the DVI double demand asynchronous (underdrive) mode, a technique not recommended fo ventricular tachycardia. For supraventricular tachycardia, a salvo of atrial impulses may be delivered.

Recent experience on implantable pacemakers for ventricular tachycardia termination

A recent review of the literature has shown that although implantable pacing for tachycardia termination devices have been the subject of great interest [30], the number of patients treated by this technique is relatively small. Ohm et al. [2] have found, over a period of 4 years (1979–1982), only 38 with ventricular tachycardia treated by pacing techniques out of a total of 199 patients who received an antitachycardia pacemaker. We updated such review by analysing 11 published series over a period of 2 years (1984–1985) and found 143 additional patients with ventricular tachycardia in whom an antitachycardia device was implanted. In 75 patients, an automatic antitachycardia device was implanted. Such a number might reflect an increased interest for pacing in this specific indication. Most reports consist of case reports or small series except for two papers [26, 27] which relate to the US and British experiences.

Griffin and Sweeney [26] have reported 52 patients who represent the USA experience of the Cybertach 60, an automatic pacemaker using overdrive burst. Over a mean follow-up period of 13 months, 18 patients died (34.6%) including 14 unrelated deaths and 4 sudden deaths in which the pacemaker might have played a part. Sowton [27] reported the British experience of the Tachylog (Siemens-Elema), a pacemaker which uses a single or several extrastimuli, a burst or combination of both techniques. Four out of 9 patients died over a mean follow-up period of 12 months. These deaths were stated to be unrelated to the pacemaker.

Our personal experience of pacing for ventricular tachycardia termination is restricted to physician-activated systems. The potential risk of ventricular tachycardia acceleration [32] or ventricular fibrillation has made us reluctant to use automatic or patient-activated devices. The physician may use such systems under electrocardiographic surveillance and wih a defibrillator nearby should a complication occur. We used the Medtronic Interactive system (described above) in 3 patients with recurrent ventricular tachycardias in whom a pacemaker was indicated for rate-support. One patient died in the hospital of electromecanical dissociation unrelated to the device. In one patient controlled by amiodarone, the rate support function was definitely useful as he developped A-V block. In the patient in whom antitachycardic function was useful it was necessary to re-programme the activator. One inconvenience of such a device is the need to send back the activator to the manufacturer should a new programme be required by changes in the pacing-parameters for tachycardia termination.

Indications of pacing for ventricular tachycardia termination

Pacing for tachycardia temination is a painless and rapid method requiring a small amount of energy. It should have been an ideal method in the absence of the following disadvantages. As mentioned above, this method is only applicable to a selected group of patients with ventricular tachycardia having a cycle length outside the physiologic range. Detection systems at present are unable to differentiate ventricular tachycardia from sinus tachycardia or atrial fibrillation [34, 35]. Such detection problems might result in tachycardia induction instead of termination. An important fact which is underestimated is the lack of reproducibility of the pacing parameters. It has been suggested that termination of a large number of episodes (50–100) in the electrophysiologic laboratory should allow a certain degree of safety; in fact, remote changes of the successful pacing formula are possible. Antiarrhythmic agents given for ventricular tachycardia prevention may, at least by their effect on the cycle length, modify the programmed pacing parameters. The major problem of pacing for ventricular tachycardia termination remains the risk of acceleration and of ventricular fibrillation. There is no way to eliminate such risk at the present time. Therefore we believe at the present time that permanent pacing is not a safe method for ventricular tachycardia termination unless it is used with a back-up defibrillator (see Dr Mirowski's chapter). Such a perspective leads to pursue active research in this field, as a programmable pacing-device capable of various pacing modalities and using back-up defibrillation may represent the solution in the near future [36].

References

1. Barold SS, Falkoff MD, Ong LS. 1985. Cardia pacing for the treatment of tachycardia. Barold S. Ed. Mount Kisco, NY, Futura Publishing: 693–724.
2. Ohm OJ, Michelson EJ, Dreifus LS. 1984. Role of pacing in the treatment of tachycardias. In Tachycardias. Surawicz B, Reddy PC, Prystowsky EN, eds. Martinus Nijhoff Publishing, Boston: 513–533.
3. Lévy S. 1984. Role of pacing in treatment of supraventricular tachycardia (supraventricular tachycardia, Wolff-Parkinson-White, Flutter). In Tachycardias: Mechanism, Diagnosis, Treatment. Josephson ME, Wellens HJJ eds, Lea and Fibiger Philidelphia: 223–240.
4. Fisher JD, Kim SG, Furman S, Matos JA. 1982. Role of implantable pacemakers in control of recurrent ventricular tachycardia. Am J Cardiol 49: 194–206.
5. Furman S, Pannizzo MS. 1985. The role of implantable pacemakers in the therapy of tachycardias. Arch Mal Coeur 78 no spécial: 29–34.
6 Aroesty JM, Cohen SI, Morkin E. 1974. Bradycardia-Tachycardia syndrome: résults in 28 patients treated by combined pharmacology therapy and pacemaker inplantation. Chest 66: 257.
7. Hauser RG, Jones J, Denes P, Messer JV. 1983. Prognosis of patients who are paced for bradyarrhythmias complicated by ventricular tachycardia in Recent Advanced in Cardiac Arrhythmias (I). Lévy S, Gérard R, eds. J. Libbey Londres: 228–232.
8. Camm J, Ward D. 1983. Pacing for tachycardia control. Telectronics. Butler and Tanner, Frome and London.
9. El-Sherif N, Gough WB, Restivo M. 1986. Mechanism of 'entrainment', acceleration or termination of reentrant ventricular tachycardia by programmed electrical stimulation. North American Society of Pacing and Electrophysiology. PACE Abstract. no 28, p 281.
10. Josephson ME, Waxman HL, Buxton AE, Marchlinski FE, Doherty JU. 1984. Recurrent ventricular tachycardias: Role of intracardiac recording and pacing for therapeutic indications. Cardiac arrhythmias. Ed.: Levy S, and Scheinman MM. Futura Pub New York. p. 22: 391–419.
11. Nathan A, Hellestrand K, Bexton R, Nappholz T, Spurrell RAJ, Camm AJ. 1982. Clinical evaluation of an adaptive tachycardia intervention pacemaker with automatic cycle length adjustment. Pace 5: 201.
12. Charos GS, Haffajee CI, Gold RL, Bishop RL, Berkovits BV, Alpert JS. 1986. A theoretically and practically more effective method for interruption of ventricular tachycardia: self-adapting autodecremental overdrive pacing. Circulation 73: 309–315.
13. Fisher JD, Ostrow E, Kim SG, Matos JA. 1983. Ultrarapid single-capture train stimulation for termination of ventricular tachycardia. Amer J Cardiol 51: 1334–1338.
14. Fisher JD, Kim SG, Matos A, Waspe LE. 1984. Pacing for ventricular Tachycardia. Pace 7: 1277–1290.

15. Osborn MJ, Holmes DR. 1985. Antitachycardia pacing. Clin Prog Electrophysiol and Pacing 3: 239–267.
16. Waxman HL, Cain ME, Greenspan AM, Josephson ME. 1982. Termination of ventricular tachycardia with ventricular stimulation: Salutary effect of increased current strength. Circulation 65: 800–804.
17. Roy D, Waxman HL, Buxton AE,, Marchlinski FE, Cain ME, Gardner MJ, Josephson ME. 1982. Termination of ventricular tachycardia: Role of Tachycardia cycle length. Amer J Cardiol 50: 1346–1350.
18. Nacarelli GV, Zipes DP, Rahilly GT, Heger JJ, Prystowsk EN. 1983. Influence of tachycardia cycle length and antiarrhythmic drugs on pacing termination and acceleration of ventricular tachycardia. Amer Heart J 105: 1–5.
19. Rothman MT, Keefe JM. 1984. Clinical results with Omni-Orthocor, an implantable antitachycardia pacing system. Pace 7: 1306–1312.
20. Tanabe A, Ikeda H, Fujiyama M, Furuta Y-I, Matsumura J, Ohbayashi J, Utsu F, Toshima H. 1985. Termination of ventricular tachycardia by an implantable atrial pacemaker and external pacemaker activator. Pace 8: 532–538.
21. Aonuma K, Rozanski JJ, Barold S, Dewitt PL, Gosselin AJ, Lester JW. 1985. Externally activated antitachycardia pacemaker with noninvasive electrophysiologic re-testing capability. Pace 8: 215–224.
22. Friday KJ, Jackman WM, Olson EG, Reynolds DW, Schechter E, Lazzara R. 1984. Limitations of synchronized burst ventricular pacemakers as primary therapy for recurrent sustained ventricular tachycardia. Pace 7: 459.
23. Saksena S, Pantopoulos D, Parsonnet V, Lombardo S, Tothbart ST, Hussain SM, Gielchinsky I. 1984. Clinical evaluation of an implantable antitachycardia system. Pace 5 (Abstr.): 476.
24. Pop T, Treese N, Henkel B, Erbel R, Meyer J. 1985. Two years experience with the Medtronic interactive tachy system in patients with ventricular tachycardia. Pace 8 (Abstr.) 8: 342. A 86.
25. Peters RW, Scheinman MM, Morady F, Jacobson L. 1985. Long-term management of recurrent paroxysmal tachycardia by cardiac burst pacing. Pace 8: 35–44.
26. Griffin JC, Sweeney M. 1984. The management of paroxysmal tachycardias using the Cybertach-60. Pace 7: 1291–1295.
27. Sowton E. 1984. Clinical results with the Tachylog antitachycardia pacemaker. Pace 7: 1313–1317.
28. Higgins JR, Swartz JF, Dehmer GJ, Beddingfield GW. 1985. Automatic scanning extrastimulus pacemaker to treat ventricular tachycardia. Pace 8: 101–109.
29. Zipes DP, Prystowsky EN, Milles WM, Heger JJ. 1984. Initial experience with Symbios Model 7008 Pacemaker. Pace 7: 1301–1305.
30. Fisher JD, Kim SG, Furman S, Matos J. 1982. Role of implantable pacemakers in control of recurrent ventricular tachycardia. Amer J Cardiol 49: 194–206.
31. Jenkins J, Bump t, Munkenbeck F, Brown J, Arzbaecher R. 1984. Tachycardia detection in implantable antitachycardia devices. Pace 7: 1273–1277.
32. Jentzer JH, Hoffman RM. 1984. Acceleration of ventricular tachycardia by rapid overdrive pacing combined with extrastimuli. Pace 7: 922–924.
33. Den Dulk K, Brugada P, Wellens HJJ. 1984. A case report demonstrating spontaneous change in tachycardia terminating window. Pace 7: 867–870.
34. Arzbaecher R, Bump, T, Jenkins J, Glick K, Munkenbec F, Brown J, Nandhakumar N. 1984. Automatic tachycardia recognition. Pace 7: 541–547.
35. Pless BD, Sweeney MB. 1984. Discrimination of supraventricular tachycardia from sinus tachycardia of overlapping cycle length. Pace 7: 1318–1324.
36. Mirowski M. 1982. Prevention of sudden arrhythmic death with implanted automatic defibrillators. Ann Intern Med 98: 585.

28. Prevention of arrhythmic death with the automatic implantable cardioverter-defibrillator

M. MIROWSKI, MORTON M. MOWER, ENRICO P. VELTRI, and JUAN M. JUANTEGUY
Departments of Medicine and Surgery, Sinai Hospital of Baltimore, Baltimore, Maryland 21215, U.S.A. and The Johns Hopkins Medical Institutions, Baltimore, Maryland 21205, U.S.A.

Because the treatment of ventricular fibrillation and many hemodynamically unstable ventricular tachycardias with electrical countershock is critically dependent on rapid availability of medical personnel and equipment, its implementation outside the hospital is rarely successful. This situation has prompted the development of a fully implantable automatic device designed for continuous monitoring of the heart rhythm and prompt recognition and treatment of life-threatening ventricular tachyarrhythmias [1]. Since the first implantation of such a device in a human being at The Johns Hopkins Hospital [1], the automatic implantable cardioverter-defibrillator (AICD*) is being used with increased frequency to prevent sudden cardiac death in high-risk patients [2–8]. The growing clinical experience has demonstrated that this therapeutic intervention dramatically lowers the prohibitive arrhythmic mortality of this population [3, 8, 9].

Description of the devices

The AICD is a self-contained automatic system with extensive monitoring, diagnostic, and therapeutic capabilities. This device is an advanced version of the original automatic implantable defibrillator (AID), which was designed to correct only ventricular fibrillation; the AICD has added cardioverting capabilities, i.e., it also treats ventricular tachycardias with an R-wave synchronised countershock.

The AICD consists of a pulse generator and three electrode leads (Figure 1). The pulse generator weighs 292 grams and has a volume of 162 cc. It is housed in an hermetically-sealed titanium case containing the electronic components and the power sources; the batteries and capacitors are expected to provide nearly three years of monitoring life or the delivery of approximately 100 discharges. Two transcardiac electrodes deliver the electrical countershock directly to the

---

* Manufactured by Cardiac Pacemakers, Inc., St. Paul, Minnesota, U.S.A.

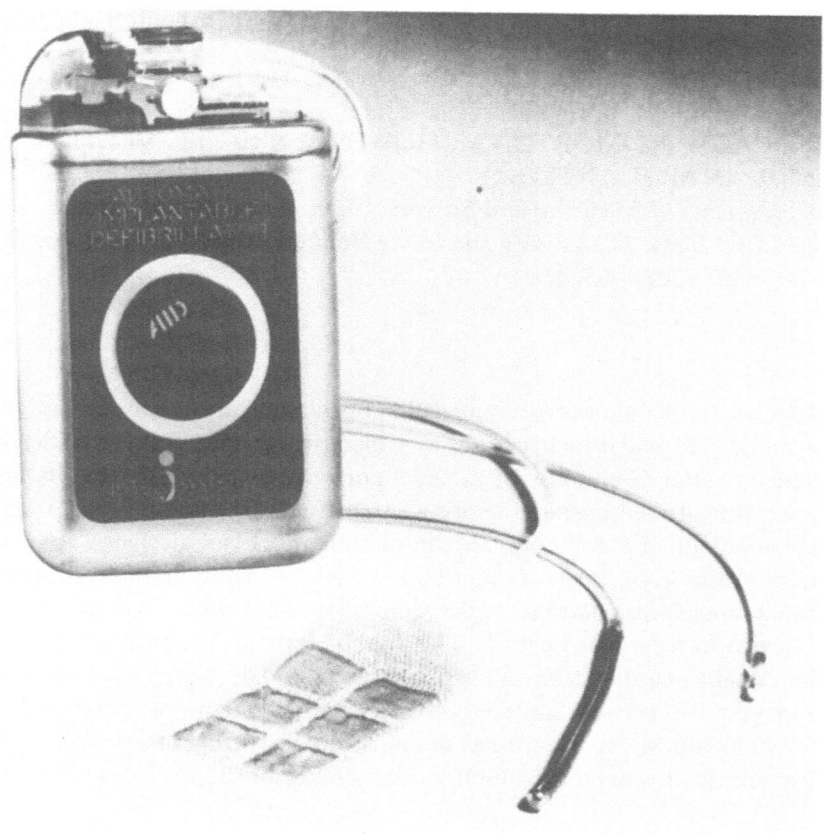

Figure 1. The automatic implantable cardioverter-defibrillator with, right to left, its bipolar right ventricular, superior vena cava, and apical patch electrodes. For more details, see text.

heart: one catheter-electrode is incorporated into an intravascular catheter positioned in the superior vena cava, while the second, a flexible rectangular patch, covers the apex of the heart; these defibrillating electrodes also serve for sensing the morphology of the cardiac electrogram. The third lead, a separate catheter containing two closely spaced electrodes on its tip, is wedged into the right ventricular apex and serves for heart rate determination and R-wave synchronization. If the implantation procedure involves a thoracotomy, two epicardial screw-in electrodes can be substituted for the right ventricular rate lead.

The device continuously analyses the patient's heart rate and waveform morphology. The latter is expressed in terms of the probability density function (PDF), which reflects the time spent by the electrical signal between two limits located near the isoelectric line. When both the heart rate and PDF exceed critical values, the capacitor charging cycle is activated, the capacitors are charged to approximately 720 volts and a truncated exponential pulse of 25 J is then delivered to the heart. In the presence of ventricular tachycardia, the pulse delivery is synchronous with the onset of ventricular depolarization. If the initial discharge does not restore normal rhythm, the device recycles and can deliver up to three additional pulses of 30 J each. The pulse generator can be deactivated and reactivated noninvasively with the proper use of a magnet.

In addition to the standard AICD device characterized by the dual detection algorithm, a variant of the device featuring a sensing system that relies only on the analysis of heart rate is also available. The 'rate only' version of the AICD is more sensitive than the standard unit and is less likely to miss ventricular tachycardias with narrow QRS complexes. However, it is also more likely to deliver pulses during those supraventricular arrhythmias which are faster than the device's present rate cut-off value.

Techniques have also been developed for noninvasively communicating with the implanted device. By magnetically triggering coded audio-signals generated by a built-in piezo-electric transducer and by using a specially designed device – the AIDCHECK* – (Figure 2) it is possible to interrogate the AICD and to obtain information about the sensing function, the status (active or inactive) of the pulse generator, the degree of battery depletion, any changes in the capacitor, and the cumulative number of pulses that the unit has delivered to the patient. These tests are performed prior to, during, and following implantation.

Clinical trials

The clinical evaluation studies of this new therapeutic intervention began in February 1980 at The Johns Hopkins Hospital in Baltimore [1]. Shortly thereafter, the trials expanded to several additional centers, following rigidly defined criteria. This effort provided important clinical and technological information which led to the incorporation of critical improvements into the device, better patient-selection criteria, and more sophisticated procedures and testing techniques. By February 1986, the number of implantees worldwide had reached 855; 12,798 pulse generator implant-months had been accumulated; the longest follow-up was 72 months and the mean follow-up was 16 months.

Patient population

Initially, the potential implantees were required to have suffered at least two previous cardiac arrests not associated with acute myocardial infarction; one such episode had to occur despite drug therapy and with the malignant arrhythmia documented at least once. Patients were excluded if their life expectancy was

---

* Manufactured by Cardiac Pacemakers, Inc., St. Paul, Minnesota, U.S.A.

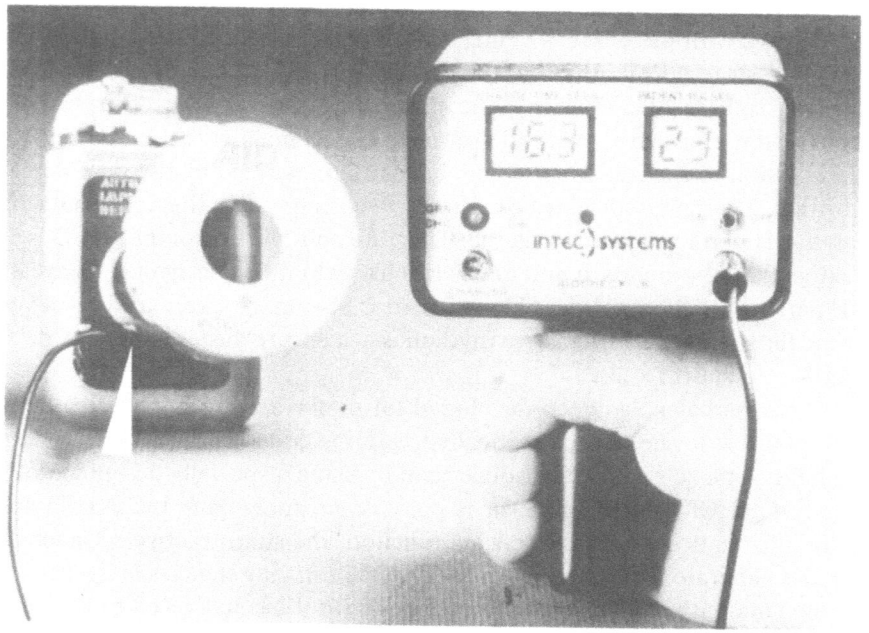

Figure 2. The defibrillator analyzer with a magnet and electromagnetic transducer placed (at arrowhead) over the automatic defibrillator pulse generator. The digital display on the left indicates the capacitor charging times, and that on the right shows the number of discharges delivered by the device to the patient.

significantly limited by non-cardiac disease, if they were on drugs (other than antiarrhythmic) known to influence electrical activity of the heart, or if they exhibited psychological disabilities. However, evidence of advanced left ventricular dysfunction was never a contraindication for the procedure.

As a result of the encouraging clinical results, only a single episode of ventricular fibrillation or hemodynamically unstable ventricular tachycardia occurring outside the context of acute myocardial infarction is now required as a precondition for the AICD implantation. However, there must also be evidence that the patient is incompletely protected by antiarrhythmic drugs, as determined by inducibility during electrophysiologic or stress testing, or the inability to suppress complex ventricular arrhythmias on Holter recordings.

Survivors of recurrent cardiac death form the great majority of the implantees. Thus, the average number of arrhythmic cardiac arrests in 112 patients operated upon at The Johns Hopkins and Sinai Hospitals in Baltimore through September 1984 is 3.5. There were 85 men and 27 women with ages ranging between 16 and 76 years (mean: 53). The average ejection fraction was 32%. Eighty-five patients had coronary artery disease, 23 had nonischemic cardiomyopathy, prolonged QT interval was present in two, and the remaining two patients had primary electrical disease. Prior to implantation, these patients had failed aggressive medical and surgical management and had not responded on average to 4.5 antiarrhythmic drugs; fifteen had been treated with coronary bypass grafting, one patient had undergone a myectomy for relief of hypertrophic sub-aortic stenosis, and ten had been implanted with permanent electronic pacemakers. The clinical profile of patients operated upon at other centers were quite similar to those in the Baltimore series.

Surgical techniques

While the superior vena cava and the right ventricular electrode catheters are introduced into their intended locations with the conventional pervenous techniques, proper placement of the apical patch-electrode requires a surgical approach [10–13]. Originally, a median sternotomy or a left lateral thoracotomy was employed for this purpose. Subsequently, simpler techniques were developed. For example, the subxiphoid approach uses a small incision below the xiphoid process to enter the pericardial space anteriorly, allowing the patch-electrode to be extended laterally over the apex and sutured proximally to the pericardium. More recently, a subcostal approach, combining the advantages of a relatively minor surgical procedure with excellent exposure of the left ventricle, has been suggested as an attractive alternative. Whichever technique is selected, the leads are channeled under the skin and connected to the pulse generator placed in a paraumbilical pocket.

In some centers, a thoracotomy is the preferred surgical approach because it provides the best possible exposure for placement of the patch or, occasionally, of two patches which may be necessary to achieve effective defibrillation. At this institution, the choice of the implantation technique is determined by clinical circumstances; median sternotomy is performed when the implantation procedure is associated with corrective open heart surgery, while subxiphoidal and subcostal approaches are reserved for patients in whom concomitant cardiac surgery is not indicated. Lateral thoracotomy is used to avoid scar tissue in patients who previously underwent cardiac surgery via sternotomy.

Whenever indicated, the AICD can be implanted concurrently with other cardiac and, particularly, with antiarrhythmic surgery. In the above mentioned series of 112 implantees, 26 patients underwent mapping-directed endocardial resection, associated in 17 with an aneurysmectomy and in 13 with coronary artery bypass grafting. Another 13 patients had only coronary artery bypass grafting, and one of these had mitral valve replacement. The primary reason for combining implantation of the device with other cardiac procedures is to provide the implantee with optimal protection against sudden cardiac death. For example, endocardial resection markedly reduces the number of subsequent arrhythmic events but does not eliminate them entirely in all cases, either because of incomplete ablation of the arrhythmogenic foci or because of the progression of the underlying disease process. Approximately 20% of the Hopkins patients who underwent antiarrhythmic surgery had recurrences of malignant arrhythmias; however, the AICD provided them with a unique back-up system to ensure their long-term safety [14].

There is no hard evidence to indicate that coronary artery bypass grafting prevents sudden arrhythmic death. However, improved vascularization of the heart could be expected to decrease or eliminate myocardial ischemia capable of triggering a lethal arrhythmia.

Electrophysiologic testing

Prior to implantation, electrophysiologic testing is performed to determine the patient's inducibility and the characteristics of induced ventricular arrhythmias [7, 15–17]. During implantation, output signals from the transcardiac leads and from the rate channel are recorded and analyzed; at some institutions, lead impedance is routinely calculated. Malignant arrhythmias are then induced with low-level alternating current [18] and the amount of energy required for their termination is measured with an external, non-automatic pulse generator which uses a waveform identical to that of the AICD. The determination of the defibrillation threshold is a safe procedure, extremely helpful for proper selection of the type of leads to be used, their optimal locations, and of the characteristics of the device to be implanted. Following implantation, the patient's malignant arrhythmia is reinduced and the device's automatic functions are tested. No patient is discharged from the hospital with an AICD unless its life-saving capabilities have been demonstrated.

Functional performance

The functional performance of the AICD has been studied extensively, with attention particularly focused on the monitoring capabilities of the system, the reliability of arrhythmia detection, and the effectiveness and ease of arrhythmia termination.

The diagnostic accuracy of the AICD has been found to be excellent. In the controlled conditions of the electrophysiology laboratory, induced ventricular fibrillation and ventricular tachycardia were correctly identified in 99% of the cases. When the proper diagnosis was not made, the cause was easily recognised and corrected. The handful of false-negative diagnoses was usually due to lead malposition, 60-cycle interference, or interaction with an implanted unipolar pacemaker.

Conversion of the malignant arrhythmias to sinus rhythm was usually accom-

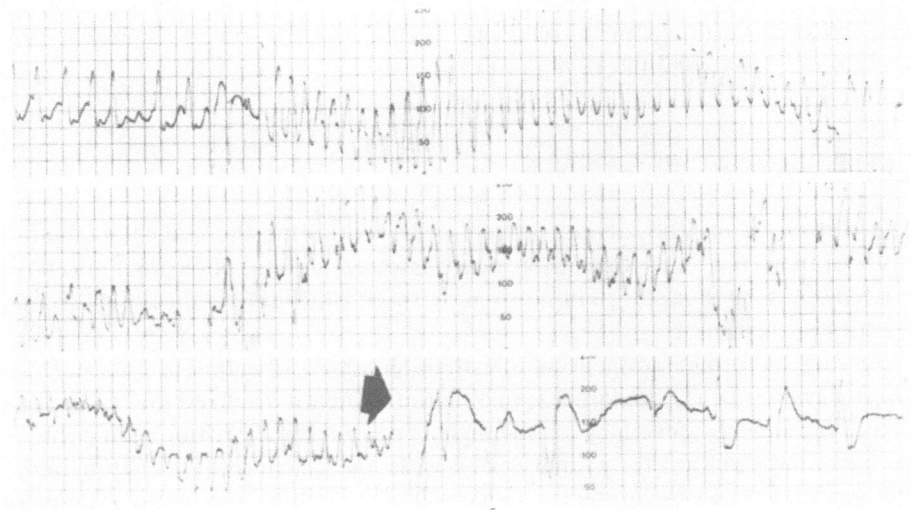

Figure 3. Record of a patient who developed atrial flutter with rapid and irregular ventricular response of 28 minutes' duration during which the implanted automatic defibrillator remained quiescent. The last few beats of this rhythm are seen in the left part of the upper strip. Two spontaneous premature ventricular contractions then induced ventricular flutter-fibrillation, and 23 seconds later (arrow), the malignant arrhythmia was automatically terminated by a single 25-joule discharge. The strips are continuous.

plished with a single 25-J internal discharge; one or more recyclings were necessary for this purpose in only a few patients. The time from the induction of the arrhythmia until its termination ranged between 11 seconds and 36 seconds, averaging 17 seconds. Post-discharge bradycardias were rare. A representative example of automatic conversion of ventricular fibrillation to sinus rhythm is shown in Figure 3.

In approximately 12% of patients, and as a result of high defibrillation threshold, standard 25-J discharges delivered through the superior vena cava patch-lead configuration were unable to restore sinus rhythm. The increase in threshold could not clearly be related to the underlying cardiac disease process, size of the heart, or the extent of the left ventricular dysfunction. However, when high threshold was associated with hypokalemia or amiodarone therapy, an appropriate electrolyte or pharmacologic adjustment could lower the energy requirements. If these simple approaches are unsuccessful, the superior vena cava electrode can be replaced with a second patch-electrode and/or a search for more effective lead positions should be undertaken. In particularly difficult cases, implantation of a high-energy output pulse generator is required.

While most implanted pulse generators achieved their predicted monitoring life in accordance with specifications, accelerated battery depletion occurred in

9% of the devices. This problem was traced to corrosion of the glass insulator in the feedthrough connectors of the battery, and was corrected by application of a protective Teflon coating.

Complications and adverse effects

The complications and adverse effects observed during the clinical evaluation study of the AICD have been thoroughly assessed and can be divided into those related to the methodology employed or to those which reflect the design characteristics of the device.

Among the former, surgical complications command the most attention. In the Hopkins series of 112 implantees, one operative death occurred due to perforation of the subclavian vein by a polyethylene central catheter. Infection occurred in six patients: in four, the primary site was the pulse generator pocket; in one, it was located at the antecubital cut-down; while in another, the origin of infection was unknown. In two cases of infection, complete explantation of the system was required. Post-operative bleeding necessitated transfusions in two patients. Occasional accumulation of sterile fluid in the pulse generator pocket was always uneventfully reabsorbed. Transient pericardial rubs were the rule following implantation. One episode of superior vena cava thrombosis responded well to anticoagulants and no embolic phenomena were noted. Lead dislodgement requiring repositioning occurred in seven patients; recently, improved fixation techniques have reduced the incidence of this complication. No untoward effects related to electrophysiologic testing were observed.

Infrequently, malfunctions of the AICD have been reported, including hermeticity loss, breakdown of the gaseous dielectric, misdirection of the battery testing pulse toward the patient, and random component failure. These complications never resulted in permanent harm.

Particularly significant from a clinical viewpoint are false-positive discharges. In the early stages of the study, spurious signals generated by fractured leads or miscounting of the heart rate caused most of the oversensing. With improvements in lead construction and the introduction of a separate rate channel, spurious discharges due to these causes have been virtually eliminated.

Currently, oversensing may still occur as a response to the interaction of an implanted unipolar pacemaker with the AICD, or in the presence of particularly rapid supraventricular arrhythmias which satisfy the device's sensing algorithm. Pulse delivery during sinus rhythm can also be caused by nonsustained ventricular tachycardias. Although the sensing function in these instances is entirely proper, once the diagnosis is made and the capacitor charging cycle has begun, the device is committed to discharge, even if sinus rhythm has been restored in the interim. The incidence of spurious discharges can be decreased by implementing a number of simple clinical measures. For example, the AICD should have a cut-off rate that is above the patient's fastest sinus rhythm and below the rate of his or her ventricular arrhythmia. Moreover, pharmacologic interventions can be used following implantation to modify the patient's rhythm favorably. In AICD patients who also require implantation of a pacemaker, only a bipolar rather than a unipolar pacemaker should be used. Frequent nonsustained ventricular tachycardias should also be controlled with antiarrhythmic medication. During intraoperative electrocautery and in the immediate post-operative period when supraventricular tachyarrhythmias frequently occur, the device should be temporarily deactivated.

Even when the patient was in a conscious state, the internal electrical discharges were generally well tolerated except when they were experienced too often. Serious emotional problems were reported by Stanford investigators regarding patients who had endured multiple discharges within a very short period of time. Overall, however, the subjective reaction ranged from a lack of any perceptible sensation to a very painful one; most of the implantees described the shock as a moderate blow to the chest and complained only of momentary discomfort. In the event of frequent discharge, it is our policy to temporarily deactivate the unit and stabilize the rhythm in a hospital setting with pharmacologic or other means.

The AICD is also capable of dealing effectively with the phenomenon of acceleration which can occur whenever ventricular tachycardia is treated with electrical discharges, i.e., during external or transvenous cardioversion and antitachycardia pacing. When acceleration occurs, the ventricular tachycardia, rather than being terminated, may become faster and less organized and may even degenerate into ventricular fibrillation. These complications are independent of the energy levels used. The AICD thus controls acceleration automatically through recycling: the device recognizes the accelerated rhythm de novo and corrects it with one or more subsequent discharges.

Clinical results: mortality

The impact of the AICD on the prevention of sudden arrhythmic death has been reported by several investigators [3, 8].

The initial data [3] were derived from the analysis of the first 52 implantees, 42 from Hopkins and 10 from Stanford, the great majority of whom were treated with the original AID device. Kaplan-Meier survival curves in this group indicated a total one-year mortality of 22.9% and an arrhythmic one-year mortality of 8.5%.

With the increase in the number of implantees, it was soon possible to compare the respective effectiveness of the original AID defibrillator with the AICD, the presently used device that treats both ventricular fibrillation and ventricular tachycardia [9]. At one year, the arrhythmic mortality of the 32 patients who received the AID was 10.6%, and in the 67 implantees treated with the AICD it was only 2%; the total-one-year mortality was 26% and 16.6%, respectively. Virtually identical figures were subsequently found in the larger Hopkins series of 112 patients.

Survival analysis was also performed in a series of 70 patients treated mainly with the 'rate only' type of AICD at Stanford University Hospital [8]. In this series, Kaplan-Meier curves revealed arrhythmic one-year mortality of 1.8%. Intec Systems, Inc., the developer of the device, has reported to the U.S. Food and Drug Administration data from a group of 323 implantees (a group which overlaps with the above described Hopkins and Stanford series). These data were also analyzed in accordance with the type of device the patients received: the one-year arrhythmic mortality was 11.9% in 37 AID patients, 1.9% in 209 patients treated with the standard AICD, and 1.3% in 95 patients who received the 'rate only' units.

All of these results are remarkably concordant. While various historical controls indicated that the expected mortality of these high-risk patients ranged between 27% and 66% [19, 20], the AID model that treated only ventricular fibrillation decreased the one-year arrhythmic mortality to approximately 11%. On the other hand, the improved, presently used version of the device – the AICD – reduced this mortality to 2% or less, virtually eradicating sudden arrhythmic death during the year following implantation.

Conclusion

During the past six years, automatic implantable defibrillating systems have been shown to be both safe and effective for prevention of sudden arrhythmic death. The risks and complications associated with the use of the device have been small and acceptable.

References

1. Mirowski M, Reid PR, Mower MM, Watkins L, Gott VL, Schauble JR, Langer A, Heilman MS, Kolenik SA, Fischell RE, Weisfeldt ML. 1980. Termination of malignant ventricular arrhythmias with an implanted automatic defibrillator in human beings. N Engl J Med 303: 322–324.
2. Mirowski M, Reid PR, Watkins L, Weisfeldt ML, Mower MM. 1981. Clinical treatment of life-threatening ventricular tachyarrhythmias with the automatic implantable defibrillator. Amer Heart J 102: 265–270.
3. Mirowski M, Reid PR, Winkle RA, Mower MM, Watkins L, Stinson EB, Griffith LSC, Kallman CH, Weisfeldt ML. 1983. Mortality in patients with implanted automatic defibrillators. Ann Inter Med 98: 585–588.
4. Mirowski M, Reid PR, Mower MM, Watkins Jr L, Platia EV, Griffith LSC, Juanteguy JM. 1984. The automatic implantable cardioverter-defibrillator. PACE 7: 534–540.
5. Reid PR, Mirowski M, Mower MM, Platia EV, Griffith LSC, Watkins Jr L. 1983. Clinical

evaluation of the internal automatic cardioverter-defibrillator in survivors of sudden cardiac death. Amer J Cardiol 51: 1608–1613.

6. Reid PR, Mower MM, Mirowski M. 1984. Pathophysiology of ventricular tachyarrhythmias amenable to electric control. PACE 7: 505–513.

7. Reid PR, Griffith LSC, Mower MM, Platia EV, Watkins Jr L, Juanteguy J, Mirowski M. 1984. Implantable cardioverter-defibrillator: Patient selection and implantation protocol. PACE 7: 1338–1344.

8. Echt DS, Armstrong K, Schmidt P, Oyer PE, Stinson EB, Winkle RA. 1985. Clinical experience, complications, and survival in 70 patients with the automatic implantable cardioverter/defibrillator. Circulation 71 (No. II): 291–296.

9. Reid PR, Mower MM, Griffith LSC, Platia EV, Watkins Jr L, Juanteguy J, Guarnieri T, Mirowski M. 1984. Comparative effects on mortality of the first and second generation implantable defibrillators (abstr). Circulation 70: II–401.

10. Watkins Jr L, Mirowski M, Mower MM, Reid PR, Griffith LSC, Vlay SC, Weisfeldt ML, Gott VL. 1981. Automatic defibrillation in man: The initial surgical experience. J Thorac Cardiovasc Surg 82: 492–500.

11. Watkins Jr L, Mirowski M, Mower MM, Reid PR, Freund P, Thomas A, Weisfeldt ML, Gott VL. 1982. Implantation of the automatic defibrillator: The subxiphoidal approach. Ann Thorac Surg 34: 515–520.

12. Lawrie GM, Griffin JC, Wyndham CRC. 1984. Epicardial implantation of the automatic implantable defibrillator by left subcostal thoracotomy. PACE 7: 1370–1374.

13. Brodman R, Fisher JD, Furman S, Johnston DR, Kim SG, Matos JA, Waspe LE. 1984. Implantation of automatic cardioverter-defibrillators via median sternotomy. PACE 7: 1363–1369.

14. Platia EV, Griffth LSC, Watkins Jr L, Mower MM, Guarnieri T, Mirowski M, Reid PR. 1986. Treatment of malignant ventricular arrhythmias with endocardial resection and implantation of the automatic cardioverter-defibrillator. N Engl J Med 314: 213–216.

15. Winkle RA, Bach SM, Echt DS, Swerdlow CD, Imran M, Mason JW, Oyer PE, Stinson EB. 1983. The automatic implantable defibrillator: Local ventricular bipolar sensing to detect ventricular tachycardia and fibrillation. Am J Cardiol 52: 265–270.

16. Winkle RA, Stinson EB, Bach Jr SM, Echt DS, Oyer PE, Armstrong K. 1984. Measurement of cardioversion/defibrillation thresholds in man by a truncated exponential waveform and an apical patch-superior vena caval spring electrode configuration. Circulation 69: 766–771.

17. Winkle RA, Stinson EB, Echt DS, Mead RH, Schmidt P. 1984. Practical aspects of automatic cardioverter/defibrillator implantation. Am Heart J 108: 1335–1346.

18. Mower M, Reid PR, Watkins Jr L, Mirowski M. 1983. Use of alternating current during diagnostic electrophysiologic studies. Circulation 67: 69–72.

19. Graboys TB, Lown B, Podrid PJ, DeSilva R. 1982. Long-term survival of patients with malignant ventricular arrhythmia treated with antiarrhythmic drugs. Am J Cardiol 50: 437–443.

20. Schulze RA Jr, Strauss HW, Pitt B. 1977. Sudden death in the year following myocardial infarction: Relation to ventricular premature contractions in the late hospital phase and left ventricular ejection fraction. Am J Med 62: 192–199.

29. Catheter endocardial mapping in fulguration

R. FRANK, G. FONTAINE, M. BARAKA, S. KOUNDE, G. FARENQ,
and Y. GROSGOGEAT
*Service de Rythmologie et de Stimulation Cardiaque, Hopital Jean Rostand,
39, rue Le Galleu, 94200 Ivry, France*

Abstract

The aim of catheter endocardial mapping is to approach the earliest endocardial
zon activated. This zone is defined by the earliest endocardial potential that can
be recorded during VT. Indirect methods as potential morphology or pacemapping are the only ones available if VT is not triggerable or absent at the time of
fulguration but have far less specificity.

Keywords

Mapping; ventricular tachycardia; fulguration.

Catheter endocardial mapping was first used to understand the mechanism of
tachycardias, atrial flutter [1] or Wolff-Parkinson-White syndrome [2]. With the
development of surgery for arrhythmias, it has become a pre-operative study to
localize the surgical zone, as in the WPW syndrome, and in ventricular tachycardias. This last application has been particularly developed and studied by Josephson [3]. Endocardial mapping is now of primary importance in the catheter
ablative techniques where it is the only way to direct the therapeutic agents inside
the arrhythmia zone.

The protocol used in catheter endocardial mapping for fulguration in ventricular tachycardias was derived from two previously existing techniques, surgical
treatment of ventricular tachycardias and His bundle fulguration. Since 1973, the
experience of surgical treament of ventricular tachycardias has demonstrated that
a selective destruction of each site of origin, sometimes a very limited incision,

This study was sponsored by Centre de Recherche sur les Maladies Cardiovasculaires de l'Association
Claude Bernard.

could prevent tachycardia recurrence [4]. This site is localized by per-operative mapping as the place where can be recorded the earliest potential in tachycardia, occurring before the onset of the surface QRS [5]. In 1982 the His bundle fulguration procedure proved that once a site is localized by its activation potential, an electric shock on that site will destroy the tissues from which that potential originates [6] and therefore prevent local conduction. It was then assumed that localizing the site of origin of VT as the earliest endocardial potential that could be recorded, allowed an electric shock to be delivered in this zone capable of preventing the reinitiation of VT [7]. The aim of the catheter endocardial mapping in fulguration is not to really map the whole right and left endocardium as in surgical mapping, but to approach the earliest endocardial zone activated in tachycardia.

Method

Bipolar or multipolar catheters with 1 cm interelectrode distance are inserted transcutaneously in the subclavian and the femoral vein, and placed in different part of the right atrium, coronary sinus, right ventricular apex, His bundle site and right ventricular outflow tract. These catheters serve as reference or as pacing electrodes. The other catheters already selected to withstand the fulguration shock [8] are moved into different parts of the ventricles to record bipolar endocardial potentials. A long sheath* is inserted via the femoral artery, inside the left ventricle, to allow easier catheter positioning (Fig. 1). Filters are set between 10 and 300 Hertz. Signals are amplified between 1000 and 10.000 times. One millivolt calibration mark and time marks are automatically generated on the tracing. All the data are recorded on an analogic tape**. The position of the catheters is monitored on a bidirectional fluoroscopy and stored on a video tape. Haemodynamic monitoring is made using radial arterial pressure, pulmonary wedge pressure through a Swan-Ganz catheter, and serial cardiac output by thermo-dilution.

To minimize the time in which the patient remains in ventricular tachycardia and the risk of haemodynamic compromise, the study starts by pacemapping. This is done by pacing the ventricle at the tachycardia rate, at different endocardial sites. 12 lead ECG recordings are made, and compared with the spontaneous VT morphology. When a good matching is obtained, VT is triggered by programmed pacing, and the endocardial potentials are analysed. Time measurements are made on the rapid portion of the signal, corresponding to the moment when the activation wave passes under the recording electrode, as suggested by previous simulation studies [6] (Fig. 2). The catheter is slightly moved in the same

---

* (Cordis femoral ventricular catheter/sheath set).
** (EMI tape recorder).

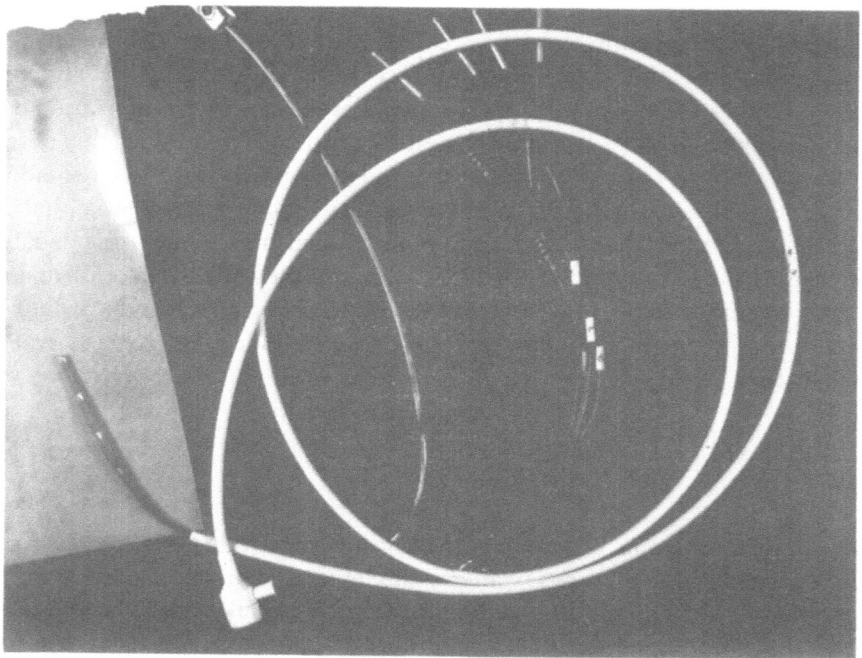

Figure 1. Left ventricular endocardial catheter inserted in its sheath.

region, and when the earliest occurring potential has been determined, fulguration is sent to that site. After 10 minutes programmed pacing may reinititate the VT and if this is the case, the mapping procedure is started again.

Mapping may take any time between 30 minutes and several hours according to the ease with which the leads can be manipulated. VT has to be haemodynamically tolerated during long periods of time, and for this purpose, the patients are left under chronic amiodarone therapy (400 mg a day) to have a slower tachycardia. All Class I antiarrhythmic drugs which have a more depressive inotropic effect have been stopped for five half-lives. Hemodynamic monitoring is continuous through the whole procedure and VT is interrupted in case of deterioration of heart function.

Direct mapping

Interpretation of the tracings has to be careful and pitfalls are multiple and not always easily dealt with.

Potential morphology in tachycardia may be misleading: an onset with low amplitude, followed by a high amplitude potential (Fig. 3) has to be interpreted as the recording of two activation fronts. The fast potential is occurring just under

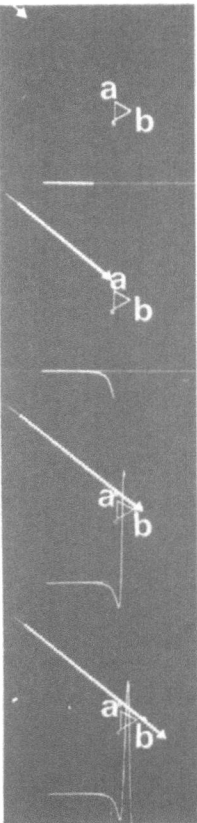

Figure 2. Computerised simulation of the deflection generated by a dipole parallel to two recording electrodes 'a' and 'b'. The interelectrode distance is of the same size as the dipole. The first sharp deflection occurs when the dipole passes on the first lectrode 'a' and the return to the baseline when it passes on the second electrode 'b'. This situation mimics recording obtained with 1 mm spaced electrodes, as in surgical mapping.

the electrode, while the low amplitude potential, although more premature tan the other, should be interpreted as the reflect of an earlier, but more distant activation (Fig. 4), and the catheter position has to be slightly changed. However, a pathologic tissue with slow conduction may generate the same low amplitude potential just under the electrode.

Recording of mid diastolic potentials or of continuous activity may be related to the reentry circuit involved in the tachycardia (Fig. 5). However, it may also be a delayed activation in another pathological zone, not related with the arrhythmia [10, 11]. A constant relationship must be found between spontaneous or induced change in the tachycardia cycle and morphology, and modifications in that continuous activity. We may then assume its direct relation with the reentry circuit which originates the VT (Fig. 6).

394

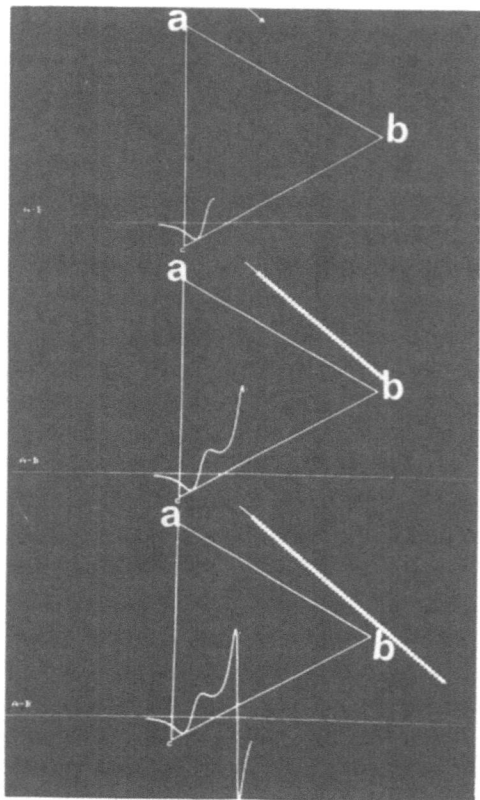

Figure 3. Computerised simulation of the deflection generated by a dipole ten times smaller than the interelectrode distance (ab). The dipole direction makes a small angle with the ab direction. The generated wave is of much larger duration. The first generated deflection is of low amplitude because of the distance between the recording electrode 'a' and the dipole. The second deflection is sharp because the dipole passes near the electrode 'b'. This situation mimics recordings obtained with 10 mm spaced electrodes, as in catheter mapping.

We have compared the timing of the earliest endocardial potential in tachycardia with the result of fulguration in 15 VT which relapsed after the session, and in 15 other VT where the arrhythmia was abolished (Fig. 7). Fulguration on a potential occurring during the QRS complex was never successful but could also be unsuccessful on premature potentials as early as −60 ms. By contrast, effective shocks have always been delivered on presystolic potentials, with a great variety of prematurities, between −10 to −80 ms. These results demonstrate that endocardial mapping allows the effective site for fulguration to be found within the earliest endocardial potential occurring before the onset of the surface QRS, but the timing of this potential by itself has a poor specificity.

The lack of multiple simultaneous recording is an important handicap in the

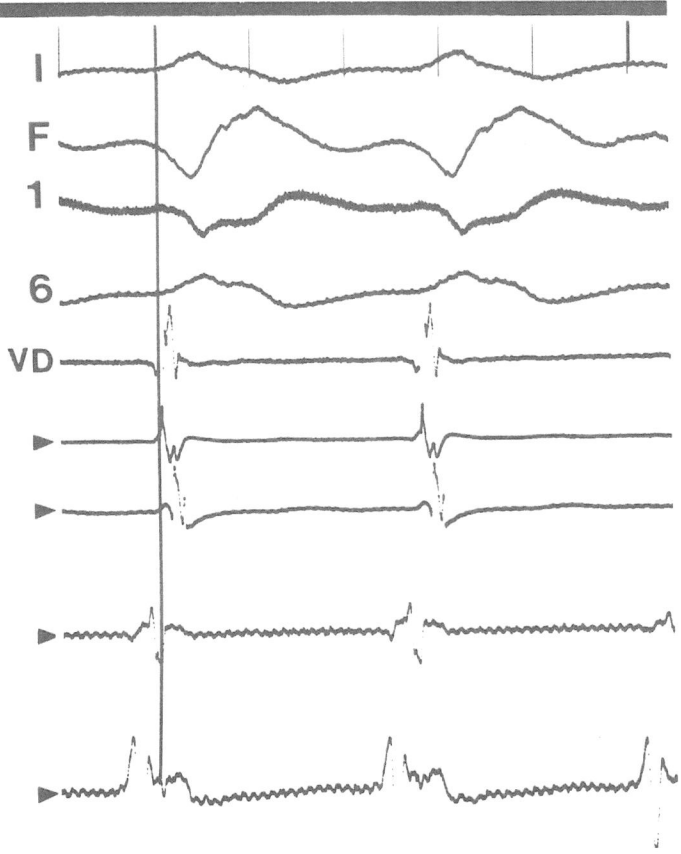

Figure 4. Recording of 5 different right ventricular sites (VD) in ventricular tachycardia. Recording 4 shows an initial premature potential of low amplitude occurring 50 ms before the onset of the QRS surface followed by a greater potential. However, moving slightly the catheter allows to find a potential of much higher amplitude with the same prematurity. The low potential was only the remote recording of the high potential. Note the similarity between recording 4 and Fig. 3.

interpretation of the data, as with the actual technique the number of catheters is necessarily limited inside the ventricles. As manipulation of the intracardiac leads is not easy, it is on some occasions nearly impossible to aim for a specific site, and to get a stable position. For this reason, interpretation of the potential prematurity must be very cautious. A more premature potential one cm apart from the recorded earliest potential may exist, but a catheter just won't go there. The search for an earlier potential has also to take into account the fact that the distance between the origin of the tachycardia and the actual catheter location may vary for the same prematurity according to the conduction disturbances between two sites. Therefore, a great timing difference may be found in adjacent

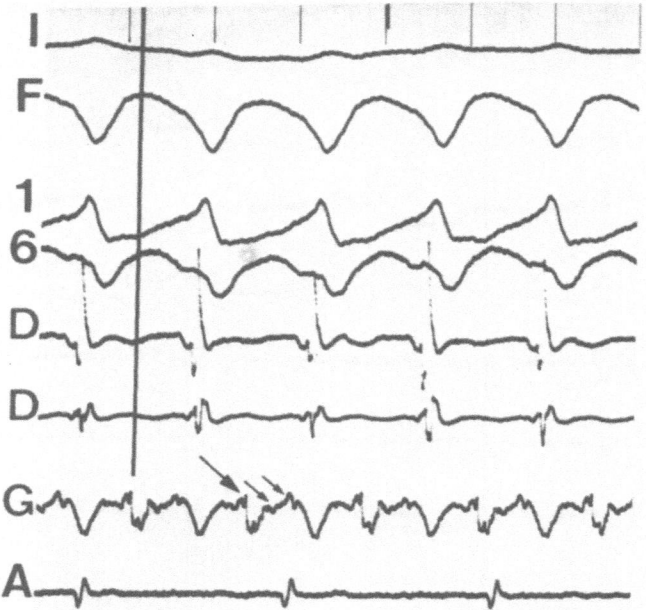

Figure 5. Surface electrocardiogram and endocardial mapping of a patient in ventricular tachycardia. D represents two different right ventricular sites and G a left ventricular site near a ventricular anevrysm. On that side, diastolic and fractionated potentials were recorded. However, the pacemapping in that site did not reproduce the tachycardia morphology.

sites in a slow conduction zone, when similar timings may occur in widely separated zones when recorded in normal conducting areas (Fig. 8).

Indirect methods

We call indirect methods approaches to the origin of VT not using local potential times. They involve potential morphology and pacemapping in sinus rhythm and in VT. Indirect methods in sinus rhythm are the only ones available when the tachycardia is not triggerable or when the triggered tachycardia is haemodynamically ill-tolerated.

Morphology

Potential morphology, duration and amplitude do not allow the site of origin of ventricular tachycardia to be recognised [11]. In our present series, we recorded in 8 out of 10 cases of right ventricular dysplasia an earliest potential which was wide,

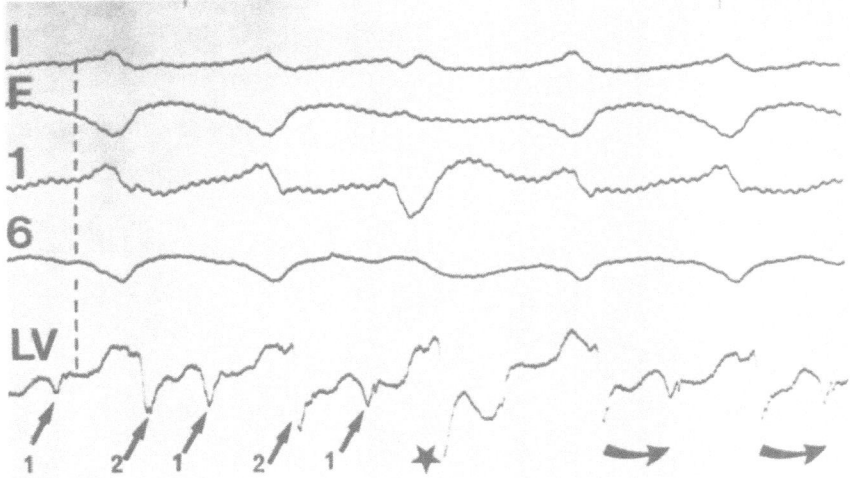

Figure 6. Same patient as in Fig. 5. In another site the surface QRS is correlated with a double endocardial activation. Potential is occurring before the onset of the QRS, potential 2 after its end. A spontaneous ventricular extrasystole occurs (marked by a star) and the tachycardia resumes with the potential no 2 followed by potential no 1. It may be deduced that potential no 1 was not an early potential for the next cycle, but was a late potential from the previous cycle.

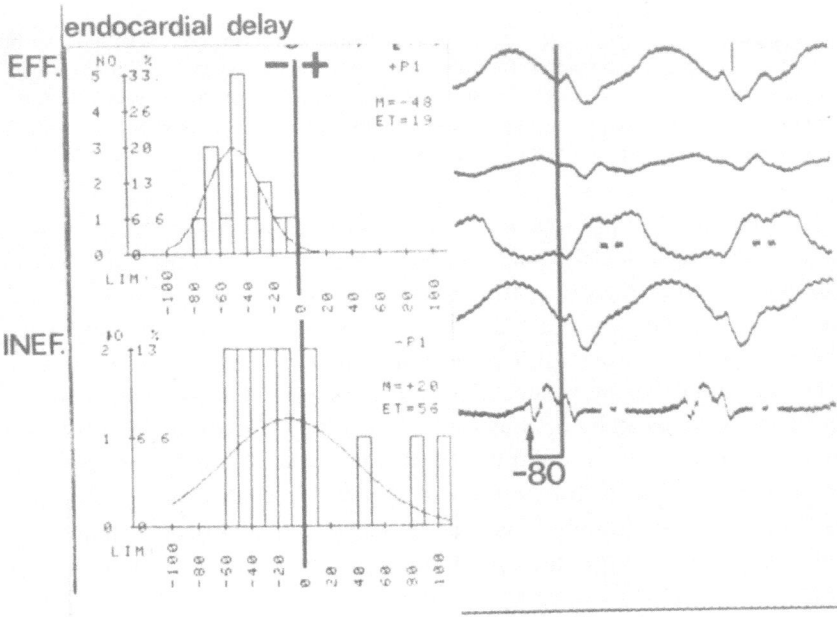

Figure 7. Histogram of the prematurity of the potential in the fulgurated zone, in 15 patients (upper panel) in whom the fulguration modified the ventricular tachycardia, and in 15 patients, (lower panel) the fulguration did not modify the ventricular tachycardia (see text). On the right panel, a low amplitude premature potential (80 ms) with 1 mV calibration marks.

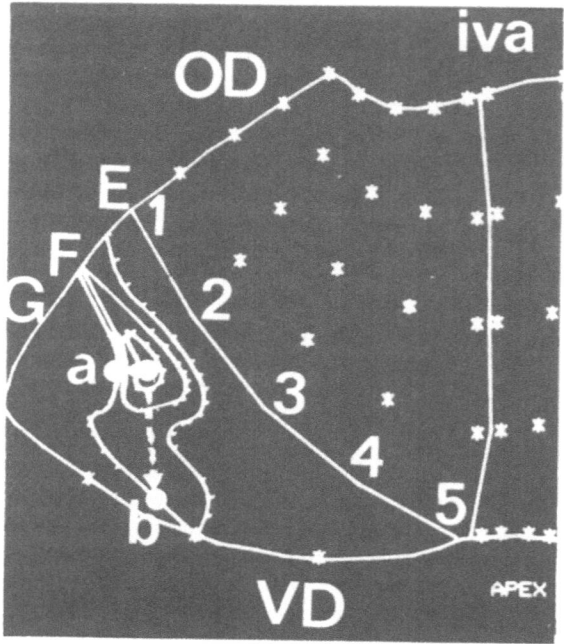

Figure 8. Epicardial mapping of the origin of ventricular tachycardia in a patient with right ventricular dysplasia. Isochrones are separated by 5 ms. The conduction velocity between the origin of the tachycardia and point 'a' is very slow, compared to the conduction velocity between the same origin and point 'b'. It is why despite having the same timing, point 'a' is very near to the origin of the tachycardia and point 'b' is at a much larger distance.

above 80 ms duration, of low amplitude, and associated with delayed activation that is occurring after the end of the surface QRS complex. In 10 cases of ventricular tachycardia originating from an old myocardial infarction, 7 earliest potentials were wide, and 4 followed by a delayed activity. But these findings have no specificity as such potentials could also be recorded in other sites with later occurrence. In fact, such delayed activation is only a marker for slow conduction, which can be demonstrated by the delay between the pacing artefact in that zone and the ventricular response (Fig. 9 and 10). Slow conduction is only one of the prerequisite for reentry and therefore cannot be used by itself s a marker for the site of origin of ventricuar tachycardia. However, that element in combination with the potential prematurity may indicate that the recorded zone is near the slow part of the reentry circuit.

Pacemapping

This is another indirect approach to the origin of VT [12], which is the only

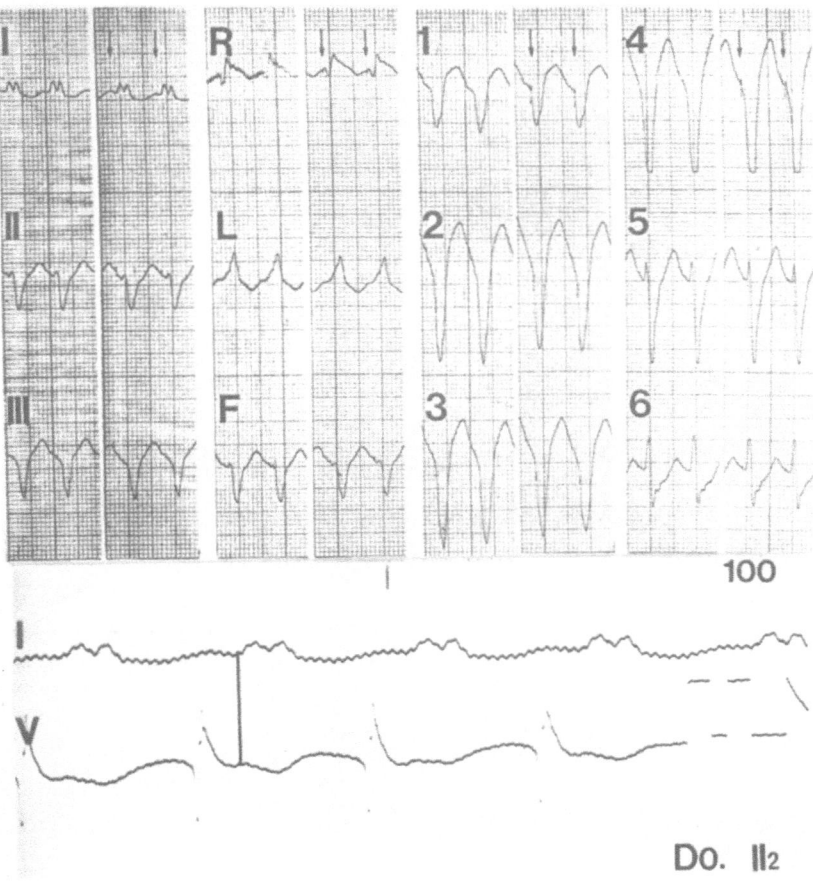

Figure 9. Pacemapping in ventricular tachycardia. Each ECG derivation is represented twice. On the left side the spontaneous ventricular tachycardia and on the right side, the paced beat which is identical to the spontaneous tachycardia. On the lower panel, potential prematurity recorded at the pacing site during tachycardia is 100 ms. Note that the distance between the pacing artefact and the onset of the QRS is short, around 20 ms.

method if VT is not triggerable or cannot be maintained. Its aim is to reproduce the exact configuration of VT on a 12 lead ECG (Fig. 9 and 10). We reviewed the results of pacemapping in our last 24 patients who underwent the fulguration procedure from a series of 38. 34 VT morphologies could be mapped and pacemapped. We could not find statistical significance correlating the accuracy of pacmapping in that subgroup of patients with the results of fulguration. However, a bad pacemapping was never correlated with a modification of VT, and two patients with idiopathic VT which could not be triggered had a successful treatment using the pacemapping data only. But in fact, different adjacent zones with

400

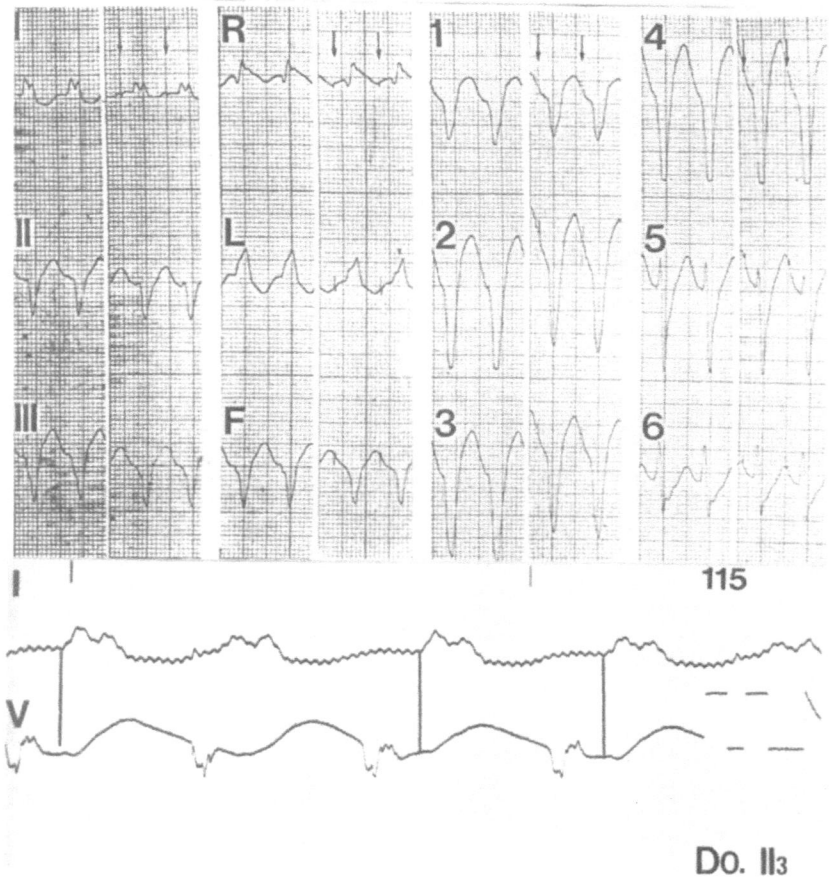

Figure 10. Pacemapping in a slightly modified ventricular tachycardia from the same patient. In that zone the earliest potential occurs 115 ms before the onset of the surface QRS. Note that the QRS configuration induced by pacemapping is not strictly identical in lead I to the spontaneous tachycardia. However, the pacing is done in a very slow conduction zone, the delay between the pacing artefact and the ventricular response is around 100 ms, nearly the same value as the delay between the potential and the onset of the surface QRS.

different potential prematurity in VT could give the same good matching between pacemapping and VT morphology. These data correlate with Josephson's studies [13] showing that pacing at the site of origin of ventricular tachycardia produces an electrocardogram and activation sequence similar to those produced by ventricular tachycardia but that pacing in close proximity to that site could produce either a similar or a grossly different electrocardiographic pattern from that during ventricular tachycardia. The pacemapping is then only used to approach the tachycardia zone, but should not be the only method.

Conclusion

Analysis of data is made difficult because of the lack of a standard for endocardial mapping. That standard could be the earliest recordable endocardial potential, associated with an exact pacemapping, but also the effectiveness of fulguration. In fact the criteria for the best side for an effective fulguration are still under investigation, and the accuracy of endocardial mapping seems to be only a part o the problem. By contrast with surgery where the surgeon can remove a large area of tissue, regardless of the accuracy of direct mapping, fulguration seems to have a very limited range of action, and this may explain why multiple shocks may be necessary to block all the exits of what may be the reentry pathway, from which VT originates.

This is why our current protocol remains to approach the zone by pacemapping, trigger the arrhythmia and look for the earliest potential that can be recorded. We then verify if pacemapping is still accurate, before we decide to send the fulguration shock.

References

1. Puech P, Latour H, Grolleau R. 1970. Le flutter et ses limites. Arch Mal Coeur 61: 116.
2. Wallace AG, Boineau JP, Davidson RM, Sealy WC. 1971. Wolff-Parkinson-White Syndrome. A New Look. Am J Cardiol 28: 509.
3. Josephson ME, Horowitz LN, Farshidi A, Spear JF, Kastor JA, Moore EN. 1978. Recurrent Sustained Ventricular Tachycardia. II-Endocardial Mapping. Circulation 57: 440.
4. Guiraudon G, Fontaine G, Frank R, Leandri R, Barra J, Cabrol C. 1981. Surgical Treatment of Ventricular Tachycardia Guided by Ventricular Mapping in 23 Patients without Coronary Artery Disease. Ann Thorac Surg 32: 439.
5. Josephson ME, Horowitz LN, Spielman SR, Greenspan AM, Vandepol CJ, Harken AH. 1980. Comparison of Endocardial Catheter Mapping with Intraoperative Mapping of Ventricular Tachycardia. Circulation 61: 395.
6. Scheinman MM, Evans-Bell T. 1984. Catheter Ablation of the Atrioventricular Junction: a Report of the Percutaneous Mapping and Ablation Registry. Circulation 70: 1024–1029.
7. Hartzler GO. 1983. Electrode Catheter Ablation of Focal Ventriular Tachycardia. J Am Coll Cardiol 1: 595.
8. Fontaine G, Cansell A, Lechat Ph, Frank R, Tonet JL, Grosgogeat Y. 1984. Les chocs electriques endocavitaires. Problemes lies au materiel. Arch Mal Coeur 77: 1307–1314.
9. Fontaine G, Pierfitte M, Tonet JL, Fillette F, Frank R, Grosgogeat Y. 1981. Interpretation of Afterpotentials Registered from Epicardium, Endocardium and Body Surface in Patients with Chronic Ventricular Tachycardia. In: Signal Averaging Technique in Clinical Cardiology. Hombach V, Hilger HH (ed). F.K. Schattauer Pub. Stuttgart: p 177.
10. Brugada P, Abdollah H, Wellens HJJ. 1985. Continuous Electrical Activity during Sustained Monomorphic Ventricular Tachycardia: Observations on its Dynamic Behavior during the Arrhythmia. Am J Cardiol 55: 402–412.
11. Josephson ME, Horowitz LN, Spielman SR, Waxman HL, Greenspan AM. 1982. Role of Catheter Mapping in the Preoperative Evaluation of Ventricular Tachycardia. Am J Cardiol 49: 207.

12. Curry PVL, O'Keefe DB, Pitcher D, Sowton E, Deverall PB, Yates AK. 1979. Localisation of Ventricular Tachycardia by a New Technique: Pace Mapping (Abstract). Circulation 60, Supp II: 11–25.

13. Josephson ME, Waxman HL, Cain ME, Gardner MJ, Buxton AE. 1982. Ventricular Activation during Ventricular Endocardial Pacing. II Role of Pacemapping to Localize Origin of Ventricular Tachycardia. Am J Cardiol 50: 11.

30. Catheter ablation of ventricular tachycardia foci

JESSE C. DAVIS, MELVIN M. SCHEINMAN, MICHAEL W. DAE,
JOSEPH A. ABBOTT, and ELIAS H. BOTVINICK

The use of endocardial catheters to localize the site of origin of ventricular tachycardia has assumed increasing clinical relevance. Map directed endocardial resection [1, 2], has been shown to produce more effective long-term response compared with blind aneurysm resection in patients with ventricular tachycardia [3, 4]. Newer techniques have allowed the use of electrode catheters for both tachycardia localization and ablation.

Delivery of high-energy direct-current shocks through electrode catheters for treatment of patients with cardiac arrhythmias was first introduced in 1981 [5]. Since that time, this experimental technique has become established as a therapeutic tool for selected patients.

In this chapter, we will present an overview of the technical considerations for performing the endocardial mapping procedure, review the catheter ablaive technique along with the biophysical effects of direct-current shocks, and summarise the present clinical indications for this therapy.

Endocardial mapping

Endocardial mapping is performed in the catheterization laboratory in the course of electrophysiologic studies. One electrode catheter is inserted into the left ventricle and two or more multipolar electrode catheters into the right ventricle. Tachycardia is induced using standard stimulation techniques. If the patient remains hemodynamically stable the catheters are manipulated to explore as many endocardial sites as possible.

The recordings may be obtained in either unipolar or bipolar configuration. A unipolar recording uses the distal electrode of the catheter coupled to remote ground. A bipolar recording uses two closely coupled electrodes and represents the potentia differences between the electrodes. The bipolar signal is preferable for localization because the signal is sharper, more discrete, and less contaminated by far field noise.

The recording is filtered (usually 30–500 Hz) and a calibration signal is inscribed. During tachycardia, the earliest very rapid deflection, or the point where the earliest rapid deflection crosses baseline, preceeding the surface electrocardiogram, is noted. At least three orthogonal surface leads must be used as reference sources. The amplitude and duration of the electrograms, as well as the presence of fragmented potentials, are also noted. A normal endocardial signal is 3 mV or greater in amplitude and less than 60 msec in duration [6]. A fragmented electrogram that appears to be critically dependent on tachycardia initiation is at present the best proof that the subjacent area is involved in the tachycardia circuit. In addition, finding diastolic potentials that bridge ventricular diastole constituts strong support for both a reentrant mechanism as well as localization of the source of tachycardia.

Catheter mapping has allowed fairly accurate localization of ventricular tachycardia foci, usually with 4 cm [2, 7]. In our laboratory, two additional techniques are used to confirm tachycardia localization. One technique is 'pace-mapping' [8] which involves pacing the ventricle in the area thought to be the origin of tachycardia. The QRS contour during ventricular pacing should be identical to that of the spontaneous tachycardia. The second technique is radionuclide phase imaging [9] to confirm the general area of tachycardia origin. Phase maps are computer generated from the gated blood pool scintigram whch is acquired during ventricular tachycardia, in multiple projections, if the patient is hemodynamically stable. For the analysis, time versus radioactivity curves for each pixel in the ventricular blood pool image are fit with a cosine function. The location of the peak of the resulting fitted curve is related to a time reference (ECG R wave), and is the called phase angle. The phase angle relates to the point in the cardiac cycle where the sampling region (pixel) looses counts, or conceptually is a measure of the time of onset of contraction. Because of excitation contraction coupling, the earliest area of activation (i.e. the ventricular tachycardia focus) is assumed to be the earliest area of contraction. In general, this relationship holds true in normal ventricles, and ventricles with compromised function as well. Usually a minimum of 1 to 1.5 million counts requiring approximately 1 to minutes of data acquisition, are necessary for a statistically valid map, however, we have generated good phase maps with 50 seconds of acquisition.

Thus far we have studied 25 patients during ventricular tachycardia by phase analysis. Each had electrophysiologic study demonstrating 28 foci, 18 of which were completely mapped. The phase image during ventricular tachycardia localized 6 right ventricular, 10 septal and 12 left ventricular foci which corresponded to the same or adjacent electrophysiologic site in 14, and matched ECG findings in 10 others, including 2 patients with multiple foci. Phase imaging was a useful adjunct to catheter mapping.

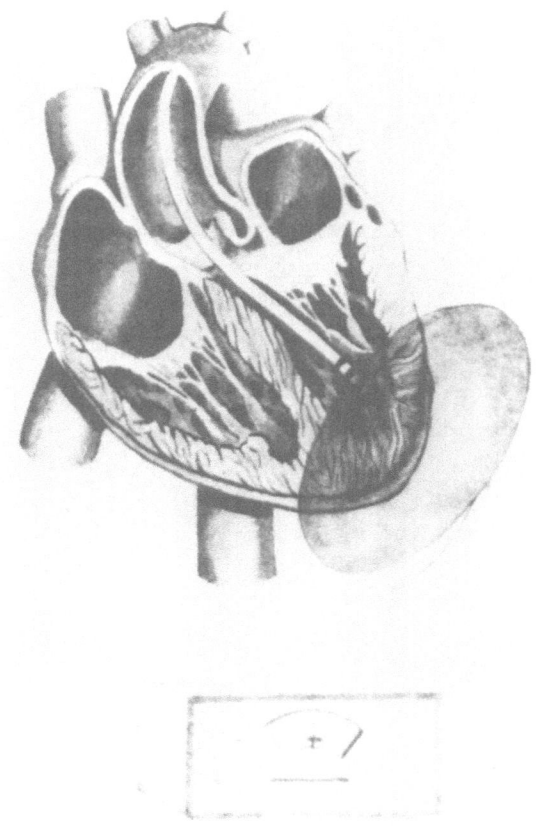

Figure 1. Catheter ablation of a left ventricular tachycardia focus. Direct-current shocks are delivered from the distal electrode to a patch on the chest wall using a standard defibrillator.

Catheter ablative technique

After tachycardia is induced, the ventricles are mapped and the earliest endocardial potentials referable to multiple surface leads are obtained. The catheter is then manipulated against the endocardium showing earliest activation, and a patch lubricated with conducting gel is placed on the chest wall in closest approximation to the electrode catheter (Fig. 1). A series of direct-current shocks are delivered from the distal electrode on the catheter (current source) to the chest patch (current sink). For septal foci, a catheter to catheter arrangement is used (Fig. 2). The patient must be anaesthetized with a shortacting agent since the shocks are quite painful.

After stablization, the patient is retested with the same stimulation protocol found to induce ventricular tachycardia in he control state. We avoid very aggressive stimulation protocols in the immediate postshock period as we have

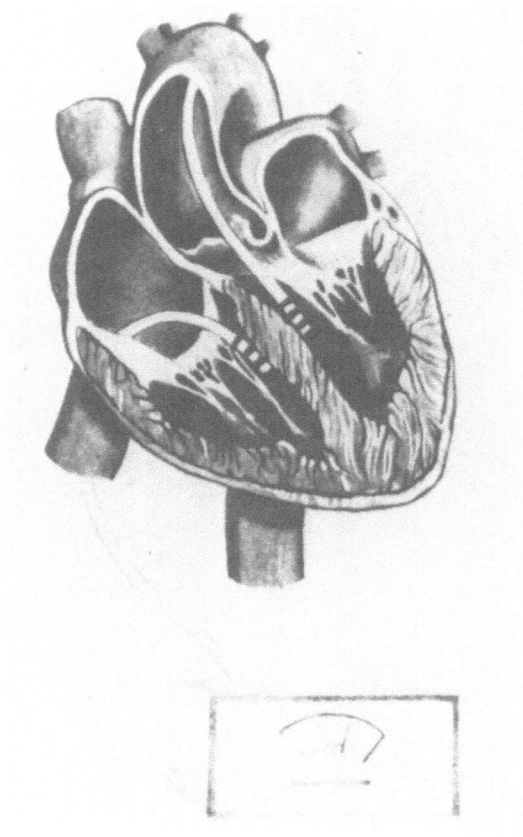

Figure 2. Catheter ablation of a septal ventricular tachycardia focus. Shocks are delivered between the distal poles of the right and left catheters across the septum.

found that they may induce rapid nonclinical arrhythmias. We prefer to use the more aggressive stimulation protocols several days after attempted catheter ablation. If the clinical ventricular tachycardia is inducible, then serial drug testing is used to find an effective regimen. Patients who have failed a clinical drug trial may become drug responsive after catheter ablation.

Biophysical effects of catheter electroshocks

The delivery of 200 to 400 J of stored energy through the electrode catheter results in 2000 to 3000 V potentials at the electrode surface. If the discharge is delivered into a saline solution, an explosive flash develops [10]. This electrical energy is at least partially converted to heat. In addition, the explosion produces concussion waves exceeding 1 to 2 atmospheres of pressure [10]. Finally, the intense electrical charge may disrupt cellular integrity [11]. Thus, local injury after delivered shocks may result from thermal electrocoagulation of tissue [5], strong concussive shock waves [10], or membrane damage due to the intense electrical field [11]. One other factor should be emphasised. The structural integrity of the electrode catheter materials to withstand shocks of this magnitude must be assured [12]. Most conventional direct-current defibrillators deliver capacitor discharge over 5 to 10 msec, with peak voltage achieved within 1 to 2 msec. Delivery of 1000 to 3000 V to one electrode of a multipolar electrode catheter may result in insulation breakdown with shunting of current to other electrodes and hence less delivered energy to the tissues. These factors will obviously influence the safety and efficacy of this approach.

The histologic effects of catheter-delivered shocks have been described [13, 14], and we have previously described the evolutionary histology after catheter-delivered shock in the normal canine heart. Anodal and cathodal discharge produce qualitatively similar spherical lesions that are 1 to 2 cm in diameter when total defibrillator energy is limited to 5 J/kg body weight or less. Histologic change is present within 20 min after the shock. The central foci show cellular deformation to heterogeneous globules with loss of cellular detail and pynknotic nuclei. The early lesions have interstitial red blood cells and edema but no inflammatory cell infiltration. Electron micrographs obtained 1 hr after shock show disrupted sarcomeres and numerous mitochondria containing electron-dense clumps within their intercristal spaces. After 1 to 2 days, the injured regions are invaded by acute inflammatory cells and after 5 to 7 days, there is replacement of necrotic myocytes by an intense organizing reaction involving fibrocytic spindle cells, multinucleated histocytes, and round cells. Lesions in atrial and ventricular myocardium are histologically identical.

Proarrhythmic effects of catheter discharge have been described at the time of shock [14] and 12 to 48 hr later [13]. In canines, tachyarrhythmias or bradyarrhythmias may occur immediately after shock. Jones et al. [11] found a characteristic response to increasingly intense stimulation of cultured myocardial pacemaker cells. Threshold stimuli caused a single activation but stimulus intensities 24 times threshold values caused transient tachyarrhythmias. With stimuli 42 times threshold, there was arrest of rhythmic activity due to membrane depolarization to zero ('dielectric breakdown') and delayed repolarization. 'Cellular fibrillation' or asynchronous contraction of sarcomeres followed application of stimuli 80 times the threshold value. Lerman et al. [13] reported spontaneos ventricular tachycardia 24 hr after catheter ablation of canine ventricular endocardium. These tachyarrhythmias were not lethal when delivered energy was 50 J or less. Programmed stimulation does not induce ventricular tachyarrhythmias 3 or more days after endocardial shock [13].

Clinical experience

Hartzler [16] was the first to report attempted catheter ablation of ventricular tachycardia foci. Although a number of subsequent reports have been published, the experience to date is still quite limited. The largest experience has been reported by Fontaine et al. [17] and their initial results have been excellent. Our own experience has been somewhat less favourable. Sixteen patients have undergone ablation for ventricular tachycardia. Of the 16 patients, 12 had left ventricular catheter ablation, and 4 had right ventricular catheter ablation. The cumulative energies used to ablate left ventricular tachycardias averaged $517 + 219$ joules. The range was from 400 to 900 joules, with median, 400 joules. Left ventricular catheter to patch was attempted on 10 occasions and catheter to catheter on six. The right ventricular ablation energies averaged cumulative doses of $575 + 303$ joules with a range of 400 to 1100 joules and a median doses of 400 joules. With right ventricular ablation, catheter to patch was used in all four patients. Ablation results in the 16 patients were excellent in three who remain ventricular tachycardia free without any antiarrhythmic drug therapy. Two of these patients had left ventricular ablations (one, interventricular septal) and the other a right ventricular ablation. In six, good results were obtained from the catheter ablation. These patients responded to a combination of ablation and an antiarrhythmic drug to remain ventricular tachycardia free. Their antiarrhythmic medications include a type I antiarrhythmic, beta-blockers, amiodarone, and/or mexiletine. Three patients in this group ultimately have died of causes unrelated to their ventricular tachycardia ablation. Seven patients failed a combination of catheter ablation and antiarrhythmic drug therapy. Six of these seven patients expired of their clinical ventricular tachycardia after their hospital discharge. One patient continues to maintain a controlled slow rate ventricular tachycardia while receiving an antiarrhythmic regimen, and is ambulatory and asymptomatic. There were no ablation related deaths. Complications resulting from the ablation procedure were due to the associated left heart catheterizations: arterial thrombosis was present in two patients, one of whom required a Forgarty catheter removal of a brachial artery thrombosis. No echocardiographic evidence of early or late ablation induced ventricular thrombi was found. Serious side effects reported to the registry include malignant ventricular arrhythmias withn 1 week after ablation, low-output syndrome resulting in death, and one report of electromechanical dissociation and death after attempted ablation. Catheter ablation for patients wth ventricular tachycardia foci must still be considered highly experimental. Suitable candidates might be those with frequent or incessant monomorphic ventricular tachycardia who are considered high-risk surgical candidates.

Future perspectives

The ideal catheter ablative technique involves ability to quickly and precisely locate the target area. The damage should be localized to the area with minimal destruction of surrounding normal myocardium, cardiac valves, or coronary vessels. Presently available techniques fall far short of the ideal in many respects. For atrioventricular junctional ablation, while current techniques appear adequate for precise localization of the atrioventricular junctional ablation, the damage induced by direct-current shocks results in damage to surrounding myocardium as well as to the support structures of the tricuspid and aortic valves. The long-term significance of these lesions is yet to be defined. Clearly many improvements are required before catheter ablation of ventricular tachycarda foci becomes clinically acceptable. Firstly, a better understanding of the ventricular tachycardia pathways is required. Current ablative techniques essentially produce a subendocardial lesion. While earliest activation over the subendocardium appears to be the rule in man, detailed animal studies have shown that ventricular tachycardia reentrant pathways are commonly localized to epicardial or intramural sites. Second, current techniques of endocardial mapping are laborious and lack the precisionrequired for localization of ventricular tachycardia foci. Future advances in catheter ablative techniques will depend on a fruitful exchange between physicians and industry engineers and scientists. Physicians are in critical need of readily maneuverable multielectrode catheters designed to allow for rapid simultaneous endocardial mapping of numerous ventricular sites. In addition, catheters and energy delivery systems are required that will deliver quantifiable energy via catheters specifically designed for this purpose and suitable for local cardiac ablation without adverse remote effects.

In summary, the use of catheter ablative procedures for destruction of ventricular tachycardia foci is still considered highly experimental and the role of these procedures remains undefined. These procedures should be performed by physicians who are experienced both in the technical requirements and more importantly, in evaluating the risks and benefits of all available therapeutic options.

References

1. Josephson ME, Harken AH, Horowitz LN. 1979. Endocardial excision – A new surgical technique for the treatment of recurrent ventricular tachycardia. Circulation 60: 1430.
2. Horowitz LN, Josephson ME, Harken AH. 1980. Ventricular resection guided by epicardial and endocardial mapping for treatment of recurrent ventricular tachycardia. N Engl J Med 302: 589.
3. Harken AH, Horowitz LN, Josephson ME. 1980. Comparison of standard aneurysmectomy with directed endocardial resection for the treatment of recurrent sustained ventricular tachycardia. J Thorac Cardiovasc Surg 80: 527.
4. Waldo AL, Arciniegas JG, Klein H. 1981. The role of intraoperative mapping and consideration of the presently available surgical techniques. Prog Cardio Vasc Dis 23: 247.

5. Scheinman MM, Morady F, Hess DS, Gonzalez R. 1982. Catheter induced ablation of the atrioventricular function to control refractory supraventricular arrhythmia. JAMA 248: 851.

6. Josephson ME, Horowitz LN, Spielman SR, Waxman HL, Greenspan AM. 1982. Role of catheter mapping in the preoperative evaluation of ventricular tachycardia. Am J Cardiol 49: 207.

7. Josephson ME 1984. Catheter ablation of arrhythmias. Annals of Int Med 10: 234.

8. Curry PVL, O'Keeffe DB, Pritcher D et al. 1979. Localization of ventricular tachycardia by new technique-pace mapping. Circulation 60 (Suppl II): II-25.

9. Botvinick E, Schechtman N, Dae M. 1986. Scintigraphy provides a thorough evaluation of 'electrical' and mechanical events druring ventricular tachycardia. J Am Coll Cardiol 7 (2): 235A.

10. Boyd EGCA, Hoh PM. 1985. An investigation into the electrical ablation technique and a method of electrode assessment. PACE 8: 815.

11. Jones JL, Proskaver CC, Paul WK, Lepeschkin E, Jones RE. 1980. Ultrastructural injury to chick myocardial cells in vitro following 'electric countershock'. Circ Res 46: 387.

12. Fisher JD, Brodmn R, Johnston DR, Waspe LE, Kim SG, Matos JA, Scavin G. 1984. Non-surgical electrical ablation of tachycardias: Importance of prior in vitro testing of catheter leads. PACE 7: 74.

13. Lerman BB, Weiss JL, Bulkey BH, Becker LS, Weisfeldt ML. 1984. Myocardial injury and induction of arrhythmia by direct current shock delivered via endocardial catheters in dogs. Circulation 69: 1006.

14. Winston SA, Davis JC, Morady F, DiCarlo LA, Matsubara T, Wexman M, Scheinman M. 1984. A new approach to electrode catheter ablation arising from the interventricular septum. Circulation 70 (Suppl II): II-412.

15. Jones JL, Lepeschkiw E, Jones RE, Rush S. 1978. Response of cultured myocardial cells to countershock-type electric field stimulation. Am J Physiol 235: H214.

16. Hartzler GO. 1983. Electrode catheter ablation of refractory focal vetricular tachycardia. J Am Coll Cardiol 2: 1107.

17. Fontaine G, Tonet JL, Frank R, Gallas Y, Fereng G, Grosgogeat Y. 1984. La fulguration endocavitaire. Une nouvele methode de traitement des troubles du rhythme? Am Cardiol Angeul 33: 543.

31. Intraoperative mapping of ventricular tachycardia associated with coronary artery disease

MARK E. JOSEPHSON*, JOHN M. MILLER, W. CLARK HARGROVE, III,
With the technical assistance of T. FRANZ ORISHIMO
*Clinical Electrophysiology Laboratory, Hospital of the University of
Pennsylvania, Cardiovascular Section, and Cardiothoracic Surgery Section,
Departments of Medicine and Surgery, University of Pennsylvania School of
Medicine, Philadelphia, Pennsylvania*

Over the past ten years electrophysiologically directed surgical techniques to ablate sustained ventricular tachycardia (VT) associated with coronary artery disease have been developed. The success rate of these procedures has primarily resulted from the increased knowledge concerning the pathophysiologic substrate of the arrhythmia in this disorder. Activation mapping, both pre- and intraoperatively, has been extensively utilized to define both the pathophysiologic substrate and localize the site of origin of VT. Prior to the use of these electrophysiologic techniques to localize arrhythmogenic areas, surgery was empiric and was often a failure. The current manuscript will detail the results of intraoperative mapping of VT associated with coronary artery disease at the University of Pennsylvania.

Methods and rationale

The purposes of intraoperative mapping are twofold: (1) to localize the site of origin of VT if possible; and (2) to define abnormalities of activation which are consistent with the known pathophysiologic substrate of VT so that if activation mapping of the tachycardia itself is impossible a surgical attack on a 'potentially' arrhythmogenic substrate can be undertaken. At the outset it must be said that we consider preoperative endocardial catheter mapping an integral part of the surgical procedure since multiple VT morphologies are often present and more time can be spent mapping than could be allowed intraoperatively [1, 2]. Furthermore, some VT may not be inducible intraoperatively or degenerate to ventricular fibrillation.

For the first 60 patients in our series both epicardial and endocardial activation

* Dr Josephson is the Robinette Foundation Professor of Medicine (Cardiovascular Diseases).

412

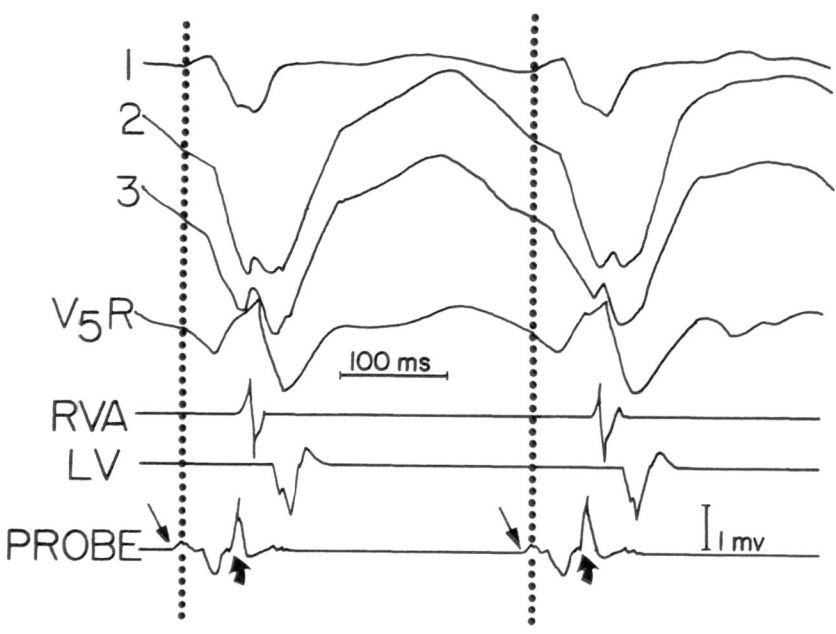

Figure 1. Local electrocardiographic measurement during ventricular tachycardia. Four surface electrocardiographic leads (1, 2, 3, nd V$_5$R), right (RVA), and left (LV) ventricular reference electrograms and an electrogram from a roving probe are shown. The vertical dotted lines mark the onset of the QRS complex, the thin arrow marks the onset of the local electrogram, and the curved arrow marks the rapid deflection. A 1 mV calibration reference is shown on the right. (From Miller et al., with permission.) [6]

mapping of VT were obtained. The results uniformly demonstrated an endocardial origin of VT which led us to curtail our intraoperative study by concentrating on the endocardium both in sinus rhythm and in VT. The results of all of our studies are detailed below.

The intraoperative procedure consists of simultaneously recording four ECG leads (1, 2, 3, and V$_{5R}$ or V$_5$), a bipolar reference from both the left and right ventricles, and mapping with a hand-held ring or stick probe (Fig. 1) [3–5]. Recently we have undertaken more detailed mapping using plaque electrodes with 20 simultaneously recorded narrow bipoles and/or multipolar plunge electrodes (Fig. 2) [6, 7].

In the first 78 patients epicardial sinus rhythm mapping was initially performed using a schema of 54 predetermined sites (Fig. 3). The tachycardia was then induced by programmed stimulation and mapped epicardially. Following epicardial mapping of procedures ventriculotomy or aneurysmectomy was performed and endocardial mapping of the tachycardia was performed using two patterns: (1) a clockwise grid as described previously with increasing radii at 1 cm intervals to obtain 3 to 5 rows (36 to 60 sites) covering most of the left ventricular

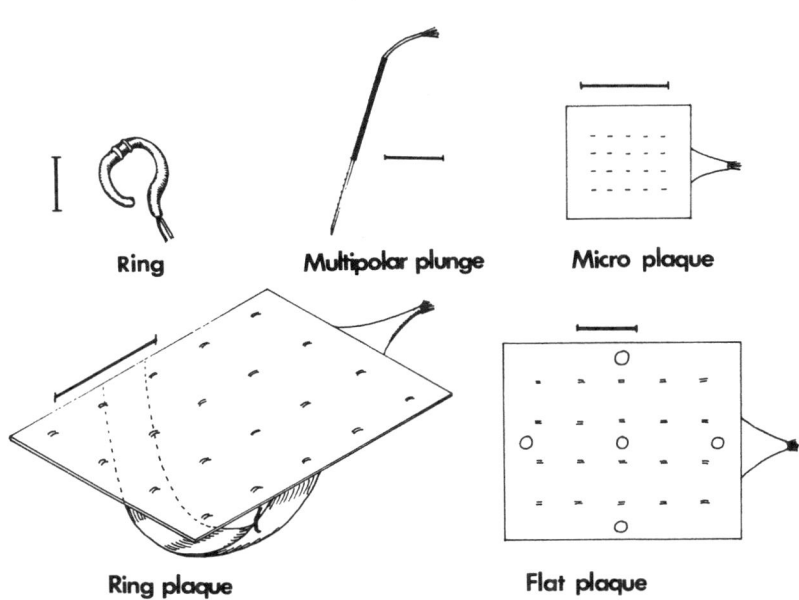

Ring   Multipolar plunge   Micro plaque

Ring plaque   Flat plaque

Figure 2. Electrodes for intraoperative mapping. Shown here are the ring electrode which along with a stick electrode (not shown) were used in all cases and require a stable tachycardia and only record a signal a point at a time. Other electrodes shown are plunge electrodes which have ten poles, several plaque electrodes with 10 bipolar pairs and/or 20 bipolar pairs.

endocardium (Fig. 4). More recently we have additionally used a specific map for the septum separating it into 9 regions. In the last 100 patients no epicardial mapping of VT has been performed. The procedure now consists of placing the patient on normothermic cardiopulmonary bypass after which access to the left ventricular endocardium is obtained via ventriculotomy or aneurysmectomy. Following this, endocardial sinus rhythm mapping is performed in selected patients; thereafter VT is induced and is mapped.

Recordings are stored on a 28-channel Honeywell 5600 FM tape recorder and displayed in real time using an Elema Mingograf 16-channel ink jet recorder at a paper speed of 200 mm/second. The timing of local electrograms is compared to the onset of the surface QRS with particular attention paid to the two bipolar references to confirm the presence of the same tachycardia regardless of changes in QRS morphology due to varying position of the heart in the chest. Once the site of origin (see definition) is determined for one or more tachycardias, the patient's body temperature is lowered, cardioplegia perfused, and surgical resection of 2 or 3 mm of subendocardium, including the site of origin and a 1 to 1½ cm surrounding margin is accomplished [4, 5, 8, 9]. When multiple sites of origin are determined an attempt is made to include all these areas in one single sheet.

Detailed data analysis is performed following the surgical procedure. The mapping data are analyzed as follows. The timing of the onset and rapid deflec-

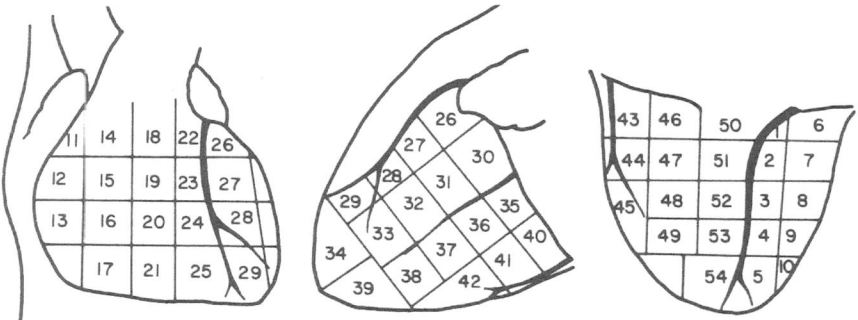

Figure 3. Epicardial mapping schema. The heart is shown in the anterior, left lateral, and inferior views. Fifty-four predetermined sites were used as a guide to the surgeon for both sinus rhythm mapping and mapping during ventricular tachycardia from the epicardium. (From Josephson et al., with permission.) [2]

tion, if present, of electrograms at each site are measured by hand relative to the onset of the surface QRS. The onset of the surface QRS was taken at the earliest reproducible deflection from the baseline in any of the surface ECG leads. The end of the QRS complex was similarly determined. In cases in which onset and offset of the QRS could not be accurately determined, assessment of QRS onset was made after a premature stimulus or a train of rapid pacing producing a pause in the tachycardia. Subsequent measurement in these cases was then made relative to one of the constant reference electrograms with appropriate adjustment to the onset of the QRS. The reproducibility of the measurements is ± 5 msec. Isochronic maps at 20 msec intervals are drawn for each VT using the difference between the onset of the ECG and the onset and rapid deflection of the local electrogram from each site.

Definitions which were used included:

1) *Site of origin* of VT is defined as the endocardial site from which the earliest electrogram in the latter half of diastole is recorded during that VT. Another specific characteristic of the site of origin is that the eletrogram, particularly the presystolic electrogram component, remains constant in timing relative to the onset of the QRS despite oscillations in cycle length that are spontaneous, or, if necessary, induced by extrastimuli.

2) *Electrograms* are classified as follows: (a) normal – discrete spike having amplitude >2 mV and duration <70 msec, (b) fractionated electrograms – abnormal electrograms with multiple high frequency components having amplitudes <0.5 mV and a duration >90 msec, (c) split electrograms – abnormal electrograms with at least two discrete spikes separated by an isoelectric interval of 30 msec. (d) a late electrogram – an electrogram in which electrical activity extends beyond the end of the surface QRS (Fig. 5). An individual electrogram could theoretically be classified as more than one type; i.e., fractionated and late.

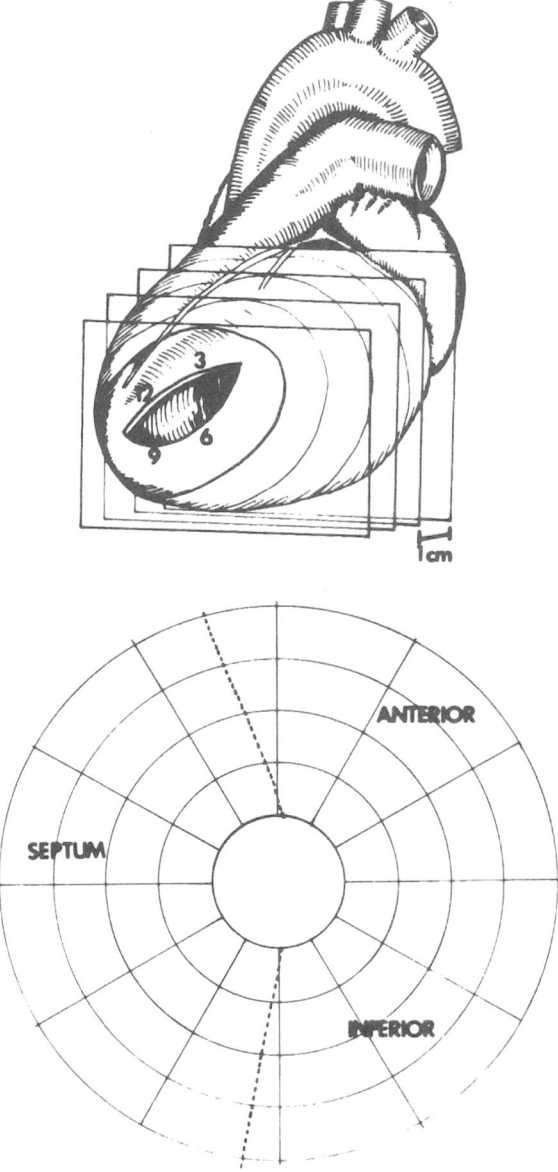

Figure 4. Endocardial mapping schema. The left ventricle is shown in a slight left anterior oblique view after aneurysmectomy or ventriculotomy. The 12 points of a clock face are arranged around the edge of the aneurysmectomy or ventriculotomy, and 4 imaginary vertical planes recessed at 1 cm intervals are shown above. In the bottom panel, the central hole represents the aneurysmectomy or ventriculotomy and the base of the heart is shown towards the outer edge of the concentric circles. The septum is to the left, the anterior free wall to the upper right, and the inferior wall to the lower right. (From Miller et al., with permission.) [6]

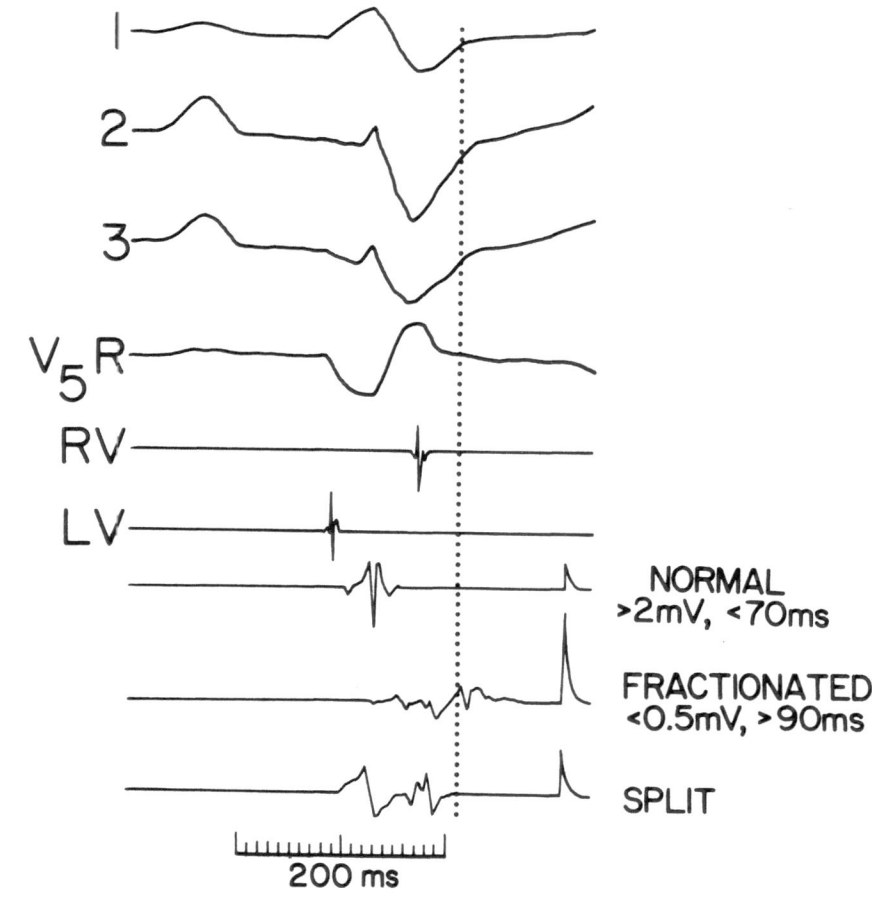

Figure 5. Types of electrograms. See text for discussion.

Activation mapping during ventricular tachycardia

To date, 161 patients with sustained VT related to prior infarction have undergone surgery for their arrhythmias at the Hospital of the University of Pennsylvania. Four hundred thirty seven morphologically distinct VT were observed in these patients. Fifteen percent of these VT were localized by catheter mapping only, 30% were mapped in the operating room only, 48% were mapped both in the catheterization laboratory and operating room, and 7% were transient and were never completely mapped either in the operating room or the catheterization laboratory. At least one tachycardia was completely mapped on the endocardium and/or epicardium in each patient. Only the first 60 patients had detailed epicardial as well endocardial mapping of VT [5]. In these 60 patients epicardial activation typically began following the onset of the QRS, except in one patient in

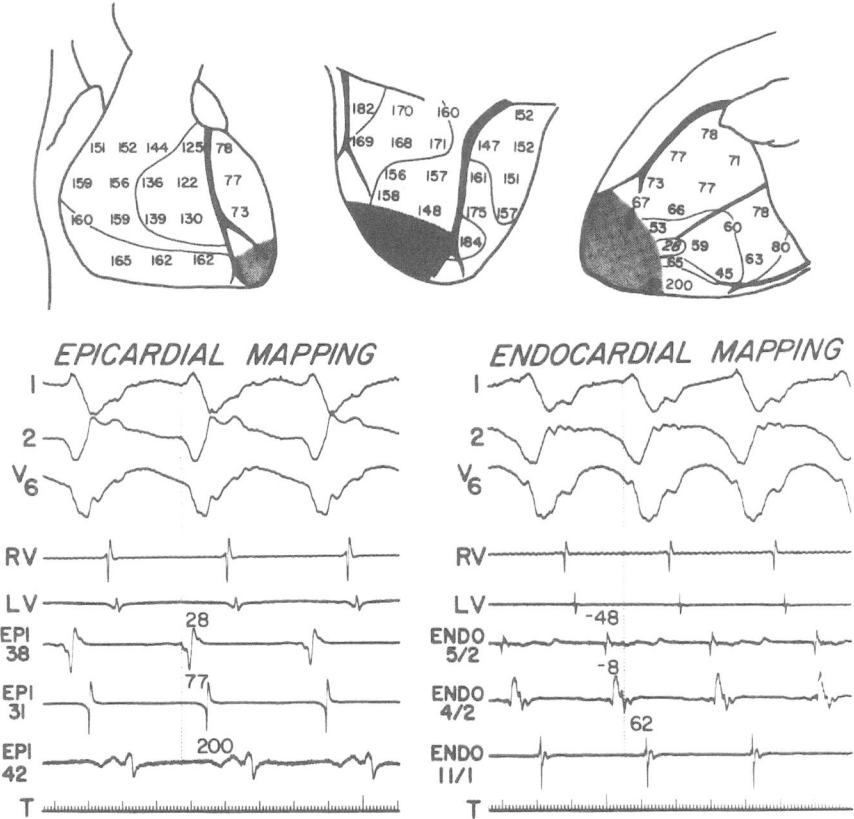

Figure 6. Epicardial and endocardial activation of VT with right bundle branch block morphology. A schematic representatio of the epicardial surface is shown in the anterior, inferior and left lateral positions in the top part of the figure. The aneurysm is shaded. Activation times at selected epicardial sites are shown using 20 msec isochronic lines. The epicardiac breakthrough occurred 28 msec after the onset of the QRS complex, the anterolateral edge of the aneurysm. Analog records for both the epicardial and endocardial mapping of this tachycardia are shown on the bottom part o the tracing. Surface ECG leads 1, 2, and V_6 are shown with the right and left ventricular reference electrodes. In each panel, three additional mapping electrograms are shown along with time lines. The dotted lines mark the onset of the QRS and the activation times are referenced to this. On the left, the epicardial electrograms recorded at the site of earliest epicardial breakthrough (38) and two other epicardial sites on the left ventricle (sites 31 and 42) are shown. Note the marked difference in epicardial activation times between sites 38 and 42 which are only three cm apart from each other. In the right hand panel, endocardial electrograms were recorded at the site of earliest activity (5 o'clock, second row in) and immediately adjacent sites (endocardial site 4/2 and anteroseptal site, endocardial site 11/1). The numbering system for these endocardial sites indicates the position around the margin of the aneurysm on the face of the clock (first number) and the concentric ring from the edge of the aneurysmectomy (second number). Note the earliest endocardial electrogram occurred 48 msec prior to the onset of the QRS and 76 msec before epicardial breakthrough.

whom the epicardial breakthrough coincided with the onset of the surface QRS during the tachycardia. In the remaining patients the epicardial breakthrough was 10 to 76 msec following onset of the QRS. In tachycardias which manifested a right bundle branch block pattern epicardial breakthrough was always earliest on the left ventricle, while in those with left bundle branch block configuration epicardial breakthrough was on the right ventricle adjacent to the anterior or inferior interventricular groove in all but three cases. In these three VT early epicardial breakthrough was on the left ventricle adjacent to the anterior (2 patients) or inferior (1 patient) intraventricular groove. In tachycardias with a right bundle branch block pattern, activation of the left ventricle was usually completed prior to the right ventricle and the opposite was true in left bundle branch block pattern tachycardias. Endocardial activation always preceded epicardial activation and was the reason which led us to discontinue epicardial mapping (Fig. 6).

All 161 patients underwent some form of endocardial mapping. In the last 100 patients the procedure consisted solely of endocardial mapping. Presystolic endocardial activity was recorded in all tachycardias. Electrograms at the site of origin were almost always abnormal or fractionated, frequently having systolic and diastolic components. Two hundred VT were mapped in detail using a large number of sites [6, 7]. Several interesting phenomena were observed. The pattern of endocardial activation was characterized as focal, in which there was centrifugal spread of endocardial activation from a small area ($1-3$ cm^2), or a continuous loop pattern in which an orderly progression of activation throughout the cardiac cycle was observed with activation at any given site dependent upon activation of the preceding site [6]. One of these two patterns of activation was observed in 83% of VTs; in the remainder, no pattern of activation could be determined because of too few mapping sites. Ninety percent of completely mapped tachycardias appeared to have centrifugal spread of activation and 10% appeared to have a continuous loop of activation. Tachycardias with continuous loop patterns had shorter cycle lengths (260 vs 338 msec, $p<.002$) than tachycardias with centrifugal spread. Of the 17 patients with a continuous loop pattern of activity, 9 were observed from the anterior wall and 8 from the inferior wall. This 'macroreentrant' type of activity was occasionally associated with two VT morphologies which were dependent upon the direction of wavefront propagation (Fig. 7). An isochronic map of such a patient is shown in Figure 8. The 'focal' tachycardias could also give rise to multiple morphologies arising from the same area (Fig. 9). In other patients with multiple morphologies, the tachycardia origins were focal but widely separated from another. An isochronic map of a focal tachycardia is shown in Figure 10.

Electrical activity could be recorded throughout the cardiac cycle in a small area in 36 tachycardias. In 28 VT an electrogram from a single site showed continuous activity which spanned systole and diastole in a repetitive fashion. In 8 tachycardias, adjacent sites showed systolic and diastolic electrical activity com-

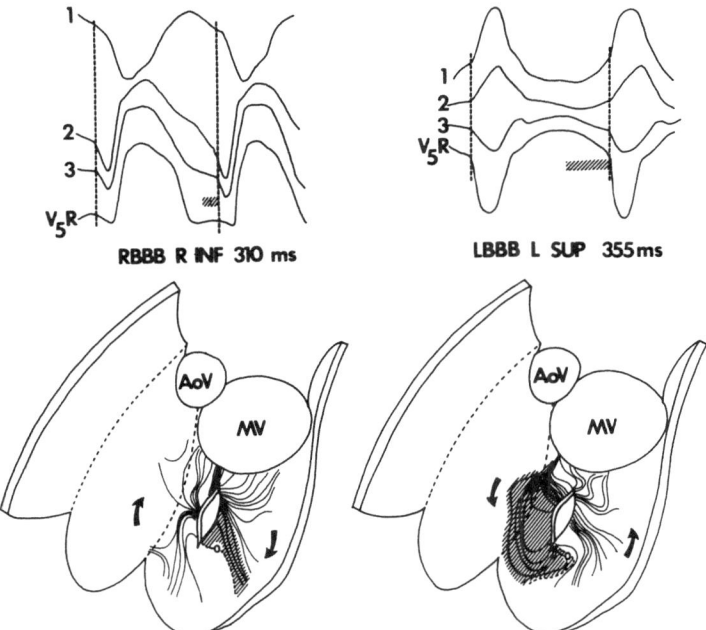

Figure 7. Continuous loop pattern during two morphological lead distinct tachycardias associated with an inferior infarction. On the left, the activation pattern of a right bundle branch block, right inferior axis tachycardia with a cycle length of 310 msec is shown. The activation pattern is clockwise around the ventriculotomy scar. The shaded area is the area from which presystolic activity was recorded. On the right is shown the activation pattern of a left bundle branch block, left superior axis tachycardia with a cycle length of 355 msec with continuous spread in a counterclockwise direction around the same ventriculotomy scar. The shaded area here is the presystolic area during this tachycardia. The shaded area relative to the QRS is shown on top with th ECGs. The vertical dashed lines mark the onset of the QRS. See text for discussion.

pleting the cardiac cycle. In these 36 cases, and in those 17 VT with a continuous loop pattern, the data were consistent with recording a reentrant circuit. Detailed mapping of some focal additional tachycardias manifested very complex activation patterns suggesting that the reentrant circuit occupied at least two levels of activation albeit probably shallow in depth (Fig. 11).

In many instances it was difficult at first glance to determine whether presystolic electrical activity was 'early' or late (and not an essential component of the tachycardia). Two methods were routinely used to help distinguish early from late sites. The first employed stimulation during the tachycardia to see what effect this had on the relationship between the presystolic electrogram and the first beat of VT following pacing. An example of this stimulation technique is shown in Figure 12, in which what appears to be a presystolic electrogram, that would normally have been considered the site of origin, is clearly shown to be late and unrelated to the VT (Fig. 12). Comparison of the relationship of the presystolic

420

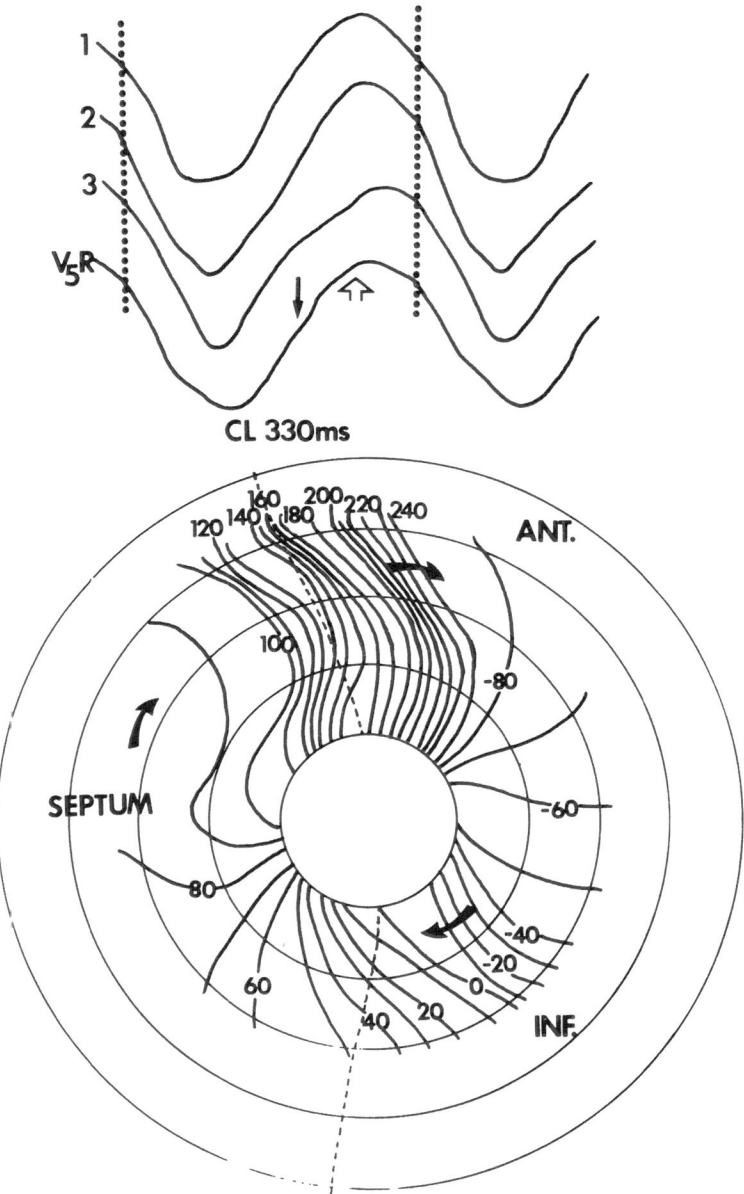

Figure 8. Detailed analysis of continuousloop pattern of activation in an anterior infarction. On top four surface ECG leads (1, 2, 3 and V_5R) are shown. The vertical dotted line denotes the onset of the QRS, the small black arrow denotes the end of the QRS, and the open arrow represents mid-electrical diastole. Electrical activity could be recorded throughout the cardiac cycle. The defined site of origin occurred at approximately 2 o'clock (see Fig. 4) where electrical activity was recorded just after the midpoint of diastole. Activation spread from this area in a clockwise direction with the cycle length of the tachycardia equalling the time required to complete one loop of endocardial activation around the aneurysmm. ANT = anterior; INF = inferior. (From Miller et al., with permission.) [6]

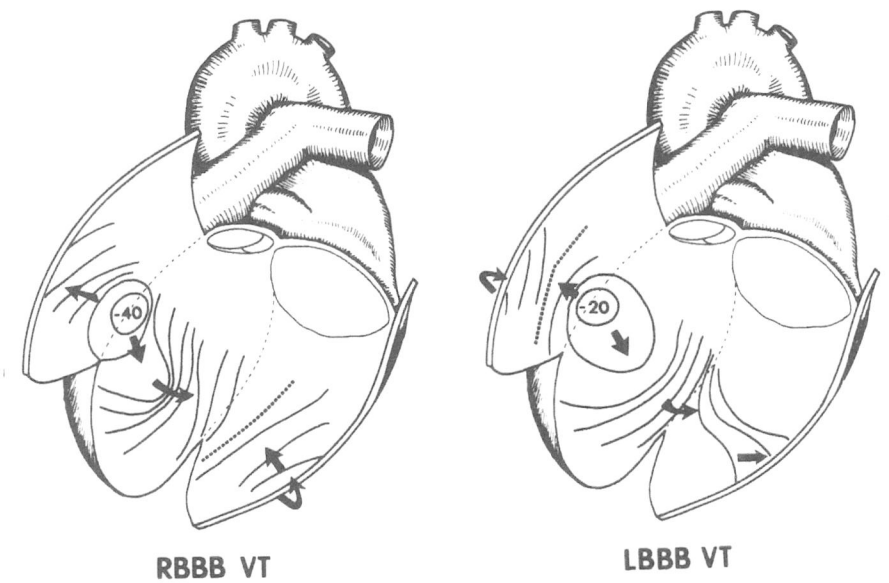

RBBB VT **LBBB VT**

Figure 9. Focal tachycardias with multiple morphologies. Shown in this figure are the isochronic maps of a right bundle branch block and a left bundle branch block tachycardia. Both have focal patterns of activation with a single breakthrough site at the junction of the superior midseptum and free wall with centrifugal spread from that point.

electrogram on the first post pacing beat and the second post pacing beat (bottom panel) demonstrates that the electrogram has moved into the QRS on the first post pacing beat as a result of delay secondary to the rapid pacing. In the second post pacing beat the presystolic electrogram is again observed prior to the QRS onset but it is clear from the prior complex that this actually represents very delayed activation. The documented site of origin of this VT was noted 4 cm from this site.

The second method of assessing presystolic activity is the demonstration that focal pressure at that site can terminate the tachycardia. An example of this is shown in Figure 13. We have applied digital pressure systematically at presumed sites of VT origin in the last 57 tachycardias which had more detailed mapping. Fifty-one tachycardias were either slowed or terminated by focal digital pressure. Digital pressure was also used at 'control' sites (those not having presystolic activity) in 15 tachycardias, but slowing or termination was observed only in response to pressure at the presumed site of origin. This suggests that the area designated as the site of origin was indeed a critical part of the reentrant circuit.

These two techniques help resolve an obvious pitfall in mapping, the misidentification of late sites as early. Another phenomenon which also demonstrates the lack of necessity of a presumed early electrogram is the manifestation of sudden failure of conduction in an electrogram. This phenomenon is clearly demon-

422

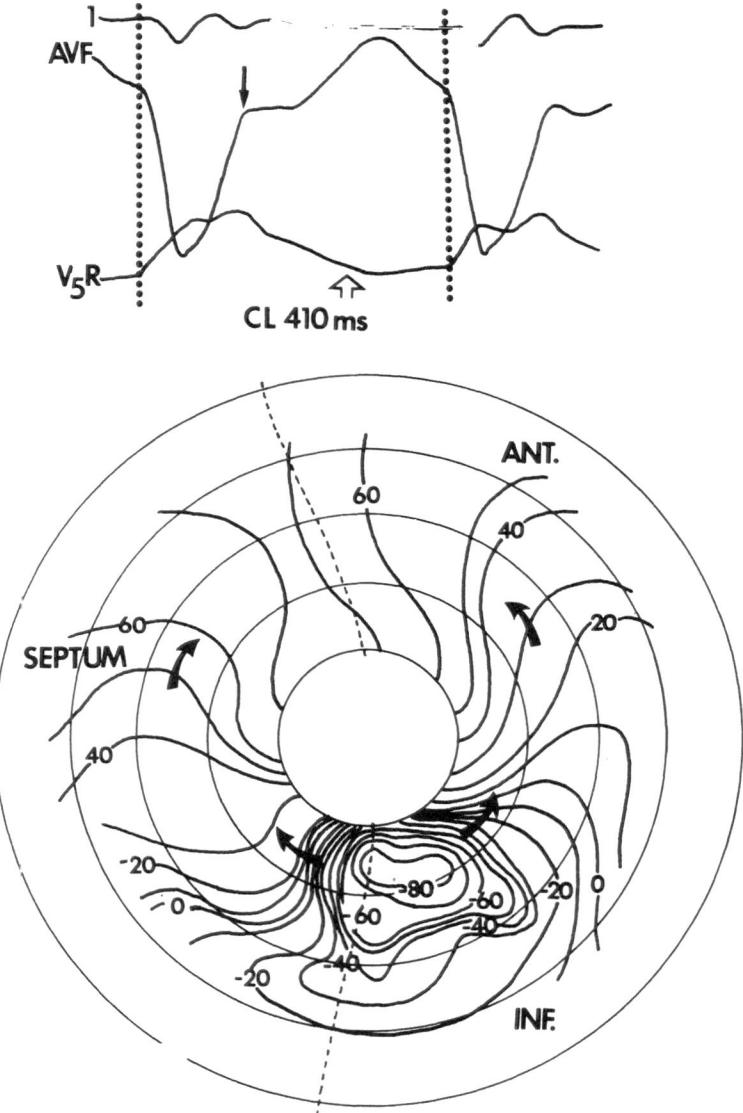

Figure 10. Centrifugal spread pattern from ventricular tachycardia. The surface leads (1, AVF, and V₅R) are shown with arrows demarcating the end of the QRS (small, dark arrow), the mid diastole (open arrow), and dotted lines marking the onset of the QRS. The tachycardia has a right bundle branch block right superior axis morphology. The endocardial activation sequence shows that early activity began near the junction of the inferior wall and septum with centrifugal spread from that site to activate the rest of the ventricles. Note the areas of closest isochrones and therefore slowest conduction occurred around the earliest site of activation. (From Miller et al., with permission.) [6]

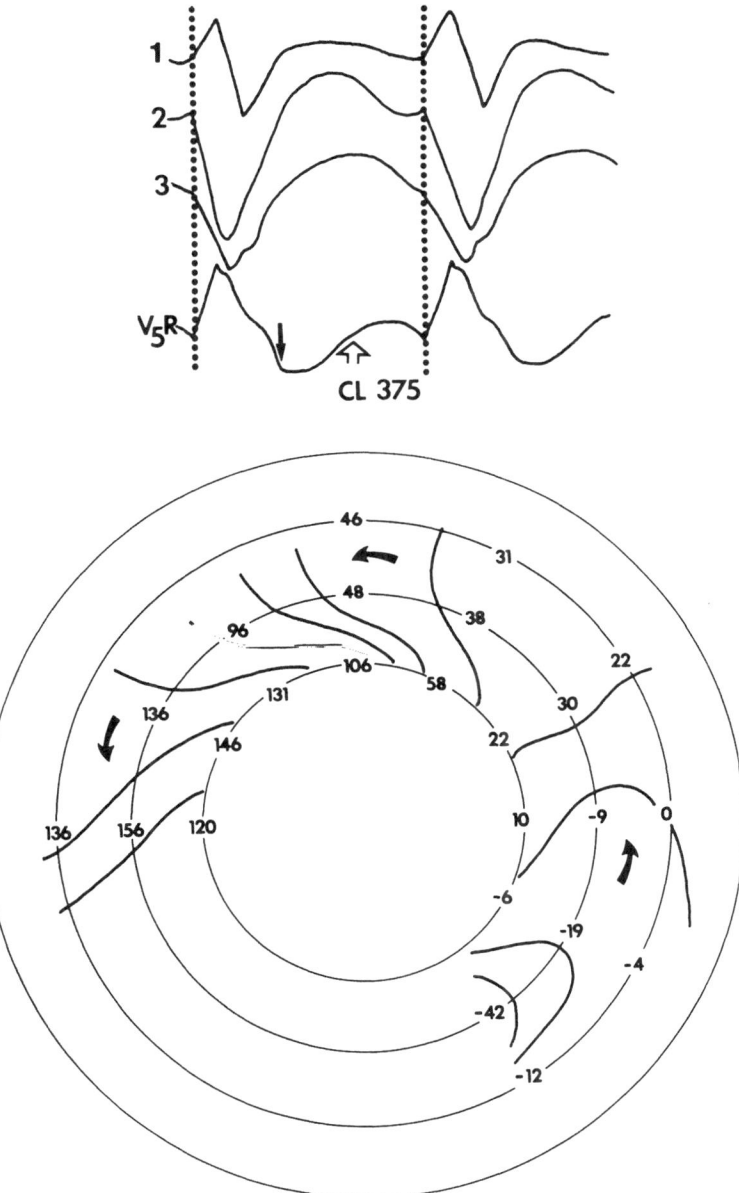

Figure 11. Incomplete pattern of activation. Leads 1, 2, 3, and V₅R are shown during a right bundle branch block ventricular tachycardia with a cycle length of 375 msec. The activation map is complete; thus, one cannot distinguish local or macroreentrant patterns. (See text for further discussion.)

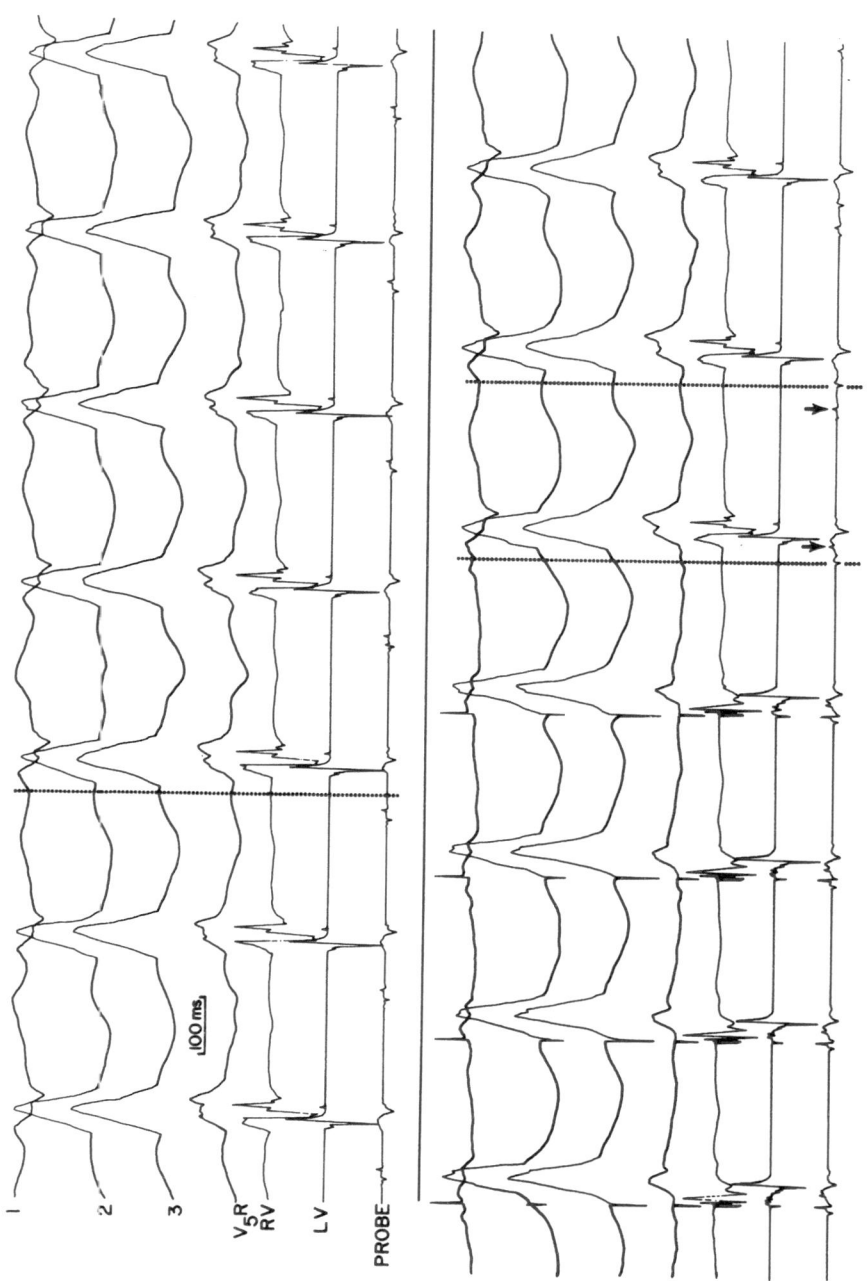

425

Figure 12. Use of pacing to distinguish early from late activity of presystolic electrogram. Both panels are displayed with surface leads 1, 2, 3, and V₅R, reference electrograms from the right and ventricles (RV, LV) and electrogram reported from a roving probe. The vertical dashed line represents the onset of the surface QRS. During the tachycardia on top, a two component presystolic electrogram is observed 50 msec prior to the onset of the QRS. Pacing during the tachycardia is begun and terminated in the bottom tracing. During the first post-pacing beat, the complex electrogram that was presystolic is now recorded inside the QRS, and it subsequently returns to a presystolic position in the following beats. This suggests that this presystolic electrogram is not early but actually late and unnecessary for the tachycardia. See text for discussion.

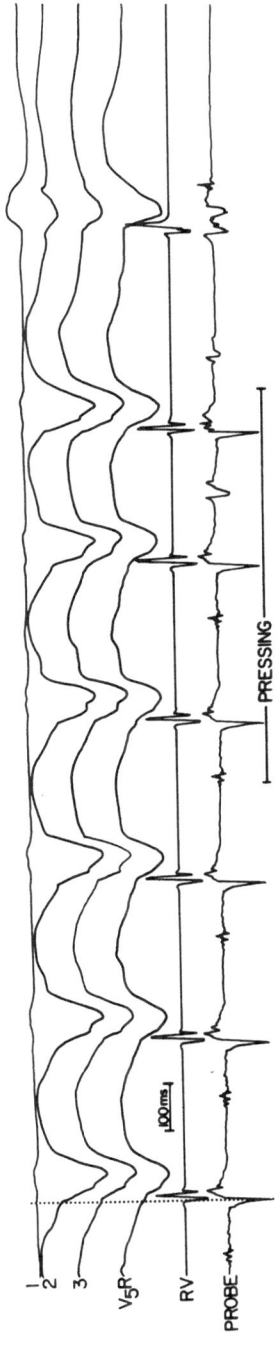

Figure 13. Use of digital pressure to verify site of origin. Ventricular tachycardia is present. Surface leads 1, 2, 3, and V₅R are shown along with a right ventricular reference and an electrogram showing presystolic activity recorded from a roving probe. Pressure is applied resulting in termination of the tachycardia.

strated in Figure 14. A presystolic electrogram is noted to be consistently present in the top tracing. In the bottom part of this continuous tracing one can see the disappearance of this electrogram although the tachycardia continues. Thus, if only the first few complexes were recorded by computer or hand, a misleading diagnosis of the site of origin would be made. It is only by observation of this site for long periods of time, or observing a change in the electrogram following pacing or digital pressure, that one can determine that the presystolic electrogram is not necessary for the maintenance of the arrhythmia. Impressively, sudden failure of conduction is a very common phenomenon. It has been observed in 68 of 78 patients (87%) in whom detailed mapping was undertaken and this phenomenon was evaluated. This included 131 of 200 tachycardias (66%). The usual form of conduction failure was 2:1 or an otherwise fixed pattern; however, Wenckebach type patterns have been observed [7]. It usually occurs in areas which manifest abnormal electrograms during sinus rhythm. This phenomenon may be extremely focal and be present in one bipolar lead and absent in an adjacent bipolar lead 4 mm away. Seventy-five percent of sites demonstrating intermittent local conduction failure were found within 2 cm of a site of origin of VT.

There have been no detailed reports of intraoperative mapping of significant number of tachycardias except that of DeBakker et al. [10] and Mason et al. [11]. This group has done detailed endocardial mapping of VT and have shown that all tachycardias had a focal origin. There have also been isolated reports of epicardial and/or endocardial mapping which are consistent with our data [4, 12–16]. In those series which have compared surgery guided by mapping to that unguided by mapping, there has been a general consensus that map guided surgery produces better results [9, 17–19]. It must be stated, however, that the interpretation of the maping data is critical to the success of the surgical procedure if it is solely based on this mapping. The potential problems with mapping and benefits from mapping have been reported by Mason et al. and Miller et al. [11, 20].

Sinus rhythm mapping in patients with ventricular tachycardia

Sinus rhythm mapping has been suggested to be a method of localizing arrhythmogenic areas responsible for VT. Abnormal fractionated electrograms and late potentials were initially observed by Fontaine et al. [16, 21, 22] in patients with VT and arrhythmogenic right ventricular dysplasia. In many of these patients the induced VT appeared to arise in areas where late potentials occurred, although they often appeared after the onset of the QRS. Fontaine, therefore, suggested that these abnormal late potentials were markers of slow conduction arising in abnormal tissue responsible for the arrhythmia. Subsequent work by Fontaine [22], Wittig and Boineau [13], Moran et al. [17] as well as our prior data suggested that the epicardium was not the source of the ventricular arrhythmias in

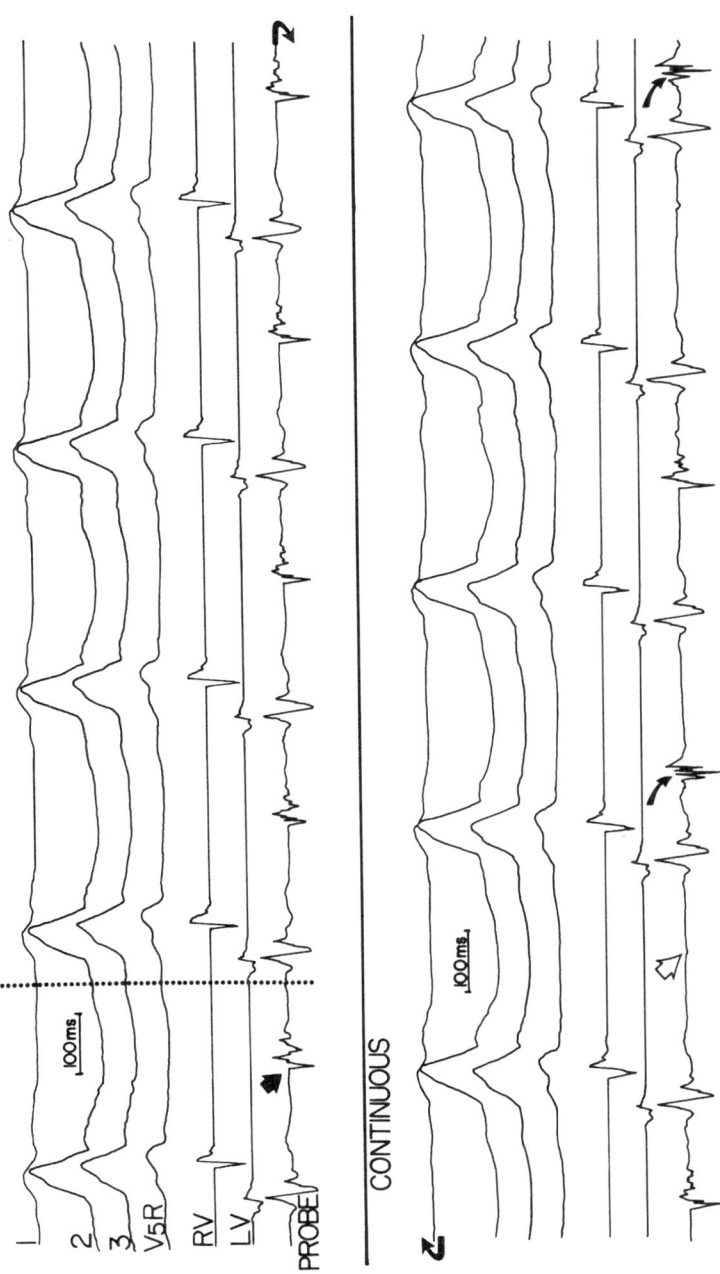

Figure 14. Failure of conduction proving lack of significance for a presystolic electrogram. RV and LV as well as a presystolic electrogram from a roving probe are shown during a tachycardia with a right bundle branch block, left inferior axis. In the top panel, the vertical line represents the onset of the QRS. On the top, the presystolic electrogram shown by the dark, short arrow appears consistently related to the onset of the QRS. However in the bottom panel, the presystolic electrogram suddenly disappears (open, broad arrow) and then reappears (curved arrow) but in a Wenckebach fashion from the prior systolic electrogram. Thus, the electrogram which was presystolic on top is clearly shown to be caused by delayed activation and is not an early site nor is it requisite for maintenance of the tachycardia.

428

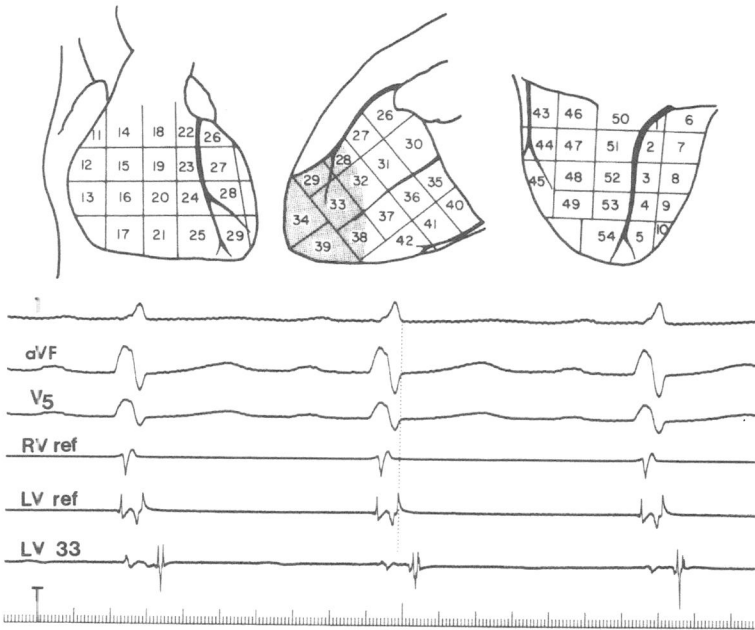

Figure 15. Epicardial late potential. On top is the schematized epicardial grid of 54 predetermined sites. The solid black circle near site 33 presents the site of late potential. The shaded area represents an apical aneurysm. Surface leads 1, aVF, and V_5 are shown with the right and left ventricular reference electogram in the bottom and from the left ventricular epicardial site 33. At this site, discrete late potential is observed 45 msec after the inscription of the QRS is completed (dotted line) T = time lines. (From Josephson et al., with permission.) [23]

Figure 16. Lack of relationship between late potential, epicardial breakthrough during VT, and site of origin of VT. From top to bottom are epicardial maps during sinus rhythm, an epicardial isochronic map during VT, and analog mapping data during VT from the site of origin and the site of epicardial late potential during sinus rhythm. The cardiac silhouettes in the top two tracings in the anterior, left lateral, and inferior (left-to-right) views with the epicardial mapping sites shown. The stippled area on top represents the apical aneurysm. The late potential (solid black circle) is seen at site 29 alongside the edge of the left ventricular aneurysm. In the middle series, the isochronic map during ventricular tachycardia shows epicardial breakthrough at the right ventricular apex at 5 msec. No discrete electrical activity could be recorded at sites 28, 29 and half of sites 33 and 34 which were on the epicardial surface of the apical aneurysm. On the bottom, surface leads 1, aVF, and V_5 are shown during the tachycardia which has a left bundle branch block, left axis deviation morphology. In addition, reference electrograms from the right and left ventricles are shown along with the electrogram recorded at the site of the late potential on the epicardium and from the endocardial site of origin of the midseptum. The site of epicardial late potential (EPI-LV 29) was activated 47 msec after the onset of the QRS of the tachycardia which was 69 msec after the earliest recorded activity along the midseptum. (From Josephson et al., with permission.) [23]

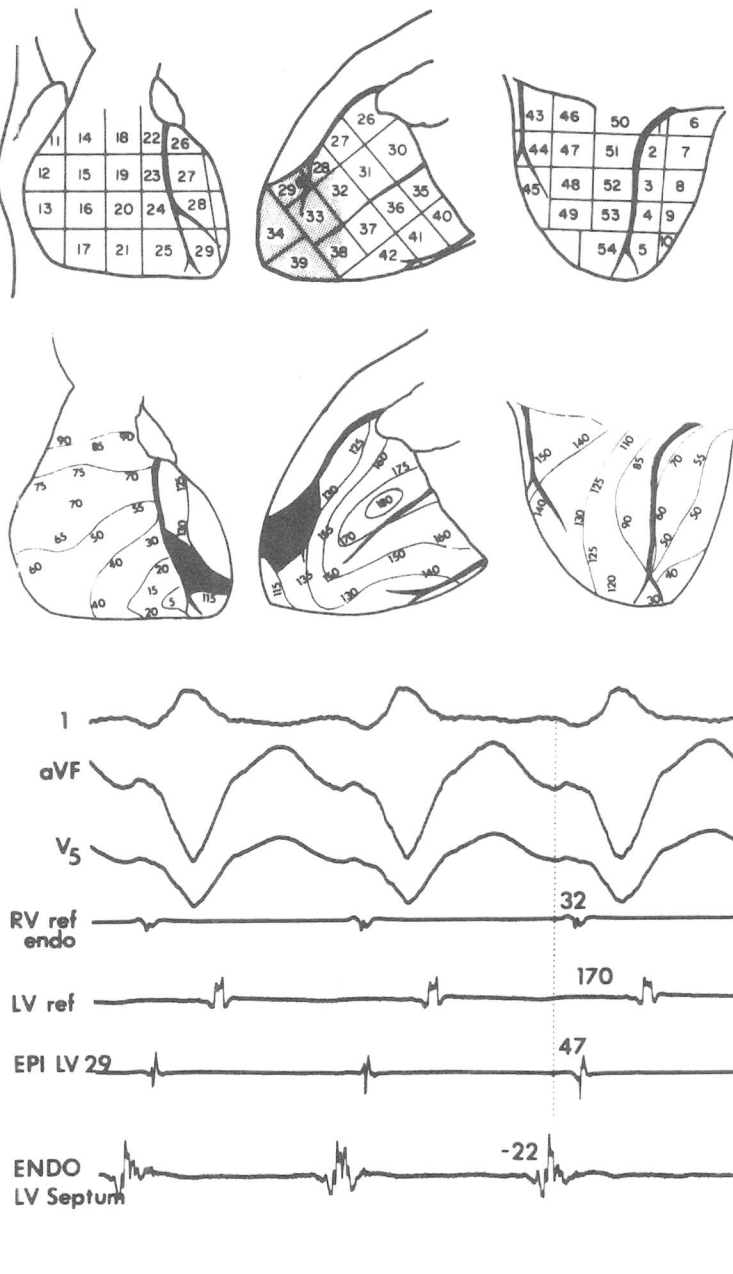

coronary artery disease [1–4]. This observation limited the likelihood that epicardial late potentials could identify the specific arrhythmogenic substrate responsible for the arrhythmia. It was not surprising, therefore, that Fontaine's experience using sinus rhythm mapping and late potentials in coronary artery disease was negative [22]. He found late potentials in only 6 of 19 patients with VT associated with coronary artery disease and in only 2 of these 6 cases was there a relationship between the earliest epicardial breakthrough and the late potential. In many patients data was considered uninterpretable.

We also evaluated the clinical significance of epicardial late potentials in patients with sustained VT and coronary artery disease [23]. We studied 78 patients using the 54 site epicardial grid shown in Figure 3. One to 4 late potentials observed in 9 of the 78 patients (11.5%), an example of which is shown in Figure 15. Eight of these patients had anterior apical aneurysms and one had an inferior infarction without an aneurysm. The patients with late potentials did not differ hemodynamically from those without late potentials, nor did the tachycardias with late potentials differ from those without late potentials. In 4 patients the site of the VT was left ventricular septum, whereas late potentials were observed in the free wall of the left ventricle over the apical aneurysm, quite distant from the site of origin of the tachycardia. An example of the disparity of the late potential, epicardial mapping and the endocardial site of origin of the tachycardia is shown in Figure 16. In the remaining 5 patients the late potential occurred near the earliest site of activation during the tachycardia, which arose on the endocardium of the left ventricular free wall at the border of the aneurysm. In these patients the late potential and the endocardial site of origin occurred within 3 cm of each other. However, in 3 of these 5 patients additional tachycardias were observed which arose on the intraventricular septum, significantly distant from the epicardial late potentials. Thus, even in patients in whom one tachycardia morphology was associated with a late potential, the site of the late potential could not be used as the sole guide for surgical intervention since other tachycardias arose at distant sites.

Because we had previously shown tachycardias arose at or near the subendocardium, we also analyzed the potential role for endocardial sinus rhythm mapping as a guide to the localization of VT. We performed this both in the catheterization laboratory and intraoperatively. The intraoperative studies compared detailed mapping of VT and sinus rhythm in 13 patients [24]. Fractionated electrograms were observed in all patients and were observed in up to a third of the mapped sites. Split potentials were seen in 10 of the 13 patients and were only observed in approximately 6% of mapped sites while distinct late potentials (isolated electrograms beyond the termination of the QRS) were only seen in 4 patients. These abnormal electrograms were widely distributed, as shown in Figure 17. It can be seen that the absolute number of clock segments and rows which abnormal electrograms could be found was extensive. Moreover, as can be seen in Figure 18, the number of fractionated electrograms and sites of frac-

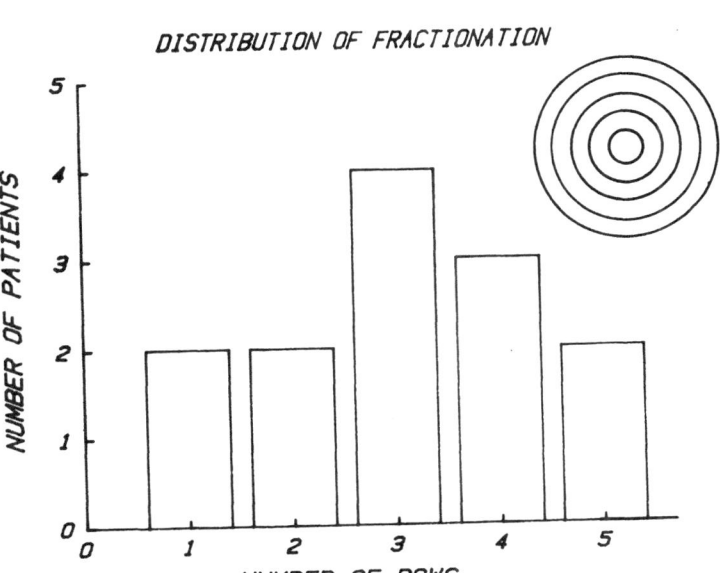

Figure 17. Distribution of abnormal electrograms during sinus rhythm endocardial mapping. Top. The absolute number of clock segments in which fractionated electrograms could be found are shown on the horizontal axis and the number of patients is displayed on the vertical axis. The majority of patients had seven to nine clock segments in which fractionated electrograms could be found. Bottom. The absolute number of rows (as measured from apex to base) in which fractionated electrograms could be found is displayed in the horizontal axis and the number or patients is on the vertical axis. Most patients had three to five rows in which fractionated electrograms could be detected. (From Kienzle et al., with permission.) [24]

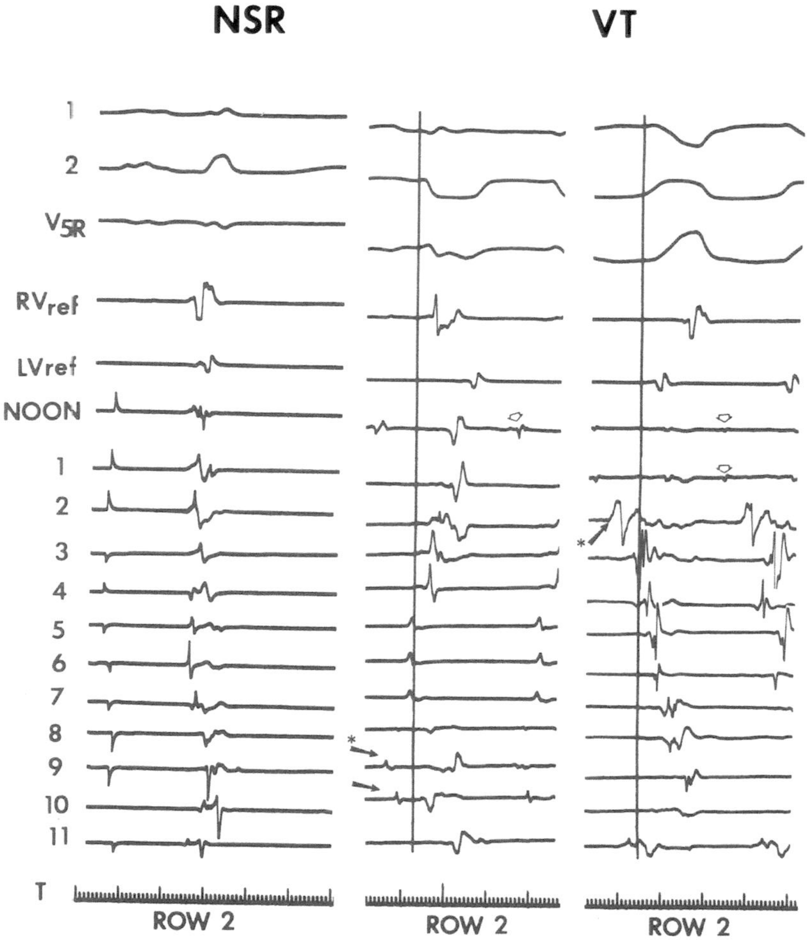

NSR
VT
1
2
V5R
RVref
LVref
NOON
1
2
3
4
5
6
7
8
9
10
11
T
ROW 2
ROW 2
ROW 2

AoV
MV
4cm
3cm
2cm
1cm
12
3
9
6

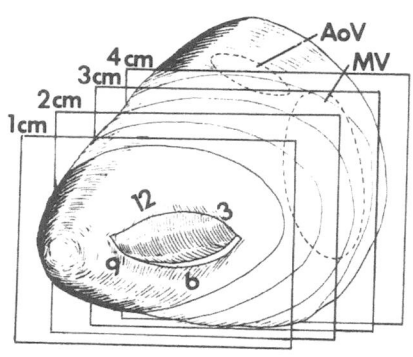

←

Figure 18. Analog records demonstrating lack of relationship of fractionated electrograms to site of origin of VT. Three panels of analog records are shown including maps during sinus rhythm (NSR) and two ventricular tachycardias (VT): one (middle panel) has a left bundle, left axis configuration, and the second (right panel) one has a right bundle right inferior axis morphology. Leads 1, 2, V_{SR} are shown with references from the right and left ventricle and electrograms recorded from the second row in from the edge of the aneurysmectomy around the entire clockface. Calibration signals are shown in the sinus rhythm tracing. A schema of the endocardial map is shown on the bottom. The recordings as noted above were taken from the 2 cm vertical plane in a clockwise fashion. In normal sinus rhythm, abnormal electrograms are noted in most of the sites. During ventricular tachycardia with a left bundle branch block pattern, the earliest site of activation was site 9 o'clock (asterisk, arrow). In the right bundle branch block tachycardia, the earliest site was 2 o'clock (asterisk, arrow). Thus, the sites of origin were disparate from each other. Several areas that were not sites of origin had fractionated electrograms, while the area from which the right bundle branch block tachycardia arose was relatively normal during sinus rhythm. That area from which the left bundle branch block tachycardia (site 9) had a late and split electrogram during sinus rhythm. See text for discussion. Open arrows = late potentials.

tionated electrograms did not necessarily correlate with the sites of origin of tachycardias. In Figure 18 two tachycardias were observed, one with a left bundle branch block pattern and one with a right bundle branch block pattern. Nine o'clock was the earliest site of the left bundle branch block type tachycardia which had a split electrogram, while site 2, which had a virtually normal electrogram, was the earliest in the right bundle branch block type tachycardia. Several other sites had abnormal fractionated electrograms which were not early in either tachycardia. The mean width of fractionated electrograms near the VT origin ($\pm 1\frac{1}{2}$ rows or one clock number) was similar to the width of the fractionated electrograms distant from the VT site (91 ± 17 vs 90 ± 18 msec, p = NS).

These findings have been more recently corroborated by comparing sinus rhythm catheter maps in 52 patients with 102 morphologically distinct tachycardias in those patients [25, 26]. These studies showed no correlation of the VT site of origin with any morphologic, duration, or timing characteristic of electrograms noted during the left ventricular catheter mapping. In addition, there was no relationship of any of these electrogram characteristics to tachycardia cycle length. These data suggest that sinus rhythm electrograms are neither sensitive nor specific markers of sites of origin of VT. Peliminary data suggest that they are likely related to a pathologic substrate of scar tissue surrounding viable myocardial scars. Electrophysiologic-pathologic correlates suggest that this anatomy generally does not distinguish between areas of prior infarction which are associated with the site of origin of tachycardia and those which are not [27]. These data are somewhat at variance with those of Waldo and Arciniegas et al. [15] who noted fractionated epicardial and/or endocardial electrograms occurred in 20 of 21 patients with ventricular arrhythmias (only 17 of whom had sustained VT) and recorded late potentials in only 12 of 21 patients. They did not, however, correlate these findings with mapping of VT so it is impossible to interpret their data other

434

than they may have selectively mapped certain areas that had fractionated electrograms. Thus, the bulk of data suggests that sinus rhythm mapping can only identify a particular anatomic substrate but not the site of origin of VT. This may, however, be useful in patients who have tachycardias that cannot be mapped. In such patients, widespread excision can be done based on this anatomic electrophysiologic correlate since 90% of tachycardias will arise in such an area.

Conclusion

Activation mapping has become an important part of the surgical approach to malignant ventricular arrhythmias. While activation mapping during VT remains the gold standard regarding therapy, sinus rhythm mapping can identify a pathophysiologic substrate which is compatible with but not specific for a site of origin of VT. It is only with higher density mapping using multiple simultaneous electrograms that we may more accurately characterize the extent of the reentrant circuit. This is probably a shallow 3-dimensional circuit since it can generally be obliterated by a 1–3 mm subendocardial resection. The use of computers with simultaneous high density data acquisition will hopefully allow for more rapid and accurate localization of these circuits and the development of more successful surgical procedures. Physician-computer interaction will, however, always be necessary because of the pitfalls of mapping, regardless of the technique of data acquisition.

References

1. Josephson ME, Horowitz LN, Spielman SR, Waxman HL, Greenspan AM. 1982. Role of catheter mapping in the preoperative valuation of ventricular tachycardia. Am J Cardiol 49: 207–221.
2. Josephson ME, Horowitz LN, Spielman SR, Greenspan AM, Vandepol C, Harken AH. 1980. Comparison of endocardial catheter mapping with intraoperative mapping of ventricular tachycardia. Circulation 61: 395–404.
3. Horowitz LN, Josephson ME, Harken AH. 1980. Epicardial and endocardial activation during sustained ventricular tachycardia in man. Circulation 61: 1227–1238.
4. Horowitz LN, Harken AH, Kastor A, Josephson ME. 1980. Ventricular resection guided by epicardial and endocardial mapping for treatment of recurrent ventriclar tachycardia. N Engl J Med 302: 589–593.
5. Josephson ME, Horowitz LN, Harken AH. 1982. Surgery for recurrent sustained ventricular tachycardia associated with coronary artery disease: the role of subendocardial resection. Ann NY Acad Sci 382: 381–395.
6. Miller J, Harken AH, Hargrove WC, Josephson ME. 1985. Pattern of endocardial activation during sustained ventricular tachycardia. JACC 6: 1280–1287.
7. Miller JM, Vassallo JA, Hargrove WC, Josephson ME. 1985. Intermittent failure of local conduction during ventricular tachycardia. Circulation 72: 1286–1292.
8. Josephson ME, Harken AH, Horowitz LN. 1979. Endocardial excision. A new surgical technique

for the treatment of recrrent ventricular tachycardia. Circulation 60: 1430–1439.

9. Josephson ME, Harken AH. 1983. Surgical therapy of arrhythmias. In: Cardiac Therapy. Edited by Rosen MR, Hoffman BF. Boston, Martinus Nijhoff, pp 337–385.

10. DeBakker JMT, Janse MJ, vanCapelle FJL, Durrer D. 1983. Endocardial mapping by simultaneous recording of endocardial electrograms during cardiac surgery for ventricular aneurysm. JACC 2: 947–953.

11. Mason JW, Stinson EB, Oyer PE, Winkle RA, Hunt S, Anderson KP, Derby GC. 1985. The mechanisms of ventricular tachycardia in humans determined by intraoperative recording of the electrical activation sequence. Int J Cardiol 8: 163–172.

12. Klein H, Kard RB, Kouchoukos NT, Zorn Jr GL, James TN, Waldo AL. 1982. Intraoperative electrophysiologic mapping of the ventricles during sinus rhythm in patients with a previous myocardial infarction. Circulation 66: 847–853.

13. Wittig JG, Boineau JP. 1975. Surgical treatment of ventricular arrhythmias using epicardial, transmural and endocardial mapping. Ann Thorac Surg 20: 117.

14. Guiraudon G, Fontaine G, Frank R, Pavie A, Grosgogeat Y, Cabrol C. 1980. Is the reentry concept a guide to the surgical treatment of chronic ventricular tachycardia? In: Medical and Surgical Management of Tahyarrhythmias. Edited by Bircks W, Loogen F, Schulte HD, Seipel L. Berlin, Springer-Verlag, pp 155–172.

15. Waldo AL, Arciniegas JG, Klein H. 1981. Surgical treatment of life-threatening ventricular arrhythmias. The role of intraoperative mapping and consideration of the presently available surgical techniques. Prog Cardiovasc Dis 23: 247–264.

16. Fontaine G, Guiraudon G, Frank R. 1979. Mechanism of ventricular tachycardia with and without associated chronic myocardial ischemia: surgical management based on epicardial mapping. In: Cardiac Arrhythmias. Electrophysiology, Diagnosis, and Management. Edited by Narula OS. Baltimore, Williams & Wilkins, p 516.

17. Moran JM, Talano JV, Euler D, Moran JF, Montoya A, Pifarre R. 1977. Refractory ventricular arrhythmia. The role of intraoperative electrophysiological study. Surgery 82: 809.

18. Mason JW, Stison EB, Winkle RA, Griffin JC, Oyer PE, Ross DL, Derby G. 1982. Surgery for ventricular tachycardia: efficacy of left ventricular aneurysm resection compared with operation guided by electrical activation mapping. Circulation 65: 1148–1155.

19. Harken AH, Horowitz LN, Josephson ME. 1980. Comparison of standard aneurysmectomy and aneursymectomy with directed endocardial resection for the treatment of recurrent sustained ventricular tachycardia. J Thorac Cardiovasc Surg 80: 527–534.

20. Miller JM, Josephson ME. 1985. Intraoperative mapping ventricular tachycardia: utility and pitfalls. Int J Cardiol 8: 173–175.

21. Fontaine G, Guiraudon G, Frank R, Vedel J, Grosgogeat Y, Cabrol C, Facquet J. 1977. Stimulation studies and epicardial mapping ventricular tachycardia. Study of mechanisms and selection for surgery. In: Re-entrant Arrhythmias: Mechanisms and Treatment. Edited by Kulbertus HE, Baltimore, University Park Press, pp 334–350.

22. Fontaine G, Guiraudon G, Frank R, Fillette F, Tonet J, Grosgogeat Y. 1980. Correlations between latest delayed potentials in sinus rhythm and earliest activation during chronic ventricular tachycardia. In: Medical and Surgical Management of Tachyarrhythmias. Edited by Bircks W, Loogen F, Schulte HD, Seipel L. Berlin, Springer-Verlag, pp 138–154.

23. Josephson ME, Simson MB, Harken AH, Horowitz LN, Falcone RA. 1982. The incidence and clinical significance of epicardial late potentials in patients with recurrent sustained ventricular tachycardia and coronary artery disease. Circulation 66: 1199–1204.

24. Kienzle MG, Miller JM, Falcone RA, Harken AH, Josephson ME. 1984. Intraoperative endocardial mapping during sinus rhythm: relation to site of origin of ventricular tachycardia. Circulation 70: 957–965.

25. Cassidy DM, Vassallo JA, Buxton AE, Doherty JU, Marchlinski FE, Josephson ME. 1984. The value of catheter mapping during sinus rhythm to localize site of origin of ventricular tachycardia. Circulation 69: 1103–1110.

26. Cassidy DM, Vassallo JA, Buxton AE, Doherty JU, Marchlinski FE, Josephson ME. 1985. Catheter mapping during sinus hythm: relation of local electrogram duration to ventricular tachycardia cycle length. Am J Cardiol 55: 713–716.
27. Fenoglio JJ, Pham TD, Harken AH, Horowitz LN, Josephson ME, Wit AL. 1983. Recurrent sustained ventricular tachycardia: structure and ultrastructure of subendocardial regions in which tachycardia originates. Circulation 68: 518–533.

32. Surgery for ventricular arrhythmias: a review

GERARD M. GUIRAUDON, GEORGE J. KLEIN,
and ARJUN D. SHARMA

Introduction

Surgery for ventricular arrhythmias is still the most challenging surgical approach in the treatment of cardiac arrhythmias. In the operating room, the pathophysiology of the lesions is still obscure, and the surgical rationale has to compromise with the imperative preservation of the left ventricular function. In this review we will try to provide some perspective on what we have learned in the clinical setting about the surgical treatment of ventricular arrhythmia based on empirical or on experimental models.

The Wolff-Parkinson-White model

W.C. Sealy first successfully operated a patient with WPW syndrome using a map guided direct surgical approach in 1967 [1]. Since then the surgery for WPW surgery has served as a unique model in surgery for arrhythmia. It suggested that the surgical rationale should take in account: (1) the mechanism of the arrhythmia, (2) the cardiac pathology (3) the pathophysiology of the anatomical lesions and (4) cardiac mapping which can localize the critical part of the lesion even if it is non visible or palpable.

Surgical approach to ventricular tachycardia

Mechanism of ventricular tachycardia

Current concepts of the mechanisms of ventricular tachycardia include reentry, abnormal or enhanced automaticity and triggered automacity [2]. Most clinical ventricular tachycardia are inducible by programmed electrical stimulation [3–4] and are thought to be due to a micro or macro reentrant circuit. Inducible ventricular tachycardia can be studied 'reliably' and 'reproducibly' in the electro-physiological laboratory and in the operating room.

Non inducible VT are elusive and difficult to assess. In addition, the few surgical attempts have been mostly unsuccessful in eradicating the tachycardia [5].

Cardiac pathology

Most inducible ventricular tachycardia are associated with myocardial structural disease [5, 6, 7]: post myocardial infarction scar, myocardiopathy, arrhyth-mogenic right ventricular dysplasia, idiopathic left ventricular aneurysm, mitral valve prolapse and a large variety of rare lesions.

All these causative lesions have one striking feature in common: a hetero-geneous myocardial structure which combines normal or abnormal myocardial fibers entwined with fatty or fibrotic streaks. Normal myocardium present with uniform anisotropy while arrhythmogenic myocardium has non-uniform aniso-tropy.

These myocardial lesions can be either discrete and well delineated or diffuse. These last features play an important role in the surgical indication as well as in the choice of surgical technique.

Intraoperative cardiac mapping

Cardiac mapping is a method by which the electrical activity of the heart is recorded directly from the heart and spatially depicted in an integrated manner as in a geographical map [8]. The site of recording can be epicardial, endocardial or intramural. The recording mode can be unipolar or bipolar. The method of display involves activation time (isochronic map) or potential amplitude (isopo-tential map) or potential morphology (post excitation map [9] or fractionation map [10]. These various maps can be obtained during sinus rhythm, or induced ventricular arrhythmia.

The crucial issue is the way the recordings are obtained from the various cardiac sites. A unique hand held roving probe can be used. That *point by point technique* [11] is feasible only if the cardiac activation is stable and each QRS complex identical to the following during the exploration. The hand held probe must be moved from one site to the other after a sufficient number of complexes have been recorded at each site. The technique is time consuming but appropriate for mapping during sinus rhythm or sustained monomorphic ventricular tachycar-dia. *Computerised mapping* [12, 13] allows the simultaneous recording of a large number of sites. The epicardial electrodes may be a fixed on a mesh which encompasses the heart like a sock [8]. The endocardial electrodes array can be attached on an inflatable balloon introduced into the left ventricle via a left ventriculotomy [13] or the aortic root [14] or the left atrium [15]. Epicardial and endocardial mapping can be carried out simultaneously [16]. Computerised mapping is of particular interest when the ventricular tachycardia are badly tolerated, and when the tachycardia are non sustained, polymorphic or multiple. It goes without saying that normothermic cardiopulmonary is used when necessary.

Cardiac mapping provides the surgeon with two critical guides [17]: (1) The site of 'origin' of the arrhythmia which corresponds to the site of the earliest activation of the QRS complex during ventricular tachycardia. In some instances the onset of the QRS can be difficult to determine, as well the activation time at various sites. (2) The area where 'abnormal' electrical activity is recorded arrhythmogenic areas. These areas can be endocardial, or epicardial. In a few patients, the surgeon may be provided with the actual macro reentrant circuit.

Despite the apparent precision, most of the information is crude and can be misleading [18] even after being corroborated by thermal mapping [19] or pace mapping [20]. The reliability of the information depends upon the site of origin (right ventricular free wall, septum, left ventricular free wall) and associated structural disease. Intraoperative cardiac mapping must be also assessed with regard to the preoperative endocardial mapping [21].

Pathophysiology of the cardiac lesion

Preoperative and intraoperative cardiac mapping allows correlation of the site of the tachycardia(s) and the arrhythmogenic area(s) with the lesion. Usually a part of the lesion is documented arrhythmogenic. However that does not imply that the rest of the lesion is not actually or has not the potential to be arrhythmogenic. This point is in favour of broad or extensive surgical interventions.

Surgical rationale

The surgical rationale is a compromise between the preservation of the cardiac function and the management of the current and/or potentially arrhythmogenic lesions. It is based on two surgical concepts: (1) The concept of exclusion and (2) the concept of ablation.

The concept of exclusion is aimed at confining the arrhythmogenic mechanism from involving the rest of the heart and producing ventricular arrhythmia. The best model of exclusion is the right ventricular free wall disconnection [22–23].

The concept of ablation is aimed at resecting or neutralizing the lesion(s) or a critical part of it. There is a large number of ablative techniques: transmural resection [24], endocardial resection [25], ventriculotomy [24], cryoablation [26], laser photocoagulation [27].

This classification is somewhat arbitrary and both concepts are combined to various extents in each technique.

The surgical implements

These two rationales can be implemented using various 'tools': (1) scalpel, (2) cryoablation (3) laser (4) caustic chemical as the lugol solution. The choice of the 'tool' is based on the assessment of its specific advantages and disadvantages. Cryosurgery and laser photocoagulation produce well demarcated mass of neutralised tissue which does not require further surgical intervention and does not impair normal surrounding myocardium. Cryosurgery requires concomitant cold cardiac arrest while laser photocoagulation can be used on the normothermic beating heart.

It is up to the surgical team to select the best surgical tactic when the strategy has been established.

Clinical experience

The surgical treatment of malignant ventricular arrhythmia was first based on indirect approaches using sympathectomy, coronary artery bypass grafting and heart wall resection [28].

The first attempted direct surgery for ventricular arrhythmia was performed by P. Puech, R. Grolleau and Negre in 1972 in Montpellier (France) [29]. The patient presented with ventricular tachycardia associated with arrhythmogenic right ventricular dysplasia.

Ventricular tachycardia in the absence of coronary artery disease

Thereafter, a similar direct approach was carried out in Paris (France) in 1973 [30] on a patient with dilated myocardiopathy. In 1981, 23 patients with ventricular tachycardia in the absence of coronary artery disease were reported by the same group [24]. Most of them had arrhythmogenic right ventricular dysplasia [31]. Four patients died during the intraoperative period. The surgery failed to interrupt the ventricular tachycardia in 3 of 4 patients with non inducible tachycardia, but was successful in all patients with inducible ventricular tachycardia. Non inducible ventricular arrhythmias were all situated in the septum. One non inducible, septal ventricular arrhythmia was successfully interrupted using cryoablation. The long-term results were dependent on the characteristics of the pathological lesions. Diffuse lesions were found prone to relapse. Consequently, a complete exclusion of the right ventricular free wall was designed and carried out in two patients with arrhythmogenic right ventricular dysplasia [22]. This Parisian experience was duplicated by others. J. Cox recently reported a similar experience with right ventricular tachycardia [32].

Ventricular tachycardia in the presence of coronary artery disease

Direct surgery for ventricular tachycardia after myocardial infarction was developed after the indirect approach (aneurysmectomy) [33] had proved unsuccessful despite early successes [34].

The first direct approach was performed in Paris in 1975: An encircling endocardial ventriculotomy [35] was aimed at excluding the 'border zone' of the arrhythmogenic scar. In Philadelphia, M.E. Josephson and A.H. Harken introduced a map guided endocardial resection [25].

In 1981, the Parisian group reported 30 patients with ventricular tachycardia after myocardial infarction treated by an encircling endocardial ventriculotomy [36, 37]. The operative mortality was 13%. Two patients (6%) had early recurrence of ventricular arrhythmia. These results were better than those obtained by simple aneurysmectomy [33]. The encircling endocardial ventriculotomy was adopted and/or modified by various groups. Ostermeyer et al. reported that map guided partial encircling endocardial ventriculotomy was effective and achieved a better preservation of the left ventricular function [38, 39] as suggested by the surgical experience in Birmingham (A1) [10].

The Philadelphia group reported the world's largest experience in 1984 [40]. One hundred and twenty-five patients had map guided endocardial resection. The surgical mortality was 10%; in 80 patients, the post-operative stimulation studies did not induce ventricular tachycardia.

Subsequently, the different surgical approaches were modified. Extensive endocardial resection was advocated [41]. A combination of different approaches were also successful [42]. Recently, cryosurgery [43] or laser photocoagulation [27] have yielded promising results.

Questions in the form of a conclusion

Despite significant improvements, the surgical treatment of ventricular arrhythmia still yields success rates far below the success rate of the Wolff-Parkinson-White surgical model [44, 45]. The reasons may be in the presence of a specific end point in the Wolff-Parkinson-White syndrome i.e. the accessory pathway, while in most cases there is no specific end point in ventricular arrhythmia. Sophisticated online ventricular mapping has failed to define a specific end point and to significantly upgrade the yield of direct surgical approaches.

Consequently, five major questions remain unanswered: The role of cardiac mapping as a surgical guide, the pathophysiology of the associated lesions, the best surgical rationale and the best surgical tool, not to mention the criteria for assessing the surgical outcome.

The surgical indications are still empirical as well as indications for alternative interventional therapies: i.e. catheter ablation, implantable cardioverter or defibrillator. Prospective randomised studies are still to be done. For the time being, the best surgical results are to be anticipated in ventricular tachycardia associated with a discrete non progressive lesion. Otherwise, the progression of the lesions and the concomitant deterioration of the left ventricular function will hamper the long-term results of surgery for ventricular arrhythmia.

References

1. Sealy WC, Hattler BG, Blumenschein SD, Cobb FR. 1969. Surgical treatment of Wolff-Parkinson-White syndrome. Ann Thorac Surg 8: 1.
2. Moe GK. 1985. Reflections on Reciprocation. Cardiac Electrophysiology and Arrhythmias, Zipes DP and Jalife J editors, Grune & Stratton, Inc.
3. Wellens HJJ, Lie KI, Durrer D. 1974. Further observations on ventriculartachycardias as studied by electrical stimulation of the heart. Circulation 49: 647.
4. Brugada P, Wellens HJJ. 1985. Comparison in the same patient of two programmed ventricular stimulation protocols to induce ventricular tachycardia. Am J Cardiol 55: 380–383.
5. Fontaine G, Guiraudon G, Frank R, Fillette F, Cabrol C, Grosgogeat Y. 1982. Surgical Management of Ventricular Tachycardia Unrelated to Myocardial Ischemia or Infarction. Am J Cardiol 49: 397–410.
6. Boineau JP, Cox JL. 1982. Rationale for a Direct Surgical Approach to Control Ventricular Arrhythmias. Am J Cardiol 49: 381–396.
7. Mallory GK, White PD, Salcedo-Salgar J. 1939. The Speed of Healing of Myocardial Infarction. Am Heart J 18, 6: 647–671.
8. Gallagher JJ, Kasell JH, Cox JL, Smith WM, Ideker RE, Smith WM. 1982. Techniques of Intraoperative Electrophysiologic Mapping. Am J Cardiol 49: 221–240.
9. Fontaine G, Guiraudon G, Frank R, Tereau Y, Pavie A, Cabrol C, Chomette G, Grosgogeat Y. 1984. Surgical Management of Ventricular Tachycardia not Related to Mocardial Ischemia. Tachycardias: Mechanisms, Diagnosis, Treatment, ME Josephson, HJJ Wellens, Lea & Febiger, Philadelphia, 451–473.
10. Klein H, Karp RB, Kouchoukos NT, Zorn GL, James TN, Waldo AL. 1982. Intraoperative Electrophysiologic Mapping of the Ventricles During Sinus Rhythm in Patients with a Previous Myocardial Infarction. Circulation 66, 4: 847–853.
11. Durrer D, van Dam RT, Freud GE, Janse MJ, Meijler FL, Arzbaecher RC. 1970. Total excitation of the isolated human heart Circulation 41: 899–912.
12. Klein GJ, Edeker RE, Smith WM, Harrison LA, Kasell J, Wallace AG. 1979. Epicardial Mapping of the Onset of Ventricular Tachycardia Initiated by Programmed Stimulation in the Canine Heart with Chronic Infarction. Circulation 60, 6: 1375–1384.
13. de Bakker JMT, Janse MJ, Van Capelle FJL, Durrer D. 1983. Endocardial Mapping by Simultaneous Recording of Endocardial Electrograms During Cardiac Surgery For Ventricular Aneurysm. JACC 2, 5: 947–953.
14. Endocardial Mapping and Cryo-ablation for the Treatment of Ventricular Bigeminy Without Left Ventriculotomy. The Transaortic Approach. In preparation.

15. Downer E, Mickleborough LL, Garris L, Parson ID. 1986. Mapping of Endocardial Activation During Ventricular Tachycardia – A 'Closed Heart' Procedure. JACC 7, 2 (Supp A): 234A.

16. Downer E, Parson ID, Mickleborough LL, Cameron DA, Yao LC, Waxman MB. 1984. On-Line Epicardial Mapping of Intraoperative Ventricular Arrhythmias: Initial Clinical Experience. JACC 4, 4: 703.

17. Guiraudon G, Fontaine G, Frank R, Pavie A, Grosgogeat Y, Cabrol C. 1980. Is the Reentry Concept a Guide to the Surgical Treatment of Chronic Ventricular Tachycardia? Medical and Surgical Management of Tachyarrhythmias, W. Bircks, F. Loogen, H.D. Schulte and L. Seipel (Ed), Springer-Verlag Berlin Heidelberg.

18. Mason JW, Stinson EB, Winkle RA, Oyer PE. 1981. Mechanisms of ventricular tachycardia: Wide, complex ignorance. Am Heart J 102, 6: 1083–1087.

19. Camm J, Ward DE, Spurrell RAJ, Rees GM. 1985. Cryothermal Mapping and Cryoablation in the Treatment of Refractory Cardiac Arrhythmias. Circulation 62, 1: 67–74.

20. Holt PM, Smallpeice C, Deverall PB, Yates AK, Curry PVL. 1985. Ventricular arrhythmias: A guide to their localization. Br Heart J 53: 417–430.

21. Josephson ME, Horowitz LN, Spielman SR, Waxman HL, Greenspan AM. 1982. Role of Catheter Mapping in the Preoperative Evaluation of Ventricular Tachycardia. Am J Cardiol 49: 207–220.

22. Guiraudon GM, Klein GJ, Sulamhusein SS, Painvin GA, Del Campo C, Gonzales JC, Ko PT. 1983. Total Disconnection of the Right Ventricular Free Wall: Surgical Treatment of Right Ventricular Tachycardia Associated with Right Ventricular Dysplasia. Circulation 67, 2: 463–470.

23. Jones DL, Guiraudon GM, Klein GJ. 1984. Total Disconnection of the Right Ventricular Free Wall: Physiological Consequences In The Dog. Am Heart J 107, 6: 1169–1177.

24. Guiraudon G, Fontaine G, Frank R, Leandri R, Barra J, Cabrol C. 1981. Surgical Treatment of Ventricular Tachycardia Guided by Ventricular Mapping in 23 Patients Without Coronary Artery Disease. Ann Thorac Surg 32, 5: 439–450.

25. Harken AH, Josephson ME, Horowitz LN. 1979. Surgical Endocardial Resection for the Treatment of Malignant Ventricular Tachycardia. Ann Surg 190, 4: 456–460.

26. Gallagher JJ, Anderson RW, Kasell J et al. 1978. Cryoablation of Drug Resistant Ventricular Tachycardia in a Patient with a Variant of Sleroderma. Circulation 57: 190.

27. Selle JG, Svenson RH, Sealy WC, Gallagher JJ, Zimmern SH, Fedor JM, Marroum M-C, Robicsek F. Successful Clinical Laser Ablation of Ventricular Tachycardia: A Promising New Therapeutic Modality. Ann Thorac Surg (accepted).

28. Sealy WC. 1978. Surgical Treatment of Malignant Ventricular Arrhythmias by Sympathectomy, Coronary Artery Grafts and Heart Wall Resection. Advances in the Management of Arrhythmias, DT Kelly, ed, Telectronics Pty. Limited, NSW Australia.

29. Puech P. 1986. Personal communication.

30. Guiraudon G, Frank R, Fontaine G. 1974. Interet des Cartographies dans le Traitement Chirurgical des Tachycardies Ventriculaire rebelles recidivantes. Nouvelle Presse Medicale 3: 321.

31. Marcus FI, Fontaine GH, Guiraudon G, Frank R, Laurenceau JL, Malergue C, Grosgogeat Y. 1982. Right Ventricular Dysplasia: A Report of 24 Adult Cases. Circulation 65, 2: 384–398.

32. Cox JL, Bardy GH, Damiano RJ, German LD, Fedor JM, Kisslo JA, Packer DL, Gallagher JJ. 1985. J Thorac Cardiovasc Surg 90: 212–224.

33. Mason JW, Stinson DB, Winkle RA, Griffin JC, Oyer PE, Ross DL, Derby G. 1982. Surgery for Ventricular Tachycardia: Efficacy of Left Ventricular Aneurysm Resection Compared with Operation Guided by Electrical Activation Mapping. Circulation 65, 6: 1148–1155.

34. Couch OA. 1959. Cardiac Aneurysm with Ventricular Tachycardia and Subsequent Excision of Aneurysm. Circulation 20: 251–253.

35. Guiraudon G, Fontaine G, Frank R, Escande G, Etievent P, Cabrol C. 1978. Encircling Endocardial Ventriculotomy: A New Surgical Treatment for Life-Threatening Ventricular Ta-

chycardias Resistant to Medical Treatment Following Myocardial Infarction. Ann Thorac Surg 26, 5: 438–444.

36. Guiraudon G, Fontaine G, Frank R, Cabrol C, Grosgogeat Y. 1982. Apports de la ventriculotomie circulaire d'exclusion dans le traitement de la tachycardie ventriculaire recidivantes apres infarctus du myocarde. Arch Mal Coeur 75, 9: 1013–1021.

37. Guiraudon GM, Klein GJ, Vermeulen FEE, Yee R, van Hemel NM. 1983. Encircling Endocardial Cryoablation: A Technique for Surgical Treatment of Ventricular Tachycardia After Myocardial Infarction. Circulation Part II, 68, 4: III-176.

38. Ostermeyer J, Breithardt G, Kolvenbach R, Borggrefe M, Seipel L, Schulte HD, Bircks W, Kirklin JW. 1982. The surgical treatment of ventricular tachycardias. J Thorac Surg 84: 704–715.

39. Ostermeyer J, Breithardt G, Borggrefe M, Godehardt E, Seipel L, Bircks W. 1984. Surgical Treatment of Ventricular Tachycardias. J Thorac Cardiovasc Surg 87: 517–525.

40. Harken AH, Josephson ME. 1984. Surgical Management of Ventricular Tachycardia. Tachycardias: Mechanism-Diagnosis-Treatment, ME Josephson, HJJ Wellens, Lea & Febiger, Philadelphia, 475–487.

41. Moran JM, Kehoe RF, Loeb JM, Lichtenthal PR, Sanders JH, Michaelis LL. 1982. Extended Endocardial Resection for the Treatment of Ventricular Tachycardia and Ventricular Fibrillation. Ann Thorac Surg 34, 5: 538–552.

42. Broadman R, Fisher JD, Johnston DR, Kim SG, Matoes JA, Waspe LE, Scavin GM, Furman S. 1984. Results of electrophysiologically guided operations for drug-resistant recurrent ventricular tachycardia and ventricular fibrillation due to coronary artery disease. J Thorac Cardiovasc Surg 87: 431–438.

43. Guiraudon GM, Klein GJ, Jones DL, McLellan DG. 1985. Encircling Endocardial Cryoablation for Ventricular Arrhythmias after Myocardial Infarction: Further Experience. Circulation Part II, 72, 4: III-222.

44. Guiraudon GM, Klein GJ, Sharma AD, Milstein S, McLellan DG. Closed Heart Technique for Wolff-Parkinson-White Syndrome: Further Experience and Potential Limitations. Ann Thorac Surg (in press).

45. Cox JL, Gallagher JJ, Cain ME. 1985. Experience with 118 consecutive patients undergoing operation for the Wolff-Parkinson-White syndrome. J Thorac Cardiovasc Surg 90: 490–501.

33. Surgery of refractory ventricular tachycardia by Nd-YAG photoablation

P. MESNILDREY, F. LABORDE, J.P. FAUCHIER, and A. PIWNICA
Cardiovascular Surgery. Hopital Lariboisière, Paris and CHU TOURS, France

Introduction

Refractory ventricular tachyarrhythmias are a frequent etiology of sudden cardiac death and many therapies have been proposed in the last years to reduce this rate: new antiarrhythmic drugs, catheter ablation, surgery, implantation of an internal defibrillator.

Our previous reports in 1983, concerning the use of Nd-YAG laser photoablation in the surgical treatment of tachyarrhythmias, were intended to ensure rapid feasibility, with minimal damage, of arrhythmogenic foci ablation [1–8] (Table 1).

The present study reviews our experience with laser therapy for the management of recurrent drug-resistant ventricular tachyarrhythmias (VT) in 29 consecutive patients between January 1984 and October 1986.

Table 1. Results of surgical treatment of tachyarrhythmias by Nd-YAG laser photoablation since January 1984.

Supra-ventricular tachycardias	11
WPW.Syndrome	5
Common Atrial flutter	4
Right atrial ectopic focus	1
Reentry within the AV node (+ WPW)	1
Ventricular tachycardias	29
Ischemic VT	24
Non ischemic VT	5

Methods

Refractory ventricular tachyarrhythmias, other than those *due* to drugs (digitalis) may be classified according to etiology into two groups in which surgical treatment differs:
– Group A (n = 24 patients): VT following myocardial infarction.
– Group B (n = 5 patients): VT not related to artery coronary disease.

Group A: Ischemic VT

1. Patient population
Twenty-four consecutive male patients age 24–66 years (mean = 55) with recurrent ventricular tachycardia following myocardial infarction underwent an encircling thermoablation with the Nd-YAG laser to eliminate tachycardia.

All patients had coronary artery disease and had had a previous myocardial infarction 2 months to 19 years prior to surgery. The resting electrocardiogram revealed a transmural myocardial infarction: antero septal in 16, posterior in 6, anterior and posterior in 1 and posterior and lateral in 1.

All patients underwent complete pre-operative angiographic and hemodynamic assessment, and an evaluation of the left ventricular (LV) function by radionuclide angiogram. Ten patients had disease of one vessel, 4 had two, and ten had three. The mean cardiac index was 2.3 liters/min per m² (SD = 0.42), mean ejection fraction was 0.27 (SD = 0.13), and mean left ventricular end-diastolic pressure at rest was 17.5 mm Hg (SD = 3.2). Eight patients had anteroapical left ventricular aneurysms (involving the septum), fourteen patients had a fibrous akinetic or dyskinetic plaque, one patient had ischemic cardiomyopathy, a last had had aneurysmectomy for congestive heart failure and angina 7 years before (at that time, no pre-operative arrhythmias had been noted).

A trial of at least 3 conventional antiarrhythmic drugs, including amiodarone, had failed in all patients.

2. Encircling thermoablation (ET): Operative procedure
In patients operated on for ischemic ventricular tachycardia, *no intra-operative mapping* is performed for several reasons: In order for reentry to occur, a zone of delayed conduction must be in close proximity to a zone of normal conduction: this situation occurs in the border zone situated at the edge of the pathological area [9–12]; Ventricular tachycardia is frequently pleomorphic [13, 14]; the changes in QRS morphology represent changing exit sites from the same re-entrant circuit, rather than changes in the site of origin and that ventricular activation from each of these exit sites produces different morphological patterns. Therefore, the procedure (ET) is the same whatever the number of QRS morphologies presented by the same patient (1 to 8, mean = 4, in our series).

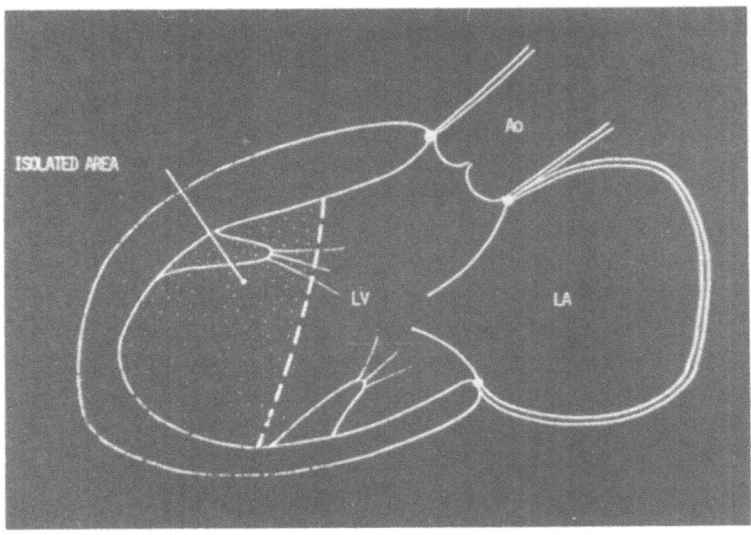

Figure 1. The left ventricle is opened from the myocardial scar. ET is indicated by dotted line. The mitral apparatus may or may not be included in the endocardial isolation.

All drugs were stopped the day before surgery. Anaesthetic techniques were uniform: high dose Fentanyl (30–50 mg/kg), Pancuronium and Flunitrazepam.

Systemic hypothermia (30° C), cold cardioplegia and topical cooling were used for myocardial preservation during ischemic arrest. Myocardial temperature was monitored and maintained below 12° C. Ancillary procedures were also performed during a single aortic cross-clamp time. Ventriculotomy was performed through the aneurysm sac or previous myocardial infarction scar.

The Nd-YAG laser (ERCELAS YM 100 – CILAS, France) was applied by continuous emission with a power of 40 watts around the endocardial scar (Figure 1) corresponding to the maximal extension of the ischemic zone. For posterior myocardial infarction (Figure 2), a double approach (ventricular and aortic) was performed to isolate the abnormal area. In one patient with posterior myocardial infarction, the superior part of the interventricular septum was only isolated via an aortotomy without a ventricular incision.

The distance between the tip of the probe and the endocardium was 5 mm. No suture is required and the maximal time for ET is 4 minutes. Under these conditions, the depth of non transmural myocardial necrosis is about 4 mm, sharply demarcated from the normal myocardium and no perforation has been observed (Figure 3). There is no danger to the mitral apparatus and when the papillary muscle is involved by myocardial infarction, an ablation is achieved around its base. The total quantity of absorbed energy is very important but this energy is distributed over about 20 centimeters and the thermal dispersion for the myocardium is rapid because of spontaneous cooling.

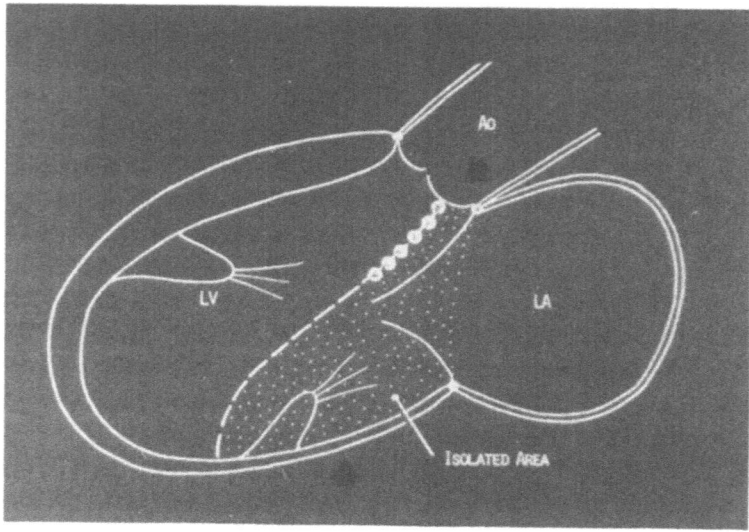

Figure 2. Location of ET positioned around the endocardial fibrosis associated with a posterior myocardial infarction: a double approach (ventricular for the lower part of the scar, aortic for the upper part of the septum) is performed to isolate the abnormal area.

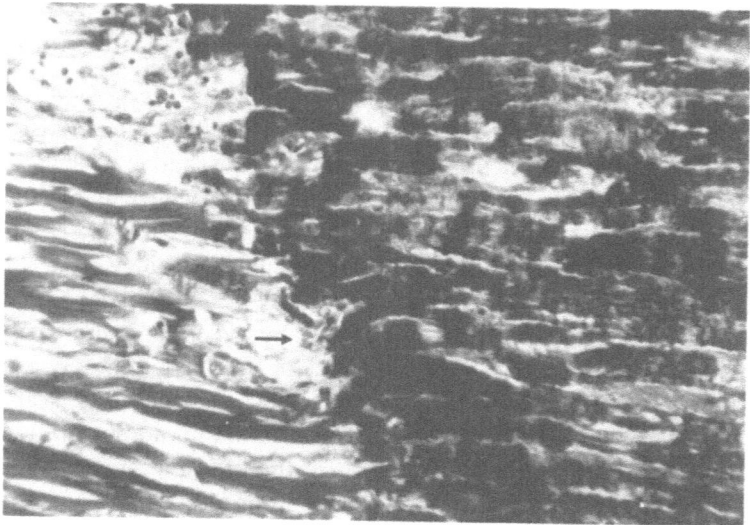

Figure 3. Morphologic effects of Nd-YAG laser photoablation: Laser injury appears as a light brown flat area without crater formation, well demarcated from the surrounding myocardium (arrow).

The left ventricle was then closed in a standard manner using Teflon pledgets (14 cases) or by imbricating aneurysmoplasty (10 cases) [15]. A concomitant aorto-coronary bypass was carried out in 9 cases, a mitral valve replacement for mitral insufficiency was performed in one. In the last five patients whose EF was lower than 0.30, circulatory support with an intraaortic balloon was begun at the end of the operation and removed after an average of two days.

Group B: VT not related to a myocardial infarction

1. Patient population

Five patients (4 men, 1 women), with an average of age of 37 (SD = 18.2), were studied between February 1985 and January 1986. Clinical data are shown in table 2.

Our cases are classified by histological examinations of intra-operative myocardial biopsy. 2 patients had non ischemic cardiomyopathy; in two, VT was a sequel of myocarditis (Fontaine G., Fontaliran F.: personal communication) and one patient had an idiopathic lef ventricular aneurysm. With the exception of pts no. 1 and 3, the other patients were classified before surgery, according to the classical knowledges (clinical, echocardiographic and angiographic data), as a right arrhythmogenic ventricular dysplasia with extension to the left ventricle. Neverthe-

Table 2. Clinical features of patients with non ischemic VT; all survived to surgery.

Patient	Age	Cardio-pathy	Origin of VT	Date of oper-ation	Oper-ative result	Post-op EPS	Drugs	Recur-rence with therapy	Follow-up (months)
1	33	ILVA	IVS (LV)	2/18/85	S	−	−	−	22
2	63	Myo-carditis	LV FW	4/10/85	S	−	−	−	20
3	24	NICM	IVS (LV)	8/ 5/85	F	+	Sotalol	−	16
4	49	NICM	IVS (LV)	12/10/85	F	+	Amio-darone and Propa-fénone	−	12
5	19	Myo-carditis	IVS (RV)	1/29/86	S	−	Propa-fénone	−	11

Abbreviations: ILVA = Idiopathic left ventricular aneurysm; NICM = Non ischemic cardiomyopathy; IVS = Interventricular septum; LV = Left ventricle; RV = Right ventricle; S = Success; F = Failure.

450

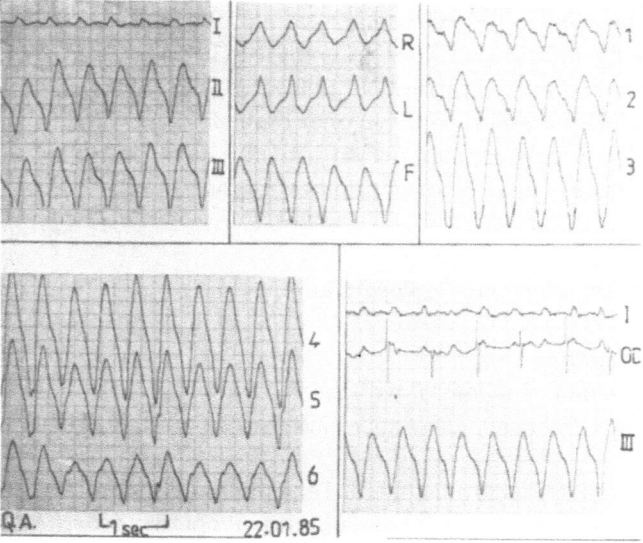

Figure 4a.

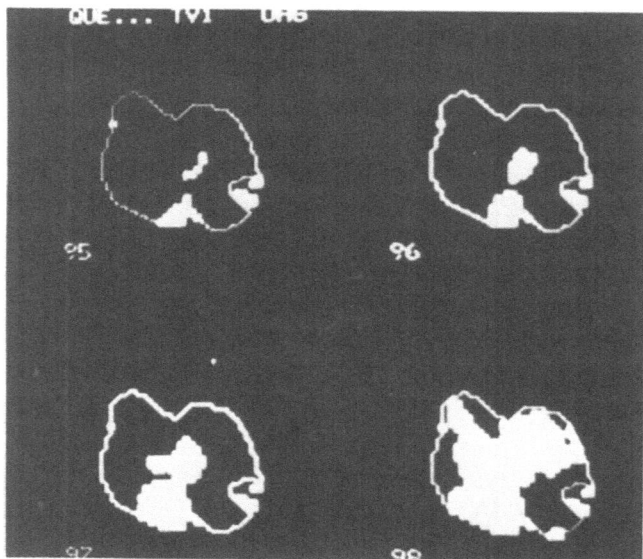

Figure 4b.

Figure 4. Patterns of ventricular activation by radionuclide angiographic phase imaging in patient no. 1. This patient presented two ECG morphologies during VT: 1. Left bundle branch block pattern (4a and 4b); 2. Right bundle banch block pattern with right axis deviation (4c and 4d). The two VT correspond to a same point of origin with different activations.

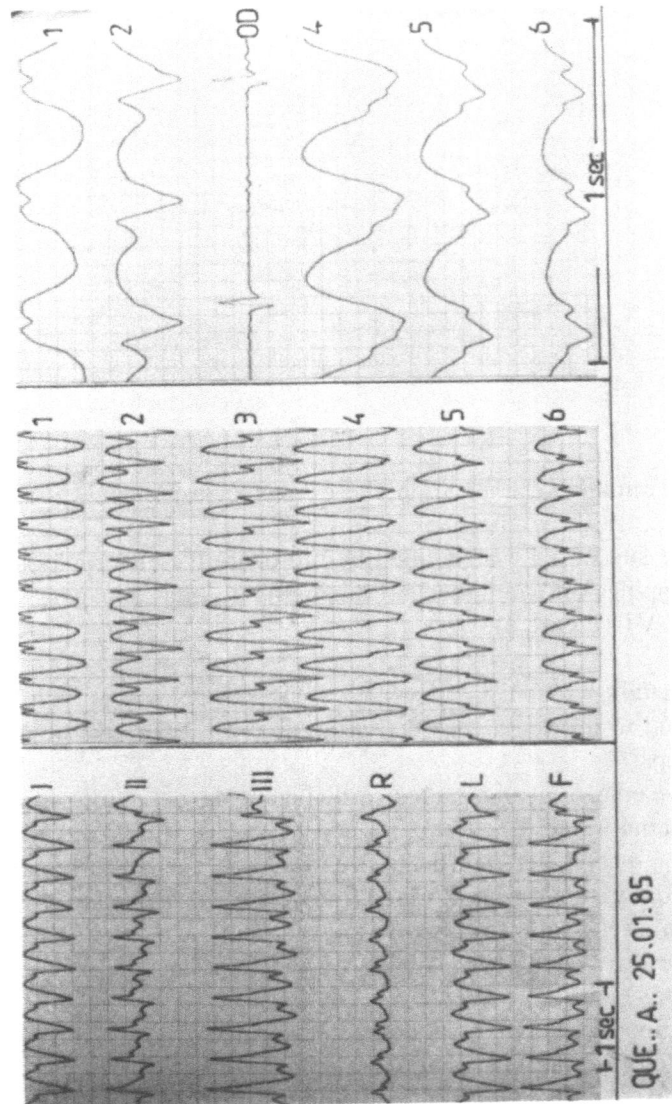

Figure 4c.

452

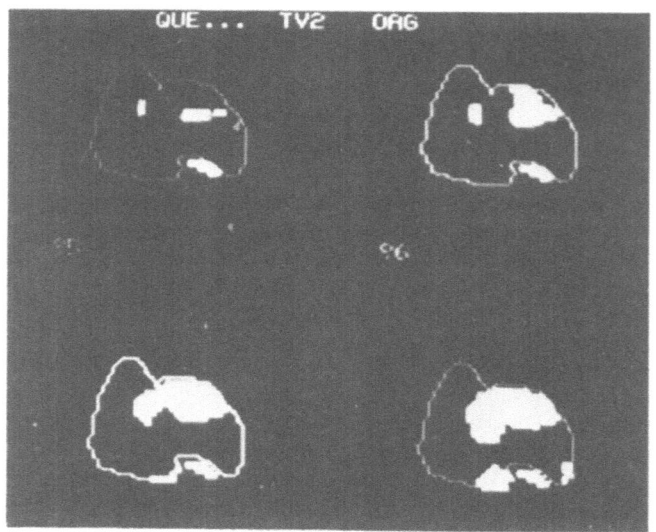

Figure 4d.

less, according to Fontaine's classification, these cases correspond now to sequels of myocarditis.

In all cases, the site of VT was defined by pre-operative electrophysiologic studies (pace-mapping) and radionuclide angiographic phase-imaging during induced sustained VT (Figure 4).

2. Operative procedure

For VT *not* related to a prior myocardial infarction, the operative procedure included three steps:

– Intra-operative epicardial and/or endocardial mapping were performed during sustained monomorphic VT. Mapping had to localize the site of earliest activation (septal = 4 cases, left ventricular free wall = 1 case) and to determine the area where surgery should be performed. In two cases, VT was not sustained or inducible (even after administration of Isoproterenol). Under these circumstances, the surgical procedure was guided by the radionuclide angiographic phase-imaging data (Figure 5).

– Photocoagulation by the Nd-YAG laser is performed to ablate the point of VT breakthrough. Laser was used in continuous emission, at a power of 40 Watts on an area of about 3 cm diameter.

– Finally, an endocardial isolation (encircling thermoablation) of the abnormal appearing zone was performed. So, the LV apex was isolated in 3 cases (pts no. 1, 3 and 4), the LV free wall in one (pt no. 2) and the right free wall in 1 (pt 5). This border is often very difficult to determine because the endocardial lesions are not always visible.

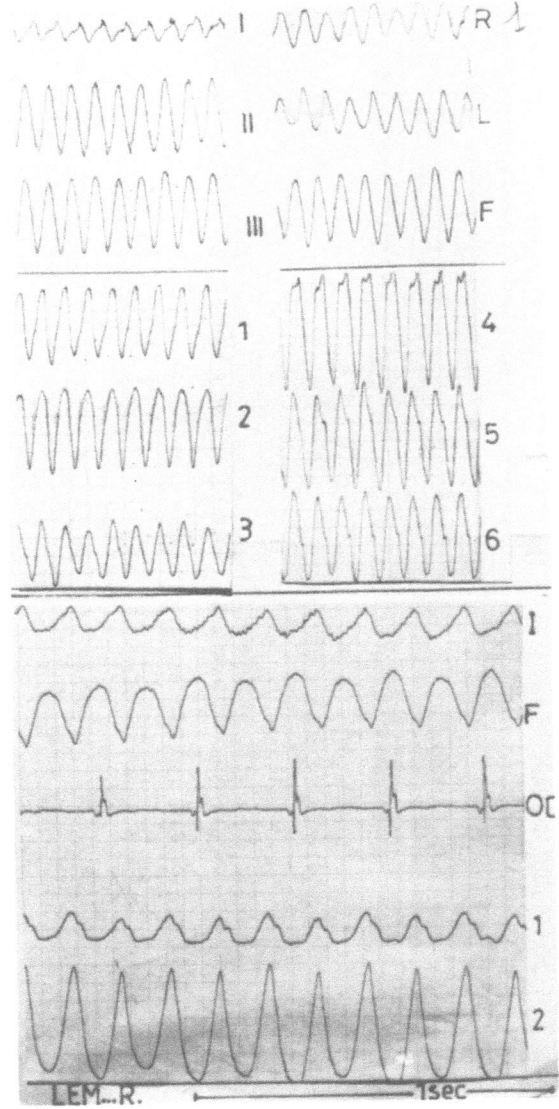

Figure 5a.

Figure 5. Correlations in pt 2 between VT morphology (a), angiographic data (b), radionucleide phase imaging (c) and intra-operative mapping (d).

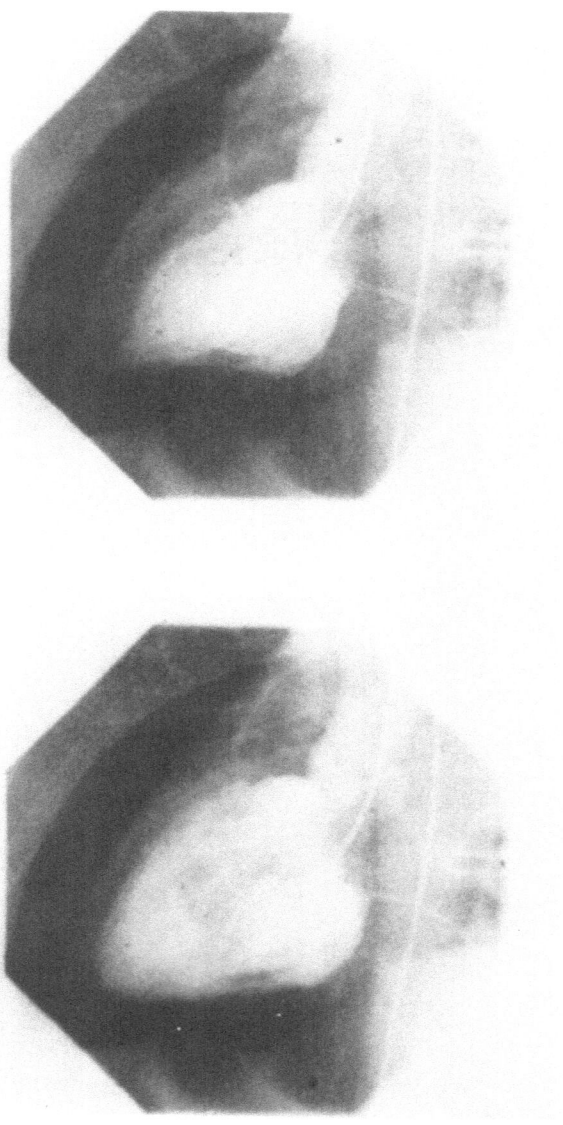

Figure 5b.

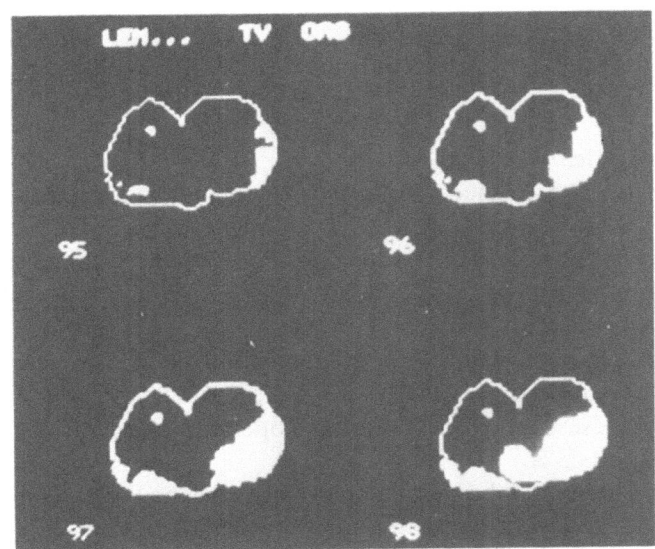

Figure 5c.

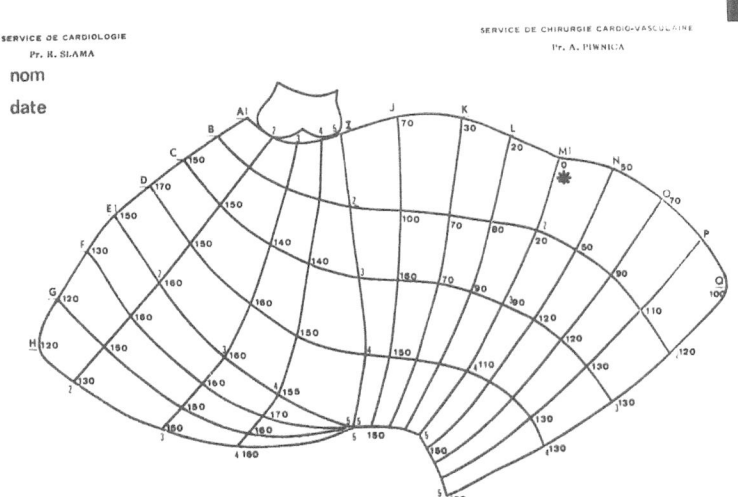

Figure 5d.

Results

Group A

1. Operative mortality

Three patients (12.5%) died during the peri-operative period of low cardiac output:

One patient with poor contractility (pre-op EF = 0.35) related to two prior myocardial infarctions and severe three-vessels disease died at operation. He was unable to come off cardiopulmonary bypass.

The second patient with diffuse cardiomyopathy died of myocardial failure on the first post-operative day. The surgical indication was syncopal VT/VF with a long period of resuscitation just before the operation. The left ventricular ejection fraction was 0.25.

The third patient, a Jehovah's Witness with incessant VT, died in electrical-mechanical dissociation 3 days after operation of a lateral myocardial infarction (early occlusion of an aorto-coronary venous graft). No recurrence of VT was noted during this short period.

2. Arrhythmogenicity in initial period (within 3 weeks)

Among the 21 survivors, there were early post-operative arrhythmias following laser photoablation. The acute rhythm response was recorded as numerous premature ventricular beats in the first post-operative days (maximal on the 5th–6th day, up to 3 weeks), unsustained VT (more than 6 repetitive complexes of less than 30 seconds duration) in 3 cases, and sustained inducible idioventricular rhythm in 2 cases with reappearance of sinus rhythm on the 7th and 8th post-operative days respectively. The tachycardias would appear and disappear sporadically. These arrhythmias disappeared with administration of indomethacin.

A lack of awareness of this phenomenon may create some confusion in the post-operative period because ventricular premature beats or VT may have a similar QRS morphology to the tachyarrhythmia for which surgery was carried out. Other QRS morphologies can also be noted. For these reasons, arrhythmias are considered recurrences if they occur after this period.

3. Follow-up data

Programmed electrophysiologic studies without antiarrhythmic therapy have been carried out in all 21 survivors to determine efficacy of surgery 2 weeks to 3 months (mean = 1 month) post-operatively. These studies consisted of introducing up to three ventricular extra-stimuli during ventricular pacing at two or more cycle lengths and rapid pacing at one or more right ventricular sites (epicardial or endocardial stimulation). In all cases, VT was not inducible. Four patients presented with recurrent VT after operation (18%).

One early recurrence was noted 1 month post-operatively (same pre-operative

QRS morphology during VT) in a patient three weeks after a posterior MI. At surgery, the lesions looked fresh, without endocardial fibrosis. A blind encircling thermoablation was performed. While he seemed well controlled with beta-blockade drugs, the patient suddenly died six months later.

A single spontaneous episode of unsustained VT, different from preoperative QRS morphology, was noted in 3 patients (3, 5 and 7 months after operation) well controlled with mexiletine and amiodarone (200 mg/day) in one case, and not treated in two cases. One of these patients died 8 months post-operatively of progressive heart failure without recurrence of VT. Seventeen patients are free of VT without medication over a mean follow-up of 19.7 months (SD = 9). A comparative hemodynamic evaluation was carried out in 15 survivors prior to discharge using radionuclide left ventricular angiogram. With the exception of the case with perioperative MI, there was an improvement in the LV function: mean EF = 0.43, SD = 0.10 (p<0.05), mean cardiac index = 2.9 l/min/m², SD = 0.53 (p = 0.38, N.S.)

Group B

No patient died in this sub-group. A permanent pacemaker was implanted in pt 2 for a combination of first degree AV block and left bundle branch block.

In all patients, pre-operative VT disappeared.

In the immediate post-operative period, two pts (3 and 4) developed spontaneous unsustained VT, of a different QRS morphology, treated by Sotalol and the association Amiodarone-Flecainide respectively. In these conditions, no recurrence was observed.

Control EPS were performed 1 month after operation.

Pts 1, 2 and 5 had negative EPS. Pt 5 is treated by Propafenone (150 mg/day) for symptomatic premature ventricular beats. The others pts are without antiarrhythmic medication (Follow-up = 11, 20 and 22 months).

Pts 3 and 4 had inducible unsustained VT but are now well-controlled by drugs (Follow-up = 12 and 16 months).

Discussion

Laser photo-ablation versus other surgical procedures

Surgical procedures have been or are being developed for treating all types of cardiac arrhythmias that are refractory to medical treatment. The most important new direction concerns the development and clinical application of various surgical procedures to ablate life-threatening ventricular tachyarrhythmias occuring with or without coronary artery disease [16–22].

Right ventricular isolation procedures [23, 24] in combination with cryoablative techniques have been employed for treating patients suffering from ventricular tachycardia associated with right ventricular arrhythmogenic foci (including dysplasia, Uhl's anomaly, cardiomyopathy, myocarditis) [25, 26]. Direct endocardial techniques guided or not by intra-operative mapping, have largely replaced the previous indirect procedures for surgical treatment of refractory ventricular tachyarrhythmias. These direct endocardial procedures include the encircling endocardial ventriculotomy, the subendocardial resection (localized or extended) [27–29], the endocardial cryoablation (localized or encircling), and laser photoablation.

Laser photo-ablation appears to avoid the disadvantages of older techniques: high risk of impairment of ventricular function [30], septal perforation [27, 29], a difficult resection when a papillary muscle is involved by MI, and prolonged time in the case of cryosurgery.

Different types of lasers are in use for the intra-operative ablation of VT [31–37]. Nd-YAG laser is the best in this indication. We and others [31, 32] have previously reported the reasons for this choice based on physical principles:

With the carbon dioxide laser, energy absorption is higher; the cutting effect is prevalent, comparable with a scalpel.

With the argon laser, the absorption and scattering coefficients of the wave length by the myocardium are similar. A coagulation necrosis, associated with an effect of cutting, can occur, leading to perforation [36]. Moreover, the maximum power delivered by argon laser is lower than 15 watts, and requires a longer time.

With Nd-YAG laser, forward scattering is higher than absorption; the obtained effect is a coagulation necrosis without cutting. The Nd-YAG laser has other advantages: high maximum power (up to 50 watts in continous emission), rapidity of action (4 minutes for encircling thermoablation), ease of manipulation of the optical probe, absence of embolism of the created lesion, absence of long-term arrhythmogenic potential, and preservation of ventricular function.

The Excimer laser [38, 39] remains a laboratory tool. Available fibers for the transmission of concurrent light in ulraviolet frequencies will not conduct the shorter wave lengths. Possible carcinogenicity of ultraviolet radiation must also be considered.

Mapping and surgery of VT

Svenson [40] described the use of the Nd-YAG laser for photo-ablation for the treatment of refractory VT in 14 patients (12 ischemic VT, 1 due to sarcoïdosis, one idiopathic). The technique differs from ours because, in their experience, intra-operative mapping is always necessary. In our opinion, mapping is only indicated for non ischemic VT in which an organic lesion is not seen in all cases.

For ischemic VT, the exact reentry mecanism is well-known and previous procedures have demonstrated their efficacy in control of arrhythmias. The anatomic basis for chronic reentrant VT following myocardial infarction is well recognized, and is observed in the 1 to 3 mm subendocardial layer of tissue surrounding the border of the endocardial scar. Endocardial mapping is not always feasible for a number of reasons [41–44], inability to initiate VT, appearance of multiple VT morphologies, or degeneration of VT to VF. On the other hand, the amount of coagulated myocardium is similar with encircling thermo-ablation. The exact mechanism of action is unknown; perhaps it is due to ablation of a reentry circuit or interruption of the subendocardium between the normal myocardium and the border zone. Total isolation of the arrhythmogenic area is more advisable than a localized procedure such as subendocardial resection or cryosurgery for which the risk of recurrence is high (up to 30% for subendocardial resection) [45].

Conclusion

Recent advances in the understanding of the mechanisms and anatomic bases of VT related or not to myocardial infarction have led to the development of new surgical procedures to treat this arrhythmia. We have utilised the technique of photoablation by a Nd-YAG laser, and have demonstrated a good success rate (overall rate of arrhythmia control = 96% with and without antiarrhythmic drugs, 77% without any drug) with excellent hemodynamic results and an acceptable mortality rate (overall rate = 10%, 0% for VT not related to a coronary artery disease).

References

1. Mesnildrey P, Goudot B, Dubois C, Schlumberger S, Bachet J, Brodaty D, Barbagelata M, Guilmet D. 1984. Destruction du faisceau de His par un laser néodyme-YAG: étude expérimentale préliminaire. Presse Med 13: 1627–1629.
2. Mesnildrey P, Goudot B, Dubois C, Schlumberger S, Bachet J, Brodaty D, Guilmet D. 1984. Encircling thermosurgery with Nd-YAG laser beam: an experimental study. Eur Heart J 5: 259.
3. Mesnildrey P, Laborde F, Mayolini P, Piwnica A. 1985. Interventions sur les voies de conduction intra-cardiaques par le laser Nd-YAG. Angeiologie 37: 45–49.
4. Bruneval P, Mesnildrey P, Camilleri JP. Nd-YAG laser induced injury in dog myocardium: optical and ultrastructural study of early lesions. Eur Heart J (in press).
5. Mesnildrey P, Laborde F, Beloucif S, Mayolini P, Piwnica A. 1986. Tachycardies ventriculaires d'origine ischémique: traitement chirurgical par thermo-exclusion circonférentielle au laser Nd-YAG.
6. Mesnildrey P, Laborde F, Bruneval P, Camilleri JP, Mayolini P, Piwnica A. Therapeutic and prophylactic surgical treatment of ventricular tachycardia by Nd-YAG laser irradiation. In: Scheiman MM, Fontaine G: Ablation in cardiac arrhythmias. Futura Publishing Comp, Mount Kisco (in press).

7. Mesnildrey P Laborde F, Piwnica A. 1985. Encircling themoexclusion by the Nd-YAG laser without mapping: a new surgical technique for ischemic ventricular tachycardia. Circulation 72 (supp III): III-389.

8. Mesnildrey P, Laborde F, Piwnica A. 1986. Surgery of ischemic ventricular tachycardias: a further experience with the Nd-YAG laser beam. Circulation 74 (supp II): II-134.

9. Josephson ME, Horowitz LN, Farshidi A, Kastor JA. 1978. Recurrent sustained ventricular tachycardia. I. Mechanisms. Circulation 57: 431–440.

10. Horowitz LN, Spear JF, Neil Moore E. 1976. Subendocardial origin of ventricular arrhythmias in 24-hour-old experimental myocardial infarction. Circulation 53: 56–63.

11. Lazzara R, Scherlag BJ. 1984. Electrophysiologic basis for arrhythmias in ischemic heart disease. Am J Cardiol 53: 1B–7B.

12. Pham TD, Fenoglio JJ, Harken AH, Ursell PC, Josephson ME, Horowitz LN, Wit AL. 1981. Structural basis for recurrent sustained ventricular tachycardia. Circulation 64 (Supp IV): IV-87.

13. Josephson ME, Horowitz LN, Farshidi A, Spielman SR, Michelson EL, Greenspan AM. 1979. Recurrent sustained ventricular tachycardia. 4. Pleomorphism. Circulation 59: 459–468.

14. Miller JM, Kienzle MG, Harken AH, Josephson ME. 1984. Morphologically distinct sustained ventricular tachycardias in coronary artery disease: significance and surgical results. J Am Coll Cardiol 4: 1073–1079.

15. Guilmet D, Popoff G, Dubois C, Tawil N, Bachet J, Goudot B, Guermonprez JL, Brodaty D, Schlumberger S. 1984. Nouvelle technique chirurgicale pour la cure des anévrysmes du ventricule gauche: l'anévrysmoplastie en paletot (résultats préliminaires). Arch Mal Coeur 77: 953–958.

16. Cox JL. 1983. Anatomic-electrophysiologic basis for the surgical treatment of refractory ischemic ventricular tachycardia. Ann Surg 198: 119–129.

17. Guiraudon G, Fontaine G, Frank R, Escande G, Etievent P, Cabrol C. 1978. Encircling endocardial ventriculotomy: a new surgical treatment for life-threatening ventricular tachycardias resistant to medical treatment following myocardial infarction. Ann Thorac Surg 26: 438–440.

18. Harken AH, Josephson ME, Horowitz LN. 1979. Surgical endocardial resection for the treatment of malignant ventricular tachycardia. Ann Surg 190: 456–460.

19. Gallagher JJ, Anderson RW, Kasell J, Rice JR, Pritchett EL, Gault JH, Harrison L, Wallace AG. 1978. Cryoablation of drug-resistant ventricular tachycardia in a patient with a variant of scleroderma. Circulation 57: 190–197.

20. Camm J, Ward De, Cory-Pearce R, Rees GM, Spurell RA. 1979. The successful cryosurgical treatment of paroxysmal ventricular tachycardia. Chest 75: 621–624.

21. Guiraudon GM, Klein GJ, Vermeulen FE, Yee R, Van Hemel NM. 1983. Encircling endocardial cryoablation: a technique for surgical treatment of ventricular tachycardia after myocardial infarction. Circulation 68 (supp. III): III-176.

22. Fontaine G, Guiraudon G, Frank R, Tereau Y, Pavie A, Cabrol C, Chomette G, Grosgogeat Y. 1984. Management of ventricular tachycardia not related to myocardial infarction. Cli Prog Pacing and Electrophysiol 2: 193–219.

23. Guiraudon GM, Klein GJ, Gulamhusein SS, Painvin GA, Del Campo C, Gonzales JC, Ko PT. 1983. Total disconnection of the right ventricular free wall: surgical treatment of right ventricular tachycardia associated with right ventricular dysplasia. Circulation 67: 463–470.

24. Cox JL, Bardy GH, Damiano RJ, German LD, Fedor JM, Kisslo JA, Packer DL, Gallagher JJ. 1985. Right ventricular isolation procedures for nonischemic ventricular tachycardia. J Thorac Cardiovasc Surg 90: 212–224.

25. Fontaine G, Fontaliran F, Chomette G. 1986. Il ventricolo destro aritmogeno. G Ital Cardiol 16: 1–3.

26. Bharati S, Lev M. 1983. Arrhythmogenic ventricles. PACE 6: 1035–1049.

27. Moran JM, Kehoe RF, Loeb JM,, Lichtenhal PR, Sanders JH, Michaelis LL. 1982. Extended endocardial resection for the treatment of ventricular tachycardia and ventricular fibrillation. Ann Thorac Surg 34: 538–552.

28. Kron IL, Lerman BB, Dimarco JP. 1985. Extended subendocardial resection: a surgical approach to ventricular tachyarrhythmias that cannot be mapped intra-operatively. J Thorac Cardiovasc Surg 90: 586–591.

29. Landymore RW, Kinley CE, Gardner M, Murphy DA. 1985. Encircling endocardial resection with complete removal of endocardial scar without intraoperative mapping for ablation of drug-resistant ventricular tachycardia. J Thorac Cardiovasc Surg 89: 18–24.

30. Ungerleider RM, Holman WL, Calcagno D, Williams JM, Lofland GK, Smith PK, Stanley III TE, Quick G, Cox JL. 1982. Encircling endocardial ventriculotomy for refractory ischemic ventricular tachycardia. III. Effects on regional left ventricular function. J Thorac Cardiovasc Surg 83: 857–864.

31. Obelenius V, Bredikis J, Knepa A. 1986. Nd-YAG lasers in the treatment of cardiac arrhythmias. In: Waidelich W, Kiefhaber P: Laser/Optoelectronics in Medicine. Berlin, Springer-Verlag, 462–465.

32. Obelenius V, Knepa A, Lubite Y, Ambartzumian R, Isakov V, Koshelev E, Markin E. 1985. Histological studies of myocardium zones irradiated with Nd-YAG laser. Lasers Surg Med 5: 475–483.

33. Selle JG, Svenson RH, Sealy WC, Gallagher JJ, Simmern SH, Fedor JM, Marroum MC, Robicsek F. 1986. Successful clinical laser ablation of ventricular tachycardia: a promising new therapeutic method. Ann Thorac Surg 42: 380–384.

34. Lee G, Ikeda RM, Theis J, Stobe D, Ogata C, Lui H, Reis RL, Mason DT. 1983. Effects of laser irradiation delivered by flexible fiberoptic system on the left ventricular internal myocardium. Am Heart J 106: 587–590.

35. Isner JM, Michlewitz H, Clarke RH, Mark Estes NA, Fortin Donaldson R, Salem DN, Bahn I, Payne DD, Cleveland RJ. 1985. Laser photoablation of pathological endocardium: In vitro findings suggesting a new approach to the surgical treatment of refractory arrhythmias and restrictive cardiomyopathy. Ann Thorac Surg 39: 201–206.

36. Saksena S, Gadhoke A. 1986. Laser therapy for tachyarrhythmias: a new frontier. PACE 9: 531–550.

37. Ciccone J, Saksena S, Pantopoulos D. 1986. Comparative efficacy of continous and pulsed argon laser ablation of human diseased ventricle. PACE 9: 697–704.

38. Isner JM, Fortin Donaldson R, Deckelbaum LI, Clarke RH, Laliberte SM, Ucci AA, Salem DN, Konstam MA. 1985. The Excimer laser: gross, light microscopic and ultrastructural analysis of potential advantages for use in laser therapy of cardiovascular disease. J Am Coll Cardiol 6: 1102–1109.

39. Downar E, Butany J, Jares A, Stoicheff BP. 1986. Endocardial photoablation by Excimer laser. J Am Coll Cardiol 7: 546–550.

40. Svenson RH, Gallagher JJ, Selle JG, Zimmern SM, Fedor JM. 1986. Intraoperative laser photoablation of ventricular tachycardia. Circulation 74 (supp. II): II-461.

41. Spielman SR, Michelson EL, Horowitz LN, Spear JF, Neil Moore E. 1978. The limitations of epicardial mapping as a guide to the surgical therapy of ventricular tachycardia. Circulation 57: 666–670.

42. Boineau JP, Cox JL. 1982. Rationale for a direct approach to control ventricular arrhythmias: relation of specific intra-operative techniques to mechanism and location of arrhythmic circuit. Am J Cardiol 49: 381–396.

43. Gallagher JJ, Kasell JH, Cox JL, Smith WM, Ideker RE, Smith WM. 1982. Techniques of intra-operative electrophysiologic mapping. Am J Cardiol 49: 221–240.

44. Kron IL, Lerman B, Dimarco JP. 1986. Surgical management of sustained ventricular arrhythmias presenting within eight weeks of acute myocardial infarction. Ann Thorac Surg 42: 13–16.

45. Platia EV, Griffith LS, Watkins L, Mower MM, Guarnieri T, Mirowski M, Reid PR. 1986. Treatment of malignant ventricular arrhythmias with endocardial resection and implantation of the automatic cardioverter-defibrillator. N Engl J Med 314: 213–216.

Index